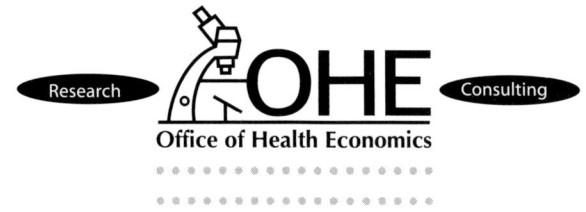

Office of Health Economics

Research  Consulting

# COMPENDIUM

# OF HEALTH

# STATISTICS

## 2008

### 19TH EDITION

# EMMA HAWE

**Radcliffe Publishing Ltd**
18 Marcham Road
Abingdon
Oxon OX14 1AA
United Kingdom

www.radcliffe-oxford.com
Electronic catalogue and worldwide online ordering facility.

---

British Library Cataloguing in Publication Data

A catalogue record for this book is available from the British Library.

ISBN-13: 978 1 84619 280 7

## Acknowledgements

The Office of Health Economics is particularly grateful to the Department of Health, the Common Services Agency for the NHS Scotland, the Welsh Assembly Government, the Central Services Agency in Northern Ireland, the Government Actuary's Department, HM Treasury, the Office for National Statistics, the Organisation for Economic Co-operation and Development (OECD), The Information Centre for Health and Social care, QResearch, NHS Finance directorate, World Health Organisation, Northern Ireland Cancer Registry and the Association of the British Pharmaceutical Industry (ABPI) for providing information, and to Mrs Lesley Baillie for her considerable assistance in the preparation of this edition of the Compendium.

**Office of Health Economics**
www.ohe.org

The Office of Health Economics provides independent research, advisory and consultancy services on policy and economic issues within the pharmaceutical, health care and biotechnology industries. Its main areas of focus are: the pharmaceutical and biotechnology industry, health care systems – their financing and organisation – and the economics of health technology assessment.

Printed and bound by TJ International Ltd, Padstow, Cornwall.

# Contents

| | | Page |
|---|---|---|
| Introduction | | i |
| List of Tables and Figures | | ii |
| Section 1 | Population, Mortality, Morbidity and Lifestyle | 1 |
| | - Population | 8 |
| | - Mortality | 33 |
| | - Morbidity | 59 |
| | - Lifestyle | 67 |
| Section 2 | UK Health Care Expenditure and Cost of the NHS | 76 |
| | - Total Health Care Expenditure in the UK | 76 |
| | - Cost of the NHS | 98 |
| | - Private Health Care | 127 |
| Section 3 | Hospital Services | 135 |
| | - Cost of Hospital Services | 140 |
| | - Hospital Workforce | 146 |
| | - Hospital Activities | 158 |
| Section 4 | Family Health Services | 191 |
| | - General Medical Services | 200 |
| | - General Pharmaceutical Services | 222 |
| | - General Dental Services | 272 |
| | - General Ophthalmic Services | 280 |
| Glossary | | 285 |
| References | | 288 |
| Index | | 291 |

# Introduction

This is the 19th edition (2008) of the Compendium of Health Statistics published by the Office of Health Economics. It aims to provide in a single volume a wide range of statistical information on health and health care in the UK and its four constituent countries, including long time series and comparisons with other economically developed nations. It has been designed to be of particular value to individuals and organisations with an interest in the UK health care sector and the National Health Service (NHS).

An internet on-line version of the Compendium (the i-Compendium) is also available, providing instant access and retrieval of information. Built-in powerful full text search capability enables the user to carry out searches across a wide range of fields. In addition to the search facility, functions available include hypertext links between narrative text, tables and graphs, and viewable Excel and PowerPoint files for editing and exporting to other applications. Further information about the i-Compendium is available at its website

www.ohecompendium.org

The Compendium comprises four main sections plus a glossary and references. The contents have been fully updated and revised since the 18th edition (2007).

- Section 1 gives a summary of UK demographic statistics, including the mortality and morbidity experience of the population. Selected Lifestyle statistics are also included. Comparisons are made with European Union and OECD countries.

- Section 2 examines the financing of the NHS and draws international comparisons. In addition, it brings together information on the main areas of private health care in the UK.

- Section 3 provides a detailed account of NHS hospital activity together with information on the hospital workforce and cost of treatment.

- Section 4 gives detailed coverage of the activities of the NHS Family Health Services: general medical, pharmaceutical, dental and ophthalmic.

Throughout the Compendium, information and comparisons are provided at national and international levels where appropriate and available. Total UK data have been compiled and are shown alongside data for the individual constituent countries. In many cases time series are presented including annual data as far back as 1949, the first full year of the NHS's life.

### Notes on tables and charts:

1. Statistical data relate mainly to the UK. Where figures are for Great Britain or for individual countries of the UK only, this is indicated in the relevant table or chart.

2. Rounding of numbers may lead to minor inconsistencies between the sum of constituent parts and the total in some tables.

3. Throughout the Compendium, "billion" means one thousand million.

4. Symbols and abbreviations used:

   -      not available or not classified at that time.

   0      nil unless otherwise stated.

   e      OHE estimate(s), unless otherwise stated.

   AGR   Annual average growth rate (per cent).

   ICD   International Classification of Diseases.

The Office of Health Economics welcomes comment on the Compendium of Health Statistics. Please write to Emma Hawe at:

12 Whitehall, London SW1A 2DY

fax     +44(0)20 7747 8851

email ehawe@ohe.org

# List of Tables and Figures

## Section 1 Population, mortality, morbidity and lifestyle statistics

### Population                                                                                            Page

| | | |
|---|---|---|
| Table 1.1 | UK resident population and projections by age group, 1948 – 2051 | **8** |
| Figure 1.1 | Trends in UK resident population and projections and age distribution of UK population, 1948 – 2051 | **9** |
| Figure 1.2 | Growth in UK elderly population and projections as a percentage of UK population, 1948 – 2051 | **10** |
| Figure 1.3 | Trends and projections for UK population aged under 65, 1948 – 2051 | **11** |
| Figure 1.4 | Trends and projections for characteristics of the UK population, 1951 – 2051 | **12** |
| Table 1.2 | UK resident population and projections by sex and country, 1951 – 2051 | **13** |
| Table 1.3 | Population by age group and sex, mid-year estimates, UK, 1951 – 2006 | **14** |
| Table 1.4 | Population by age group and sex, mid-year estimates, England, 1951 – 2006 | **15** |
| Table 1.5 | Population by age group and sex, mid-year estimates, Wales, 1951 – 2006 | **16** |
| Table 1.6 | Population by age group and sex, mid-year estimates, Scotland, 1951 – 2006 | **17** |
| Table 1.7 | Population by age group and sex, mid-year estimates, Northern Ireland, 1951 – 2006 | **18** |
| Table 1.8 | Mid-year population estimates, total, aged 65 and over and aged 75 and over by country, UK, 1991 – 2006 | **19** |
| Table 1.9 | Total populations and projected populations of OECD and EU countries, 1950 – 2020 | **20** |
| Table 1.10 | Dependency ratios and projected dependency ratios (number aged under 15 or 65 and over, per 100 working population) in OECD and EU countries, 1950 – 2020 | **21** |
| Table 1.11 | Population aged 65 and over in OECD and EU countries, 1950 – 2020 | **22** |
| Table 1.12 | People aged 65 and over as a percentage of total population in OECD and EU countries, 1950 – 2020 | **23** |
| Table 1.13 | Population aged 75 and over in OECD and EU countries, 1950 – 2020 | **24** |
| Table 1.14 | People aged 75 and over as a percentage of total population in OECD and EU countries, 1950 – 2020 | **25** |
| Figure 1.5 | Median ages in OECD and EU countries, 2005 | **26** |
| Table 1.15 | Life expectancy at birth and aged 65 by sex, by country, UK, 1981 – 2004 | **27** |
| Table 1.16 | Residual life expectancy in years, England and Wales, 1841 – 2004 | **28** |
| Figure 1.6 | Trends in life expectancy in England and Wales, 1841 – 2051 | **29** |
| Table 1.17 | Life expectancy at birth in OECD and EU countries, males, 1950/55 – 2020/25 | **30** |
| Table 1.18 | Life expectancy at birth in OECD and EU countries, females, 1950/55 – 2020/25 | **31** |
| Figure 1.7 | Projected life expectancy at birth in OECD and EU countries, 2005 – 2010 | **32** |

### Mortality

| | | |
|---|---|---|
| Figure 1.8 | Trends in birth rate, infant, childhood and age standardised mortality rates, UK, 1950 – 2005 | **33** |
| Figure 1.9 | Trends in all causes mortality for males in the countries of the UK, 1950 – 2005 | **34** |
| Figure 1.10 | Trends in all causes mortality for females in the countries of the UK, 1950 – 2005 | **35** |
| Table 1.19 | Birth rates, infant and childhood mortality rates, UK, 1870 – 2005 | **36** |
| Table 1.20 | Crude mortality rates in OECD and EU countries, 1960 – 2003 | **37** |
| Table 1.21 | Infant mortality rates in OECD and EU countries, 1960 – 2005 | **38** |
| Figure 1.11 | Infant mortality rates in selected OECD and EU countries, circa, 2005 | **39** |
| Table 1.22 | Infant and neonatal mortality in selected OECD and EU countries, circa 2004 | **40** |
| Table 1.23 | Infant and neonatal mortality rates per 1,000 live births in selected OECD and EU countries, circa 2004 | **41** |
| Table 1.24 | Childhood mortality in selected OECD and EU countries, circa 2004 | **42** |
| Table 1.25 | Childhood mortality rates per 100,000 population in selected OECD and EU countries, circa 2004 | **43** |

# List of Tables and Figures

| | | |
|---|---|---|
| Table 1.26 | Age specific mortality rates per 1,000 population, UK, 1870 – 2005 | **44** |
| Figure 1.12 | Trends in age specific mortality rates, UK, 1948 – 2005 | **45** |
| Table 1.27(a) | Deaths and crude death rates by main cause, UK, 1970 – 2005 | **46** |
| Table 1.27(b) | Crude death rates by main cause, rates per 100,000 population, UK, 1970 – 2005 | **46** |
| Table 1.28 | Number of deaths and age standardised mortality rates by main cause, sex and country, UK, 2005 | **47** |
| Table 1.29 | Years of potential working life lost due to premature deaths by selected causes, England and Wales, 1980 – 2005 | **48** |
| Table 1.30 | Deaths by main cause in selected OECD and EU countries, circa 2004 | **49** |
| Table 1.31 | Age standardised mortality rates for all persons by main cause in selected OECD and EU countries, circa 2004 | **50** |
| Table 1.32 | Age standardised mortality rates for males by main cause in selected OECD and EU countries, circa 2004 | **51** |
| Table 1.33 | Age standardised mortality rates for females by main cause in selected OECD and EU countries, circa 2004 | **52** |
| Table 1.34 | Crude death rates per 100,000 population for leading causes of death, UK, 1970 – 2005 | **53** |
| Table 1.35 | Age standardised mortality rates from coronary heart disease, cerebrovascular disease, lung cancer and breast cancer, men and women aged 15-74, in selected OECD and EU countries, circa 2004 | **54** |
| Figure 1.13 | Age standardised mortality rates from coronary heart disease, men and women aged 15-74, in selected OECD and EU countries, circa 2004 | **55** |
| Figure 1.14 | Age standardised mortality rates from cerebrovascular disease, men and women aged 15-74, in selected OECD and EU countries, circa 2004 | **56** |
| Figure 1.15 | Age standardised mortality rates from lung cancer, men and women aged 15-74, in selected OECD and EU countries, circa 2004 | **57** |
| Figure 1.16 | Age standardised mortality rates from breast cancer, women aged 15-74, in selected OECD and EU countries, circa 2004 | **58** |

### *Morbidity*

| | | |
|---|---|---|
| Table 1.36 | Registrations of newly diagnosed cases of cancer, selected sites, by sex and country, UK, 2004 | **59** |
| Table 1.37 | Age standardised registration rates of newly diagnosed cases of cancer, selected sites, by sex and country, UK, 2004 | **60** |
| Table 1.38(a) | Prevalence of longstanding illness by age and sex, Great Britain, 1975 – 2005 | **61** |
| Table 1.38(b) | Prevalence of limiting longstanding illness by age and sex, Great Britain, 1975 – 2005 | **61** |
| Figure 1.17 | Trends in prevalence of longstanding illness by age group, Great Britain, 1972 – 2005 | **62** |
| Figure 1.18 | Prevalence of longstanding illness by socio-economic classification, Great Britain, 2005 | **63** |
| Table 1.39(a) | Percentage of population consulting a NHS GP in a two-week period, Great Britain, 1975 – 2005 | **64** |
| Table 1.39(b) | Average number of NHS GP consultations per person per year, Great Britain, 1975 – 2005 | **64** |
| Table 1.40 | Longstanding chronic sickness rates by age and condition groups, Great Britain, 2005 | **65** |
| Table 1.41 | Estimated days off work due to self-reported illness caused or made worse by work, by complaint type, Great Britain, 2001/02 – 2005/06 | **66** |

### *Lifestyle*

| | | |
|---|---|---|
| Table 1.42 | Prevalence of cigarette smoking by sex and age, Great Britain, 1974 - 2005 | **67** |
| Figure 1.19 | Prevalence of cigarette smoking by country, 1978 – 2005 | **68** |
| Figure 1.20 | Prevalence of smoking males and females aged 15 and over in selected OECD and EU countries, circa 2005 | **69** |
| Table 1.43 | Weekly consumption of alcohol (in units) by sex and age, Great Britain, 1988/89 – 2005 | **70** |

# List of Tables and Figures

Figure 1.21 Percentage who drank more than 3 or 4 units on at least one day in the last week by sex and country, 1998 – 2005 **71**

Figure 1.22 Annual consumption of pure alcohol (in litres) per person aged 15 and over in selected OECD and EU countries, circa 2005 **72**

Table 1.44(a) Percentage of men, women and children who are overweight , 1995 – 2005 **73**

Table 1.44(b) Percentage of men, women and children who are obese, 1995 – 2005 **73**

Figure 1.23 Percentage of population who are overweight or obese by sex and country, 2004 **74**

Figure 1.24 Prevalence of obesity, males and females in OECD and EU countries, 2005 **75**

## Section 2 UK Health Care Expenditure and Cost of the NHS

### Total Health Care Expenditure in the UK

Table 2.1 Total health care expenditure, UK, 1972/73 – 2007/08 **77**

Figure 2.1 Total health care expenditure, UK, 1972/73 – 2007/08 **78**

Figure 2.2 Relationship between total UK health care expenditure and GDP, 1972/73 – 2007/08 **79**

Figure 2.3 NHS pay and prices index and GDP deflator index, 1975/76 – 2005/06 **80**

Figure 2.4 Indices of total UK NHS expenditure at constant prices, 1975/76 – 2005/06 **81**

Figure 2.5 Indices of UK spending on public and private health care at constant prices, 1973/74 – 2006/07 **82**

Table 2.2 Total health care expenditure (£ billion) in OECD and EU countries, 1960 – 2005 **83**

Table 2.3 Total health care expenditure per capita (£ cash) in OECD and EU countries, 1960 – 2005 **84**

Figure 2.6 Total annual health care expenditure per capita in OECD and EU countries, circa 2005 **85**

Table 2.4 Total health care expenditure as per cent of GDP in OECD and EU countries, 1960 – 2005 **86**

Table 2.5 Index (2000=100) of total health care expenditure as per cent of GDP in OECD and EU countries, 1960 – 2005 **87**

Table 2.6 GDP per capita in OECD and EU countries (£ cash), 1960 – 2005 **88**

Table 2.7 Index of GDP per capita at £ cash prices (2000=100) in OECD and EU countries, 1960 – 2005 **89**

Table 2.8 Public health spending as a percentage of total health care expenditure in OECD and EU countries, 1960 – 2005 **90**

Table 2.9 Private health spending as a percentage of total health care expenditure in OECD and EU countries, 1960 – 2005 **91**

Figure 2.7 Public and private health spending as a percentage of total health care expenditure, OECD and EU countries, circa 2005 **92**

Figure 2.8 Total, public and private health care expenditure as a percentage of GDP in OECD and EU countries, circa 2005 **93**

Figure 2.9 Relationship between total health care spending per capita and GDP per capita in OECD and EU countries, circa 2005 **94**

Table 2.10 Total health care expenditure, infant mortality and life expectancy in OECD and EU countries, 1960 and 2005 **95**

Table 2.11 Relative indices (UK=100) for total health care expenditure, infant mortality and life expectancy in OECD and EU countries, 1960 and 2005 **96**

Figure 2.10 Relationship between total health care expenditure per capita and infant mortality rate in OECD and EU countries, circa 2005 **97**

### Cost of the NHS

Table 2.12 GDP and NHS expenditure, UK, 1949/50 – 2006/07 **100**

Table 2.13 GDP and NHS expenditure per capita, UK, 1949/50 – 2006/07 **101**

# List of Tables and Figures

| | | |
|---|---|---|
| Figure 2.11 | Gross cost of NHS, in cash and real terms and NHS cost as a per cent of GDP, UK, 1949/50 – 2006/07 | **102** |
| Figure 2.12 | Relationship between gross NHS cost and GDP, UK, 1949/50 – 2006/07 | **103** |
| Figure 2.13 | Relationship between NHS cost as a percentage of GDP and GDP, UK, 1949/50 – 2006/07 | **104** |
| Table 2.14 | Public health expenditure as a percentage of GDP at market prices, in OECD and EU countries, 1960 – 2005 | **105** |
| Table 2.15 | Index (2000=100) of public health expenditure as a percentage of GDP at market prices in OECD and EU countries, 1960 – 2005 | **106** |
| Figure 2.14 | Public health expenditure as a percentage of GDP in selected OECD and EU countries, 1960 and 2005 | **107** |
| Table 2.16 | Public health expenditure per capita (£ cash) in OECD and EU countries, 1960 – 2005 | **108** |
| Table 2.17 | Index of (£) public health expenditure per capita (2000=100) in OECD and EU countries, 1960 – 2005 | **109** |
| Figure 2.15 | Relationship between per capita public health spending and per capita GDP, OECD and EU countries, circa 2005 | **110** |
| Table 2.18 | Hospital and Community Health Services gross expenditure by age, England, 1980/81 – 2003/04 | **111** |
| Table 2.19 | Percentage distribution of HCHS gross expenditure by age, England, 1980/81 – 2003/04 | **111** |
| Figure 2.16 | Estimated Hospital and Community Health Services expenditure per capita by age group, England, 2003/04 | **112** |
| Table 2.20 | Revenue expenditure of strategic health authorities, NHS trusts and primary care trusts , England, 1984/85 – 2004/05 | **113** |
| Figure 2.17 | Revenue expenditure of strategic health authorities, NHS trusts and primary care trusts, England, 1984/85 – 2004/05 | **114** |
| Table 2.21 | UK public employees in selected sectors, 1961 – 2007 | **115** |
| Figure 2.18 | Indices of UK public employees in selected sectors, 1975 – 2007 | **116** |
| Table 2.22 | NHS net expenditure (revenue and capital) per capita and per household, UK, 1975/76 – 2005/06 | **117** |
| Table 2.23 | UK NHS gross expenditure (£) per capita, by service, 1950 – 2004/05 | **118** |
| Table 2.24 | NHS gross expenditure – proportion spent on each service, UK, 1949 – 2005/06 | **119** |
| Table 2.25 | UK NHS sources of finance, 1949 – 2006 | **120** |
| Table 2.26 | NHS patient charges, UK, 1950/51 – 2006/07 | **121** |
| Table 2.27 | Distribution of UK public expenditure by selected sectors, 1950 – 2006/07 | **122** |
| Figure 2.19 | Indices of UK public expenditure at constant prices, 1986/87 – 2006/07 | **123** |
| Table 2.28 | The Government's Expenditure Plans for the NHS, England, 1999/2000 – 2007/08 | **124** |
| Table 2.29 | Gross NHS expenditure by Programme budget categories, England, 2002/03 – 2005/06 | **125** |
| Table 2.30 | Gross NHS expenditure by Programme budget categories, Wales, 2003/04 – 2005/06 | **126** |

## *Private Health Care*

| | | |
|---|---|---|
| Table 2.31 | Number of private medical insurance subscribers, people covered and payments, UK, 1955 – 2005 | **128** |
| Figure 2.20 | Number of private medical insurance subscribers and people insured, UK, 1955 – 2005 | **129** |
| Table 2.32 | Private health care and gross NHS expenditure per household, UK, 1973 – 2006 | **130** |
| Figure 2.21 | UK consumer expenditure on private health care at 2006 prices, 1973 – 2006 | **131** |
| Table 2.33 | Private health care expenditure as a percentage of GDP in OECD and EU countries, 1960 – 2005 | **132** |
| Table 2.34 | Private health care expenditure per capita (£ cash) in OECD and EU countries, 1960 – 2005 | **133** |
| Figure 2.22 | Private health care expenditure per capita in OECD and EU countries, 2005 | **134** |

## Section 3 Hospital Services

### Cost of Hospital Services

| | | |
|---|---|---|
| Table 3.1 | Gross cost of hospital services and Family Health Services (FHS), UK, 1949/50 – 2005/06 | **140** |
| Table 3.2 | NHS hospital gross expenditure (revenue and capital) per capita and household, UK, 1975/76 – 2005/06 | **141** |
| Figure 3.1 | Gross cost of hospital services £ cash and as a percentage of NHS cost, UK, 1949/50 – 2005/06 | **142** |
| Figure 3.2 | Relationship between NHS expenditure on Family Health Services (FHS) and on hospital services, UK, 1975/76 – 2005/06 | **143** |
| Figure 3.3 | Hospital expenditure as a percentage of total health spending and hospital expenditure per capita (£) in selected OECD countries, circa 2005 | **144** |
| Figure 3.4 | Comparison of volume and real growth in NHS hospital gross expenditure, UK, 1975/76 – 2005/06 | **145** |

### Hospital Workforce

| | | |
|---|---|---|
| Table 3.3 | Number of staff employed in NHS hospitals and community services by category, UK, 1951 – 2005 | **146** |
| Figure 3.5 | Index of NHS hospital and community workforce per 100,000 population, UK, 1951 – 2005 | **147** |
| Table 3.4 | Medical and dental staff employed in NHS hospitals, UK, 1951 – 2005 | **148** |
| Table 3.5 | NHS available hospital beds and FCEs per medical and dental staff, UK, 1951 – 2005/06 | **149** |
| Table 3.6 | NHS hospital and community nursing and midwifery staff, UK, 1951 – 2005 | **150** |
| Figure 3.6 | Trends in NHS medical and nursing staff numbers, FCEs and available beds, UK, 1951 – 2005 | **151** |
| Table 3.7 | NHS available hospital beds and FCEs per nursing and midwifery staff, 1951 – 2005/06 | **152** |
| Table 3.8 | Number of hospital and community medical and dental staff (full-time equivalents), by grade England, 1996 – 2006 | **153** |
| Table 3.9 | Number of full-time equivalent hospital and community medical staff by selected specialty, England, 1990 – 2006 | **154** |
| Table 3.10 | Full-time equivalent hospital and community medical staff by selected specialty and country, number and per 10,000 population, Great Britain, 2005 | **155** |
| Table 3.11 | Number of full-time equivalent hospital and community medical consultants by selected specialty, England, 1990 – 2006 | **156** |
| Table 3.12 | Full-time equivalent hospital and community consultants by selected specialty and country, number and per 10,000 population, Great Britain, 2005 | **157** |

### Hospital Activities

| | | |
|---|---|---|
| Table 3.13 | Average daily number of available NHS hospital beds, UK, 1951 – 2005/06 | **158** |
| Table 3.14 | Average daily available acute beds in NHS hospitals, Great Britain, 1959 – 2005/06 | **159** |
| Table 3.15 | Average daily available NHS beds: number, per 100,000 population and occupancy, England, 1996/97 – 2006/07 | **160** |
| Table 3.16 | Average daily occupied beds in NHS hospitals by country, UK, 1951 – 2005/06 | **161** |
| Figure 3.7 | Hospital inpatient acute beds per 1,000 population in selected OECD countries, circa 2005 | **162** |
| Table 3.17 | Number of NHS hospital finished consultant episodes (FCEs)/discharges and deaths, UK, 1951 – 2005/06 | **163** |
| Table 3.18 | Inpatient finished consultant episodes (FCEs), discharges and deaths in NHS hospitals, by selected specialties, Great Britain, 1959 – 2005/06 | **164** |
| Figure 3.8 | Relationship between acute bed provision and hospital discharge rate in selected OECD countries, circa 2005 | **165** |
| Table 3.19 | Average inpatient length of stay in NHS hospitals, all specialties, UK, 1951 – 2005/06 | **166** |
| Figure 3.9 | Average inpatient length of stay in NHS acute hospitals, England, 1959 – 2005/06 | **167** |

# List of Tables and Figures

| | | |
|---|---|---|
| Table 3.20 | Hospital finished consultant episodes (FCEs) by primary diagnosis, England, 1995/96 – 2005/06 | **168** |
| Table 3.21(a) | Hospital finished consultant episodes per 1,000 population by primary diagnosis, England, 1995/96 – 2005/06 | **169** |
| Table 3.21(b) | Estimated number of hospital finished consultant episodes, UK, 1995/96 – 2005/06 | **169** |
| Table 3.22 | Hospital ordinary admissions (excluding day cases) by main cause, England, 1995/96 – 2005/06 | **170** |
| Table 3.23 | Mean length of stay of hospital ordinary admissions and index (1995/96=100), by main cause, England, 1995/96 – 2005/06 | **171** |
| Table 3.24 | Number and percentage distribution of hospital bed days for ordinary admissions by main cause, England, 1995/96 – 2005/06 | **172** |
| Table 3.25 | Estimated ordinary admissions by top major diagnostic group, England, 2000/01 – 2005/06 | **173** |
| Table 3.26 | Inpatient bed days and lengths of stay by top major diagnostic group, England, 2000/01 – 2005/06 | **174** |
| Table 3.27 | Number and rate of surgical operations by main site, England, 1995/96 – 2005/06 | **175** |
| Table 3.28 | Number and rate of NHS hospital surgical operations by site and age, England, 2005/06 | **176** |
| Table 3.29 | Number and rate of the most frequent surgical operations, England, 2000/01 – 2005/06 | **177** |
| Table 3.30 | Patients waiting for elective admission, by selected specialties, England, 1997 – 2007 | **178** |
| Figure 3.10 | Patients waiting for elective admission, England, 1992 – 2007 | **179** |
| Table 3.31 | Top 50 Healthcare Resource Groups (HRGs) with high mean waiting time, number of admissions and percentage admitted from waiting lists, England, 2005/06 | **180** |
| Table 3.32 | Waiting time for first outpatient appointment by the top 30 specialties, England, 31 March 2007 | **181** |
| Table 3.33 | Number of hospital day cases by main specialty, England, 2000/01 – 2005/06 | **182** |
| Table 3.34 | Reference costs per FCE and average length of stay of top 40 Healthcare Resource Groups (HRGs) ranked by total cost, NHS Trusts, elective inpatients, England, 2005/06 | **183** |
| Table 3.35 | Reference costs per FCE and average length of stay of top 40 Healthcare Resource Groups (HRGs) ranked by total cost, NHS Trusts, non-elective inpatients, England, 2005/06 | **184** |
| Table 3.36 | Reference costs per case of top 40 Healthcare Resource Groups (HRGs) ranked by total cost, NHS Trusts, day cases, England, 2005/06 | **185** |
| Table 3.37 | Reference costs per FCE of top 40 Healthcare Resource Groups (HRGs) ranked by total cost, non-NHS providers, elective inpatients, England, 2005/06 | **186** |
| Table 3.38 | Reference costs per case of top 40 Healthcare Resource Groups (HRGs) ranked by total cost, non-NHS providers, day cases, England, 2005/06 | **187** |
| Table 3.39 | Hospital outpatient clinics: total attendances, by country, UK, 1952 – 2005/06 | **188** |
| Table 3.40 | Hospital outpatient clinics: new cases, by country, UK, 1952 – 2005/06 | **189** |
| Table 3.41(a) | Percentage of population attending NHS hospital outpatient departments by age group, in 3 months prior to survey interview, Great Britain, 1985/86 – 2005 | **190** |
| Table 3.41(b) | Estimated number of annual NHS hospital outpatient department attendances by age group, UK, 1985/86 – 2005 | **190** |

## Section 4 Family Health Services

| | | |
|---|---|---|
| Table 4.1 | Cost of Family Health Services (FHS) at 2005/06 prices, UK, 1949/50 – 2005/06 | **193** |
| Figure 4.1 | Family Health Services (FHS) expenditure as a percentage of gross NHS cost, UK, 1949/50 – 2005/06 | **194** |
| Table 4.2 | Family Health Services (FHS) expenditure distribution by service, UK, 1949/50 – 2005/06 | **195** |
| Figure 4.2 | Primary health care as a percentage of total health expenditure in selected OECD countries, circa 2005 | **196** |
| Figure 4.3 | Real growth in expenditure on Family Health Services (FHS) and hospital services, UK, 1949/50 – 2005/06 | **197** |

# List of Tables and Figures

Table 4.3    Real cost of Family Health Services (FHS) per capita, UK, 1949/50 – 2005/06    **198**

Table 4.4    Family Health Services (FHS) gross expenditure (revenue and capital) per capita and per household, UK, 1975/76 – 2005/06    **199**

### *General Medical Services*

Table 4.5    Cost of General Medical Services (GMS) per capita and per household, UK, 1975/76 – 2005/06    **203**

Figure 4.4    Cost of General Medical Services (GMS) at 2005/06 prices, UK, 1949/50 – 2005/06    **204**

Table 4.6    NHS medical workforce (GPs, hospital and community medical staff), UK, 1951 – 2006    **205**

Figure 4.5    Number of GPs per 1,000 population in selected OECD and EU countries, circa 2005    **206**

Table 4.7    Number of general medical practitioners (GPs including registrars) in general practice and per 100,000 population, by country, UK, 1985 – 2006    **207**

Table 4.8    Number of medical practitioners (excluding registrars and retainers), in general practice, UK, 1951– 2006    **208**

Table 4.9(a)    Number of GP registrars by country, UK, 1996 – 2006    **209**

Table 4.9(b)    Number of medical practitioners in general practice (excluding GP retainers) per GP registrar by country, UK, 1996 – 2006    **209**

Table 4.10    Resident population per medical practitioner (excluding GP registrars and retainers) in general practice, UK, 1951 – 2006    **210**

Table 4.11    Average list size of medical practitioners (excluding GP registrars and retainers) in general practice by country, UK, 1964 – 2006    **211**

Figure 4.6    Average list size of medical practitioners (excluding GP registrars and retainers) in general practice by country, UK, 1964 – 2006    **212**

Table 4.12    Number of patients per medical practitioner (excluding GP registrars and retainers) in general practice, by patient age group, UK, 1951 – 2006    **213**

Table 4.13(a) People aged 65 and over per medical practitioner (excluding GP registrars and retainers) in general practice, by country, UK, 1996 – 2006    **214**

Table 4.13(b) People aged 75 and over per medical practitioner (excluding GP registrars and retainers) in general practice, by country, UK, 1996 – 2006    **214**

Table 4.14    Number of all general medical practitioners (excluding GP retainers) in general practice by age and sex, England, 1996 – 2006    **215**

Table 4.15    Distribution of medical practitioners (excluding GP registrars and retainers) in general practice by size of practice, UK, 1975 – 2005    **216**

Table 4.16(a) Number of medical practitioners (excluding GP registrars and retainers) in general practice by size of practice, England and Wales, 1975 – 2006    **216**

Table 4.16(b) Number of medical practitioners (excluding GP registrars and retainers) in general practice by size of practice, Scotland, 1975 – 2005    **217**

Table 4.16(c) Number of medical practitioners (excluding GP registrars and retainers) in general practice by size of practice, Northern Ireland, 1975 – 2005    **217**

Figure 4.7    Index (1959=100) of number of medical practitioners (excluding GP registrars and retainers) in general practice, by size of practice, England and Wales, 1959 – 2006    **218**

Table 4.17    Estimated number and index (1975=100) of NHS GP consultations by age group, UK, 1975 – 2005    **219**

Table 4.18    Estimated number and index (1975=100) of NHS consultations per medical practitioner (excluding GP registrars and retainers), in general practice, UK, 1975 – 2005    **220**

Table 4.19(a) Number of dispensing doctors by country, UK, 1995 – 2005    **221**

Table 4.19(b) Number of NHS prescription items dispensed by dispensing doctors by country, UK, 1995 – 2005    **221**

*General Pharmaceutical Services*

| | | |
|---|---|---|
| Table 4.20 | Cost of General Pharmaceutical Services (GPS) per capita and per household, UK, 1989/90 – 2005/06 | **227** |
| Figure 4.8 | Gross cost of General Pharmaceutical Services (GPS), UK, 1951/52 – 2005/06 | **228** |
| Figure 4.9 | Pharmaceutical expenditure as per cent of GDP in selected OECD countries, circa 2005 | **229** |
| Figure 4.10 | Pharmaceutical expenditure per capita in selected OECD countries, circa 2005 | **230** |
| Table 4.21 | Number of chemists and appliance contractors and number per 100,000 population by country, UK, 1996 – 2006 | **231** |
| Figure 4.11 | Practising pharmacists per 1,000 population in selected OECD and EU countries, circa 2005 | **232** |
| Table 4.22 | Number and index (1995=100) of prescription items dispensed per chemist by country, UK, 1996 – 2006 | **233** |
| Table 4.23 | Number of NHS prescriptions (R$_x$s) (based on fees) dispensed by chemists and appliance contractors, UK, 1948 – 2006 | **234** |
| Figure 4.12 | Index of number of prescriptions (R$_x$s) (based on fees) dispensed by chemists and appliance contractors, by country, UK, 1949 – 2006 | **235** |
| Table 4.24 | Total number of NHS prescriptions (based on items) dispensed by country, UK, 1995/96 – 2005/06 | **236** |
| Table 4.25 | Number of prescription items dispensed, and per capita, by age group, England, 1978 – 2006 | **237** |
| Figure 4.13 | Prescription items dispensed per capita among elderly people, England, 1978 – 2006 | **238** |
| Table 4.26 | Total cost of NHS prescriptions (R$_x$s) dispensed, UK, 1948 – 2006 | **239** |
| Figure 4.14 | Total cost of NHS prescriptions (R$_x$s) dispensed as a percentage of total NHS cost and total costs per prescription, UK, 1949 – 2006 | **240** |
| Figure 4.15 | NHS prescription charges and items dispensed by chemists and appliance contractors, UK, 1949 – 2006 | **241** |
| Figure 4.16 | Basic rate of prescription charges at constant prices and as a percentage of total prescription costs, UK, 1978 – 2006 | **242** |
| Figure 4.17 | Revenue from prescription charges and as a percentage of General Pharmaceutical Services (GPS) cost, UK, 1951/52 – 2005/06 | **243** |
| Figure 4.18 | Proportion of NHS prescriptions exempt from the prescription charge, England, 1984 – 2006 | **244** |
| Table 4.27 | Net ingredient cost (NIC) of NHS prescriptions (R$_x$s) dispensed, UK, 1949 – 2006 | **245** |
| Table 4.28 | Net ingredient cost per prescription dispensed and at constant prices (1995=100) by country, UK, 1996 – 2006 | **246** |
| Table 4.29 | Net ingredient cost (NIC) of prescriptions per capita and per household, UK, 1975 – 2006 | **247** |
| Table 4.30 | Net ingredient cost of prescriptions and cost per capita by age group, England, 1978 – 2006 | **248** |
| Figure 4.19 | Net ingredient cost (NIC) per elderly person, England, 1978 – 2006 | **249** |
| Figure 4.20 | Prescription items per capita dispensed by chemists, by major therapeutic group, UK, 1996 – 2006 | **250** |
| Figure 4.21 | Net ingredient cost (NIC) per capita, by major therapeutic group, UK, 1996 – 2006 | **251** |
| Table 4.31 | Number and net ingredient cost (NIC) of prescriptions by therapeutic group, UK, 1996 – 2006 | **252** |
| Table 4.32 | Number and net ingredient cost (NIC) of prescriptions by therapeutic group, England, 1996 – 2006 | **253** |
| Table 4.33 | Number and net ingredient cost (NIC) of prescriptions by therapeutic group, Wales, 1996 – 2006 | **254** |
| Table 4.34 | Number and net ingredient cost (NIC) of prescriptions by therapeutic group, Scotland, 1996 – 2006 | **255** |
| Table 4.35 | Number and net ingredient cost (NIC) of prescriptions by therapeutic group, Northern Ireland, 1996 – 2006 | **256** |
| Table 4.36 | Percentage of total number and net ingredient cost (NIC) of prescriptions by therapeutic group, UK, 1996 – 2006 | **257** |

Table 4.37    Percentage of total number and net ingredient cost (NIC) of prescriptions by therapeutic group, England, 1996 – 2006   **258**

Table 4.38    Percentage of total number and net ingredient cost (NIC) of prescriptions by therapeutic group, Wales, 1996 – 2006   **259**

Table 4.39    Percentage of total number and net ingredient cost (NIC) of prescriptions by therapeutic group, Scotland, 1996 – 2006   **260**

Table 4.40    Percentage of total number and net ingredient cost (NIC) of prescriptions by therapeutic group, Northern Ireland, 1996 – 2006   **261**

Table 4.41    Net ingredient cost (NIC) per prescription item at 2005 prices by therapeutic group, UK, 1996 – 2006   **262**

Table 4.42    Net ingredient cost (NIC) per prescription item at 2005 prices by therapeutic group, England, 1996 – 2006   **263**

Table 4.43    Net ingredient cost (NIC) per prescription item at 2005 prices by therapeutic group, Wales, 1996 – 2006   **264**

Table 4.44    Net ingredient cost (NIC) per prescription item at 2005 prices by therapeutic group, Scotland, 1996 – 2006   **265**

Table 4.45    Net ingredient cost (NIC) per prescription item at 2005 prices by therapeutic group, Northern Ireland, 1996 – 2006   **266**

Figure 4.22    Market share of branded and generic prescription items dispensed by chemists, England, 1949 – 2006   **267**

Figure 4.23    Relationship between generic prescribing and generic dispensing, England, 2006   **268**

Table 4.46    Estimated total NHS expenditure on pharmaceuticals at manufacturers' prices, UK, 1969 – 2006   **269**

Figure 4.24    Estimated total NHS expenditure on medicines (at manufacturers' prices) and per cent of gross NHS cost, UK, 1969 – 2006   **270**

### *General Dental Services*

Table 4.47    General Dental Services (GDS) gross expenditure per capita and per household, UK, 1975/76 – 2005/06   **273**

Figure 4.25    Gross cost of General Dental Services (GDS) and per cent of gross NHS cost, UK, 1949/50 – 2005/06   **274**

Figure 4.26    Patient dental charges and as a percentage of the gross cost of General Dental Services (GDS), UK, 1951/52 – 2005/06   **275**

Figure 4.27    Courses of dental treatment and per 1,000 people, UK, 1951 – 2004/05   **276**

Table 4.48    Number of NHS dental practitioners, UK, 1951 – 2006   **277**

Figure 4.28    Number of practising dentists per 1,000 population in OECD countries, circa 2005   **278**

### *General Ophthalmic Services*

Figure 4.29    Gross cost of General Ophthalmic Services (GOS) and per cent of gross NHS cost, UK, 1949/50 – 2005/06   **280**

Table 4.49    General Ophthalmic Services (GOS) expenditure per capita and per household, UK, 1975/76 – 2005/06   **281**

Figure 4.30    Numbers of NHS sight tests and pairs of glasses supplied per 1,000 population, UK, 1965 – 2006/07   **282**

Table 4.50    Number of opticians and per 100,000 population, UK, 1949 – 2005/06   **283**

# Population, Mortality, Morbidity and Lifestyle Statistics

## Main points

- Life expectancy at birth in England and Wales has increased over the last two decades by 5.0 years for men and 3.3 years for women.

- Partly as a consequence of that, the UK population is ageing. Of the 60.6 million in population 2006, 16.0% were aged 65 and over and 7.7% were aged 75 and over.

- Within the UK, life expectancy is highest in England and lowest in Scotland with a difference between them of about two years for both sexes.

- Circulatory diseases remain the most common cause of death in the UK, accounting for almost 36% of all deaths.

- The UK has higher death rates from coronary heart disease and breast cancer than most EU countries, with Scotland also having relatively high mortality from lung cancer and stroke.

### Population

In 2006 the UK population was 60.6 million, of whom 83.8% lived in England, 8.4% in Scotland, 4.9% in Wales and 2.9% in Northern Ireland (**Table 1.2** and **1.4** to **1.7**). The UK total has increased by 2.4 million (4.2%) over the past decade (**Table 1.1**). The UK is not alone in its growth; many OECD[1] and EU[2] countries continue to experience an increase in population size (**Table 1.9**), with some countries, such as Turkey and Mexico, growing appreciably faster than the UK. Current predictions suggest that by 2051, the UK population will rise to 77.2 million (**Table 1.2**).

**Table 1.8** shows that population growth has not been equal within the UK over the last decade. The population in England increased by 4.6 per cent, Northern Ireland by a similar 4.8 per cent, Wales by only 2.6 per cent and Scotland only 0.5 per cent.

Changes in population size are driven by the net difference between the birth and death rate, known as natural change, net migration and other changes such as the number of armed forces and their dependents resident in the UK. Since the 1990s, migration has become a major factor affecting the UK population size (**Box 1**).

Box 1 **Components of change in population size, UK 1951-2021**

| Decade | Start population | Annual averages (000's) | | | |
|---|---|---|---|---|---|
| | | Live births | Deaths | Natural Change | Migration and other factors |
| 1951-61 | 50,287 | 839 | 593 | 246 | 6 |
| 1961-71 | 52,807 | 962 | 638 | 324 | -12 |
| 1971-81 | 55,928 | 736 | 666 | 69 | -27 |
| 1981-91 | 56,357 | 757 | 655 | 103 | 5 |
| 1991-01 | 57,439 | 731 | 631 | 100 | 68 |
| 2001-11[1] | 59,113 | 741 | 580 | 160 | 201 |
| 2011-21[1] | 62,761 | 802 | 551 | 252 | 191 |

*Note:* 1 Projections are 2006-based.
*Sources:* Government Actuary's Department (GAD). Population Estimates and Projections (ONS).

The live birth rate has generally declined since its postwar peak in 1964 at the height of the baby boom. There were 723,000 UK births in 2005, the highest number since 1997 (**Table 1.19**). In parallel, the total period fertility rate for the UK has also increased in recent years, reaching 1.79 in 2005, compared to an all time low of 1.63 in 2001. However, this is still below the typically quoted fertility level required for population replacement of 2.1.

**Box 2** shows the changing distribution of the UK population. In 2006, the number of individuals in the elderly age groups was considerably greater than half a century earlier, and the number of children somewhat lower.

Box 2. **Age distribution of UK population, by age and gender, 1956 and 2006**.

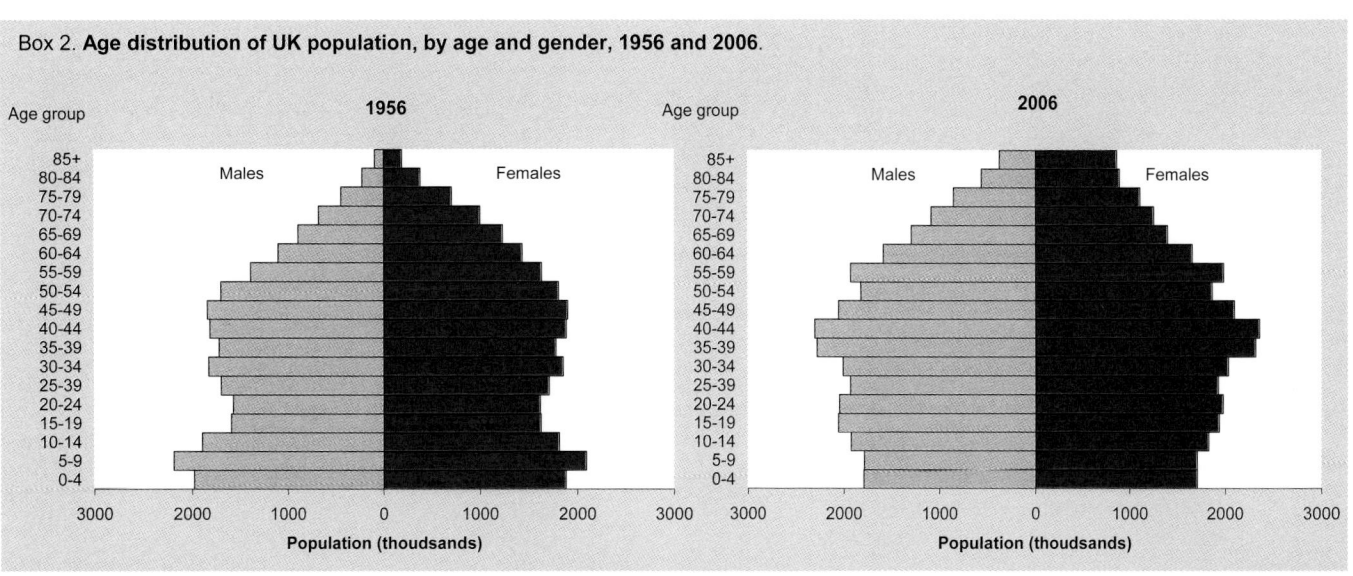

# Population, Mortality, Morbidity and Lifestyle Statistics

| Decade | Total change | <15 | 15 - 64 | >= 65 | >= 75 | >= 85 |
|---|---|---|---|---|---|---|
| 1951-61 | 5.2 | 9.7 | 2.4 | 12.7 | 22.2 | 50.0 |
| 1961-71 | 5.9 | 8.9 | 2.3 | 19.4 | 18.2 | 66.7 |
| 1971-81 | 0.9 | -14.1 | 3.7 | 14.9 | 26.9 | 20.0 |
| 1981-91 | 1.8 | -5.1 | 3.0 | 6.6 | 21.0 | 45.6 |
| 1991-2001 | 2.9 | 0.9 | 3.4 | 3.5 | 10.9 | 29.4 |
| 2001-11[1] | 6.2 | -1.7 | 7.0 | 12.0 | 12.4 | 27.1 |
| 2011-21[1] | 7.1 | 9.5 | 2.4 | 22.9 | 26.8 | 35.6 |
| 2021-31[1] | 5.8 | 0.2 | 2.4 | 22.3 | 30.3 | 47.7 |

Note:     1 Projections are 2006-based.
Sources: Monitor PP2 (ONS).
            Government Actuary's Department (GAD).
            Population Estimates and Projections (ONS).

The elderly population has been increasing throughout this period (**Box 3**). In 2006 approximately one in six individuals in the UK were 65 or older, compared to just one in nine 50 years earlier (**Table 1.1**). This is predicted to rise yet further, to an estimated one in five by 2021. There has also been a dramatic increase in those 85 or older, with 1.2 million in 2006 (**Figure 1.1** and **Table 1.1**). Within the UK, Wales has the largest proportion of elderly people and Northern Ireland the smallest (**Table 1.8**). In contrast there has been a decline in the proportion of children in the UK population over the past decade. Those aged 0-14 represented 17.7% of the UK population in 2006, compared to 23.2% 50 years earlier (**Table 1.1**).

In 2005 the dependency ratio, the number of individuals aged ≥65 or <15 per 100 people aged 15 to 64, stood at 52 in the UK (**Table 1.10**). This is in line with the dependency ratios observed for the majority of other EU and OECD countries. However, there is considerable spread in dependency ratios, ranging from 39 in Korea to 58 in Mexico.

The median age[3] in the UK rose to 38.9 in 2005, this is in line with the majority of other EU and OECD countries. However, in Japan the median age observed is considerably higher, at 43. The lowest median age observed is for Mexico, standing at just 26 (**Figure 1.5**). It is predicted that the median age in the UK will rise to nearly 42.9 by 2051 (**Box 4**).

In 2006 49.0% of the UK population were male (**Table 1.2**). The number of boys was greater than the number of girls in all age groups up to age 20, reflecting the greater number of male births, whereas females outnumber males in all age groups above 30. For those aged 85+, just 30.5% are males, due to the greater life expectancy of women (**Table 1.3**).

| Year | Median age | Working age population[1] (millions) |
|---|---|---|
| 1950 | 33.8 | 37.9 |
| 1960 | 35.3 | 38.6 |
| 1970 | 33.4 | 38.2 |
| 1980 | 33.5 | 36.3 |
| 1990 | 35.0 | 37.4 |
| 1995 | 35.8 | 37.5 |
| 2000 | 36.9 | 38.4 |
| 2001 | 38.0 | 38.6 |
| 2011 | 39.7 | 41.4 |
| 2021 | 40.2 | 42.3 |
| 2031 | 41.8 | 43.0 |
| 2041 | 42.9 | 43.3 |
| 2051 | 42.9 | 44.6 |

Notes:    Figures from 2011 to 2051 are based on 2006 population projections.
            1 Men and women aged 16 to 64 years.
Sources: Government Actuary's Department.
            Population Estimates and Projections (ONS).

## Life Expectancy

In 1841 life expectancy at birth in England and Wales was 40.2 years for males and 42.2 years for females. This has risen steadily through the years, reaching 76.9 and 81.1, for males and females born in 2004 (**Table 1.16** and **Figure 1.6**). Females who had reached age 65 in 2004 were expected to live for a further 19.6 years, and males for an additional 16.8 years. Life expectancy in Scotland is well below that in the rest of the UK. (**Box 5** and **Table 1.15**).

Box 5  Residual life expectancy in years, UK, 2004

**Males**

| | At birth | Aged 45 | Age 65 |
|---|---|---|---|
| UK | 76.62 | 33.58 | 16.63 |
| England | 76.91 | 33.81 | 16.78 |
| Wales | 76.32 | 33.29 | 16.36 |
| Scotland | 74.23 | 31.75 | 15.46 |
| Northern Ireland | 76.01 | 33.21 | 16.35 |

**Females**

| | At birth | Aged 45 | Age 65 |
|---|---|---|---|
| UK | 80.95 | 37.24 | 19.44 |
| England | 81.17 | 37.43 | 19.58 |
| Wales | 80.65 | 36.87 | 19.17 |
| Scotland | 79.27 | 35.74 | 18.38 |
| Northern Ireland | 80.83 | 37.15 | 19.34 |

Note:    Figures are based on population and deaths for a three year period centered on the year shown (i.e. figures for 2004 cover 2003-2005).
Source: Government Actuary's Department.

# Population, Mortality, Morbidity and Lifestyle Statistics

Life expectancy in the UK was above the average for males and approximately average for females compared with other high income countries in 2000-2005 (**Tables 1.17** and **1.18**). Iceland currently has the highest life expectancy for males: 79.3 (**Table 1.17**), whereas Japan has the greatest life expectancy for women: 85.2 (**Table 1.18**). For all countries in the OECD and EU, and for the world as a whole, life expectancy for both sexes is expected to rise over the next 20 years. Life expectancy for the world as a whole was over 11 years less than that of the average observed for OECD countries in 2004. However, this marks a considerable improvement on 50 years ago when the difference in life expectancy between developed and less developed countries exceeded 25 years.[4]

## Mortality

There has been a significant decline in the mortality rates for England and Wales, Scotland, and Northern Ireland over the past 50 years, particularly after adjusting for the changing age distribution[5] (**Figures 1.9** and **1.10**). Of the 582,663 deaths within the UK in 2005 (**Table 1.27**), more deaths per population occurred in Scotland than in the rest of the UK, with the lowest mortality rate being for England and Wales (**Table 1.28** and **Figures 1.9** and **1.10**). The UK mortality rate remains above the averages observed across the EU15 and OECD countries (**Table 1.20**).

Mortality in all age groups and for both sexes has significantly declined in the UK over the past 50 years, though the decrease is particularly marked for both the young and the elderly (**Box 6**). In 2004 the crude death rate for the UK fell below 10 per 1,000 population for the first time and remained at 9.7 deaths per thousand population in 2005 (**Table 1.26**).

Infant mortality is often used as a measure of living standards and the effectiveness of health care provision. In the UK there has been a marked reduction in infant and childhood mortality over the 20th century, with 5.1 deaths under a year per 1,000 live births in 2005 compared to 31.2 in 1950 and 142.5 in c1900 (**Table 1.19**). The infant mortality rate in the UK is currently similar to that observed for the majority of EU and OECD countries. However, there is a considerable spread reported in the rates for individual countries, ranging from 2.3 per 1,000 live births in 2005 for Iceland to 23.6 for Turkey (**Table 1.21**). As for all international comparisons, differences should be interpreted with caution.[6] In 2005, UK neonatal and postnatal mortality rates for both sexes combined stood at 3.9 and 1.8 per 1,000 live births respectively. Rates were higher for boys than for girls in all infant age groups (**Table 1.23**).

**Box 6  UK mortality rates (deaths per 1,000 population in each age group)**

**Males**

| Year | Infant deaths | 1-14 | 15-44 | 45-64 | 65-84 | >=85 |
|---|---|---|---|---|---|---|
| 1950 | 35.0 | 0.9 | 2.0 | 14.6 | 76.3 | 272.0 |
| 1960 | 25.1 | 0.6 | 1.6 | 14.0 | 74.9 | 251.0 |
| 1970 | 20.9 | 0.5 | 1.4 | 13.9 | 69.2 | 246.1 |
| 1980 | 13.4 | 0.4 | 1.2 | 12.5 | 63.9 | 227.0 |
| 1990 | 10.0 | 0.3 | 1.2 | 9.4 | 57.8 | 202.1 |
| 1995 | 6.9 | 0.2 | 1.1 | 7.9 | 54.3 | 188.0 |
| 2000 | 6.1 | 0.2 | 1.1 | 7.0 | 46.9 | 188.0 |
| 2001 | 6.0 | 0.2 | 1.1 | 6.8 | 45.3 | 186.9 |
| 2002 | 5.9 | 0.2 | 1.1 | 6.8 | 44.8 | 188.4 |
| 2003 | 5.7 | 0.2 | 1.1 | 6.7 | 44.3 | 192.2 |
| 2004 | 5.5 | 0.2 | 1.1 | 6.4 | 42.3 | 177.1 |
| 2005 | 5.7 | 0.2 | 1.1 | 6.3 | 40.9 | 173.3 |

**Females**

| Year | Infant deaths | 1-14 | 15-44 | 45-64 | 65-84 | >=85 |
|---|---|---|---|---|---|---|
| 1950 | 26.0 | 0.7 | 1.5 | 8.7 | 54.9 | 239.2 |
| 1960 | 19.0 | 0.6 | 1.0 | 7.5 | 50.0 | 212.1 |
| 1970 | 16.0 | 0.4 | 0.8 | 7.5 | 44.0 | 189.5 |
| 1980 | 10.0 | 0.3 | 0.7 | 6.9 | 40.6 | 179.5 |
| 1990 | 7.7 | 0.2 | 0.6 | 5.8 | 37.4 | 158.7 |
| 1995 | 5.4 | 0.2 | 0.6 | 4.9 | 36.3 | 161.4 |
| 2000 | 5.0 | 0.1 | 0.6 | 4.4 | 32.6 | 155.8 |
| 2001 | 5.0 | 0.1 | 0.6 | 4.3 | 32.0 | 155.8 |
| 2002 | 4.5 | 0.1 | 0.6 | 4.3 | 31.9 | 160.2 |
| 2003 | 4.9 | 0.1 | 0.6 | 4.2 | 32.1 | 166.3 |
| 2004 | 4.6 | 0.1 | 0.6 | 4.1 | 30.5 | 155.1 |
| 2005 | 4.5 | 0.1 | 0.6 | 4.0 | 29.9 | 153.1 |

*Note:* All rates are age specific death rates per 1,000 in each age group, except "infant deaths" which are per 1,000 live births.
*Sources:* Population Trends (ONS); Annual Abstract of Statistics (ONS).

Amongst the UK working age population there has been a reduction in the potential years of working life lost over the past 50 years, from 2.24 million in 1950 to 1.23 in 2005 (**Box 7**). In England and Wales, 20% of working years of life lost in males were due to cancer and 19% to circulatory diseases in 2005. Among women, cancer accounted for 35% and circulatory diseases 12% of years of potential working life lost in 2005 (**Table 1.29**).

| Box 7 Years of working life lost due to mortality from all causes, UK | | | |
|---|---|---|---|
| Year | Mean death age (15-65) | Total years of life lost[1] (millions) | Working years lost[2] (millions) |
| 1950 | 51.2 | 2.98 | 2.24 |
| 1960 | 52.7 | 2.99 | 1.86 |
| 1970 | 53.2 | 3.14 | 1.81 |
| 1980 | 52.8 | 3.00 | 1.60 |
| 1990 | 52.1 | 2.75 | 1.39 |
| 1995 | 51.6 | 3.63 | 1.37 |
| 2000 | 51.3 | 3.31 | 1.32 |
| 2001 | 51.3 | 3.24 | 1.31 |
| 2002 | 51.4 | 3.21 | 1.30 |
| 2003 | 51.6 | 3.19 | 1.28 |
| 2004 | 51.6 | 3.08 | 1.24 |
| 2005 | 51.7 | 3.05 | 1.23 |

*Notes:* 1 Total years life lost relates to those aged up to age 75.
2 Working years lost for those up to age 65.
*Sources:* OHE calculation based on data supplied by the Government Actuary's Office and the Office for National Statistics.

The UK's crude death rate has decreased over the past 25 years for most leading causes (**Table 1.34**). Deaths from diseases of the circulatory system, including hypertensive disease, coronary heart disease and cerebrovascular disease, have seen a dramatic decrease of 37% since 1980 (**Table 1.27**). Despite this, 209,059 deaths, 36% of all deaths registered in the UK in 2005, were due to diseases of the circulatory system.

## Coronary Heart Disease

Coronary Heart Disease (CHD) is the single leading cause of death for both sexes in the UK, accounting for 101,310 deaths in 2005, and representing 17.4% of all mortality (**Table 1.28**). Within the UK, Scotland consistently has the highest age standardised rate of mortality from CHD, followed by Northern Ireland, then England and Wales. Of the total years of working life lost, 11.0% and 4.1% were as the result of ischaemic heart disease in men and women respectively (**Table 1.29**).

The rate of deaths from CHD in the UK has declined over past 25 years, primarily due to improvements in lifestyles (such as a reduction in the rate of smoking, see the section on lifestyle below) and in treatments (such as increased use of thrombolytics). In 1980 the rate of deaths due to CHD stood at 314 per 100,000, but by 2005 this rate had declined to 168 (**Table 1.34**). Despite this decrease, the UK CHD rate still remains higher than that in most other western European countries (see **Table 1.35** and **Figure 1.13**).

In 1999 the UK Government set out a committment to reduce the death rate from CHD and stroke and related diseases in people under 75 by at least 40% (to 83.8 deaths per 100,000 population) by 2010. Even if the target rate is attained in the UK, it will still be higher than rates already achieved by a number of OECD and EU countries. Factors which might halt or even reverse the falling trend in deaths from CHD include the rise in inactivity and obesity in the UK population, and the consequent rise in type 2 diabetes.

## Cerebrovascular Disease

Cerebrovascular disease (mainly strokes), killed 21,966 men and 35,902 women in the UK in 2005, and is the second leading cause of mortality in the UK. Although for some decades there has been a decline in the cerebrovascular mortality rate in the UK (**Table 1.34**). As for CHD, there is considerable variation in mortality rates from cerebrovascular disease amongst OECD and EU countries, with rates in some Eastern European countries being exceedingly high (**Figure 1.14**). The mortality rate in 2005 for cerebrovascular disease in Scotland was higher than in England and Wales and Northern Ireland (**Table 1.35**).

## Cancer

In the UK in 2005, there were 157,688 deaths due to cancer and 1.2 million in the EU27 countries combined (**Table 1.30**). Mortality is generally the most reliable source of statistical information on cancer as it is collected from the death certificate which is a legally required document. The drawback is that mortality rates are the result of both incidence and survival rates and mortality rates alone may mask important trends in incidence and survival. In the UK there were 284,569 newly diagnosed cancers in 2004, with almost equal numbers of men and women being diagnosed. Although mortality from breast cancer has declined of late, incidence rates have increased and breast cancer is now the most common cancer in the UK amongst women, with 44,333 registrations of new cases diagnosed in 2004 (**Table 1.36**). The incidence of many cancers is higher in Scotland than for England and Wales. This is particularly apparent for cancer of the trachea, bronchus and lung, where age standardised registration rates for cancer in Scotland are over one third higher for men and approaching two thirds higher in women compared to England (**Table 1.37**).

Cancer Research UK lists the four most common cancers in the UK as lung cancer, bowel cancer, breast cancer and prostate cancer.

## Lung Cancer

In the UK, cancer of the lung was the third most common cause of death in males, accounting for 7.1% of deaths in 2005; in women it accounted for 4.6% of deaths (**Table 1.28**). Compared to other OECD and EU countries, the UK now has one of the highest rates of lung cancer in women, with 28 deaths per 100,000 population in 2005 after age standardisation. In contrast, the rate for males is below the average observed in other OECD and EU countries with 45 deaths per 100,000 population (**Table 1.35** and **Figure 1.15**). The rate is considerably higher for Scotland than England and Wales and Northern Ireland for both sexes (**Table 1.28**).

## Breast Cancer

Breast cancer is the most common cancer in women worldwide. In the UK in 2005, 12,488 women died from breast cancer (**Table 1.28**). Deaths from breast cancer do occur in men, but are rare. In England and Wales cancers account for 35% of total years of potential working life lost in women, with 10% (5 thousand years) due to breast cancer (**Table 1.29**). Breast cancer mortality rates in the UK are higher than in the majority of OECD and EU countries (**Figure 1.16**).

## Morbidity

There are limitations to using mortality statistics as a measure of the health of a population or the burden of a disease, particularly as life expectancy increases. As life expectancy increases, the focus has shifted toward measures such as the prevalence of chronic diseases, and the maintenance of good health, both of which impact significantly on the usage of health care resources. Healthy life expectancy at birth has been approximately 10 years less than life expectancy per se. Of the constituent countries of the UK, Wales has the lowest healthy life expectancy for both males and females, standing at 65.6 and 68.7 years respectively in 2003, compared to 67.6 and 70.1 years for males and females in the UK as a whole (**Box 8**).

**Box 8  Residual healthy life expectancy in years, UK, 2003**

**Males**

|  | At birth | Aged 65 |
|---|---|---|
| UK | 67.6 | 12.3 |
| England | 67.9 | 12.5 |
| Wales | 65.5 | 10.9 |
| Scotland | 66.1 | 11.7 |
| Northern Ireland | 65.7 | 11.9 |

**Females**

|  | At birth | Aged 65 |
|---|---|---|
| UK | 70.1 | 14.3 |
| England | 70.2 | 14.4 |
| Wales | 68.7 | 13.5 |
| Scotland | 69.7 | 13.8 |
| Northern Ireland | 67.9 | 13.2 |

*Sources*: Office of National Statistics, Government Actuary's Department.

The prevalence of self-reported chronic ill health in the community has been stable since the 1990's in Great Britain according to the *General Household Survey*.[7] Although the prevalence has been stable of late, from 1975 to 1990 the proportions reporting ill health increased somewhat across all age groups (**Figure 1.17** and **Box 9**), but this may represent people's changing expectations rather than "real" change.

**Box 9  Prevalence[1] longstanding illness in Great Britain, 1975 -2005 (per cent)**

| Year | Age group (years) | | |
|---|---|---|---|
|  | < 16 | 16 to 64 | >= 65 |
| 1975 | 9 | 23 | 55 |
| 1980 | 12 | 30 | 60 |
| 1990 | 17 | 33 | 63 |
| 1995 | 17 | 30 | 58 |
| 2000 | 18 | 31 | 60 |
| 2001 | 17 | 30 | 60 |
| 2002 | 19 | 32 | 67 |
| 2003 | 16 | 29 | 62 |
| 2004 | 16 | 30 | 59 |
| 2005 | 16 | 29 | 62 |

*Note:* 1 Percentages of respondents reporting long-standing illness.
*Source:* Living in Britain: Results from the General Household Survey (ONS).

In 2005, considering all ages combined, approximately one third (33%) reported having an illness that had troubled them, or was likely to trouble them over a period of time, and one fifth (19%) said that they had a long standing disability that limited their activities in some way. The prevalence of longstanding illness and limiting longstanding illness significantly increases with age for both sexes. Of those over 75, 64% registered a longstanding illness, and 47% a limiting long standing illness (**Table 1.38(a)** and **Table 1.38(b)**). In comparison, 16% of those aged under 16 reported a longstanding illness and 6% a limiting long standing illness (**Table 1.38** and **Table 1.38(b)**).

There is no consistent pattern of differences in the prevalence of sickness between the sexes for any age groups (**Table 1.38**) and only minor differences between the constituent countries of Great Britain (**Box 10**). There is a tendency for the reported prevalence of both chronic and acute illness to increase with decreasing socio-economic status (**Figure 1.18**).

The prevalence of self reported sickness in adults in Great Britain in 2005 was highest for the musculoskeletal system, affecting approximately 1 in 7 adults. For those aged 75 and over, conditions related to the heart and circulatory system were reported to be the predominant longstanding condition, affecting nearly 1 in 3 individuals (**Table 1.40**).

# Population, Mortality, Morbidity and Lifestyle Statistics

Box 10 **Prevalence[1] of long-standing illness in Great Britain, 2005 (per cent)**

|  | Male | Female |
|---|---|---|
| England | 32 | 33 |
| Wales | 32 | 35 |
| Scotland | 33 | 34 |
| Great Britain | 32 | 33 |

*Note:* 1 Percentages of respondents reporting long-standing illness.
*Source:* Living in Britain: Results from the General Household Survey (ONS).

The extent to which these levels of morbidity lead to demands on the health services is illustrated in detail in Sections 3 and 4 of the Compendium. However, **Tables 1.39(a) and 1.39(b)** show that, in 2005, about one in 7 of the population had consulted a GP in the two weeks before the *General Household Survey* interview. Women are more likely than men to consult a GP. This difference is especially noticeable for women of child-bearing age. In the 16-44 age group, 17% of women had visited a GP in the preceding fortnight, compared with only 8% of men. However, considering both sexes combined, the heaviest users of the primary care health services are the elderly: 21% of the over 75s had consulted a GP during the preceding fortnight. This age group reported an average of seven GP attendances per person per year.

The estimated number of GP consultations in England, has risen by 31% during the last decade, from 221 million in 1996 to 290 million in 2006 (**Box 11**).

Box 11 **Estimated[1] number of GP consultations in England, 1996-2006 (millions)**

| Year | Estimated number of consultations (millions) | 95% Confidence Interval (CI)[2] | |
|---|---|---|---|
| 1996 | 221.0 | 204.7 | 237.3 |
| 1997 | 219.7 | 202.7 | 236.8 |
| 1998 | 219.2 | 203.3 | 235.2 |
| 1999 | 218.3 | 204.4 | 232.1 |
| 2000 | 221.7 | 208.6 | 234.8 |
| 2001 | 236.2 | 223.8 | 248.7 |
| 2002 | 240.8 | 229.9 | 251.6 |
| 2003 | 260.1 | 249.7 | 270.6 |
| 2004 | 267.8 | 258.0 | 277.5 |
| 2005 | 281.1 | 271.9 | 290.3 |
| 2006 | 289.8 | 280.8 | 298.9 |

*Note:* 1 Estimates of volume of consultations are based on regression modeling conducted by QRESEARCH.
2 As the number of consultations is based on a sample of GP practices it has been presented along with QRESREARCH 95% CI. The 95% CI represents the range within which we can be 95% confident the true national volume of consultations lies.
*Source:* Reproduced with permission of the copyright owner. QRESEARCH (version 13)

The number of days lost from work due to self-reported illness caused or made worse by work, has declined in recent years (**Table 1.41**). An estimated 24.3 million days were lost as a result of work related illnesses in 2005/06, according to calculations based on the Labour Force Survey,[8] down by a third from 36.4 million days in 2001/02. The greatest single cause of days lost was musculo-skeletal problems followed by mental health problems.

Statistics from the Confederation of British Industry (CBI) suggest that the primary causes of short term illness were reported as minor illnesses, followed by back pain, other musculoskeletal and non-work related stress, anxiety and depression. Whereas for long-term absences, non-work related stress was reported as the leading cause. In contrast to working days lost due to work-related illnesses, absence levels have remained fairly constant in recent years, following a general pattern of decline through the 1990s.[9]

## Lifestyle

Lifestyle choices are known to contribute significantly to the health of a nation. Factors such as alcohol and tobacco intake and diet have been shown to be related to health.

## Smoking

Smoking is known to be the principal avoidable cause of premature deaths in the UK. The Department of Health has set up a series of programmes aimed at reducing the prevalence of smoking, ranging from a government ban on smoking in enclosed public places and the workplace in the UK, to the setting up of NHS stop smoking services. The prevalence of cigarette smoking in Great Britain has declined considerably over the past 30 years, with 24% of individuals smoking in 2005 compared to 45% in 1974 (**Table 1.42** and **Figure 1.19**). The percentages of males and females that smoke have reached similar proportions, being 25% and 23% respectively in 2005. Since 2001, of those 16-19 years of age, a greater proportion of females than males smoked. The highest smokers prevalence is for those in their early 20s, with around 1 in 3 smoking compared to approximately 1 in 7 of those aged 60 and over.

Smoking prevalence has declined in England, Scotland and Wales. With the exception of 2004, the recorded rates of smoking were higher in Scotland than in England and Wales (**Figure 1.19**). There was considerable variation in the ranking of smoking prevalence in 2005 between males and females across OECD and EU countries (**Figure 1.20**). For males, the percentage smoking tobacco is relatively low in the UK compared to other OECD and EU countries but, in contrast, the rate for females is relatively high.

# Population, Mortality, Morbidity and Lifestyle Statistics

## Alcohol

Guidelines set down by Government suggest that sensible limits for weekly consumption of alcohol are 21 units for men and 14 units for females. In 2005, about 1 in 4 men drank over the recommended weekly limit and 1 in 7 females exceeded their recommended limit. Across the age groups, young adults were the most likely to exceed this limit (**Table 1.43**).

While the focus for alcohol consumption was previously set using weekly limits, the Department of Health now advises that men should not regularly drink more than 3 - 4 units of alcohol per day, and women should not regularly drink more than 2 - 3 units of alcohol per day, with the aim, in part, to reduce binge drinking. According to the 2005 General Household Survey, approximately 1 in 5 females in Great Britain drank in excess of 3 units in a day during the week prior to interview, and 1 in 3 males drank in excess of 4 units in a day (**Figure 1.21**).

The UK consumer higher levels of alcohol than most other EU and OECD countries (**Figure 1.22**). In 2005, the country with the highest annual alcohol consumption per capita was Luxembourg.

## Obesity

Improvement in diet and levels of physical activity both lead to improvements in obesity. Following a rise in Great Britain in the percentage of overweight males and females (defined as having a body mass index (BMI) in excess of 25) over the last 10 years, the prevalence appears to have levelled off among adults, if not declined slightly in 2005 (**Table 1.44(a)**). The increase in overweight and obese children under 11 years appears to have persisted, with 1 in 6 obese in 2005 compared to 1 in 10 in 1995. In 2005, 24% of all women over 16 years would be defined as clinically obese (BMI >30), and over 22% of male adults (**Table 1.44(b)**).

The lowest percentage of obese individuals in Great Britain in 2004 was for Wales, standing at approximately 1 in 6, followed by England and Scotland (**Figure 1.23**). Compared to other EU and OECD countries, the UK has relatively high levels of obesity for both males and females. The country with the greatest prevalence of obesity is the United States, with over 1 in 3 Males and females defined as clinically obese in 2005. In contrast fewer than 1 in 50 were clinically obese in Japan (**Figure 1.24**).

## Notes

1. The Organisation for Economic Co-operation and Development (OECD) was formed in 1960. The 20 original member countries are: Austria, Belgium, Canada, Denmark, France, Germany, Greece, Iceland, Ireland, Italy, Luxembourg, the Netherlands, Norway, Portugal, Spain, Sweden, Switzerland, Turkey, the UK and the USA. The following 10 countries became members subsequently: Japan (in 1964), Finland (1969), Australia (1971), New Zealand (1973), Mexico (1994), the Czech Republic (1995), Hungary (1996), Poland (1996), Republic of Korea (1996) and the Slovak Republic (2000).

2. The European Union (EU) was comprised of 15 members (EU15) in 2003: Austria, Belgium, Denmark, Finland, France, Germany, Greece, Ireland, Italy, Luxembourg, The Netherlands, Portugal, Spain, Sweden and the UK. On 1 May 2006 10 new members joined: Cyprus (Greek Cypriot part), the Czech Republic, Estonia, Hungary, Latvia, Lithuania, Malta, Poland, Slovakia and Slovenia, Bulgaria and Romania joined in January 2007. In this Compendium EU15 is the group of 15 countries which formed the EU in 2003 and EU27 represents the full current membership.

3. The median age is the age that 50% of the population lies above and 50% below.

4. Yaukey, David, and Douglas L. Anderton. *Demography: The Study of Human Population*, Prospect Heights, IL: Waveland, 2001.

5. In comparing mortality experience across different populations, use of crude death rates is affected by the age structure of populations. Direct age standardisation (Breslow NE, Day NE. *Statistical Methods in Cancer Research. Volume 2. The Design of Analysis of Cohort Studies*. Lyon: IARC Scientific Publications, 1987) can be used to control for such confounding age effects, allowing meaningful comparisons to be made between countries. In our calculations, we use the European Standard Population (Waterhouse J. *Cancer Incidence in Five Continents*. Lyon: IARC, 1976) to produce the age standardised mortality rates. Details of the calculations can be found in the references cited above.

6. Jennifer Zeitlin et al, PERISTAT. Indicators for monitoring and evaluating perinatal health in Europe, The European Journal of Public Health 2003 13(Supplement 1):29-37

7. The *General Household Survey* – an annual survey based on a sample of the general population resident in private households in Great Britain – is an important source of information which provides a broad picture of the pattern of morbidity in the UK. It must be emphasised that these survey data are based on people's subjective assessments of their health. Any change over time may therefore reflect changes in their expectations of good health as well as changes in the incidence or duration of chronic illness. The survey data are also subject to sampling error, which must be taken into account when looking at differences between subgroups of the sample and at changes over time.

8. The Labour Force Survey (LFS) collects data on a sample of the population. To convert this information to give estimates for the population, the sample data are weighted. The LFS gives estimates of the number of people who have conditions which they think have been caused or made worse by work (regardless of whether they have been seen by doctors). Information is presented as estimated prevalence and rates of self-reported illness and estimated incidence and rates of self-reported illness. *Working days lost* are expressed as full-day equivalent (FDE) days to allow for variation in daily hours worked. Survey estimates are subject to uncertainty or sampling error.

9. CBI in association with AXA,.Attending to absence – Absence and labour turnover survey 2007.

# Population Statistics

Table 1.1 **UK resident population and projections by age group, 1948 - 2051**

Millions

| Year | Age group | | | | | | | | All ages | As % of all ages | | | |
|------|-----|-----|-------|-------|-------|-------|------|------|------|-------|------|------|------|
| | <5 | <15 | 15-29 | 30-44 | 45-64 | 65-74 | =>75 | =>85 | | 15-64 | =>65 | =>75 | =>85 |
| 1948 | 4.3 | 10.8 | 10.4 | 11.3 | 11.6 | 3.6 | 1.7 | 0.2 | 49.4 | 67.4 | 10.7 | 3.4 | 0.4 |
| 1950 | 4.4 | 11.3 | 10.6 | 11.1 | 11.9 | 3.6 | 1.8 | 0.2 | 50.3 | 66.8 | 10.7 | 3.6 | 0.5 |
| 1955 | 3.9 | 11.7 | 10.1 | 11.0 | 12.7 | 3.8 | 2.0 | 0.3 | 51.2 | 65.9 | 11.3 | 3.9 | 0.5 |
| 1956 | 3.9 | 11.9 | 10.0 | 10.9 | 12.8 | 3.8 | 2.0 | 0.3 | 51.4 | 65.6 | 11.3 | 4.0 | 0.5 |
| 1957 | 3.9 | 12.0 | 10.0 | 10.8 | 13.0 | 3.8 | 2.1 | 0.3 | 51.7 | 65.4 | 11.5 | 4.1 | 0.6 |
| 1958 | 4.0 | 12.0 | 10.0 | 10.7 | 13.1 | 3.9 | 2.1 | 0.3 | 51.9 | 65.2 | 11.5 | 4.1 | 0.6 |
| 1959 | 4.1 | 12.1 | 10.1 | 10.6 | 13.2 | 3.9 | 2.2 | 0.3 | 52.2 | 65.2 | 11.6 | 4.1 | 0.6 |
| 1960 | 4.2 | 12.2 | 10.3 | 10.6 | 13.3 | 3.9 | 2.2 | 0.3 | 52.6 | 65.1 | 11.7 | 4.2 | 0.6 |
| 1961 | 4.3 | 12.4 | 10.3 | 10.5 | 13.4 | 4.0 | 2.2 | 0.3 | 52.8 | 64.8 | 11.7 | 4.2 | 0.6 |
| 1962 | 4.4 | 12.3 | 10.8 | 10.6 | 13.4 | 4.0 | 2.3 | 0.4 | 53.4 | 65.2 | 11.7 | 4.2 | 0.7 |
| 1963 | 4.5 | 12.4 | 11.1 | 10.7 | 13.3 | 4.1 | 2.3 | 0.4 | 53.8 | 65.2 | 11.8 | 4.2 | 0.7 |
| 1964 | 4.6 | 12.5 | 11.3 | 10.7 | 13.3 | 4.1 | 2.3 | 0.4 | 54.2 | 65.0 | 11.9 | 4.3 | 0.7 |
| 1965 | 4.8 | 12.7 | 11.4 | 10.5 | 13.4 | 4.2 | 2.4 | 0.4 | 54.5 | 64.8 | 12.0 | 4.3 | 0.7 |
| 1966 | 4.8 | 12.8 | 11.5 | 10.3 | 13.5 | 4.3 | 2.4 | 0.4 | 54.8 | 64.5 | 12.1 | 4.3 | 0.7 |
| 1967 | 4.8 | 13.0 | 11.6 | 10.2 | 13.5 | 4.4 | 2.4 | 0.4 | 55.1 | 64.1 | 12.3 | 4.4 | 0.8 |
| 1968 | 4.8 | 13.2 | 11.6 | 10.1 | 13.5 | 4.4 | 2.5 | 0.4 | 55.4 | 63.8 | 12.5 | 4.4 | 0.8 |
| 1969 | 4.7 | 13.3 | 11.7 | 10.1 | 13.5 | 4.5 | 2.5 | 0.4 | 55.6 | 63.4 | 12.6 | 4.5 | 0.8 |
| 1970 | 4.6 | 13.4 | 11.6 | 9.8 | 13.4 | 4.6 | 2.6 | 0.4 | 55.4 | 62.9 | 13.0 | 4.6 | 0.8 |
| 1971 | 4.6 | 13.5 | 11.8 | 9.8 | 13.4 | 4.8 | 2.6 | 0.5 | 55.9 | 62.6 | 13.2 | 4.7 | 0.9 |
| 1972 | 4.4 | 13.4 | 11.9 | 9.7 | 13.3 | 4.8 | 2.7 | 0.5 | 55.8 | 62.5 | 13.4 | 4.8 | 0.9 |
| 1973 | 4.3 | 13.4 | 12.0 | 9.8 | 13.2 | 4.9 | 2.7 | 0.5 | 55.9 | 62.5 | 13.6 | 4.8 | 0.9 |
| 1974 | 4.1 | 13.3 | 12.1 | 9.9 | 13.1 | 5.0 | 2.8 | 0.5 | 56.2 | 62.5 | 13.8 | 4.9 | 0.9 |
| 1975 | 3.9 | 13.1 | 12.2 | 9.9 | 13.1 | 5.1 | 2.8 | 0.5 | 56.2 | 62.6 | 14.0 | 5.0 | 0.9 |
| 1976 | 3.7 | 12.9 | 12.4 | 10.0 | 13.0 | 5.1 | 2.9 | 0.5 | 56.2 | 62.9 | 14.2 | 5.1 | 1.0 |
| 1977 | 3.5 | 12.6 | 12.3 | 10.3 | 13.0 | 5.1 | 3.0 | 0.5 | 56.3 | 63.2 | 14.4 | 5.2 | 1.0 |
| 1978 | 3.4 | 12.3 | 12.4 | 10.5 | 12.9 | 5.2 | 3.0 | 0.6 | 56.3 | 63.6 | 14.6 | 5.4 | 1.0 |
| 1979 | 3.4 | 12.1 | 12.5 | 10.7 | 12.7 | 5.2 | 3.1 | 0.6 | 56.4 | 63.9 | 14.7 | 5.5 | 1.0 |
| 1980 | 3.4 | 11.8 | 12.7 | 10.9 | 12.6 | 5.2 | 3.2 | 0.6 | 56.4 | 64.1 | 14.9 | 5.7 | 1.0 |
| 1981 | 3.5 | 11.6 | 12.8 | 11.0 | 12.5 | 5.2 | 3.3 | 0.6 | 56.4 | 64.4 | 15.1 | 5.9 | 1.1 |
| 1982 | 3.5 | 11.4 | 13.0 | 11.0 | 12.5 | 5.1 | 3.4 | 0.6 | 56.3 | 64.8 | 15.1 | 6.0 | 1.1 |
| 1983 | 3.6 | 11.2 | 13.1 | 11.1 | 12.5 | 5.0 | 3.5 | 0.6 | 56.3 | 65.2 | 15.0 | 6.1 | 1.1 |
| 1984 | 3.6 | 11.0 | 13.2 | 11.2 | 12.6 | 4.9 | 3.5 | 0.7 | 56.4 | 65.7 | 14.9 | 6.3 | 1.2 |
| 1985 | 3.6 | 10.9 | 13.3 | 11.3 | 12.4 | 5.0 | 3.6 | 0.7 | 56.6 | 65.6 | 15.2 | 6.4 | 1.2 |
| 1986 | 3.6 | 10.8 | 13.4 | 11.5 | 12.3 | 5.0 | 3.7 | 0.7 | 56.7 | 65.6 | 15.4 | 6.5 | 1.3 |
| 1987 | 3.7 | 10.7 | 13.4 | 11.6 | 12.2 | 5.1 | 3.8 | 0.7 | 56.8 | 65.6 | 15.5 | 6.6 | 1.3 |
| 1988 | 3.7 | 10.7 | 13.4 | 11.7 | 12.2 | 5.1 | 3.8 | 0.8 | 56.9 | 65.5 | 15.6 | 6.7 | 1.4 |
| 1989 | 3.8 | 10.8 | 13.2 | 11.8 | 12.3 | 5.1 | 3.9 | 0.8 | 57.1 | 65.4 | 15.7 | 6.9 | 1.4 |
| 1990 | 3.8 | 10.9 | 13.1 | 12.0 | 12.3 | 5.0 | 4.0 | 0.8 | 57.2 | 65.3 | 15.7 | 6.9 | 1.5 |
| 1991 | 3.9 | 11.0 | 12.9 | 12.1 | 12.4 | 5.1 | 4.0 | 0.9 | 57.4 | 65.1 | 15.8 | 6.9 | 1.5 |
| 1992 | 3.9 | 11.1 | 12.6 | 12.1 | 12.7 | 5.1 | 4.0 | 0.9 | 57.6 | 64.8 | 15.8 | 6.9 | 1.6 |
| 1993 | 3.9 | 11.2 | 12.3 | 12.1 | 12.9 | 5.2 | 4.0 | 0.9 | 57.7 | 64.7 | 15.8 | 6.9 | 1.6 |
| 1994 | 3.9 | 11.3 | 12.1 | 12.3 | 13.1 | 5.2 | 3.9 | 1.0 | 57.9 | 64.7 | 15.8 | 6.8 | 1.7 |
| 1995 | 3.8 | 11.3 | 11.9 | 12.4 | 13.2 | 5.1 | 4.1 | 1.0 | 58.0 | 64.7 | 15.8 | 7.0 | 1.7 |
| 1996 | 3.7 | 11.3 | 11.7 | 12.6 | 13.3 | 5.1 | 4.2 | 1.0 | 58.2 | 64.7 | 15.9 | 7.1 | 1.8 |
| 1997 | 3.7 | 11.3 | 11.5 | 12.8 | 13.5 | 5.0 | 4.2 | 1.0 | 58.3 | 64.8 | 15.9 | 7.3 | 1.8 |
| 1998 | 3.6 | 11.3 | 11.4 | 13.0 | 13.6 | 5.0 | 4.3 | 1.1 | 58.5 | 64.8 | 15.9 | 7.3 | 1.8 |
| 1999 | 3.6 | 11.3 | 11.2 | 13.1 | 13.8 | 4.9 | 4.3 | 1.1 | 58.7 | 65.0 | 15.8 | 7.4 | 1.9 |
| 2000 | 3.6 | 11.2 | 11.2 | 13.3 | 13.9 | 4.9 | 4.4 | 1.1 | 58.9 | 65.2 | 15.8 | 7.4 | 1.9 |
| 2001 | 3.5 | 11.1 | 11.2 | 13.4 | 14.1 | 4.9 | 4.4 | 1.1 | 59.1 | 65.4 | 15.9 | 7.5 | 1.9 |
| 2002 | 3.4 | 11.0 | 11.2 | 13.5 | 14.2 | 5.0 | 4.5 | 1.1 | 59.3 | 65.5 | 15.9 | 7.5 | 1.9 |
| 2003 | 3.4 | 10.9 | 11.3 | 13.5 | 14.4 | 5.0 | 4.5 | 1.1 | 59.6 | 65.7 | 16.0 | 7.6 | 1.9 |
| 2004 | 3.4 | 10.9 | 11.4 | 13.5 | 14.5 | 5.0 | 4.5 | 1.1 | 59.8 | 65.9 | 16.0 | 7.6 | 1.9 |
| 2005 | 3.4 | 10.8 | 11.6 | 13.4 | 14.7 | 5.0 | 4.6 | 1.2 | 60.2 | 66.1 | 16.0 | 7.6 | 1.9 |
| 2006 | 3.5 | 10.7 | 11.9 | 13.3 | 15.0 | 5.0 | 4.7 | 1.2 | 60.6 | 66.3 | 16.0 | 7.7 | 2.1 |
| **Projections based on 2006 mid-year population** | | | | | | | | | | | | | |
| 2011 | 3.9 | 10.9 | 12.6 | 12.7 | 16.0 | 5.5 | 5.0 | 1.4 | 62.8 | 65.9 | 16.7 | 7.9 | 2.3 |
| 2016 | 4.0 | 11.4 | 12.5 | 12.7 | 16.5 | 6.4 | 5.5 | 1.7 | 65.0 | 64.2 | 18.2 | 8.4 | 2.5 |
| 2021 | 4.0 | 11.9 | 12.0 | 13.5 | 16.8 | 6.6 | 6.3 | 1.9 | 67.2 | 63.0 | 19.2 | 9.4 | 2.9 |
| 2051 | 4.3 | 12.6 | 13.2 | 14.8 | 17.9 | 7.6 | 11.2 | 4.9 | 77.2 | 59.4 | 24.3 | 14.5 | 6.3 |

*Notes:* Mid-year population estimates from 1982 have been revised based on the results of the 2001 Census.

Data from 2002 has been revised due to improved methodology on international migration.

*Sources:* Annual Abstract of Statistics (ONS).

Population Projections Database (GAD).

Population Estimates and Projections (ONS).

Figure 1.1 **Trends in UK resident population and projections and age distribution of UK population**[1]**,
1948 - 2051**

**Index (log scale) 1948=100**

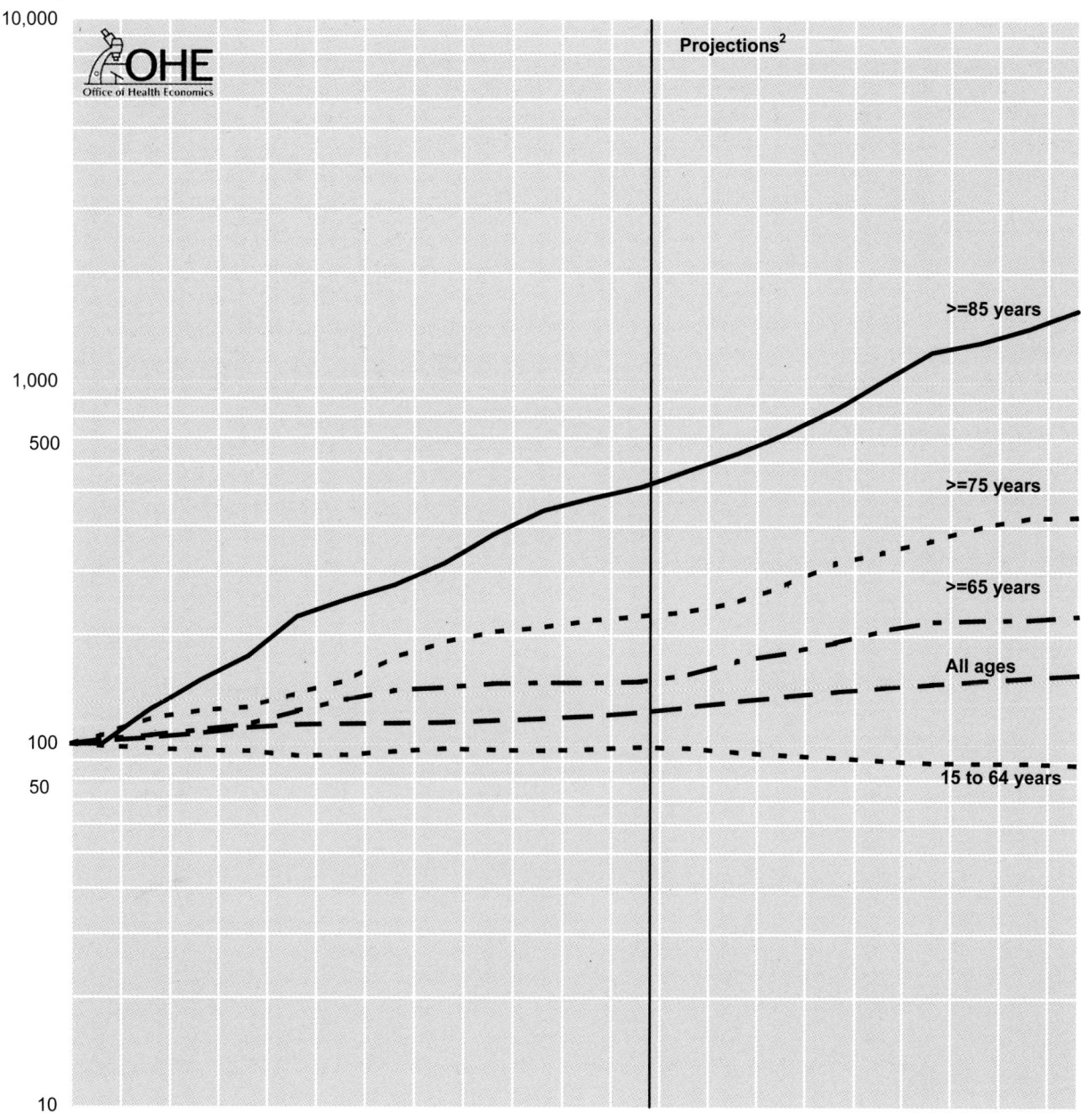

*Notes:* 1 Trends by age group represent changes in the percentage of individuals within the specified age group as a proportion of the
total population.

2 Projections from 2007 are based on 2006 mid-year estimates.

*Sources:* Annual Abstract of Statistics (ONS).

Population Projections Database (GAD).

Population Estimates and Projections (ONS).

Figure 1.2 **Growth in UK elderly population and projections as a percentage of UK population, 1948 - 2051**

**Per cent of UK population**

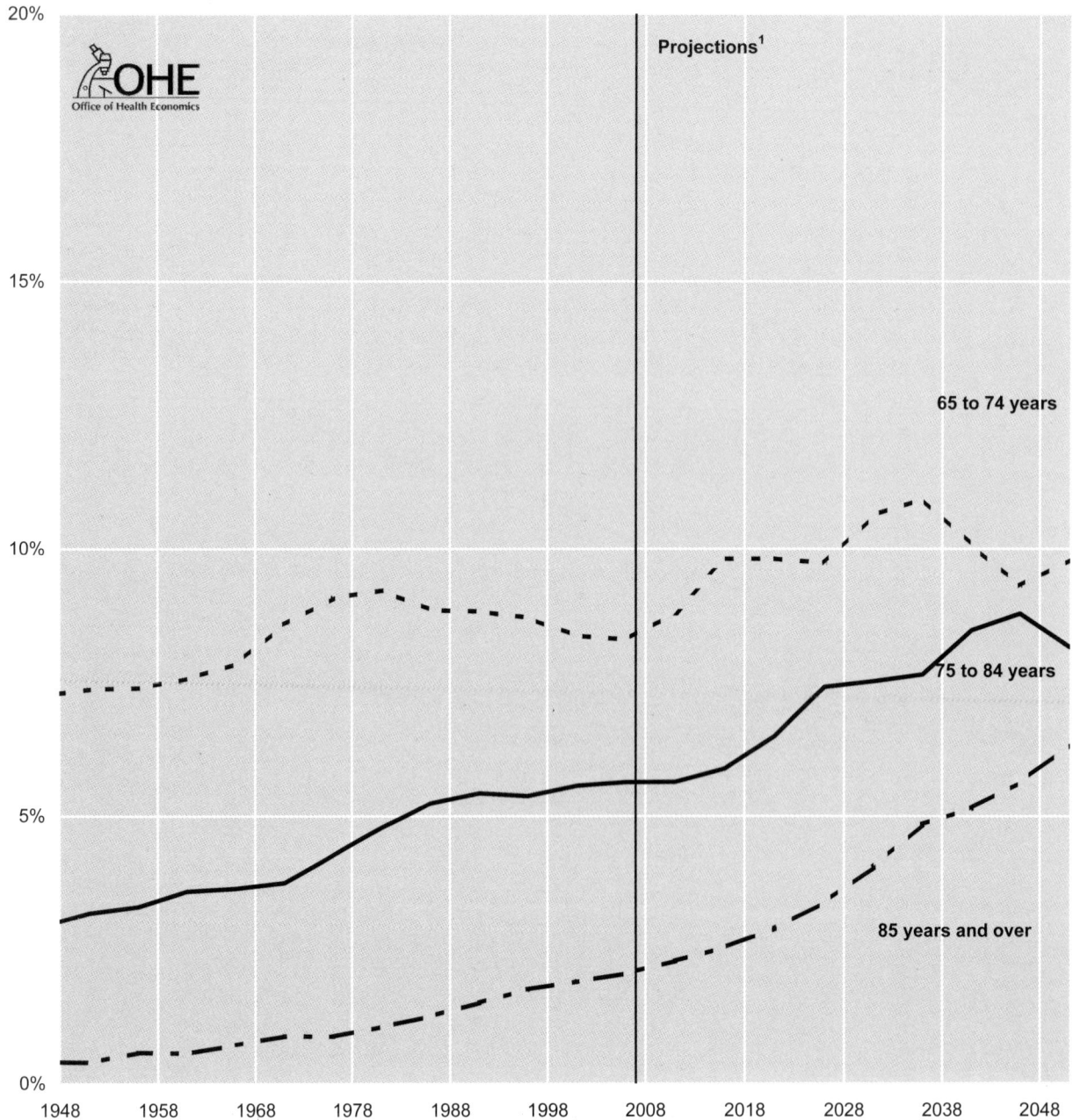

*Note:* 1 Projections from 2007 are based on 2004 mid-year estimates.
*Sources:* Annual Abstract of Statistics (ONS).
Population Projections Database (GAD).
Population Estimates and Projections (ONS).

Figure 1.3  **Trends[1] and projections for UK population aged under 65, 1948 - 2051**

**Index 1948 = 100**

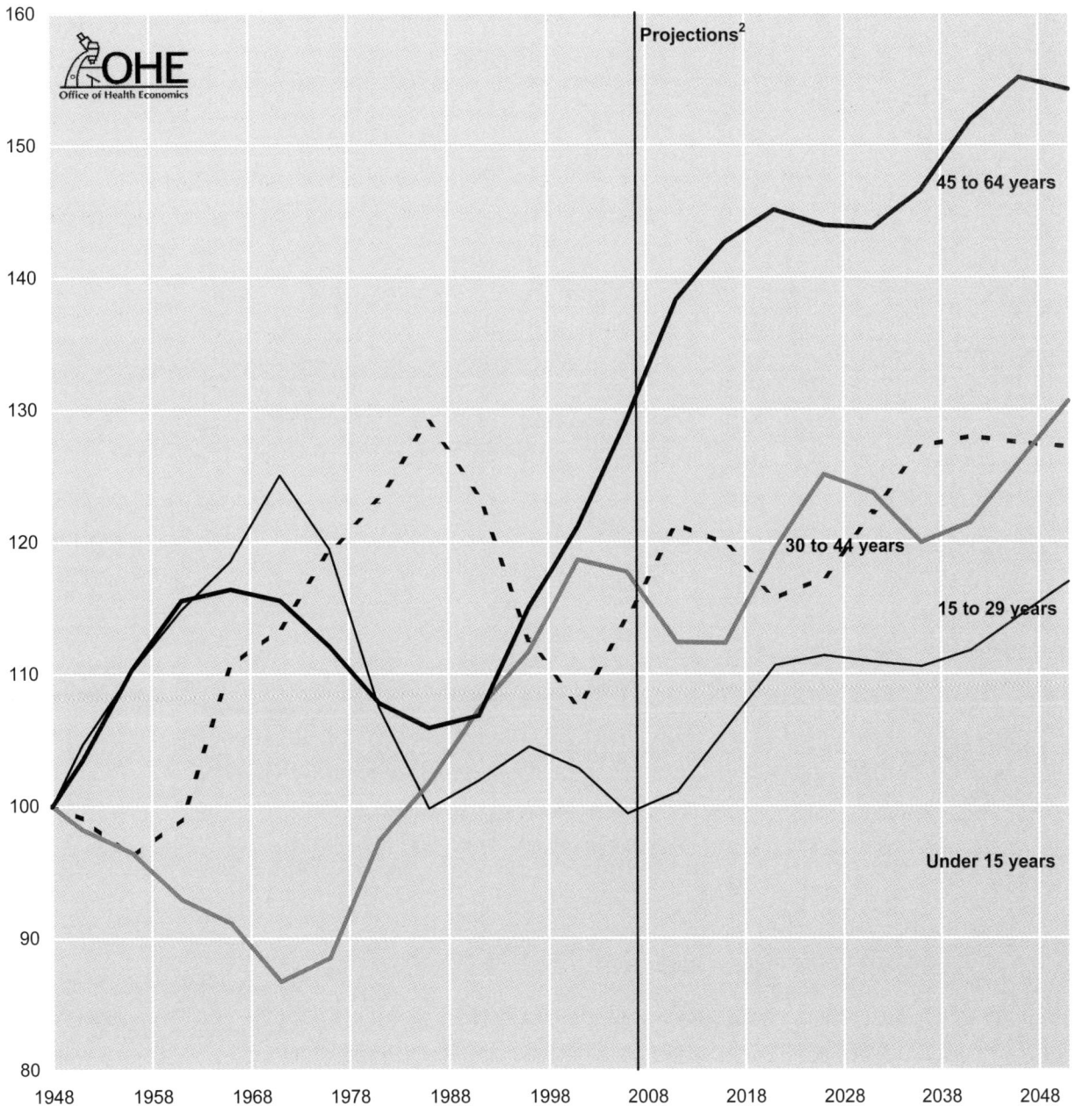

Notes:    1 Trends in population by age group correspond to changes in the number of individuals in each age group.
          2 Projections from 2007 are based on 2006 mid-year estimates.
Sources:  Annual Abstract of Statistics (ONS).
          Population Projections Database (GAD).
          Population Estimates and Projections (ONS).

Figure 1.4 **Trends and projections for characteristics of the UK population, 1951 - 2051**

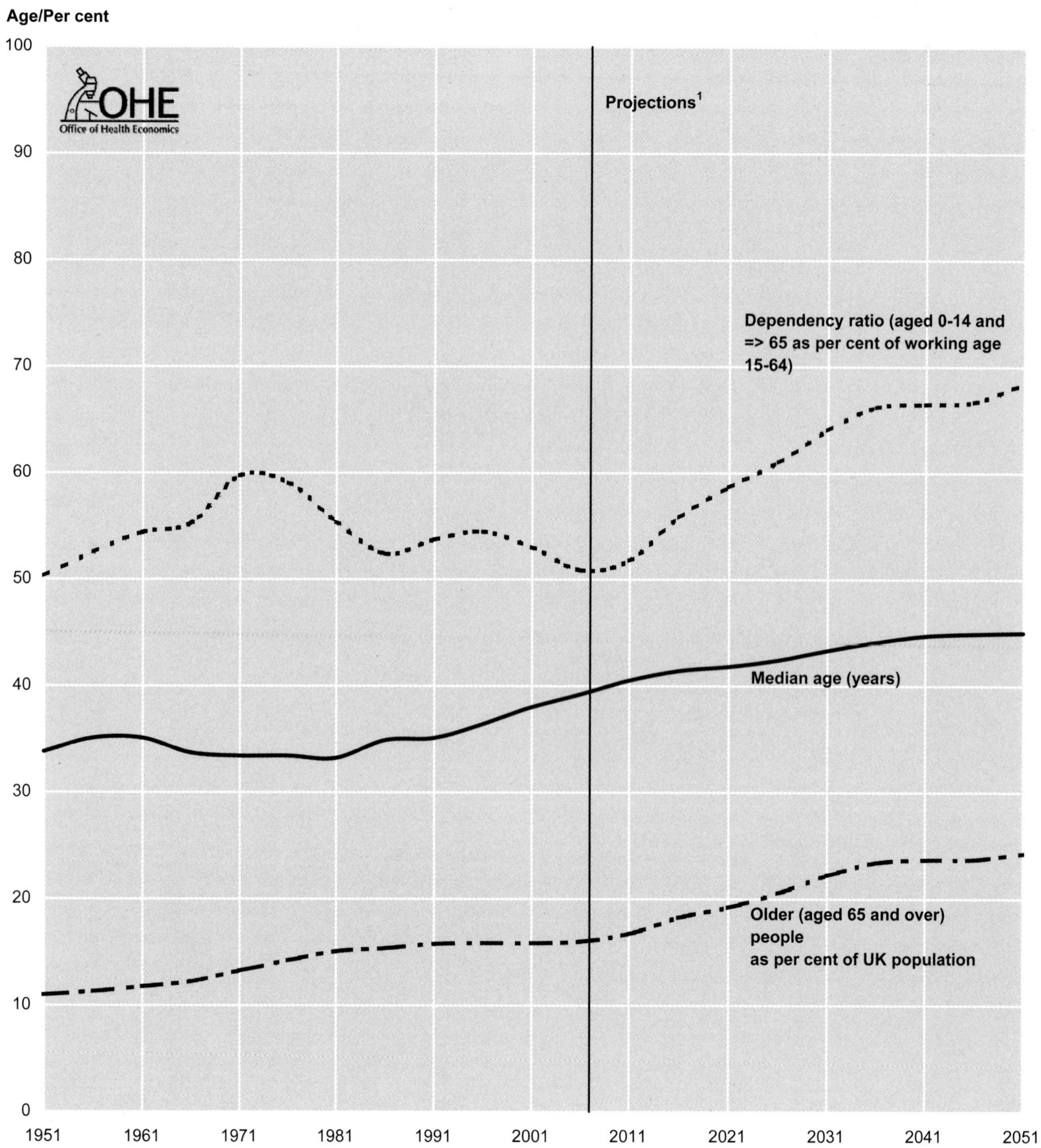

**Age/Per cent**

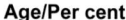

Figure shows trends with lines for:
- **Projections[1]**
- **Dependency ratio (aged 0-14 and => 65 as per cent of working age 15-64)**
- **Median age (years)**
- **Older (aged 65 and over) people as per cent of UK population**

X-axis years: 1951, 1961, 1971, 1981, 1991, 2001, 2011, 2021, 2031, 2041, 2051

*Note:* 1 Projections from 2007 are based on 2006 mid-year estimates.
*Sources:* Annual Abstract of Statistics (ONS).
Population Projections Database (GAD).
Population Estimates and Projections (ONS).

# Population Statistics

Table 1.2 **UK resident population and projections by sex and country, 1951 - 2051**

Millions

| Year | England & Wales | | Scotland | | N Ireland | | Great Britain | | | United Kingdom | | |
|---|---|---|---|---|---|---|---|---|---|---|---|---|
| | Male | Female | Male | Female | Male | Female | Male | Female | Total | Male | Female | Total |
| 1951 | 21.04 | 22.77 | 2.44 | 2.66 | 0.67 | 0.70 | 23.48 | 25.44 | 48.92 | 24.15 | 26.14 | 50.29 |
| 1955 | 21.39 | 23.05 | 2.44 | 2.67 | 0.68 | 0.72 | 23.83 | 25.72 | 49.55 | 24.51 | 26.44 | 50.95 |
| 1960 | 22.10 | 23.68 | 2.48 | 2.70 | 0.69 | 0.73 | 24.58 | 26.37 | 50.95 | 25.27 | 27.10 | 52.37 |
| 1961 | 22.35 | 23.85 | 2.49 | 2.70 | 0.70 | 0.73 | 24.83 | 26.55 | 51.38 | 25.53 | 27.28 | 52.81 |
| 1962 | 22.63 | 24.03 | 2.50 | 2.70 | 0.70 | 0.74 | 25.13 | 26.73 | 51.86 | 25.83 | 27.47 | 53.29 |
| 1963 | 22.79 | 24.19 | 2.50 | 2.71 | 0.71 | 0.74 | 25.29 | 26.89 | 52.18 | 25.99 | 27.63 | 53.62 |
| 1964 | 22.98 | 24.35 | 2.50 | 2.71 | 0.71 | 0.75 | 25.48 | 27.05 | 52.53 | 26.19 | 27.80 | 53.99 |
| 1965 | 23.15 | 24.52 | 2.50 | 2.71 | 0.72 | 0.75 | 25.65 | 27.23 | 52.88 | 26.37 | 27.98 | 54.35 |
| 1966 | 23.30 | 24.67 | 2.50 | 2.70 | 0.72 | 0.76 | 25.79 | 27.38 | 53.17 | 26.51 | 28.13 | 54.64 |
| 1967 | 23.45 | 24.82 | 2.50 | 2.70 | 0.73 | 0.76 | 25.95 | 27.52 | 53.47 | 26.67 | 28.29 | 54.96 |
| 1968 | 23.55 | 24.96 | 2.50 | 2.70 | 0.73 | 0.77 | 26.05 | 27.66 | 53.71 | 26.79 | 28.43 | 55.21 |
| 1969 | 23.67 | 25.07 | 2.50 | 2.71 | 0.74 | 0.78 | 26.17 | 27.78 | 53.95 | 26.91 | 28.55 | 55.46 |
| 1970 | 23.74 | 25.15 | 2.51 | 2.71 | 0.75 | 0.78 | 26.25 | 27.86 | 54.11 | 26.99 | 28.64 | 55.63 |
| 1971 | 23.90 | 25.26 | 2.52 | 2.72 | 0.76 | 0.79 | 26.41 | 27.98 | 54.39 | 27.17 | 28.76 | 55.93 |
| 1972 | 23.99 | 25.34 | 2.51 | 2.72 | 0.76 | 0.78 | 26.50 | 28.06 | 54.56 | 27.26 | 28.84 | 56.10 |
| 1973 | 24.06 | 25.40 | 2.52 | 2.72 | 0.76 | 0.77 | 26.58 | 28.12 | 54.69 | 27.33 | 28.89 | 56.22 |
| 1974 | 24.07 | 25.39 | 2.52 | 2.72 | 0.76 | 0.77 | 26.59 | 28.12 | 54.71 | 27.35 | 28.89 | 56.24 |
| 1975 | 24.09 | 25.38 | 2.52 | 2.72 | 0.75 | 0.77 | 26.61 | 28.09 | 54.70 | 27.36 | 28.87 | 56.23 |
| 1976 | 24.09 | 25.37 | 2.52 | 2.72 | 0.75 | 0.77 | 26.61 | 28.09 | 54.69 | 27.36 | 28.86 | 56.22 |
| 1977 | 24.08 | 25.36 | 2.52 | 2.71 | 0.75 | 0.77 | 26.59 | 28.08 | 54.67 | 27.35 | 28.85 | 56.19 |
| 1978 | 24.07 | 25.38 | 2.51 | 2.70 | 0.75 | 0.77 | 26.58 | 28.08 | 54.66 | 27.33 | 28.85 | 56.18 |
| 1979 | 24.11 | 25.40 | 2.51 | 2.70 | 0.76 | 0.77 | 26.62 | 28.09 | 54.71 | 27.37 | 28.87 | 56.24 |
| 1980 | 24.16 | 25.45 | 2.50 | 2.69 | 0.76 | 0.78 | 26.66 | 28.14 | 54.80 | 27.41 | 28.92 | 56.33 |
| 1981 | 24.16 | 25.47 | 2.50 | 2.69 | 0.75 | 0.78 | 26.66 | 28.16 | 54.81 | 27.41 | 28.94 | 56.35 |
| 1982 | 24.12 | 25.46 | 2.49 | 2.68 | 0.76 | 0.79 | 26.61 | 28.14 | 54.75 | 27.36 | 28.93 | 56.29 |
| 1983 | 24.13 | 25.48 | 2.48 | 2.67 | 0.76 | 0.79 | 26.61 | 28.15 | 54.77 | 27.37 | 28.94 | 56.32 |
| 1984 | 24.18 | 25.53 | 2.47 | 2.66 | 0.76 | 0.80 | 26.66 | 28.19 | 54.96 | 27.42 | 28.99 | 56.41 |
| 1985 | 24.25 | 25.61 | 2.47 | 2.66 | 0.76 | 0.80 | 26.72 | 28.26 | 54.99 | 27.49 | 29.07 | 56.55 |
| 1986 | 24.31 | 25.69 | 2.46 | 2.65 | 0.77 | 0.81 | 26.77 | 28.34 | 55.11 | 27.54 | 29.14 | 56.68 |
| 1987 | 24.37 | 25.75 | 2.46 | 2.64 | 0.77 | 0.81 | 26.83 | 28.40 | 55.43 | 27.60 | 29.21 | 56.80 |
| 1988 | 24.43 | 25.82 | 2.44 | 2.63 | 0.77 | 0.81 | 26.88 | 28.45 | 55.33 | 27.65 | 29.26 | 56.92 |
| 1989 | 24.51 | 25.90 | 2.44 | 2.64 | 0.78 | 0.81 | 26.95 | 28.53 | 55.78 | 27.73 | 29.35 | 57.08 |
| 1990 | 24.60 | 25.96 | 2.44 | 2.64 | 0.78 | 0.82 | 27.04 | 28.60 | 55.64 | 27.82 | 29.42 | 57.24 |
| 1991 | 24.68 | 26.07 | 2.44 | 2.64 | 0.78 | 0.82 | 27.13 | 28.71 | 55.83 | 27.91 | 29.53 | 57.44 |
| 1992 | 24.74 | 26.14 | 2.45 | 2.64 | 0.79 | 0.83 | 27.18 | 28.78 | 55.96 | 27.98 | 29.61 | 57.58 |
| 1993 | 24.79 | 26.19 | 2.45 | 2.64 | 0.80 | 0.84 | 27.24 | 28.84 | 56.08 | 28.04 | 29.67 | 57.71 |
| 1994 | 24.85 | 26.26 | 2.45 | 2.65 | 0.80 | 0.84 | 27.31 | 28.91 | 56.22 | 28.11 | 29.75 | 57.86 |
| 1995 | 24.95 | 26.33 | 2.45 | 2.65 | 0.80 | 0.85 | 27.40 | 28.98 | 56.38 | 28.20 | 29.82 | 58.02 |
| 1996 | 25.03 | 26.38 | 2.45 | 2.65 | 0.81 | 0.85 | 27.48 | 29.03 | 56.50 | 28.29 | 29.88 | 58.16 |
| 1997 | 25.11 | 26.45 | 2.44 | 2.64 | 0.82 | 0.86 | 27.56 | 29.09 | 56.64 | 28.37 | 29.94 | 58.31 |
| 1998 | 25.20 | 26.52 | 2.44 | 2.64 | 0.82 | 0.86 | 27.64 | 29.16 | 56.80 | 28.46 | 30.02 | 58.47 |
| 1999 | 25.32 | 26.61 | 2.44 | 2.64 | 0.82 | 0.86 | 27.76 | 29.25 | 57.01 | 28.58 | 30.11 | 58.68 |
| 2000 | 25.44 | 26.70 | 2.43 | 2.63 | 0.82 | 0.86 | 27.87 | 29.33 | 57.20 | 28.69 | 30.20 | 58.89 |
| 2001 | 25.57 | 26.79 | 2.43 | 2.63 | 0.82 | 0.86 | 28.01 | 29.42 | 57.42 | 28.83 | 30.28 | 59.11 |
| 2002 | 25.70 | 26.87 | 2.43 | 2.62 | 0.83 | 0.87 | 28.14 | 29.49 | 57.63 | 28.96 | 30.36 | 59.32 |
| 2003 | 25.84 | 26.96 | 2.43 | 2.62 | 0.83 | 0.87 | 28.28 | 29.58 | 57.85 | 29.11 | 30.45 | 59.56 |
| 2004 | 26.00 | 27.06 | 2.45 | 2.63 | 0.84 | 0.87 | 28.44 | 29.69 | 58.14 | 29.28 | 30.57 | 59.85 |
| 2005 | 26.20 | 27.22 | 2.46 | 2.64 | 0.84 | 0.88 | 28.65 | 29.86 | 58.51 | 29.50 | 30.74 | 60.24 |
| 2006 | 26.37 | 27.36 | 2.47 | 2.65 | 0.85 | 0.89 | 28.84 | 30.01 | 58.85 | 29.69 | 30.89 | 60.59 |
| **Projections based on 2006 mid-year estimates** | | | | | | | | | | | | |
| 2011 | 27.48 | 28.26 | 2.52 | 2.69 | 0.89 | 0.92 | 30.00 | 30.95 | 60.95 | 30.89 | 31.87 | 62.76 |
| 2016 | 28.61 | 29.23 | 2.56 | 2.71 | 0.92 | 0.95 | 31.17 | 31.94 | 63.11 | 32.09 | 32.89 | 64.98 |
| 2021 | 29.72 | 30.23 | 2.59 | 2.74 | 0.95 | 0.97 | 32.30 | 32.97 | 65.27 | 33.25 | 33.94 | 67.19 |
| 2036 | 32.48 | 32.89 | 2.60 | 2.76 | 1.00 | 1.02 | 35.08 | 35.64 | 70.72 | 36.08 | 36.67 | 72.75 |
| 2051 | 34.85 | 35.07 | 2.55 | 2.70 | 1.03 | 1.04 | 37.40 | 37.77 | 75.17 | 38.43 | 38.81 | 77.24 |

*Notes:* Mid-year population estimates from 1982 have been revised based on the results of the 2001 Census.
England and Wales mid-year population estimates from 1992 to 2002 have been further revised in light of the local authority population studies.
Figures may not sum to totals due to rounding.

*Sources:* Annual Abstract of Statistics (ONS).
Population Projections Database (GAD).
Population Estimates and Projections (ONS).

Table 1.3 **Population by age group and sex, mid-year estimates, UK, 1951 - 2006**

## Male population by age group, UK

Millions

| Age | 1951 | 1961 | 1971 | 1981 | 1991 | 1995 | 1996 | 1997 | 1998 | 1999 | 2000 | 2001 | 2002 | 2003 | 2004 | 2005 | 2006 |
|---|---|---|---|---|---|---|---|---|---|---|---|---|---|---|---|---|---|
| Total | 24.12 | 25.53 | 27.17 | 27.41 | 27.91 | 28.20 | 28.29 | 28.37 | 28.46 | 28.58 | 28.69 | 28.83 | 28.96 | 29.11 | 29.28 | 29.50 | 29.69 |
| Under 5 | 2.22 | 2.19 | 2.34 | 1.77 | 1.97 | 1.95 | 1.92 | 1.89 | 1.87 | 1.85 | 1.82 | 1.78 | 1.75 | 1.73 | 1.74 | 1.76 | 1.79 |
| 5-9 | 1.89 | 1.96 | 2.40 | 1.89 | 1.87 | 1.96 | 1.98 | 1.99 | 1.98 | 1.97 | 1.95 | 1.91 | 1.89 | 1.87 | 1.85 | 1.82 | 1.78 |
| 10-14 | 1.68 | 2.19 | 2.18 | 2.30 | 1.78 | 1.86 | 1.88 | 1.90 | 1.93 | 1.96 | 1.97 | 1.99 | 2.01 | 2.00 | 1.99 | 1.96 | 1.92 |
| 15-19 | 1.56 | 1.90 | 1.98 | 2.42 | 1.90 | 1.74 | 1.76 | 1.80 | 1.83 | 1.84 | 1.85 | 1.88 | 1.94 | 1.99 | 2.02 | 2.03 | 2.06 |
| 20-29 | 3.51 | 3.29 | 4.02 | 4.10 | 4.58 | 4.23 | 4.12 | 3.98 | 3.87 | 3.80 | 3.77 | 3.74 | 3.71 | 3.71 | 3.77 | 3.88 | 3.98 |
| 30-44 | 5.46 | 5.24 | 4.94 | 5.51 | 6.04 | 6.18 | 6.27 | 6.35 | 6.42 | 6.50 | 6.58 | 6.64 | 6.69 | 6.70 | 6.67 | 6.65 | 6.60 |
| 45-59 | 4.49 | 5.14 | 4.97 | 4.71 | 4.73 | 5.18 | 5.24 | 5.29 | 5.34 | 5.40 | 5.46 | 5.53 | 5.59 | 5.65 | 5.69 | 5.74 | 5.80 |
| 60-64 | 1.06 | 1.25 | 1.51 | 1.38 | 1.39 | 1.36 | 1.36 | 1.37 | 1.39 | 1.41 | 1.42 | 1.41 | 1.41 | 1.44 | 1.48 | 1.52 | 1.58 |
| 65-74 | 1.56 | 1.61 | 2.00 | 2.26 | 2.27 | 2.33 | 2.31 | 2.30 | 2.29 | 2.29 | 2.29 | 2.31 | 2.32 | 2.35 | 2.37 | 2.38 | 2.38 |
| 75-84 | 0.62 | 0.68 | 0.72 | 0.92 | 1.15 | 1.15 | 1.19 | 1.22 | 1.24 | 1.26 | 1.28 | 1.31 | 1.34 | 1.37 | 1.39 | 1.40 | 1.41 |
| 85+ | 0.07 | 0.11 | 0.13 | 0.14 | 0.21 | 0.26 | 0.27 | 0.28 | 0.29 | 0.30 | 0.31 | 0.31 | 0.32 | 0.31 | 0.32 | 0.35 | 0.38 |

## Female population by age group, UK

Millions

| Age | 1951 | 1961 | 1971 | 1981 | 1991 | 1995 | 1996 | 1997 | 1998 | 1999 | 2000 | 2001 | 2002 | 2003 | 2004 | 2005 | 2006 |
|---|---|---|---|---|---|---|---|---|---|---|---|---|---|---|---|---|---|
| Total | 26.11 | 27.28 | 28.76 | 28.95 | 29.53 | 29.82 | 29.88 | 29.94 | 30.02 | 30.11 | 30.20 | 30.28 | 30.36 | 30.45 | 30.57 | 30.74 | 30.89 |
| Under 5 | 2.11 | 2.08 | 2.22 | 1.68 | 1.89 | 1.86 | 1.82 | 1.80 | 1.77 | 1.76 | 1.73 | 1.70 | 1.67 | 1.65 | 1.65 | 1.67 | 1.71 |
| 5-9 | 1.80 | 1.86 | 2.28 | 1.79 | 1.79 | 1.87 | 1.89 | 1.90 | 1.89 | 1.88 | 1.85 | 1.82 | 1.80 | 1.78 | 1.76 | 1.74 | 1.71 |
| 10-14 | 1.63 | 2.08 | 2.06 | 2.18 | 1.70 | 1.78 | 1.79 | 1.81 | 1.84 | 1.87 | 1.88 | 1.90 | 1.91 | 1.90 | 1.88 | 1.86 | 1.83 |
| 15-19 | 1.61 | 1.85 | 1.89 | 2.31 | 1.81 | 1.69 | 1.72 | 1.75 | 1.78 | 1.79 | 1.78 | 1.80 | 1.82 | 1.87 | 1.90 | 1.93 | 1.94 |
| 20-29 | 3.64 | 3.28 | 3.95 | 4.01 | 4.56 | 4.22 | 4.10 | 3.98 | 3.88 | 3.82 | 3.79 | 3.75 | 3.71 | 3.69 | 3.72 | 3.81 | 3.90 |
| 30-44 | 5.66 | 5.29 | 4.86 | 5.44 | 6.08 | 6.26 | 6.35 | 6.45 | 6.53 | 6.61 | 6.69 | 6.76 | 6.81 | 6.81 | 6.79 | 6.76 | 6.71 |
| 45-59 | 5.07 | 5.47 | 5.23 | 4.83 | 4.77 | 5.24 | 5.31 | 5.37 | 5.42 | 5.49 | 5.55 | 5.63 | 5.71 | 5.77 | 5.82 | 5.87 | 5.94 |
| 60-64 | 1.36 | 1.54 | 1.72 | 1.56 | 1.50 | 1.43 | 1.43 | 1.43 | 1.45 | 1.47 | 1.48 | 1.47 | 1.48 | 1.51 | 1.55 | 1.59 | 1.66 |
| 65-74 | 2.13 | 2.37 | 2.77 | 2.93 | 2.80 | 2.80 | 2.76 | 2.72 | 2.69 | 2.66 | 2.65 | 2.64 | 2.64 | 2.65 | 2.66 | 2.67 | 2.65 |
| 75-84 | 0.94 | 1.21 | 1.44 | 1.76 | 1.97 | 1.91 | 1.94 | 1.96 | 1.97 | 1.97 | 1.97 | 1.99 | 2.01 | 2.03 | 2.04 | 2.02 | 2.00 |
| 85+ | 0.15 | 0.24 | 0.36 | 0.46 | 0.66 | 0.75 | 0.76 | 0.77 | 0.79 | 0.80 | 0.81 | 0.82 | 0.81 | 0.79 | 0.79 | 0.82 | 0.86 |

*Notes:* Mid-year population estimates from 1982 have been revised based on the results of the 2001 Census.

Mid-year population estimates for England and Wales from 1992 to 2002 have been further revised in light of the local authority population studies.

*Sources:* Annual Abstract of Statistics (ONS).

Population Projections Database (GAD).

# Population Statistics

Table 1.4  **Population by age group and sex, mid-year estimates, England, 1951 - 2006**

**Male population by age group, England**

Millions

| Age | Year | | | | | | | | | | | | | | | | |
|---|---|---|---|---|---|---|---|---|---|---|---|---|---|---|---|---|---|
| | 1951 | 1961 | 1971 | 1981 | 1991 | 1995 | 1996 | 1997 | 1998 | 1999 | 2000 | 2001 | 2002 | 2003 | 2004 | 2005 | 2006 |
| Total | 19.75 | 21.02 | 22.36 | 22.80 | 23.29 | 23.55 | 23.63 | 23.71 | 23.79 | 23.92 | 24.03 | 24.17 | 24.29 | 24.42 | 24.56 | 24.76 | 24.93 |
| Under 5 | 1.79 | 1.74 | 1.89 | 1.45 | 1.64 | 1.63 | 1.60 | 1.58 | 1.56 | 1.55 | 1.53 | 1.50 | 1.47 | 1.46 | 1.47 | 1.48 | 1.51 |
| 5-9 | 1.52 | 1.57 | 1.96 | 1.55 | 1.54 | 1.63 | 1.65 | 1.66 | 1.65 | 1.65 | 1.63 | 1.60 | 1.58 | 1.56 | 1.55 | 1.52 | 1.49 |
| 10-14 | 1.34 | 1.80 | 1.76 | 1.88 | 1.47 | 1.54 | 1.55 | 1.57 | 1.60 | 1.62 | 1.64 | 1.66 | 1.67 | 1.67 | 1.66 | 1.64 | 1.61 |
| 15-19 | 1.26 | 1.53 | 1.60 | 2.00 | 1.57 | 1.43 | 1.46 | 1.49 | 1.51 | 1.52 | 1.53 | 1.56 | 1.61 | 1.65 | 1.68 | 1.69 | 1.72 |
| 20-29 | 2.88 | 2.72 | 3.30 | 3.40 | 3.83 | 3.54 | 3.44 | 3.33 | 3.24 | 3.19 | 3.17 | 3.15 | 3.13 | 3.13 | 3.18 | 3.27 | 3.35 |
| 30-44 | 4.53 | 4.35 | 4.10 | 4.62 | 5.06 | 5.17 | 5.25 | 5.33 | 5.39 | 5.46 | 5.53 | 5.60 | 5.64 | 5.66 | 5.64 | 5.64 | 5.59 |
| 45-59 | 3.71 | 4.30 | 4.15 | 3.94 | 3.96 | 4.34 | 4.39 | 4.43 | 4.47 | 4.52 | 4.56 | 4.62 | 4.67 | 4.71 | 4.75 | 4.79 | 4.84 |
| 60-64 | 0.88 | 1.03 | 1.25 | 1.15 | 1.16 | 1.13 | 1.13 | 1.14 | 1.16 | 1.18 | 1.18 | 1.18 | 1.18 | 1.20 | 1.23 | 1.27 | 1.32 |
| 65-74 | 1.29 | 1.33 | 1.65 | 1.90 | 1.90 | 1.95 | 1.93 | 1.92 | 1.92 | 1.91 | 1.92 | 1.93 | 1.94 | 1.96 | 1.97 | 1.98 | 1.98 |
| 75-84 | 0.51 | 0.56 | 0.59 | 0.78 | 0.97 | 0.97 | 1.00 | 1.03 | 1.05 | 1.06 | 1.08 | 1.10 | 1.13 | 1.15 | 1.17 | 1.18 | 1.19 |
| 85+ | 0.06 | 0.08 | 0.10 | 0.12 | 0.18 | 0.22 | 0.23 | 0.24 | 0.25 | 0.25 | 0.26 | 0.27 | 0.27 | 0.27 | 0.27 | 0.30 | 0.32 |

**Female population by age group, England**

Millions

| Age | Year | | | | | | | | | | | | | | | | |
|---|---|---|---|---|---|---|---|---|---|---|---|---|---|---|---|---|---|
| | 1951 | 1961 | 1971 | 1981 | 1991 | 1995 | 1996 | 1997 | 1998 | 1999 | 2000 | 2001 | 2002 | 2003 | 2004 | 2005 | 2006 |
| Total | 21.43 | 22.45 | 23.66 | 24.02 | 24.58 | 24.84 | 24.89 | 24.96 | 25.03 | 25.12 | 25.20 | 25.28 | 25.36 | 25.45 | 25.55 | 25.71 | 25.84 |
| Under 5 | 1.71 | 1.65 | 1.80 | 1.38 | 1.58 | 1.55 | 1.52 | 1.50 | 1.49 | 1.47 | 1.45 | 1.43 | 1.40 | 1.39 | 1.39 | 1.41 | 1.44 |
| 5-9 | 1.45 | 1.50 | 1.86 | 1.46 | 1.47 | 1.56 | 1.58 | 1.59 | 1.58 | 1.57 | 1.55 | 1.52 | 1.50 | 1.49 | 1.47 | 1.45 | 1.43 |
| 10-14 | 1.30 | 1.71 | 1.66 | 1.78 | 1.40 | 1.47 | 1.48 | 1.50 | 1.53 | 1.55 | 1.56 | 1.58 | 1.59 | 1.58 | 1.57 | 1.55 | 1.52 |
| 15-19 | 1.29 | 1.49 | 1.53 | 1.90 | 1.50 | 1.39 | 1.42 | 1.45 | 1.47 | 1.48 | 1.47 | 1.49 | 1.51 | 1.55 | 1.58 | 1.61 | 1.61 |
| 20-29 | 2.97 | 2.68 | 3.25 | 3.33 | 3.82 | 3.53 | 3.43 | 3.32 | 3.24 | 3.20 | 3.18 | 3.15 | 3.11 | 3.11 | 3.13 | 3.21 | 3.28 |
| 30-44 | 4.68 | 4.39 | 4.02 | 4.55 | 5.08 | 5.23 | 5.30 | 5.39 | 5.45 | 5.53 | 5.60 | 5.66 | 5.70 | 5.71 | 5.70 | 5.68 | 5.64 |
| 45-59 | 4.20 | 4.54 | 4.35 | 4.01 | 3.96 | 4.37 | 4.43 | 4.48 | 4.53 | 4.58 | 4.64 | 4.70 | 4.77 | 4.81 | 4.84 | 4.88 | 4.94 |
| 60-64 | 1.13 | 1.28 | 1.42 | 1.30 | 1.24 | 1.18 | 1.18 | 1.18 | 1.20 | 1.22 | 1.23 | 1.22 | 1.22 | 1.25 | 1.28 | 1.32 | 1.38 |
| 65-74 | 1.78 | 1.98 | 2.28 | 2.45 | 2.32 | 2.33 | 2.29 | 2.25 | 2.22 | 2.20 | 2.19 | 2.19 | 2.19 | 2.20 | 2.20 | 2.21 | 2.19 |
| 75-84 | 0.78 | 1.02 | 1.20 | 1.47 | 1.66 | 1.60 | 1.63 | 1.64 | 1.65 | 1.65 | 1.65 | 1.66 | 1.68 | 1.70 | 1.70 | 1.69 | 1.67 |
| 85+ | 0.13 | 0.20 | 0.30 | 0.39 | 0.56 | 0.63 | 0.64 | 0.65 | 0.67 | 0.68 | 0.69 | 0.69 | 0.69 | 0.67 | 0.67 | 0.70 | 0.73 |

*Notes:*  Mid-year population estimates from 1982 have been revised based on the results of the 2001 Census.

Mid-year population estimates for England from 1992 to 2002 have been further revised in light of the local authority population studies.

*Sources:*  Annual Abstract of Statistics (ONS).

Population Projections Database (GAD).

Table 1.5  **Population by age group and sex, mid-year estimates, Wales, 1951 - 2006**

**Male population by age group, Wales**

Millions

| Age | Year | | | | | | | | | | | | | | | | |
|---|---|---|---|---|---|---|---|---|---|---|---|---|---|---|---|---|---|
| | 1951 | 1961 | 1971 | 1981 | 1991 | 1995 | 1996 | 1997 | 1998 | 1999 | 2000 | 2001 | 2002 | 2003 | 2004 | 2005 | 2006 |
| Total | 1.27 | 1.28 | 1.32 | 1.37 | 1.39 | 1.40 | 1.40 | 1.40 | 1.41 | 1.41 | 1.41 | 1.41 | 1.41 | 1.42 | 1.43 | 1.44 | 1.44 |
| Under 5 | 0.11 | 0.11 | 0.11 | 0.09 | 0.10 | 0.09 | 0.09 | 0.09 | 0.09 | 0.09 | 0.09 | 0.09 | 0.08 | 0.08 | 0.08 | 0.08 | 0.08 |
| 5-9 | 0.10 | 0.10 | 0.12 | 0.10 | 0.10 | 0.10 | 0.10 | 0.10 | 0.10 | 0.10 | 0.10 | 0.09 | 0.09 | 0.09 | 0.09 | 0.09 | 0.09 |
| 10-14 | 0.09 | 0.11 | 0.10 | 0.11 | 0.09 | 0.09 | 0.10 | 0.10 | 0.10 | 0.10 | 0.10 | 0.10 | 0.10 | 0.10 | 0.10 | 0.10 | 0.10 |
| 15-19 | 0.08 | 0.09 | 0.09 | 0.12 | 0.10 | 0.09 | 0.09 | 0.09 | 0.09 | 0.09 | 0.09 | 0.09 | 0.10 | 0.10 | 0.10 | 0.10 | 0.10 |
| 20-29 | 0.18 | 0.16 | 0.19 | 0.19 | 0.21 | 0.19 | 0.19 | 0.18 | 0.18 | 0.17 | 0.17 | 0.17 | 0.16 | 0.17 | 0.17 | 0.18 | 0.18 |
| 30-44 | 0.28 | 0.26 | 0.23 | 0.27 | 0.29 | 0.29 | 0.29 | 0.29 | 0.29 | 0.30 | 0.30 | 0.30 | 0.30 | 0.30 | 0.29 | 0.29 | 0.29 |
| 45-59 | 0.25 | 0.26 | 0.25 | 0.24 | 0.24 | 0.27 | 0.27 | 0.27 | 0.27 | 0.28 | 0.28 | 0.28 | 0.29 | 0.29 | 0.29 | 0.29 | 0.29 |
| 60-64 | 0.06 | 0.06 | 0.08 | 0.07 | 0.07 | 0.07 | 0.07 | 0.07 | 0.07 | 0.07 | 0.08 | 0.08 | 0.08 | 0.08 | 0.08 | 0.08 | 0.09 |
| 65-74 | 0.09 | 0.09 | 0.11 | 0.12 | 0.13 | 0.13 | 0.13 | 0.13 | 0.13 | 0.12 | 0.12 | 0.12 | 0.12 | 0.13 | 0.13 | 0.13 | 0.13 |
| 75-84 | 0.03 | 0.04 | 0.04 | 0.05 | 0.06 | 0.06 | 0.06 | 0.07 | 0.07 | 0.07 | 0.07 | 0.07 | 0.07 | 0.08 | 0.08 | 0.08 | 0.08 |
| 85+ | 0.00 | 0.01 | 0.01 | 0.01 | 0.01 | 0.01 | 0.01 | 0.01 | 0.01 | 0.02 | 0.02 | 0.02 | 0.02 | 0.02 | 0.02 | 0.02 | 0.02 |

**Female population by age group, Wales**

Millions

| Age | Year | | | | | | | | | | | | | | | | |
|---|---|---|---|---|---|---|---|---|---|---|---|---|---|---|---|---|---|
| | 1951 | 1961 | 1971 | 1981 | 1991 | 1995 | 1996 | 1997 | 1998 | 1999 | 2000 | 2001 | 2002 | 2003 | 2004 | 2005 | 2006 |
| Total | 1.32 | 1.35 | 1.40 | 1.45 | 1.48 | 1.49 | 1.49 | 1.49 | 1.49 | 1.49 | 1.50 | 1.50 | 1.51 | 1.51 | 1.51 | 1.51 | 1.52 |
| Under 5 | 0.11 | 0.10 | 0.10 | 0.08 | 0.09 | 0.09 | 0.09 | 0.09 | 0.09 | 0.08 | 0.08 | 0.08 | 0.08 | 0.08 | 0.08 | 0.08 | 0.08 |
| 5-9 | 0.10 | 0.09 | 0.11 | 0.09 | 0.09 | 0.09 | 0.09 | 0.09 | 0.09 | 0.09 | 0.09 | 0.09 | 0.09 | 0.09 | 0.09 | 0.09 | 0.08 |
| 10-14 | 0.09 | 0.11 | 0.10 | 0.11 | 0.09 | 0.09 | 0.09 | 0.09 | 0.09 | 0.09 | 0.09 | 0.10 | 0.10 | 0.10 | 0.09 | 0.09 | 0.09 |
| 15-19 | 0.08 | 0.09 | 0.09 | 0.11 | 0.09 | 0.08 | 0.09 | 0.09 | 0.09 | 0.09 | 0.09 | 0.09 | 0.09 | 0.10 | 0.10 | 0.10 | 0.10 |
| 20-29 | 0.18 | 0.16 | 0.19 | 0.19 | 0.21 | 0.19 | 0.19 | 0.18 | 0.18 | 0.17 | 0.17 | 0.17 | 0.17 | 0.17 | 0.17 | 0.17 | 0.18 |
| 30-44 | 0.29 | 0.26 | 0.23 | 0.27 | 0.29 | 0.30 | 0.30 | 0.30 | 0.30 | 0.31 | 0.31 | 0.31 | 0.31 | 0.31 | 0.31 | 0.31 | 0.30 |
| 45-59 | 0.26 | 0.27 | 0.26 | 0.25 | 0.24 | 0.27 | 0.27 | 0.28 | 0.28 | 0.28 | 0.29 | 0.29 | 0.29 | 0.30 | 0.30 | 0.30 | 0.30 |
| 60-64 | 0.07 | 0.08 | 0.09 | 0.08 | 0.08 | 0.08 | 0.08 | 0.08 | 0.08 | 0.08 | 0.08 | 0.08 | 0.08 | 0.08 | 0.08 | 0.09 | 0.09 |
| 65-74 | 0.10 | 0.12 | 0.14 | 0.15 | 0.16 | 0.15 | 0.15 | 0.15 | 0.15 | 0.14 | 0.14 | 0.14 | 0.14 | 0.14 | 0.14 | 0.14 | 0.14 |
| 75-84 | 0.05 | 0.06 | 0.07 | 0.09 | 0.10 | 0.10 | 0.11 | 0.11 | 0.11 | 0.11 | 0.11 | 0.11 | 0.11 | 0.11 | 0.11 | 0.11 | 0.11 |
| 85+ | 0.01 | 0.01 | 0.02 | 0.02 | 0.03 | 0.04 | 0.04 | 0.04 | 0.04 | 0.04 | 0.04 | 0.04 | 0.04 | 0.04 | 0.04 | 0.04 | 0.05 |

*Notes:*  Mid-year population estimates from 1982 have been revised based on the results of the 2001 Census.
Mid-year population estimates from 1992 to 2002 have been further revised in light of the local authority population studies.
0.00: non-zero but less than 5000.

*Sources:*  Annual Abstract of Statistics (ONS).
Population Projections Database (GAD).

# Population Statistics

Table 1.6　**Population by age group and sex, mid-year estimates, Scotland, 1951 - 2006**

**Male population by age group, Scotland**

Millions

| Age | Year | | | | | | | | | | | | | | | | |
|---|---|---|---|---|---|---|---|---|---|---|---|---|---|---|---|---|---|
| | 1951 | 1961 | 1971 | 1981 | 1991 | 1995 | 1996 | 1997 | 1998 | 1999 | 2000 | 2001 | 2002 | 2003 | 2004 | 2005 | 2006 |
| **Total** | **2.43** | **2.48** | **2.51** | **2.49** | **2.44** | **2.45** | **2.45** | **2.44** | **2.44** | **2.44** | **2.43** | **2.43** | **2.43** | **2.43** | **2.45** | **2.46** | **2.47** |
| Under 5 | 0.24 | 0.24 | 0.23 | 0.16 | 0.17 | 0.16 | 0.16 | 0.15 | 0.15 | 0.15 | 0.15 | 0.14 | 0.14 | 0.13 | 0.13 | 0.14 | 0.14 |
| 5-9 | 0.20 | 0.22 | 0.24 | 0.18 | 0.16 | 0.17 | 0.17 | 0.17 | 0.16 | 0.16 | 0.16 | 0.16 | 0.15 | 0.15 | 0.15 | 0.15 | 0.14 |
| 10-14 | 0.20 | 0.23 | 0.23 | 0.22 | 0.16 | 0.16 | 0.16 | 0.16 | 0.17 | 0.17 | 0.17 | 0.17 | 0.17 | 0.16 | 0.16 | 0.16 | 0.16 |
| 15-19 | 0.17 | 0.19 | 0.20 | 0.23 | 0.17 | 0.16 | 0.16 | 0.16 | 0.16 | 0.16 | 0.16 | 0.16 | 0.16 | 0.17 | 0.17 | 0.17 | 0.17 |
| 20-29 | 0.36 | 0.32 | 0.35 | 0.39 | 0.41 | 0.38 | 0.36 | 0.35 | 0.33 | 0.32 | 0.31 | 0.31 | 0.31 | 0.31 | 0.31 | 0.32 | 0.33 |
| 30-44 | 0.52 | 0.49 | 0.45 | 0.48 | 0.54 | 0.55 | 0.55 | 0.56 | 0.56 | 0.56 | 0.56 | 0.56 | 0.56 | 0.56 | 0.55 | 0.54 | 0.53 |
| 45-59 | 0.43 | 0.48 | 0.44 | 0.42 | 0.42 | 0.45 | 0.45 | 0.46 | 0.46 | 0.47 | 0.47 | 0.48 | 0.49 | 0.50 | 0.50 | 0.51 | 0.52 |
| 60-64 | 0.10 | 0.11 | 0.13 | 0.12 | 0.12 | 0.12 | 0.12 | 0.12 | 0.12 | 0.12 | 0.13 | 0.12 | 0.12 | 0.13 | 0.13 | 0.13 | 0.14 |
| 65-74 | 0.15 | 0.14 | 0.17 | 0.19 | 0.19 | 0.20 | 0.20 | 0.20 | 0.20 | 0.20 | 0.20 | 0.20 | 0.20 | 0.20 | 0.21 | 0.21 | 0.21 |
| 75-84 | 0.06 | 0.06 | 0.06 | 0.08 | 0.09 | 0.09 | 0.09 | 0.10 | 0.10 | 0.10 | 0.10 | 0.10 | 0.11 | 0.11 | 0.11 | 0.11 | 0.11 |
| 85+ | 0.01 | 0.01 | 0.01 | 0.01 | 0.02 | 0.02 | 0.02 | 0.02 | 0.02 | 0.02 | 0.02 | 0.02 | 0.02 | 0.02 | 0.02 | 0.03 | 0.03 |

**Female population by age group, Scotland**

Millions

| Age | Year | | | | | | | | | | | | | | | | |
|---|---|---|---|---|---|---|---|---|---|---|---|---|---|---|---|---|---|
| | 1951 | 1961 | 1971 | 1981 | 1991 | 1995 | 1996 | 1997 | 1998 | 1999 | 2000 | 2001 | 2002 | 2003 | 2004 | 2005 | 2006 |
| **Total** | **2.66** | **2.70** | **2.71** | **2.69** | **2.64** | **2.65** | **2.65** | **2.64** | **2.64** | **2.64** | **2.63** | **2.63** | **2.62** | **2.62** | **2.63** | **2.64** | **2.65** |
| Under 5 | 0.23 | 0.23 | 0.22 | 0.15 | 0.16 | 0.16 | 0.15 | 0.15 | 0.14 | 0.14 | 0.14 | 0.13 | 0.13 | 0.13 | 0.13 | 0.13 | 0.13 |
| 5-9 | 0.20 | 0.21 | 0.23 | 0.17 | 0.16 | 0.16 | 0.16 | 0.16 | 0.16 | 0.16 | 0.15 | 0.15 | 0.15 | 0.14 | 0.14 | 0.14 | 0.14 |
| 10-14 | 0.19 | 0.22 | 0.22 | 0.21 | 0.15 | 0.16 | 0.16 | 0.16 | 0.16 | 0.16 | 0.16 | 0.16 | 0.16 | 0.16 | 0.16 | 0.15 | 0.15 |
| 15-19 | 0.19 | 0.19 | 0.19 | 0.23 | 0.17 | 0.15 | 0.15 | 0.16 | 0.16 | 0.16 | 0.16 | 0.16 | 0.16 | 0.16 | 0.16 | 0.16 | 0.16 |
| 20-29 | 0.39 | 0.34 | 0.35 | 0.38 | 0.41 | 0.38 | 0.37 | 0.35 | 0.34 | 0.33 | 0.33 | 0.32 | 0.31 | 0.31 | 0.31 | 0.31 | 0.32 |
| 30-44 | 0.56 | 0.51 | 0.47 | 0.49 | 0.54 | 0.57 | 0.57 | 0.58 | 0.59 | 0.59 | 0.60 | 0.60 | 0.60 | 0.59 | 0.59 | 0.58 | 0.57 |
| 45-59 | 0.49 | 0.52 | 0.49 | 0.46 | 0.44 | 0.47 | 0.47 | 0.47 | 0.48 | 0.48 | 0.49 | 0.50 | 0.50 | 0.51 | 0.52 | 0.53 | 0.54 |
| 60-64 | 0.13 | 0.15 | 0.16 | 0.14 | 0.14 | 0.14 | 0.14 | 0.14 | 0.14 | 0.14 | 0.14 | 0.14 | 0.14 | 0.14 | 0.14 | 0.14 | 0.14 |
| 65-74 | 0.19 | 0.21 | 0.25 | 0.27 | 0.25 | 0.25 | 0.25 | 0.25 | 0.25 | 0.25 | 0.25 | 0.25 | 0.25 | 0.25 | 0.25 | 0.25 | 0.25 |
| 75-84 | 0.08 | 0.10 | 0.12 | 0.16 | 0.17 | 0.16 | 0.16 | 0.17 | 0.17 | 0.17 | 0.17 | 0.17 | 0.17 | 0.17 | 0.18 | 0.17 | 0.17 |
| 85+ | 0.01 | 0.02 | 0.03 | 0.04 | 0.05 | 0.06 | 0.06 | 0.06 | 0.06 | 0.06 | 0.07 | 0.07 | 0.06 | 0.06 | 0.06 | 0.07 | 0.07 |

*Note:*　Mid-year population estimates from 1982 have been revised based on the results of the 2001 Census.
*Sources:*　Annual Abstract of Statistics (ONS).
　　　　　Population Projections Database (GAD).

# Population Statistics

Table 1.7 **Population by age group and sex, mid-year estimates, Northern Ireland, 1951 - 2006**

**Male population by age group, Northern Ireland**

Millions

| Age | Year | | | | | | | | | | | | | | | | |
|---|---|---|---|---|---|---|---|---|---|---|---|---|---|---|---|---|---|
| | 1951 | 1961 | 1971 | 1981 | 1991 | 1995 | 1996 | 1997 | 1998 | 1999 | 2000 | 2001 | 2002 | 2003 | 2004 | 2005 | 2006 |
| **Total** | **0.67** | **0.69** | **0.75** | **0.76** | **0.78** | **0.80** | **0.81** | **0.82** | **0.82** | **0.82** | **0.82** | **0.82** | **0.83** | **0.83** | **0.84** | **0.84** | **0.85** |
| Under 5 | 0.07 | 0.08 | 0.08 | 0.07 | 0.07 | 0.06 | 0.06 | 0.06 | 0.06 | 0.06 | 0.06 | 0.06 | 0.06 | 0.06 | 0.06 | 0.06 | 0.06 |
| 5-9 | 0.07 | 0.07 | 0.08 | 0.07 | 0.07 | 0.07 | 0.07 | 0.07 | 0.07 | 0.07 | 0.06 | 0.06 | 0.06 | 0.06 | 0.06 | 0.06 | 0.06 |
| 10-14 | 0.06 | 0.07 | 0.07 | 0.08 | 0.07 | 0.07 | 0.07 | 0.07 | 0.07 | 0.07 | 0.07 | 0.07 | 0.07 | 0.07 | 0.07 | 0.06 | 0.06 |
| 15-19 | 0.06 | 0.06 | 0.07 | 0.08 | 0.07 | 0.06 | 0.06 | 0.06 | 0.06 | 0.06 | 0.06 | 0.07 | 0.07 | 0.07 | 0.07 | 0.07 | 0.07 |
| 20-29 | 0.10 | 0.09 | 0.11 | 0.12 | 0.13 | 0.13 | 0.13 | 0.12 | 0.12 | 0.12 | 0.11 | 0.11 | 0.11 | 0.11 | 0.11 | 0.12 | 0.12 |
| 30-44 | 0.13 | 0.13 | 0.12 | 0.14 | 0.16 | 0.17 | 0.17 | 0.18 | 0.18 | 0.18 | 0.18 | 0.18 | 0.19 | 0.19 | 0.19 | 0.18 | 0.18 |
| 45-59 | 0.10 | 0.12 | 0.12 | 0.11 | 0.12 | 0.13 | 0.13 | 0.13 | 0.14 | 0.14 | 0.14 | 0.14 | 0.15 | 0.15 | 0.15 | 0.15 | 0.16 |
| 60-64 | 0.02 | 0.03 | 0.03 | 0.03 | 0.03 | 0.03 | 0.03 | 0.03 | 0.03 | 0.03 | 0.04 | 0.04 | 0.04 | 0.04 | 0.04 | 0.04 | 0.04 |
| 65-74 | 0.04 | 0.04 | 0.05 | 0.05 | 0.05 | 0.05 | 0.05 | 0.05 | 0.05 | 0.05 | 0.05 | 0.06 | 0.06 | 0.06 | 0.06 | 0.06 | 0.06 |
| 75-84 | 0.02 | 0.02 | 0.02 | 0.02 | 0.03 | 0.03 | 0.03 | 0.03 | 0.03 | 0.03 | 0.03 | 0.03 | 0.03 | 0.03 | 0.03 | 0.03 | 0.03 |
| 85+ | 0.00 | 0.00 | 0.00 | 0.00 | 0.00 | 0.01 | 0.01 | 0.01 | 0.01 | 0.01 | 0.01 | 0.01 | 0.01 | 0.01 | 0.01 | 0.01 | 0.01 |

**Female population by age group, Northern Ireland**

Millions

| Age | Year | | | | | | | | | | | | | | | | |
|---|---|---|---|---|---|---|---|---|---|---|---|---|---|---|---|---|---|
| | 1951 | 1961 | 1971 | 1981 | 1991 | 1995 | 1996 | 1997 | 1998 | 1999 | 2000 | 2001 | 2002 | 2003 | 2004 | 2005 | 2006 |
| **Total** | **0.70** | **0.73** | **0.78** | **0.79** | **0.82** | **0.85** | **0.85** | **0.86** | **0.86** | **0.86** | **0.86** | **0.86** | **0.87** | **0.87** | **0.87** | **0.88** | **0.89** |
| Under 5 | 0.07 | 0.07 | 0.08 | 0.07 | 0.06 | 0.06 | 0.06 | 0.06 | 0.06 | 0.06 | 0.06 | 0.06 | 0.05 | 0.05 | 0.05 | 0.05 | 0.05 |
| 5-9 | 0.06 | 0.06 | 0.08 | 0.07 | 0.06 | 0.06 | 0.06 | 0.06 | 0.06 | 0.06 | 0.06 | 0.06 | 0.06 | 0.06 | 0.06 | 0.06 | 0.06 |
| 10-14 | 0.05 | 0.07 | 0.07 | 0.07 | 0.06 | 0.06 | 0.07 | 0.07 | 0.07 | 0.07 | 0.07 | 0.06 | 0.06 | 0.06 | 0.06 | 0.06 | 0.06 |
| 15-19 | 0.05 | 0.06 | 0.06 | 0.07 | 0.06 | 0.06 | 0.06 | 0.06 | 0.06 | 0.06 | 0.06 | 0.06 | 0.06 | 0.06 | 0.06 | 0.06 | 0.06 |
| 20-29 | 0.10 | 0.09 | 0.11 | 0.11 | 0.13 | 0.12 | 0.12 | 0.12 | 0.12 | 0.12 | 0.11 | 0.11 | 0.11 | 0.11 | 0.11 | 0.11 | 0.12 |
| 30-44 | 0.14 | 0.14 | 0.13 | 0.14 | 0.16 | 0.17 | 0.18 | 0.18 | 0.18 | 0.19 | 0.19 | 0.19 | 0.19 | 0.19 | 0.19 | 0.19 | 0.19 |
| 45-59 | 0.12 | 0.13 | 0.13 | 0.12 | 0.12 | 0.13 | 0.14 | 0.14 | 0.14 | 0.14 | 0.14 | 0.15 | 0.15 | 0.15 | 0.15 | 0.16 | 0.16 |
| 60-64 | 0.03 | 0.04 | 0.04 | 0.04 | 0.04 | 0.04 | 0.04 | 0.04 | 0.04 | 0.04 | 0.04 | 0.04 | 0.04 | 0.04 | 0.04 | 0.04 | 0.04 |
| 65-74 | 0.05 | 0.05 | 0.06 | 0.07 | 0.07 | 0.07 | 0.07 | 0.07 | 0.07 | 0.07 | 0.07 | 0.07 | 0.07 | 0.07 | 0.07 | 0.07 | 0.07 |
| 75-84 | 0.02 | 0.03 | 0.03 | 0.04 | 0.04 | 0.04 | 0.04 | 0.05 | 0.05 | 0.05 | 0.05 | 0.05 | 0.05 | 0.05 | 0.05 | 0.05 | 0.05 |
| 85+ | 0.00 | 0.01 | 0.01 | 0.01 | 0.01 | 0.02 | 0.02 | 0.02 | 0.02 | 0.02 | 0.02 | 0.02 | 0.02 | 0.02 | 0.02 | 0.02 | 0.02 |

*Notes:* Mid-year population estimates from 1982 have been revised based on the results of the 2001 Census.

0.00: non-zero but less than 5000.

*Sources:* Annual Abstract of Statistics (ONS).

Population Projections Database (GAD).

# Population Statistics

Table 1.8   **Mid-year population estimates, total, aged 65 and over and aged 75 and over by country, UK, 1991 - 2006**

## Total population (millions)

|  | 1991 | 1995 | 1996 | 1997 | 1998 | 1999 | 2000 | 2001 | 2002 | 2003 | 2004 | 2005 | 2006 |
|---|---|---|---|---|---|---|---|---|---|---|---|---|---|
| **United Kingdom** | 57.44 | 58.02 | 58.16 | 58.31 | 58.47 | 58.68 | 58.89 | 59.11 | 59.32 | 59.56 | 59.85 | 60.24 | 60.59 |
| **England** | 47.88 | 48.38 | 48.52 | 48.66 | 48.82 | 49.03 | 49.23 | 49.45 | 49.65 | 49.87 | 50.11 | 50.47 | 50.76 |
| **Wales** | 2.87 | 2.89 | 2.89 | 2.89 | 2.90 | 2.90 | 2.91 | 2.91 | 2.92 | 2.93 | 2.95 | 2.95 | 2.97 |
| **Scotland** | 5.08 | 5.10 | 5.09 | 5.08 | 5.08 | 5.07 | 5.06 | 5.06 | 5.05 | 5.06 | 5.08 | 5.09 | 5.12 |
| **Northern Ireland** | 1.61 | 1.65 | 1.66 | 1.67 | 1.68 | 1.68 | 1.68 | 1.69 | 1.70 | 1.70 | 1.71 | 1.72 | 1.74 |

## Population aged 65 and over (millions)

|  | 1991 | 1995 | 1996 | 1997 | 1998 | 1999 | 2000 | 2001 | 2002 | 2003 | 2004 | 2005 | 2006 |
|---|---|---|---|---|---|---|---|---|---|---|---|---|---|
| **United Kingdom** | 9.06 | 9.20 | 9.22 | 9.24 | 9.27 | 9.28 | 9.31 | 9.37 | 9.44 | 9.50 | 9.57 | 9.64 | 9.69 |
| **England** | 7.59 | 7.70 | 7.72 | 7.73 | 7.75 | 7.76 | 7.78 | 7.84 | 7.89 | 7.94 | 7.99 | 8.05 | 8.09 |
| **Wales** | 0.49 | 0.50 | 0.50 | 0.50 | 0.50 | 0.50 | 0.50 | 0.51 | 0.51 | 0.51 | 0.52 | 0.52 | 0.52 |
| **Scotland** | 0.77 | 0.78 | 0.79 | 0.79 | 0.79 | 0.80 | 0.80 | 0.81 | 0.81 | 0.82 | 0.83 | 0.83 | 0.84 |
| **Northern Ireland** | 0.21 | 0.22 | 0.22 | 0.22 | 0.22 | 0.22 | 0.22 | 0.22 | 0.23 | 0.23 | 0.23 | 0.24 | 0.24 |

## Per cent of total population aged 65 and over

|  | 1991 | 1995 | 1996 | 1997 | 1998 | 1999 | 2000 | 2001 | 2002 | 2003 | 2004 | 2005 | 2006 |
|---|---|---|---|---|---|---|---|---|---|---|---|---|---|
| **United Kingdom** | 15.7 | 15.8 | 15.9 | 15.9 | 15.9 | 15.8 | 15.8 | 15.9 | 15.9 | 16.0 | 16.0 | 16.0 | 16.0 |
| **England** | 15.8 | 15.9 | 15.9 | 15.9 | 15.9 | 15.8 | 15.8 | 15.8 | 15.9 | 15.9 | 16.0 | 16.0 | 15.9 |
| **Wales** | 17.1 | 17.4 | 17.4 | 17.4 | 17.4 | 17.3 | 17.3 | 17.4 | 17.5 | 17.5 | 17.6 | 17.6 | 17.7 |
| **Scotland** | 15.1 | 15.3 | 15.4 | 15.5 | 15.6 | 15.7 | 15.8 | 15.9 | 16.1 | 16.2 | 16.3 | 16.4 | 16.4 |
| **Northern Ireland** | 12.7 | 12.6 | 13.0 | 13.0 | 13.1 | 13.1 | 13.1 | 13.3 | 13.4 | 13.5 | 13.6 | 13.7 | 13.7 |

## Population aged 75 and over (millions)

|  | 1991 | 1995 | 1996 | 1997 | 1998 | 1999 | 2000 | 2001 | 2002 | 2003 | 2004 | 2005 | 2006 |
|---|---|---|---|---|---|---|---|---|---|---|---|---|---|
| **United Kingdom** | 3.99 | 4.06 | 4.16 | 4.23 | 4.29 | 4.33 | 4.37 | 4.43 | 4.47 | 4.50 | 4.54 | 4.59 | 4.66 |
| **England** | 3.37 | 3.42 | 3.50 | 3.56 | 3.61 | 3.65 | 3.68 | 3.72 | 3.76 | 3.79 | 3.82 | 3.86 | 3.91 |
| **Wales** | 0.21 | 0.22 | 0.22 | 0.23 | 0.23 | 0.24 | 0.24 | 0.24 | 0.24 | 0.25 | 0.25 | 0.25 | 0.25 |
| **Scotland** | 0.33 | 0.33 | 0.34 | 0.34 | 0.35 | 0.35 | 0.35 | 0.36 | 0.36 | 0.37 | 0.37 | 0.38 | 0.38 |
| **Northern Ireland** | 0.09 | 0.09 | 0.09 | 0.10 | 0.10 | 0.10 | 0.10 | 0.10 | 0.10 | 0.10 | 0.11 | 0.11 | 0.11 |

## Per cent of total population aged 75 and over

|  | 1991 | 1995 | 1996 | 1997 | 1998 | 1999 | 2000 | 2001 | 2002 | 2003 | 2004 | 2005 | 2006 |
|---|---|---|---|---|---|---|---|---|---|---|---|---|---|
| **United Kingdom** | 6.9 | 7.0 | 7.1 | 7.3 | 7.3 | 7.4 | 7.4 | 7.5 | 7.5 | 7.6 | 7.6 | 7.6 | 7.7 |
| **England** | 7.0 | 7.1 | 7.2 | 7.3 | 7.4 | 7.4 | 7.5 | 7.5 | 7.6 | 7.6 | 7.6 | 7.7 | 7.7 |
| **Wales** | 7.3 | 7.6 | 7.8 | 7.9 | 8.0 | 8.1 | 8.2 | 8.3 | 8.4 | 8.4 | 8.4 | 8.4 | 8.5 |
| **Scotland** | 6.5 | 6.5 | 6.6 | 6.7 | 6.8 | 6.9 | 7.0 | 7.1 | 7.2 | 7.3 | 7.3 | 7.4 | 7.5 |
| **Northern Ireland** | 5.5 | 5.6 | 5.7 | 5.7 | 5.8 | 5.8 | 5.9 | 6.0 | 6.1 | 6.1 | 6.2 | 6.3 | 6.3 |

*Notes:*   Mid-year population estimates from 1982 have been revised based on the results of the 2001 Census.
Mid-year population estimates for England and Wales from 1992 to 2002 have been further revised in light of the local authority population studies.

*Sources:*   Annual Abstract of Statistics (ONS).
Population Estimates and Projections (ONS).

Table 1.9   **Total populations and projected populations of OECD and EU countries, 1950 - 2020**

Millions

| | Year | | | | | | | | |
| | 1950 | 1960 | 1970 | 1980 | 1990 | 2000 | 2005 | *2010* | *2020* |
|---|---|---|---|---|---|---|---|---|---|
| **World** | 2,519 | 3,024 | 3,697 | 4,442 | 5,280 | 6,124 | 6,515 | *6,907* | *7,667* |
| **OECD** | 683 | 779 | 878 | 969 | 1,051 | 1,134 | 1,173 | *1,208* | *1,262* |
| **EU27** | 370 | 400 | 431 | 453 | 467 | 478 | 486 | *491* | *494* |
| **EU15**[1] | 295 | 315 | 340 | 355 | 364 | 377 | 387 | *393* | *399* |
| Australia | 8.2 | 10.3 | 12.7 | 14.6 | 16.9 | 19.1 | 20.3 | *21.4* | *23.4* |
| Austria | 6.9 | 7.0 | 7.5 | 7.5 | 7.7 | 8.1 | 8.3 | *8.4* | *8.6* |
| Belgium | 8.6 | 9.2 | 9.7 | 9.9 | 10.0 | 10.2 | 10.4 | *10.5* | *10.7* |
| Bulgaria | 7.3 | 7.9 | 8.5 | 8.9 | 8.8 | 8.0 | 7.7 | *7.5* | *6.9* |
| Canada | 13.7 | 17.9 | 21.7 | 24.5 | 27.7 | 30.7 | 32.3 | *33.8* | *36.6* |
| Cyprus[2] | 0.5 | 0.6 | 0.6 | 0.6 | 0.7 | 0.8 | 0.8 | *0.9* | *1.0* |
| Czech Republic | 8.9 | 9.6 | 9.8 | 10.3 | 10.3 | 10.2 | 10.2 | *10.2* | *10.0* |
| Denmark | 4.3 | 4.6 | 4.9 | 5.1 | 5.1 | 5.3 | 5.4 | *5.5* | *5.5* |
| Estonia | 1.1 | 1.2 | 1.4 | 1.5 | 1.6 | 1.4 | 1.3 | *1.3* | *1.3* |
| Finland | 4.0 | 4.4 | 4.6 | 4.8 | 5.0 | 5.2 | 5.2 | *5.3* | *5.4* |
| France | 41.8 | 45.7 | 50.8 | 53.9 | 56.7 | 59.2 | 61.0 | *62.5* | *64.8* |
| Germany[3] | 68.4 | 72.8 | 78.2 | 78.3 | 79.4 | 82.3 | 82.7 | *82.4* | *81.2* |
| Greece | 7.6 | 8.3 | 8.8 | 9.6 | 10.2 | 11.0 | 11.1 | *11.2* | *11.3* |
| Hungary | 9.3 | 10.0 | 10.3 | 10.7 | 10.4 | 10.2 | 10.1 | *9.9* | *9.6* |
| Iceland | 0.1 | 0.2 | 0.2 | 0.2 | 0.3 | 0.3 | 0.3 | *0.3* | *0.3* |
| Ireland | 3.0 | 2.8 | 3.0 | 3.4 | 3.5 | 3.8 | 4.1 | *4.5* | *5.1* |
| Italy | 47.1 | 50.2 | 53.8 | 56.4 | 56.7 | 57.7 | 58.6 | *59.0* | *58.6* |
| Japan | 83.6 | 94.1 | 104.3 | 116.8 | 123.5 | 127.0 | 127.9 | *127.8* | *124.5* |
| Korea, Republic of | 18.9 | 25.0 | 31.9 | 38.1 | 42.9 | 46.8 | 47.9 | *48.7* | *49.2* |
| Latvia | 1.9 | 2.1 | 2.4 | 2.5 | 2.7 | 2.4 | 2.3 | *2.2* | *2.1* |
| Lithuania | 2.6 | 2.8 | 3.1 | 3.4 | 3.7 | 3.5 | 3.4 | *3.3* | *3.2* |
| Luxembourg | 0.3 | 0.3 | 0.3 | 0.4 | 0.4 | 0.4 | 0.5 | *0.5* | *0.5* |
| Malta | 0.3 | 0.3 | 0.3 | 0.3 | 0.4 | 0.4 | 0.4 | *0.4* | *0.4* |
| Mexico | 27.7 | 36.9 | 50.6 | 68.0 | 84.3 | 99.7 | 104.3 | *110.3* | *120.6* |
| Netherlands | 10.1 | 11.5 | 13.0 | 14.2 | 15.0 | 15.9 | 16.3 | *16.5* | *16.8* |
| New Zealand | 1.9 | 2.4 | 2.8 | 3.1 | 3.4 | 3.9 | 4.1 | *4.3* | *4.6* |
| Norway | 3.3 | 3.6 | 3.9 | 4.1 | 4.2 | 4.5 | 4.6 | *4.8* | *5.1* |
| Poland | 24.8 | 29.6 | 32.7 | 35.6 | 38.1 | 38.4 | 38.2 | *37.9* | *37.1* |
| Portugal | 8.4 | 8.9 | 8.7 | 9.8 | 10.0 | 10.2 | 10.5 | *10.7* | *10.8* |
| Romania | 16.3 | 18.4 | 20.3 | 22.2 | 23.2 | 22.1 | 21.6 | *21.1* | *20.1* |
| Slovak Republic | 3.5 | 4.1 | 4.5 | 5.0 | 5.3 | 5.4 | 5.4 | *5.4* | *5.4* |
| Slovenia | 1.5 | 1.6 | 1.7 | 1.8 | 1.9 | 2.0 | 2.0 | *2.0* | *2.0* |
| Spain | 28.0 | 30.5 | 33.8 | 37.5 | 39.3 | 40.2 | 43.4 | *45.1* | *46.4* |
| Sweden | 7.0 | 7.5 | 8.0 | 8.3 | 8.6 | 8.9 | 9.0 | *9.2* | *9.7* |
| Switzerland | 4.7 | 5.4 | 6.2 | 6.3 | 6.8 | 7.3 | 7.4 | *7.6* | *7.8* |
| Turkey | 21.5 | 28.2 | 36.2 | 46.3 | 57.3 | 68.2 | 73.0 | *77.7* | *86.1* |
| UK | 49.8 | 51.6 | 54.8 | 55.5 | 56.8 | 58.9 | 60.2 | *61.5* | *64.0* |
| USA | 157.8 | 186.2 | 210.1 | 230.9 | 255.5 | 284.9 | 299.8 | *314.7* | *342.5* |

*Notes:*   Figures for 2005 are UN estimates.
Figures for the years 2010 and 2020 are UN projections.
UK data is from World Population Prospects and may differ slightly from other tables, as future projections are based on calculations conducted by the United Nations, as opposed to the Office for National Statistics
1 EU15 as constituted before 1 May 2004.
2 Including Northern and Southern Cyprus.
3 Including former East Germany.

*Source:*   World Population Prospects (United Nations).

# Population Statistics

Table 1.10 **Dependency ratios and projected dependency ratios (number aged under 15 or 65 and over, per 100 working population) in OECD and EU countries, 1950 - 2020**

| | Year | | | | | | | | |
|---|---|---|---|---|---|---|---|---|---|
| | 1950 | 1960 | 1970 | 1980 | 1990 | 2000 | 2005 | *2010* | *2020* |
| World[4] | 65 | 73 | 75 | 70 | 63 | 59 | 55 | *53* | *53* |
| OECD[4] | 57 | 62 | 61 | 57 | 51 | 49 | 48 | *48* | *53* |
| EU27[4] | 54 | 57 | 57 | 54 | 51 | 49 | 47 | *47* | *53* |
| EU15[1,4] | 53 | 56 | 58 | 55 | 50 | 49 | 49 | *50* | *55* |
| | | | | | | | | | |
| Australia | 53 | 63 | 59 | 54 | 49 | 49 | 48 | *48* | *55* |
| Austria | 50 | 52 | 62 | 56 | 48 | 47 | 47 | *47* | *51* |
| Belgium | 47 | 55 | 59 | 53 | 49 | 52 | 52 | *51* | *56* |
| Bulgaria | 50 | 51 | 48 | 52 | 50 | 48 | 45 | *45* | *51* |
| Canada | 60 | 70 | 61 | 47 | 47 | 46 | 44 | *44* | *51* |
| Cyprus[2] | 68 | 74 | 70 | 53 | 58 | 51 | 47 | *45* | *49* |
| Czech Republic | 48 | 54 | 50 | 58 | 51 | 43 | 41 | *41* | *52* |
| Denmark | 55 | 56 | 55 | 54 | 48 | 50 | 51 | *53* | *58* |
| Estonia | 57 | 50 | 51 | 52 | 51 | 50 | 47 | *47* | *54* |
| Finland | 58 | 60 | 51 | 48 | 49 | 49 | 50 | *51* | *63* |
| France | 52 | 61 | 61 | 57 | 52 | 54 | 53 | *53* | *60* |
| Germany[3] | 49 | 49 | 59 | 52 | 45 | 47 | 50 | *51* | *54* |
| Greece | 55 | 53 | 56 | 56 | 49 | 47 | 48 | *49* | *53* |
| Hungary | 48 | 52 | 48 | 55 | 51 | 46 | 45 | *44* | *50* |
| Iceland | 62 | 74 | 70 | 60 | 55 | 53 | 51 | *50* | *55* |
| Ireland | 65 | 73 | 73 | 70 | 63 | 49 | 47 | *48* | *51* |
| Italy | 53 | 52 | 55 | 55 | 45 | 48 | 51 | *52* | *57* |
| Japan | 68 | 56 | 45 | 48 | 44 | 47 | 51 | *56* | *67* |
| Korea, Republic of | 81 | 83 | 83 | 61 | 45 | 39 | 39 | *37* | *40* |
| Latvia | 57 | 48 | 51 | 50 | 50 | 49 | 45 | *45* | *50* |
| Lithuania | 58 | 53 | 59 | 54 | 50 | 51 | 47 | *45* | *47* |
| Luxembourg | 42 | 47 | 53 | 48 | 44 | 49 | 49 | *47* | *48* |
| Malta | 69 | 79 | 58 | 49 | 51 | 48 | 44 | *43* | *53* |
| Mexico | 85 | 97 | 101 | 94 | 75 | 62 | 58 | *53* | *48* |
| Netherlands | 59 | 64 | 60 | 51 | 45 | 47 | 48 | *49* | *55* |
| New Zealand | 61 | 71 | 67 | 58 | 53 | 53 | 51 | *50* | *54* |
| Norway | 52 | 59 | 60 | 59 | 54 | 54 | 52 | *51* | *55* |
| Poland | 53 | 65 | 54 | 52 | 54 | 46 | 42 | *39* | *48* |
| Portugal | 57 | 59 | 61 | 57 | 51 | 48 | 48 | *49* | *53* |
| Romania | 51 | 54 | 53 | 59 | 51 | 47 | 44 | *43* | *46* |
| Slovak Republic | 55 | 65 | 57 | 58 | 55 | 45 | 40 | *38* | *44* |
| Slovenia | 53 | 54 | 51 | 53 | 47 | 43 | 42 | *43* | *51* |
| Spain | 52 | 55 | 61 | 59 | 50 | 46 | 45 | *48* | *53* |
| Sweden | 51 | 51 | 53 | 56 | 56 | 55 | 53 | *53* | *62* |
| Switzerland | 50 | 51 | 54 | 51 | 45 | 47 | 47 | *48* | *53* |
| Turkey | 76 | 85 | 85 | 82 | 66 | 55 | 51 | *47* | *44* |
| UK | 49 | 54 | 59 | 56 | 53 | 53 | 52 | *51* | *57* |
| USA | 54 | 67 | 62 | 51 | 51 | 51 | 49 | *49* | *55* |

*Notes:*     Figures for 2005 are UN estimates.
               Figures for the years 2010 and 2020 are UN projections.
               1 EU15 as constituted before 1 May 2004.
               2 Including Northern and Southern Cyprus.
               3 Including former East Germany.
               4 Unweighted averages.
*Source:*    World Population Prospects (United Nations).

Table 1.11  **Population aged 65 and over in OECD and EU countries, 1950 - 2020**

Millions

| | Year | | | | | | | 2010 | 2020 |
|---|---|---|---|---|---|---|---|---|---|
| | 1950 | 1960 | 1970 | 1980 | 1990 | 2000 | 2005 | 2010 | 2020 |
| **World** | 130.85 | 159.29 | 200.32 | 260.75 | 321.86 | 420.95 | 477.36 | 528.52 | 719.42 |
| **OECD** | 53.07 | 66.15 | 83.88 | 104.40 | 121.77 | 147.63 | 161.67 | 177.12 | 223.43 |
| **EU27** | 33.09 | 39.78 | 50.66 | 60.82 | 65.38 | 75.87 | 81.84 | 86.50 | 101.33 |
| **EU15[1]** | 28.05 | 33.42 | 41.61 | 49.35 | 53.53 | 61.86 | 67.05 | 71.39 | 82.89 |
| Australia | 0.67 | 0.87 | 1.06 | 1.40 | 1.88 | 2.38 | 2.66 | 3.04 | 4.18 |
| Austria | 0.72 | 0.85 | 1.05 | 1.16 | 1.16 | 1.26 | 1.34 | 1.48 | 1.70 |
| Belgium | 0.95 | 1.10 | 1.29 | 1.42 | 1.49 | 1.72 | 1.80 | 1.85 | 2.19 |
| Bulgaria | 0.49 | 0.59 | 0.81 | 1.05 | 1.16 | 1.33 | 1.33 | 1.32 | 1.42 |
| Canada | 1.05 | 1.34 | 1.72 | 2.31 | 3.12 | 3.87 | 4.23 | 4.78 | 6.72 |
| Cyprus[2] | 0.03 | 0.03 | 0.06 | 0.06 | 0.07 | 0.09 | 0.10 | 0.12 | 0.15 |
| Czech Republic | 0.74 | 0.89 | 1.18 | 1.38 | 1.29 | 1.41 | 1.44 | 1.59 | 2.06 |
| Denmark | 0.39 | 0.49 | 0.61 | 0.74 | 0.80 | 0.79 | 0.82 | 0.91 | 1.12 |
| Estonia | 0.12 | 0.13 | 0.16 | 0.18 | 0.18 | 0.21 | 0.22 | 0.22 | 0.23 |
| Finland | 0.27 | 0.32 | 0.42 | 0.57 | 0.67 | 0.77 | 0.84 | 0.91 | 1.21 |
| France | 4.76 | 5.32 | 6.54 | 7.53 | 7.94 | 9.63 | 9.96 | 10.34 | 13.08 |
| Germany[3] | 6.65 | 8.39 | 10.70 | 12.21 | 11.88 | 13.46 | 15.53 | 16.87 | 18.18 |
| Greece | 0.51 | 0.69 | 0.98 | 1.27 | 1.39 | 1.84 | 2.03 | 2.10 | 2.38 |
| Hungary | 0.69 | 0.90 | 1.19 | 1.44 | 1.38 | 1.50 | 1.54 | 1.60 | 1.87 |
| Iceland | 0.01 | 0.01 | 0.02 | 0.02 | 0.03 | 0.03 | 0.04 | 0.04 | 0.05 |
| Ireland | 0.32 | 0.32 | 0.33 | 0.37 | 0.40 | 0.43 | 0.46 | 0.51 | 0.69 |
| Italy | 3.89 | 4.67 | 5.86 | 7.42 | 8.69 | 10.51 | 11.58 | 12.16 | 13.60 |
| Japan | 4.14 | 5.40 | 7.37 | 10.56 | 14.81 | 21.86 | 25.26 | 28.75 | 35.32 |
| Korea, Republic of | 0.57 | 0.83 | 1.05 | 1.45 | 2.14 | 3.44 | 4.52 | 5.52 | 7.73 |
| Latvia | 0.22 | 0.22 | 0.28 | 0.33 | 0.32 | 0.37 | 0.38 | 0.39 | 0.40 |
| Lithuania | 0.24 | 0.21 | 0.31 | 0.39 | 0.40 | 0.49 | 0.53 | 0.54 | 0.56 |
| Luxembourg | 0.03 | 0.03 | 0.04 | 0.05 | 0.05 | 0.06 | 0.07 | 0.07 | 0.08 |
| Malta | 0.02 | 0.02 | 0.03 | 0.03 | 0.04 | 0.05 | 0.05 | 0.06 | 0.08 |
| Mexico | 0.96 | 1.27 | 1.90 | 2.60 | 3.56 | 5.19 | 6.08 | 7.29 | 10.81 |
| Netherlands | 0.78 | 1.04 | 1.33 | 1.63 | 1.92 | 2.17 | 2.32 | 2.55 | 3.36 |
| New Zealand | 0.17 | 0.21 | 0.24 | 0.31 | 0.38 | 0.45 | 0.50 | 0.56 | 0.76 |
| Norway | 0.32 | 0.40 | 0.50 | 0.60 | 0.69 | 0.68 | 0.68 | 0.73 | 0.93 |
| Poland | 1.30 | 1.71 | 2.69 | 3.60 | 3.83 | 4.71 | 5.06 | 5.14 | 6.85 |
| Portugal | 0.59 | 0.71 | 0.80 | 1.02 | 1.34 | 1.65 | 1.78 | 1.87 | 2.13 |
| Romania | 0.87 | 1.24 | 1.74 | 2.28 | 2.41 | 2.98 | 3.20 | 3.14 | 3.52 |
| Slovak Republic | 0.23 | 0.28 | 0.42 | 0.52 | 0.54 | 0.61 | 0.63 | 0.67 | 0.88 |
| Slovenia | 0.10 | 0.12 | 0.17 | 0.21 | 0.21 | 0.28 | 0.31 | 0.33 | 0.41 |
| Spain | 2.04 | 2.50 | 3.31 | 4.21 | 5.29 | 6.75 | 7.30 | 7.82 | 9.07 |
| Sweden | 0.72 | 0.90 | 1.10 | 1.35 | 1.52 | 1.53 | 1.56 | 1.70 | 2.04 |
| Switzerland | 0.45 | 0.54 | 0.70 | 0.88 | 0.98 | 1.06 | 1.14 | 1.28 | 1.57 |
| Turkey | 0.69 | 0.97 | 1.55 | 2.11 | 2.30 | 3.51 | 4.09 | 4.61 | 6.55 |
| UK | 5.43 | 6.12 | 7.26 | 8.41 | 9.00 | 9.31 | 9.68 | 10.24 | 12.08 |
| USA | 13.04 | 17.10 | 20.67 | 25.87 | 31.29 | 35.07 | 36.75 | 40.15 | 54.26 |

*Notes:*  Figures for 2005 are UN estimates.
Figures for the years 2010 and 2020 are UN projections.
1 EU15 as constituted before 1 May 2004.
2 Including Northern and Southern Cyprus
3 Including former East Germany.

*Source:*  World Population Prospects (United Nations).

Table 1.12 **People aged 65 and over as a percentage of total population in OECD and EU countries, 1950 - 2020**

Percent

| | Year | | | | | | | | |
|---|---|---|---|---|---|---|---|---|---|
| | 1950 | 1960 | 1970 | 1980 | 1990 | 2000 | 2005 | *2010* | *2020* |
| **World** | **5.2** | **5.3** | **5.4** | **5.9** | **6.1** | **6.9** | **7.3** | *7.7* | *9.4* |
| **OECD** | **7.8** | **8.5** | **9.6** | **10.8** | **11.6** | **13.0** | **13.8** | *14.7* | *17.7* |
| **EU27** | **8.9** | **9.9** | **11.6** | **13.3** | **13.9** | **15.7** | **16.7** | *17.5* | *20.3* |
| **EU15[1]** | **9.5** | **10.6** | **12.2** | **13.9** | **14.7** | **16.4** | **17.3** | *18.2* | *20.8* |
| | | | | | | | | | |
| Australia | 8.1 | 8.5 | 8.4 | 9.6 | 11.2 | 12.4 | 13.1 | *14.2* | *17.8* |
| Austria | 10.4 | 12.0 | 14.1 | 15.4 | 14.9 | 15.5 | 16.2 | *17.5* | *19.8* |
| Belgium | 11.0 | 12.0 | 13.3 | 14.4 | 14.9 | 16.9 | 17.3 | *17.6* | *20.5* |
| Bulgaria | 6.7 | 7.5 | 9.6 | 11.9 | 13.1 | 16.6 | 17.2 | *17.7* | *20.6* |
| Canada | 7.7 | 7.5 | 7.9 | 9.4 | 11.3 | 12.6 | 13.1 | *14.2* | *18.4* |
| Cyprus[2] | 6.1 | 5.9 | 10.1 | 10.3 | 10.9 | 11.3 | 12.1 | *13.0* | *15.5* |
| Czech Republic | 8.3 | 9.3 | 12.1 | 13.4 | 12.5 | 13.8 | 14.2 | *15.6* | *20.5* |
| Denmark | 9.1 | 10.6 | 12.3 | 14.4 | 15.6 | 14.8 | 15.1 | *16.7* | *20.2* |
| Estonia | 10.6 | 10.5 | 11.7 | 12.5 | 11.4 | 15.0 | 16.6 | *16.7* | *18.3* |
| Finland | 6.7 | 7.2 | 9.2 | 12.0 | 13.4 | 14.9 | 15.9 | *17.1* | *22.2* |
| France | 11.4 | 11.6 | 12.9 | 14.0 | 14.0 | 16.3 | 16.3 | *16.5* | *20.2* |
| Germany[3] | 9.7 | 11.5 | 13.7 | 15.6 | 15.0 | 16.4 | 18.8 | *20.5* | *22.4* |
| Greece | 6.8 | 8.3 | 11.1 | 13.1 | 13.7 | 16.7 | 18.3 | *18.8* | *21.1* |
| Hungary | 7.3 | 9.0 | 11.6 | 13.4 | 13.3 | 14.7 | 15.2 | *16.1* | *19.5* |
| Iceland | 7.7 | 8.0 | 8.8 | 10.1 | 10.6 | 11.7 | 11.8 | *12.7* | *16.1* |
| Ireland | 10.7 | 11.2 | 11.2 | 10.7 | 11.4 | 11.2 | 11.1 | *11.3* | *13.6* |
| Italy | 8.3 | 9.3 | 10.9 | 13.1 | 15.3 | 18.2 | 19.7 | *20.6* | *23.2* |
| Japan | 4.9 | 5.7 | 7.1 | 9.0 | 12.0 | 17.2 | 19.7 | *22.5* | *28.4* |
| Korea, Republic of | 3.0 | 3.3 | 3.3 | 3.8 | 5.0 | 7.4 | 9.4 | *11.3* | *15.7* |
| Latvia | 11.2 | 10.5 | 11.9 | 13.0 | 11.6 | 15.3 | 16.6 | *17.6* | *18.7* |
| Lithuania | 9.4 | 7.7 | 10.0 | 11.3 | 10.9 | 13.9 | 15.3 | *16.2* | *17.7* |
| Luxembourg | 9.8 | 10.8 | 12.7 | 13.7 | 13.5 | 14.2 | 14.2 | *14.1* | *15.2* |
| Malta | 5.8 | 7.4 | 8.9 | 9.9 | 10.6 | 12.3 | 13.2 | *14.8* | *19.7* |
| Mexico | 3.5 | 3.4 | 3.8 | 3.8 | 4.2 | 5.2 | 5.8 | *6.6* | *9.0* |
| Netherlands | 7.7 | 9.0 | 10.2 | 11.5 | 12.8 | 13.6 | 14.2 | *15.4* | *20.0* |
| New Zealand | 9.0 | 8.6 | 8.5 | 10.0 | 11.1 | 11.8 | 12.2 | *13.0* | *16.4* |
| Norway | 9.7 | 11.1 | 12.9 | 14.8 | 16.3 | 15.2 | 14.7 | *15.3* | *18.4* |
| Poland | 5.2 | 5.8 | 8.2 | 10.1 | 10.1 | 12.2 | 13.3 | *13.6* | *18.5* |
| Portugal | 7.0 | 8.0 | 9.2 | 10.5 | 13.4 | 16.1 | 16.9 | *17.5* | *19.8* |
| Romania | 5.3 | 6.7 | 8.6 | 10.3 | 10.4 | 13.5 | 14.8 | *14.9* | *17.5* |
| Slovak Republic | 6.7 | 6.7 | 9.2 | 10.4 | 10.3 | 11.4 | 11.7 | *12.3* | *16.4* |
| Slovenia | 7.0 | 7.8 | 9.9 | 11.4 | 11.1 | 14.1 | 15.6 | *16.5* | *20.8* |
| Spain | 7.3 | 8.2 | 9.8 | 11.2 | 13.5 | 16.8 | 16.8 | *17.3* | *19.5* |
| Sweden | 10.3 | 12.0 | 13.7 | 16.3 | 17.8 | 17.2 | 17.2 | *18.4* | *21.1* |
| Switzerland | 9.6 | 10.1 | 11.3 | 13.8 | 14.4 | 14.6 | 15.4 | *17.0* | *20.0* |
| Turkey | 3.2 | 3.4 | 4.3 | 4.6 | 4.0 | 5.2 | 5.6 | *5.9* | *7.6* |
| UK | 10.9 | 11.9 | 13.2 | 15.1 | 15.9 | 15.8 | 16.1 | *16.6* | *18.9* |
| USA | 8.3 | 9.2 | 9.8 | 11.2 | 12.2 | 12.3 | 12.3 | *12.8* | *15.8* |

*Notes:* Figures for 2005 are UN estimates.
Figures for the years 2010 and 2020 are UN projections.
1 EU15 as constituted before 1 May 2004.
2 Including Northern and Southern Cyprus.
3 Including former East Germany.

*Source:* World Population Prospects (United Nations).

Table 1.13 **Population aged 75 and over in OECD and EU countries, 1950 - 2020**

Millions

| | Year | | | | | | | | |
|---|---|---|---|---|---|---|---|---|---|
| | 1950 | 1960 | 1970 | 1980 | 1990 | 2000 | 2005 | 2010 | 2020 |
| **World** | **36.03** | **47.50** | **63.31** | **84.33** | **114.63** | **149.34** | **179.86** | **208.28** | **266.66** |
| **OECD** | **16.35** | **22.28** | **29.02** | **39.55** | **51.36** | **63.83** | **73.64** | **82.13** | **100.22** |
| **EU27** | **10.43** | **13.40** | **16.95** | **23.06** | **28.87** | **32.61** | **37.11** | **40.86** | **46.95** |
| **EU15[1]** | **8.87** | **11.47** | **14.24** | **19.11** | **24.08** | **27.49** | **31.07** | **34.13** | **39.75** |
| Australia | 0.21 | 0.28 | 0.38 | 0.50 | 0.74 | 1.06 | 1.27 | 1.41 | 1.82 |
| Austria | 0.21 | 0.28 | 0.35 | 0.45 | 0.53 | 0.58 | 0.64 | 0.67 | 0.82 |
| Belgium | 0.31 | 0.38 | 0.44 | 0.57 | 0.66 | 0.75 | 0.84 | 0.94 | 1.00 |
| Bulgaria | 0.13 | 0.19 | 0.25 | 0.34 | 0.43 | 0.47 | 0.54 | 0.59 | 0.57 |
| Canada | 0.33 | 0.48 | 0.66 | 0.86 | 1.25 | 1.72 | 1.99 | 2.22 | 2.81 |
| Cyprus[2] | 0.01 | 0.01 | 0.02 | 0.02 | 0.03 | 0.04 | 0.04 | 0.05 | 0.06 |
| Czech Republic | 0.22 | 0.26 | 0.35 | 0.46 | 0.54 | 0.56 | 0.63 | 0.67 | 0.79 |
| Denmark | 0.12 | 0.17 | 0.22 | 0.29 | 0.36 | 0.38 | 0.38 | 0.39 | 0.49 |
| Estonia | 0.04 | 0.05 | 0.06 | 0.07 | 0.08 | 0.08 | 0.09 | 0.10 | 0.10 |
| Finland | 0.08 | 0.10 | 0.12 | 0.20 | 0.28 | 0.34 | 0.39 | 0.42 | 0.50 |
| France | 1.63 | 1.98 | 2.39 | 3.33 | 3.78 | 4.44 | 4.98 | 5.44 | 5.79 |
| Germany[3] | 1.88 | 2.72 | 3.45 | 4.82 | 5.70 | 5.86 | 6.68 | 7.31 | 9.46 |
| Greece | 0.17 | 0.25 | 0.33 | 0.48 | 0.60 | 0.68 | 0.84 | 1.02 | 1.15 |
| Hungary | 0.19 | 0.28 | 0.37 | 0.51 | 0.57 | 0.59 | 0.66 | 0.69 | 0.75 |
| Iceland | 0.00 | 0.00 | 0.01 | 0.01 | 0.01 | 0.01 | 0.02 | 0.02 | 0.02 |
| Ireland | 0.11 | 0.12 | 0.12 | 0.13 | 0.16 | 0.19 | 0.20 | 0.22 | 0.28 |
| Italy | 1.24 | 1.58 | 2.08 | 2.67 | 3.79 | 4.58 | 5.39 | 6.01 | 6.84 |
| Japan | 1.07 | 1.65 | 2.23 | 3.62 | 5.92 | 8.91 | 11.36 | 13.83 | 18.18 |
| Korea, Republic of | 0.12 | 0.25 | 0.29 | 0.38 | 0.64 | 1.08 | 1.44 | 1.99 | 3.26 |
| Latvia | 0.08 | 0.09 | 0.10 | 0.12 | 0.15 | 0.13 | 0.16 | 0.17 | 0.19 |
| Lithuania | 0.09 | 0.07 | 0.10 | 0.15 | 0.18 | 0.18 | 0.21 | 0.24 | 0.27 |
| Luxembourg | 0.01 | 0.01 | 0.01 | 0.02 | 0.02 | 0.03 | 0.03 | 0.03 | 0.04 |
| Malta | 0.01 | 0.01 | 0.01 | 0.01 | 0.01 | 0.02 | 0.02 | 0.03 | 0.03 |
| Mexico | 0.35 | 0.51 | 0.78 | 1.00 | 1.24 | 1.92 | 2.40 | 2.94 | 4.24 |
| Netherlands | 0.25 | 0.35 | 0.48 | 0.65 | 0.81 | 0.97 | 1.05 | 1.15 | 1.41 |
| New Zealand | 0.05 | 0.08 | 0.09 | 0.11 | 0.15 | 0.20 | 0.23 | 0.25 | 0.32 |
| Norway | 0.12 | 0.14 | 0.18 | 0.24 | 0.30 | 0.35 | 0.36 | 0.35 | 0.40 |
| Poland | 0.41 | 0.51 | 0.78 | 1.27 | 1.56 | 1.72 | 2.11 | 2.41 | 2.54 |
| Portugal | 0.19 | 0.24 | 0.27 | 0.34 | 0.53 | 0.67 | 0.77 | 0.86 | 0.99 |
| Romania | 0.26 | 0.35 | 0.51 | 0.74 | 0.94 | 1.00 | 1.18 | 1.34 | 1.40 |
| Slovak Republic | 0.07 | 0.09 | 0.12 | 0.18 | 0.22 | 0.23 | 0.26 | 0.29 | 0.32 |
| Slovenia | 0.04 | 0.04 | 0.05 | 0.07 | 0.08 | 0.10 | 0.13 | 0.15 | 0.17 |
| Spain | 0.67 | 0.82 | 1.10 | 1.41 | 2.23 | 2.87 | 3.47 | 4.03 | 4.48 |
| Sweden | 0.24 | 0.31 | 0.40 | 0.54 | 0.68 | 0.79 | 0.80 | 0.80 | 0.96 |
| Switzerland | 0.14 | 0.19 | 0.24 | 0.36 | 0.45 | 0.50 | 0.54 | 0.60 | 0.76 |
| Turkey | 0.18 | 0.26 | 0.34 | 0.66 | 0.81 | 0.88 | 1.24 | 1.58 | 2.04 |
| UK | 1.75 | 2.16 | 2.48 | 3.21 | 3.95 | 4.37 | 4.64 | 4.85 | 5.55 |
| USA | 4.02 | 5.84 | 7.96 | 10.29 | 12.87 | 16.61 | 18.07 | 18.76 | 22.21 |

*Notes:*   Figures for 2005 are UN estimates.
Figures for the years 2010 and 2020 are UN projections.
0.00: non-zero but less than 5000.
1 EU15 as constituted before 1 May 2004.
2 Including Northern and Southern Cyprus
3 Including former East Germany.

*Source:*   World Population Prospects (United Nations).

Table 1.14 **People aged 75 and over as a percentage of total population in OECD and EU countries, 1950 - 2020**

Percent

| | Year | | | | | | | 2010 | 2020 |
|---|---|---|---|---|---|---|---|---|---|
| | 1950 | 1960 | 1970 | 1980 | 1990 | 2000 | 2005 | 2010 | 2020 |
| **World** | **1.4** | **1.6** | **1.7** | **1.9** | **2.2** | **2.4** | **2.8** | *3.0* | *3.5* |
| **OECD** | **2.4** | **2.9** | **3.3** | **4.1** | **4.9** | **5.6** | **6.3** | *6.8* | *7.9* |
| **EU27[1]** | **2.8** | **3.3** | **3.9** | **5.0** | **6.1** | **6.8** | **7.6** | *8.3* | *9.4* |
| **EU15[1]** | **3.0** | **3.6** | **4.2** | **5.4** | **6.6** | **7.3** | **8.0** | *8.7* | *10.0* |
| Australia | 2.6 | 2.7 | 3.0 | 3.4 | 4.4 | 5.6 | 6.2 | *6.6* | *7.8* |
| Austria | 3.1 | 4.0 | 4.7 | 6.0 | 6.9 | 7.1 | 7.7 | *7.9* | *9.6* |
| Belgium | 3.6 | 4.2 | 4.6 | 5.8 | 6.6 | 7.3 | 8.0 | *8.9* | *9.4* |
| Bulgaria | 1.8 | 2.4 | 2.9 | 3.8 | 4.9 | 5.9 | 7.0 | *7.8* | *8.3* |
| Canada | 2.4 | 2.7 | 3.0 | 3.5 | 4.5 | 5.6 | 6.2 | *6.6* | *7.7* |
| Cyprus[2] | 1.6 | 1.9 | 3.7 | 3.6 | 4.6 | 4.7 | 5.1 | *5.6* | *6.6* |
| Czech Republic | 2.5 | 2.7 | 3.6 | 4.5 | 5.2 | 5.5 | 6.2 | *6.6* | *7.9* |
| Denmark | 2.9 | 3.7 | 4.4 | 5.7 | 6.9 | 7.1 | 7.0 | *7.2* | *8.9* |
| Estonia | 4.0 | 3.9 | 4.0 | 4.6 | 5.1 | 5.5 | 6.8 | *7.5* | *8.0* |
| Finland | 2.0 | 2.2 | 2.7 | 4.2 | 5.6 | 6.5 | 7.4 | *7.9* | *9.3* |
| France | 3.9 | 4.3 | 4.7 | 6.2 | 6.7 | 7.5 | 8.2 | *8.7* | *8.9* |
| Germany[3] | 2.8 | 3.7 | 4.4 | 6.2 | 7.2 | 7.1 | 8.1 | *8.9* | *11.7* |
| Greece | 2.2 | 3.0 | 3.8 | 5.0 | 5.9 | 6.2 | 7.6 | *9.1* | *10.2* |
| Hungary | 2.0 | 2.8 | 3.5 | 4.7 | 5.5 | 5.8 | 6.5 | *7.0* | *7.8* |
| Iceland | 2.8 | 2.3 | 3.4 | 3.9 | 4.3 | 5.0 | 5.4 | *5.8* | *6.7* |
| Ireland | 3.7 | 4.2 | 4.1 | 3.9 | 4.5 | 4.9 | 4.9 | *4.9* | *5.5* |
| Italy | 2.6 | 3.1 | 3.9 | 4.7 | 6.7 | 7.9 | 9.2 | *10.2* | *11.7* |
| Japan | 1.3 | 1.8 | 2.1 | 3.1 | 4.8 | 7.0 | 8.9 | *10.8* | *14.6* |
| Korea, Republic of | 0.7 | 1.0 | 0.9 | 1.0 | 1.5 | 2.3 | 3.0 | *4.1* | *6.6* |
| Latvia | 4.2 | 4.1 | 4.2 | 4.9 | 5.3 | 5.6 | 6.7 | *7.5* | *8.8* |
| Lithuania | 3.4 | 2.7 | 3.3 | 4.4 | 4.8 | 5.1 | 6.2 | *7.3* | *8.3* |
| Luxembourg | 3.0 | 3.5 | 3.8 | 4.9 | 4.8 | 5.7 | 6.1 | *6.6* | *6.7* |
| Malta | 1.6 | 1.9 | 3.0 | 3.7 | 3.9 | 4.9 | 5.5 | *6.1* | *8.0* |
| Mexico | 1.2 | 1.4 | 1.5 | 1.5 | 1.5 | 1.9 | 2.3 | *2.7* | *3.5* |
| Netherlands | 2.4 | 3.1 | 3.7 | 4.6 | 5.4 | 6.1 | 6.4 | *6.9* | *8.4* |
| New Zealand | 2.6 | 3.3 | 3.0 | 3.5 | 4.4 | 5.2 | 5.7 | *5.9* | *7.0* |
| Norway | 3.6 | 4.0 | 4.7 | 5.9 | 7.1 | 7.8 | 7.7 | *7.3* | *7.9* |
| Poland | 1.7 | 1.7 | 2.4 | 3.6 | 4.1 | 4.5 | 5.5 | *6.4* | *6.9* |
| Portugal | 2.3 | 2.7 | 3.1 | 3.5 | 5.3 | 6.6 | 7.3 | *8.0* | *9.1* |
| Romania | 1.6 | 1.9 | 2.5 | 3.3 | 4.1 | 4.5 | 5.5 | *6.3* | *7.0* |
| Slovak Republic | 2.1 | 2.3 | 2.7 | 3.6 | 4.2 | 4.3 | 4.9 | *5.3* | *5.9* |
| Slovenia | 2.9 | 2.5 | 2.8 | 3.9 | 4.0 | 5.2 | 6.5 | *7.6* | *8.8* |
| Spain | 2.4 | 2.7 | 3.3 | 3.8 | 5.7 | 7.1 | 8.0 | *8.9* | *9.6* |
| Sweden | 3.4 | 4.2 | 4.9 | 6.5 | 8.0 | 8.9 | 8.8 | *8.6* | *9.9* |
| Switzerland | 2.9 | 3.5 | 3.9 | 5.7 | 6.6 | 6.9 | 7.3 | *7.9* | *9.6* |
| Turkey | 0.8 | 0.9 | 0.9 | 1.4 | 1.4 | 1.3 | 1.7 | *2.0* | *2.4* |
| UK | 3.5 | 4.2 | 4.5 | 5.8 | 7.0 | 7.4 | 7.7 | *7.9* | *8.7* |
| USA | 2.5 | 3.1 | 3.8 | 4.5 | 5.0 | 5.8 | 6.0 | *6.0* | *6.5* |

*Notes:*   Figures for 2005 are UN estimates.
Figures for the years 2010 and 2020 are UN projections.
1 EU15 as constituted before 1 May 2004 and EU27 as constituted since 1 January 2007.
2 Including Northern and Southern Cyprus.
3 Including former East Germany.

*Source:*   World Population Prospects (United Nations).

Figure 1.5  **Median ages in OECD and EU countries, 2005**

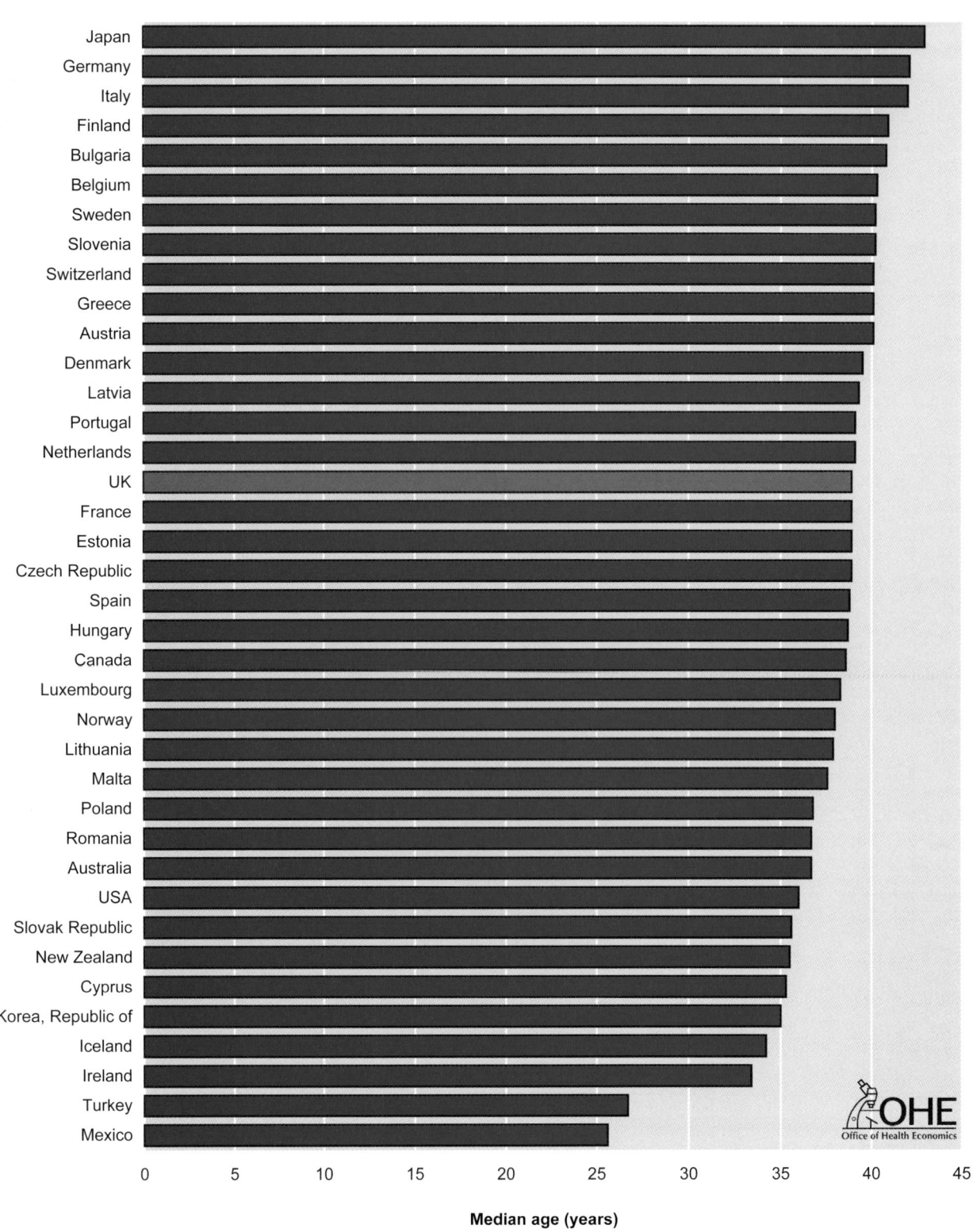

Median age (years)

*Note:*  Figures are UN estimates.
*Source:*  World Population Prospects (United Nations).

Table 1.15  **Life expectancy at birth and aged 65, by sex, by country, UK, 1981 - 2004**

### Life expectancy at Birth - Males

| | 1981 | 1985 | 1990 | 1991 | 1995 | 1996 | 1997 | 1998 | 1999 | 2000 | 2001 | 2002 | 2003 | 2004 |
|---|---|---|---|---|---|---|---|---|---|---|---|---|---|---|
| **United Kingdom** | 70.81 | 71.73 | 72.86 | 73.16 | 74.06 | 74.25 | 74.52 | 74.75 | 75.03 | 75.36 | 75.70 | 75.94 | 76.26 | 76.62 |
| **England** | 71.08 | 71.97 | 73.08 | 73.37 | 74.33 | 74.52 | 74.78 | 75.02 | 75.31 | 75.65 | 75.99 | 76.24 | 76.56 | 76.91 |
| **Wales** | 70.43 | 71.41 | 72.80 | 73.12 | 73.66 | 73.85 | 74.25 | 74.38 | 74.68 | 74.93 | 75.43 | 75.65 | 75.99 | 76.32 |
| **Scotland** | 69.11 | 70.01 | 71.06 | 71.38 | 72.08 | 72.23 | 72.40 | 72.64 | 72.84 | 73.10 | 73.31 | 73.50 | 73.79 | 74.23 |
| **Northern Ireland** | 69.17 | 70.57 | 72.14 | 72.55 | 73.51 | 73.83 | 74.16 | 74.27 | 74.48 | 74.79 | 75.20 | 75.56 | 75.83 | 76.01 |

### Life expectancy at Age 65 - Males

| | 1981 | 1985 | 1990 | 1991 | 1995 | 1996 | 1997 | 1998 | 1999 | 2000 | 2001 | 2002 | 2003 | 2004 |
|---|---|---|---|---|---|---|---|---|---|---|---|---|---|---|
| **United Kingdom** | 12.96 | 13.33 | 13.98 | 14.14 | 14.67 | 14.81 | 15.02 | 15.18 | 15.40 | 15.67 | 15.94 | 16.13 | 16.37 | 16.63 |
| **England** | 13.07 | 13.44 | 14.10 | 14.25 | 14.79 | 14.93 | 15.14 | 15.31 | 15.54 | 15.80 | 16.07 | 16.27 | 16.51 | 16.78 |
| **Wales** | 12.54 | 13.11 | 13.77 | 14.00 | 14.43 | 14.52 | 14.80 | 14.88 | 15.14 | 15.37 | 15.72 | 15.89 | 16.13 | 16.36 |
| **Scotland** | 12.28 | 12.54 | 13.05 | 13.26 | 13.76 | 13.88 | 14.05 | 14.21 | 14.42 | 14.66 | 14.92 | 15.05 | 15.23 | 15.46 |
| **Northern Ireland** | 12.46 | 13.02 | 13.68 | 13.91 | 14.44 | 14.56 | 14.72 | 14.85 | 15.03 | 15.27 | 15.66 | 15.86 | 16.12 | 16.35 |

### Life expectancy at Birth - Females

| | 1981 | 1985 | 1990 | 1991 | 1995 | 1996 | 1997 | 1998 | 1999 | 2000 | 2001 | 2002 | 2003 | 2004 |
|---|---|---|---|---|---|---|---|---|---|---|---|---|---|---|
| **United Kingdom** | 76.80 | 77.55 | 78.41 | 78.70 | 79.30 | 79.39 | 79.57 | 79.70 | 79.91 | 80.15 | 80.40 | 80.51 | 80.73 | 80.95 |
| **England** | 77.04 | 77.75 | 78.61 | 78.88 | 79.51 | 79.60 | 79.77 | 79.90 | 80.12 | 80.36 | 80.61 | 19.18 | 80.94 | 81.17 |
| **Wales** | 76.36 | 77.41 | 78.46 | 78.78 | 79.08 | 79.10 | 79.29 | 79.36 | 79.60 | 79.81 | 80.09 | 80.19 | 80.40 | 80.65 |
| **Scotland** | 75.31 | 76.00 | 76.74 | 77.11 | 77.73 | 77.85 | 78.04 | 78.18 | 78.35 | 78.56 | 78.78 | 78.87 | 79.07 | 79.27 |
| **Northern Ireland** | 75.54 | 76.89 | 78.01 | 78.39 | 78.94 | 79.16 | 79.49 | 79.46 | 79.55 | 79.75 | 80.13 | 80.43 | 80.55 | 80.83 |

### Life expectancy at Age 65 - Females

| | 1981 | 1985 | 1990 | 1991 | 1995 | 1996 | 1997 | 1998 | 1999 | 2000 | 2001 | 2002 | 2003 | 2004 |
|---|---|---|---|---|---|---|---|---|---|---|---|---|---|---|
| **United Kingdom** | 16.91 | 17.27 | 17.74 | 17.90 | 18.21 | 18.26 | 18.38 | 18.46 | 18.63 | 18.83 | 19.03 | 19.10 | 19.26 | 19.44 |
| **England** | 17.04 | 17.39 | 17.87 | 18.02 | 18.33 | 18.38 | 18.50 | 18.59 | 18.77 | 18.98 | 19.18 | 19.24 | 19.40 | 19.58 |
| **Wales** | 16.63 | 17.18 | 17.70 | 17.90 | 18.04 | 18.05 | 18.18 | 18.24 | 18.39 | 18.53 | 18.72 | 18.80 | 18.98 | 19.17 |
| **Scotland** | 16.04 | 16.34 | 16.66 | 16.88 | 17.25 | 17.31 | 17.44 | 17.49 | 17.62 | 17.80 | 18.01 | 18.10 | 18.22 | 18.38 |
| **Northern Ireland** | 16.27 | 16.82 | 17.51 | 17.76 | 18.04 | 18.12 | 18.29 | 18.29 | 18.37 | 18.49 | 18.74 | 18.92 | 19.10 | 19.34 |

*Notes:*   Figures for 1981 through to 2004 are based on population estimates the actual number of births and deaths for each three year period, centred on the years shown (i.e. figures for 1995 cover 1994-1996 etc).
Figures are based interim life tables.

*Sources:*   Population Trends (ONS).
Life Tables (GAD).

Table 1.16    **Residual life expectancy in years, England and Wales, 1841 - 2004**

| Year | At birth | | Age 1 | | Age 15 | | Age 45 | | Age 65 | |
|---|---|---|---|---|---|---|---|---|---|---|
| | Males | Females | Males | Females | Males | Females | Males | Females | Males | Females |
| 1841[1] | 40.2 | 42.2 | 46.7 | 47.6 | 43.4 | 44.1 | 23.3 | 24.4 | 10.9 | 11.5 |
| 1838-54[1] | 39.9 | 41.9 | 46.7 | 47.3 | 43.2 | 43.9 | 22.8 | 24.1 | 10.8 | 11.5 |
| 1871-80[1] | 41.4 | 44.6 | 48.1 | 50.1 | 43.4 | 45.6 | 22.1 | 24.1 | 10.6 | 11.4 |
| 1881-90[1] | 43.7 | 47.2 | 51.0 | 53.2 | 44.5 | 46.6 | 22.1 | 24.1 | 10.3 | 11.3 |
| 1891-1900[1] | 44.1 | 47.8 | 52.2 | 54.5 | 45.2 | 47.6 | 22.2 | 24.2 | 10.3 | 11.3 |
| 1901-10[1] | 48.5 | 52.4 | 55.7 | 58.3 | 47.3 | 50.1 | 23.3 | 25.5 | 10.8 | 12.0 |
| 1910-12[1] | 51.5 | 55.4 | 57.5 | 60.3 | 48.6 | 51.4 | 23.9 | 26.3 | 11.0 | 12.4 |
| 1920-22[1] | 55.6 | 59.6 | 60.1 | 63.0 | 50.1 | 53.1 | 25.2 | 27.7 | 11.4 | 12.9 |
| 1930-32[1] | 58.7 | 62.9 | 62.3 | 65.5 | 51.2 | 54.3 | 25.5 | 28.3 | 11.3 | 13.1 |
| 1948[2] | 66.4 | 71.2 | 68.0 | 72.3 | 54.9 | 59.1 | 27.4 | 31.5 | 12.8 | 15.3 |
| 1949[2] | 66.0 | 70.6 | 67.5 | 71.7 | 54.4 | 58.4 | 26.7 | 30.6 | 12.1 | 14.3 |
| 1950[2] | 66.5 | 71.2 | 67.8 | 72.1 | 54.6 | 58.8 | 26.8 | 30.7 | 12.0 | 14.4 |
| 1955[2] | 67.5 | 73.0 | 68.5 | 73.6 | 55.0 | 60.1 | 26.8 | 31.5 | 11.8 | 14.8 |
| 1960[2] | 68.3 | 74.1 | 69.0 | 74.6 | 55.5 | 61.0 | 27.3 | 32.2 | 12.2 | 15.4 |
| 1965[2] | 68.5 | 74.7 | 69.0 | 75.0 | 55.5 | 61.4 | 27.2 | 32.6 | 12.1 | 15.8 |
| 1966[2] | 68.4 | 74.7 | 68.9 | 74.9 | 55.4 | 61.3 | 27.1 | 32.5 | 12.0 | 15.7 |
| 1967[2] | 69.1 | 75.2 | 69.5 | 75.4 | 56.0 | 61.8 | 27.6 | 33.0 | 12.4 | 16.2 |
| 1968[2] | 68.6 | 74.8 | 69.1 | 75.0 | 55.6 | 61.4 | 27.1 | 32.5 | 11.9 | 15.7 |
| 1969[2] | 68.5 | 74.8 | 68.9 | 75.0 | 55.4 | 61.4 | 27.0 | 32.5 | 11.9 | 15.8 |
| 1970[2] | 68.8 | 75.1 | 69.2 | 75.3 | 55.7 | 61.6 | 27.2 | 32.7 | 12.0 | 16.0 |
| 1971[2] | 69.0 | 75.3 | 69.4 | 75.4 | 55.8 | 61.8 | 27.5 | 32.9 | 12.2 | 16.1 |
| 1972[2] | 68.9 | 75.1 | 69.2 | 75.2 | 55.7 | 61.7 | 27.3 | 32.8 | 12.1 | 16.0 |
| 1973[2] | 69.1 | 75.3 | 69.5 | 75.4 | 55.9 | 61.8 | 27.4 | 32.9 | 12.2 | 16.2 |
| 1974[3] | 69.2 | 75.6 | 69.6 | 75.7 | 56.0 | 62.0 | 27.6 | 33.1 | 12.3 | 16.3 |
| 1975[3] | 69.5 | 75.7 | 69.8 | 75.8 | 56.2 | 62.1 | 27.7 | 33.2 | 12.4 | 16.4 |
| 1976[3] | 69.6 | 75.8 | 69.8 | 75.8 | 56.2 | 62.1 | 27.8 | 33.2 | 12.4 | 16.4 |
| 1977[3] | 69.9 | 76.0 | 70.0 | 76.0 | 56.4 | 62.3 | 27.9 | 33.3 | 12.5 | 16.5 |
| 1978[3] | 70.0 | 76.2 | 70.1 | 76.1 | 56.5 | 62.4 | 28.0 | 33.4 | 12.5 | 16.6 |
| 1979[3] | 70.2 | 76.4 | 70.3 | 76.3 | 56.6 | 62.6 | 28.1 | 33.6 | 12.6 | 16.8 |
| 1980[3] | 70.4 | 76.6 | 70.4 | 76.4 | 56.8 | 62.7 | 28.3 | 33.7 | 12.8 | 16.8 |
| 1981[3] | 71.1 | 77.1 | 71.0 | 76.8 | 57.3 | 63.1 | 28.7 | 34.0 | 13.1 | 17.1 |
| 1982[3] | 71.3 | 77.2 | 71.1 | 76.9 | 57.5 | 63.1 | 28.9 | 34.1 | 13.1 | 17.1 |
| 1983[3] | 71.5 | 77.4 | 71.3 | 77.1 | 57.6 | 63.4 | 29.0 | 34.2 | 13.2 | 17.2 |
| 1984[3] | 71.9 | 77.8 | 71.7 | 77.4 | 58.0 | 63.7 | 29.4 | 34.5 | 13.5 | 17.5 |
| 1985[3] | 71.8 | 77.6 | 71.6 | 77.2 | 57.9 | 63.5 | 29.2 | 34.3 | 13.3 | 17.2 |
| 1986[3] | 72.1 | 77.9 | 71.9 | 77.5 | 58.1 | 63.7 | 29.5 | 34.6 | 13.5 | 17.4 |
| 1987[3] | 72.5 | 78.2 | 72.2 | 77.8 | 58.5 | 64.0 | 29.9 | 34.9 | 13.8 | 17.7 |
| 1988[3] | 72.6 | 78.3 | 72.4 | 77.9 | 58.6 | 64.1 | 30.0 | 34.9 | 13.9 | 17.7 |
| 1989[3] | 72.8 | 78.3 | 72.5 | 77.9 | 58.8 | 64.1 | 30.2 | 35.0 | 13.9 | 17.7 |
| 1990[3] | 73.1 | 78.7 | 72.7 | 78.3 | 59.0 | 64.5 | 30.5 | 35.3 | 14.1 | 18.0 |
| 1991 | 73.3 | 78.8 | 72.9 | 78.3 | 59.2 | 64.5 | 30.6 | 35.3 | 14.2 | 17.9 |
| 1992 | 73.7 | 79.2 | 73.3 | 78.6 | 59.5 | 64.8 | 30.9 | 35.6 | 14.4 | 18.2 |
| 1993 | 73.7 | 79.0 | 73.2 | 78.4 | 59.4 | 64.6 | 30.9 | 35.4 | 14.3 | 18.0 |
| 1994 | 74.2 | 79.5 | 73.7 | 78.9 | 60.0 | 65.1 | 31.4 | 35.9 | 14.7 | 18.4 |
| 1995 | 74.2 | 79.4 | 73.7 | 78.8 | 59.9 | 65.0 | 31.3 | 35.8 | 14.7 | 18.2 |
| 1996 | 74.5 | 79.6 | 74.0 | 79.0 | 60.2 | 65.2 | 31.7 | 36.0 | 14.9 | 18.4 |
| 1997 | 74.8 | 79.7 | 74.3 | 79.2 | 60.5 | 65.3 | 32.0 | 36.1 | 15.2 | 18.5 |
| 1998 | 75.0 | 79.9 | 74.5 | 79.3 | 60.7 | 65.5 | 32.1 | 36.3 | 15.3 | 18.6 |
| 1999 | 75.2 | 80.0 | 74.7 | 79.4 | 60.8 | 65.5 | 32.3 | 36.3 | 15.4 | 18.6 |
| 2000 | 75.7 | 80.4 | 75.1 | 79.8 | 61.3 | 65.9 | 32.7 | 36.7 | 15.8 | 19.0 |
| 2001 | 76.0 | 80.6 | 75.5 | 80.0 | 61.6 | 66.2 | 33.0 | 36.9 | 16.1 | 19.2 |
| 2002 | 76.2 | 80.7 | 75.7 | 80.1 | 61.8 | 66.2 | 33.2 | 37.0 | 16.3 | 19.2 |
| 2003 | 76.4 | 80.7 | 75.8 | 80.1 | 62.0 | 66.3 | 33.4 | 37.0 | 16.4 | 19.2 |
| 2004 | 76.9 | 81.1 | 76.3 | 80.5 | 62.5 | 66.7 | 33.8 | 37.4 | 16.8 | 19.6 |

*Notes:*      Figures for 1991 through to 2004 are based on population estimates and the actual number of births and deaths for each three year period, centred on the years shown (i.e. figures for 1995 cover 1994-1996 etc).
1 Figures are based on English Life Tables.  2 Figures are based on Abridged Life Tables.  3 Figures are based on future lifetime.

*Sources:*    Population Trends (ONS).
Life Tables (GAD).

Figure 1.6 **Trends in life expectancy in England and Wales, 1841 - 2051**

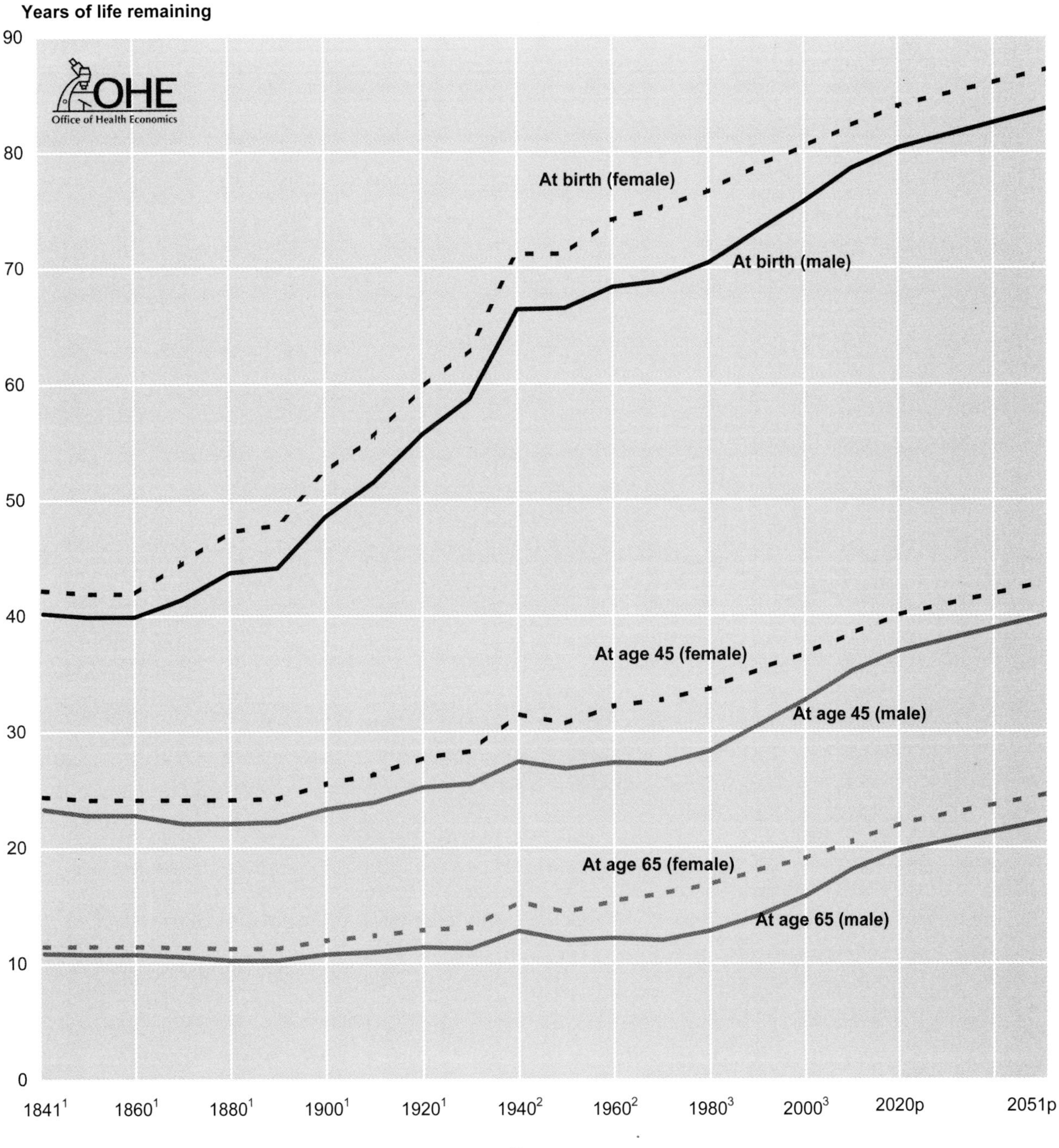
Years of life remaining
90
80
70
60
50
40
30
20
10
0
OHE
Office of Health Economics
At birth (female)
At birth (male)
At age 45 (female)
At age 45 (male)
At age 65 (female)
At age 65 (male)
1841¹
1860¹
1880¹
1900¹
1920¹
1940²
1960²
1980³
2000³
2020p
2051p
Year

*Notes:* p = 2004-based population projections. Data from 2010 onwards are projections.
1 Figures are based on English Life Tables.
2 Figures are based on Abridged Life Tables.
3 Figures are based on future lifetime.
Figures from 1981 onwards have been amended in light of the 2001 Census.

*Sources:* Population Trends (ONS).
Life Tables (GAD).

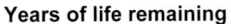

Table 1.17  **Life expectancy at birth in OECD and EU countries, males, 1950/55 - 2020/25**

**Male life expectancy at birth (years)**

| | Year | | | | | | | | |
|---|---|---|---|---|---|---|---|---|---|
| | 1950-55 | 1960-65 | 1970-75 | 1980-85 | 1990-95 | 1995-2000 | 2000-05 | 2010-15 | 2020-25 |
| **World** | **45.0** | **50.9** | **56.7** | **59.7** | **62.1** | **63.0** | **63.9** | **66.3** | **68.6** |
| **OECD[4]** | **63.2** | **66.3** | **67.8** | **70.0** | **72.2** | **73.5** | **75.0** | **76.9** | **78.2** |
| **EU27[1,4]** | **63.2** | **66.8** | **67.8** | **69.2** | **70.6** | **71.8** | **73.2** | **75.1** | **76.6** |
| **EU15[1,4]** | **65.0** | **67.5** | **68.8** | **71.1** | **73.2** | **74.4** | **75.8** | **77.5** | **78.8** |
| Australia | 66.9 | 67.8 | 68.4 | 71.9 | 74.7 | 75.9 | 77.9 | 79.8 | 81.3 |
| Austria | 63.2 | 66.1 | 67.0 | 69.6 | 72.7 | 74.2 | 75.9 | 77.6 | 78.8 |
| Belgium | 65.9 | 67.1 | 68.4 | 70.6 | 73.0 | 74.3 | 75.1 | 77.2 | 78.4 |
| Bulgaria | 62.2 | 68.4 | 68.7 | 68.4 | 67.6 | 67.5 | 68.9 | 70.4 | 72.0 |
| Canada | 66.8 | 68.5 | 69.6 | 72.5 | 74.8 | 75.9 | 77.3 | 79.2 | 80.5 |
| Cyprus[2] | 65.1 | 67.5 | 70.0 | 73.0 | 74.7 | 75.5 | 76.6 | 77.2 | 78.4 |
| Czech Republic | 64.5 | 67.3 | 66.6 | 67.2 | 69.3 | 71.1 | 72.1 | 74.3 | 75.9 |
| Denmark | 69.6 | 70.3 | 70.9 | 71.6 | 72.5 | 73.6 | 75.0 | 76.7 | 78.0 |
| Estonia | 61.7 | 65.0 | 65.7 | 64.4 | 62.6 | 63.9 | 65.1 | 66.9 | 70.1 |
| Finland | 63.2 | 65.4 | 66.6 | 70.0 | 72.0 | 73.4 | 74.9 | 77.2 | 78.6 |
| France | 63.7 | 67.6 | 68.6 | 70.8 | 73.3 | 74.6 | 76.0 | 77.8 | 79.0 |
| Germany[3] | 65.3 | 67.4 | 67.9 | 70.3 | 72.6 | 74.1 | 75.7 | 77.2 | 78.5 |
| Greece | 64.3 | 67.9 | 70.6 | 72.8 | 74.8 | 75.3 | 76.4 | 77.7 | 79.0 |
| Hungary | 61.5 | 66.4 | 66.5 | 65.3 | 64.8 | 66.4 | 68.3 | 70.4 | 72.5 |
| Iceland | 70.0 | 70.8 | 71.4 | 73.9 | 76.3 | 77.1 | 79.3 | 80.8 | 81.9 |
| Ireland | 65.7 | 68.4 | 68.9 | 70.4 | 72.6 | 73.5 | 75.3 | 77.1 | 78.4 |
| Italy | 64.3 | 67.4 | 69.2 | 71.5 | 74.0 | 75.5 | 76.9 | 78.1 | 79.3 |
| Japan | 61.6 | 66.7 | 70.6 | 74.2 | 76.2 | 77.1 | 78.3 | 79.9 | 81.0 |
| Korea, Republic of | 46.0 | 53.6 | 59.3 | 63.1 | 68.5 | 70.9 | 73.5 | 75.9 | 77.2 |
| Latvia | 62.5 | 66.3 | 65.3 | 64.5 | 61.8 | 64.0 | 65.7 | 68.8 | 71.1 |
| Lithuania | 61.5 | 67.0 | 67.0 | 66.1 | 64.1 | 65.5 | 66.4 | 68.9 | 71.2 |
| Luxembourg | 63.1 | 65.7 | 67.2 | 69.8 | 72.4 | 73.9 | 75.1 | 76.4 | 77.8 |
| Malta | 64.2 | 67.0 | 68.5 | 71.3 | 74.0 | 75.0 | 76.2 | 78.0 | 79.2 |
| Mexico | 48.9 | 56.4 | 60.1 | 64.4 | 69.0 | 71.3 | 72.4 | 74.9 | 76.6 |
| Netherlands | 70.9 | 71.1 | 71.1 | 72.8 | 74.2 | 75.1 | 76.3 | 78.2 | 79.4 |
| New Zealand | 67.5 | 68.3 | 68.7 | 70.7 | 73.3 | 75.0 | 77.0 | 79.1 | 80.7 |
| Norway | 70.9 | 71.1 | 71.4 | 72.9 | 74.3 | 75.2 | 76.7 | 78.6 | 79.9 |
| Poland | 58.6 | 65.8 | 67.0 | 67.0 | 67.0 | 68.6 | 70.4 | 72.3 | 74.0 |
| Portugal | 56.9 | 61.4 | 64.9 | 68.8 | 70.9 | 72.1 | 73.9 | 75.7 | 77.1 |
| Romania | 59.4 | 65.2 | 66.9 | 66.8 | 65.8 | 66.1 | 67.8 | 70.2 | 72.3 |
| Slovak Republic | 62.4 | 68.3 | 66.8 | 66.8 | 67.8 | 68.7 | 69.8 | 71.8 | 73.6 |
| Slovenia | 63.0 | 66.1 | 66.0 | 67.1 | 69.7 | 71.2 | 72.9 | 75.0 | 76.5 |
| Spain | 61.6 | 67.9 | 70.2 | 72.8 | 73.8 | 75.1 | 76.6 | 78.3 | 79.5 |
| Sweden | 70.4 | 71.6 | 72.1 | 73.5 | 75.5 | 76.8 | 77.8 | 79.6 | 80.8 |
| Switzerland | 67.0 | 68.9 | 70.8 | 72.9 | 74.7 | 76.3 | 77.9 | 79.6 | 80.7 |
| Turkey | 42.0 | 50.3 | 55.0 | 59.0 | 64.0 | 66.6 | 68.5 | 70.3 | 72.3 |
| UK | 66.7 | 67.9 | 69.0 | 71.2 | 73.6 | 74.7 | 76.1 | 77.8 | 79.1 |
| USA | 66.1 | 66.8 | 67.8 | 70.8 | 72.2 | 73.6 | 74.7 | 76.2 | 77.4 |

*Notes:*  Figures for 2000-05 are UN estimates.
Figures for the years 2010 and 2020 are UN projections.
1 EU15 as constituted before 1 May 2004 and EU27 as constituted since 1 January 2007.
2 Including Northern and Southern Cyprus.
3 Including former East Germany.
4 Unweighted average of life expectancies for the constituent countries.

*Source:*  World Population Prospects (United Nations).

# Population Statistics

Table 1.18 **Life expectancy at birth in OECD and EU countries, females, 1950/55 - 2020/25**

**Female life expectancy at birth (years)**

| | Year | | | | | | | | |
|---|---|---|---|---|---|---|---|---|---|
| | 1950-55 | 1960-65 | 1970-75 | 1980-85 | 1990-95 | 1995-2000 | 2000-05 | 2010-15 | 2020-25 |
| **World** | **47.8** | **53.6** | **59.9** | **63.5** | **66.3** | **67.4** | **68.3** | **70.8** | **73.2** |
| **OECD[4]** | **67.5** | **71.6** | **74.0** | **76.6** | **78.7** | **79.7** | **80.8** | **82.4** | **83.6** |
| **EU27[4]** | **67.7** | **72.1** | **74.0** | **76.1** | **77.7** | **78.8** | **79.8** | **81.4** | **82.7** |
| **EU15[1,4]** | **69.3** | **72.9** | **75.0** | **77.6** | **79.6** | **80.5** | **81.4** | **82.9** | **84.1** |
| Australia | 72.4 | 74.2 | 75.2 | 78.7 | 80.6 | 81.5 | 82.9 | 84.2 | 85.3 |
| Austria | 68.4 | 72.6 | 74.3 | 76.8 | 79.3 | 80.6 | 81.7 | 83.2 | 84.4 |
| Belgium | 70.9 | 73.1 | 74.9 | 77.2 | 79.8 | 80.6 | 81.2 | 83.0 | 84.2 |
| Bulgaria | 66.1 | 72.1 | 73.4 | 74.2 | 74.7 | 74.6 | 76.0 | 77.3 | 78.6 |
| Canada | 71.7 | 74.6 | 76.7 | 79.5 | 81.0 | 81.4 | 82.3 | 83.6 | 84.7 |
| Cyprus[2] | 69.0 | 71.0 | 72.9 | 77.5 | 79.2 | 80.5 | 81.3 | 82.3 | 83.5 |
| Czech Republic | 69.5 | 73.4 | 73.6 | 74.4 | 76.4 | 78.0 | 78.7 | 80.3 | 81.8 |
| Denmark | 72.4 | 74.4 | 76.4 | 77.6 | 77.8 | 78.6 | 79.6 | 81.4 | 82.7 |
| Estonia | 68.3 | 73.4 | 74.7 | 74.3 | 74.0 | 75.3 | 76.7 | 77.4 | 79.3 |
| Finland | 69.6 | 72.5 | 75.0 | 77.9 | 79.6 | 80.7 | 81.7 | 83.0 | 84.3 |
| France | 69.5 | 74.5 | 76.3 | 78.9 | 81.5 | 82.3 | 83.2 | 84.7 | 85.8 |
| Germany[3] | 69.6 | 72.9 | 73.8 | 76.8 | 79.1 | 80.3 | 81.5 | 82.8 | 84.0 |
| Greece | 67.5 | 71.2 | 74.2 | 77.5 | 79.7 | 80.4 | 80.1 | 82.5 | 83.8 |
| Hungary | 65.8 | 71.0 | 72.4 | 73.0 | 73.9 | 75.3 | 76.6 | 78.3 | 79.8 |
| Iceland | 74.1 | 76.1 | 77.4 | 79.8 | 80.8 | 81.4 | 82.7 | 83.9 | 85.0 |
| Ireland | 68.2 | 72.3 | 73.8 | 75.9 | 78.1 | 78.8 | 80.3 | 82.0 | 83.3 |
| Italy | 67.8 | 72.6 | 75.2 | 78.0 | 80.5 | 81.8 | 82.9 | 84.1 | 85.2 |
| Japan | 65.5 | 71.7 | 75.9 | 79.7 | 82.4 | 83.8 | 85.2 | 87.1 | 88.4 |
| Korea, Republic of | 49.0 | 56.9 | 66.1 | 71.4 | 76.5 | 78.5 | 80.6 | 83.2 | 84.4 |
| Latvia | 69.0 | 73.8 | 74.5 | 74.2 | 73.8 | 75.6 | 76.8 | 78.6 | 80.0 |
| Lithuania | 67.8 | 73.5 | 75.4 | 75.7 | 75.4 | 76.5 | 77.7 | 79.1 | 80.5 |
| Luxembourg | 68.9 | 72.1 | 74.1 | 76.6 | 79.2 | 80.4 | 81.1 | 82.3 | 83.6 |
| Malta | 67.7 | 70.8 | 72.8 | 75.8 | 78.4 | 79.8 | 80.8 | 82.0 | 83.3 |
| Mexico | 52.5 | 60.6 | 65.2 | 71.2 | 74.6 | 76.1 | 77.4 | 79.7 | 81.3 |
| Netherlands | 73.4 | 75.8 | 77.0 | 79.4 | 80.2 | 80.5 | 81.0 | 82.5 | 83.5 |
| New Zealand | 71.8 | 73.9 | 74.8 | 76.9 | 78.9 | 80.1 | 81.3 | 82.8 | 84.0 |
| Norway | 74.5 | 75.9 | 77.6 | 79.5 | 80.3 | 81.1 | 81.8 | 83.2 | 84.4 |
| Poland | 64.2 | 71.0 | 74.1 | 75.0 | 75.9 | 77.2 | 78.8 | 80.4 | 81.7 |
| Portugal | 61.9 | 67.1 | 71.3 | 75.8 | 78.1 | 79.2 | 80.5 | 81.9 | 83.2 |
| Romania | 62.8 | 68.8 | 71.5 | 72.6 | 73.2 | 73.6 | 75.0 | 77.1 | 78.8 |
| Slovak Republic | 66.2 | 73.0 | 73.5 | 74.7 | 76.2 | 76.9 | 77.8 | 79.3 | 80.7 |
| Slovenia | 68.1 | 72.0 | 73.5 | 75.2 | 77.4 | 78.7 | 80.4 | 82.2 | 83.5 |
| Spain | 66.3 | 72.7 | 75.7 | 78.9 | 81.0 | 82.2 | 83.4 | 84.8 | 85.9 |
| Sweden | 73.3 | 75.6 | 77.5 | 79.5 | 80.9 | 81.8 | 82.3 | 83.6 | 84.7 |
| Switzerland | 71.6 | 74.6 | 77.0 | 79.6 | 81.4 | 82.3 | 83.2 | 84.8 | 85.9 |
| Turkey | 45.2 | 54.0 | 59.2 | 63.2 | 68.5 | 71.2 | 73.3 | 75.2 | 77.1 |
| UK | 71.8 | 73.8 | 75.2 | 77.2 | 79.0 | 79.7 | 80.7 | 82.3 | 83.5 |
| USA | 72.0 | 73.5 | 75.4 | 77.9 | 78.9 | 79.3 | 80.0 | 81.5 | 82.7 |

*Notes:* Figures for 2000-05 are UN estimates.
Figures for the years 2010 and 2020 are UN projections.
1 EU15 as constituted before 1 May 2004.
2 Including Northern and Southern Cyprus.
3 Including former East Germany.
4 Unweighted average of life expectancies for the constituent countries.

*Source:* World Population Prospects (United Nations).

Figure 1.7  **Projected life expectancy at birth in OECD and EU countries, 2005 - 2010**

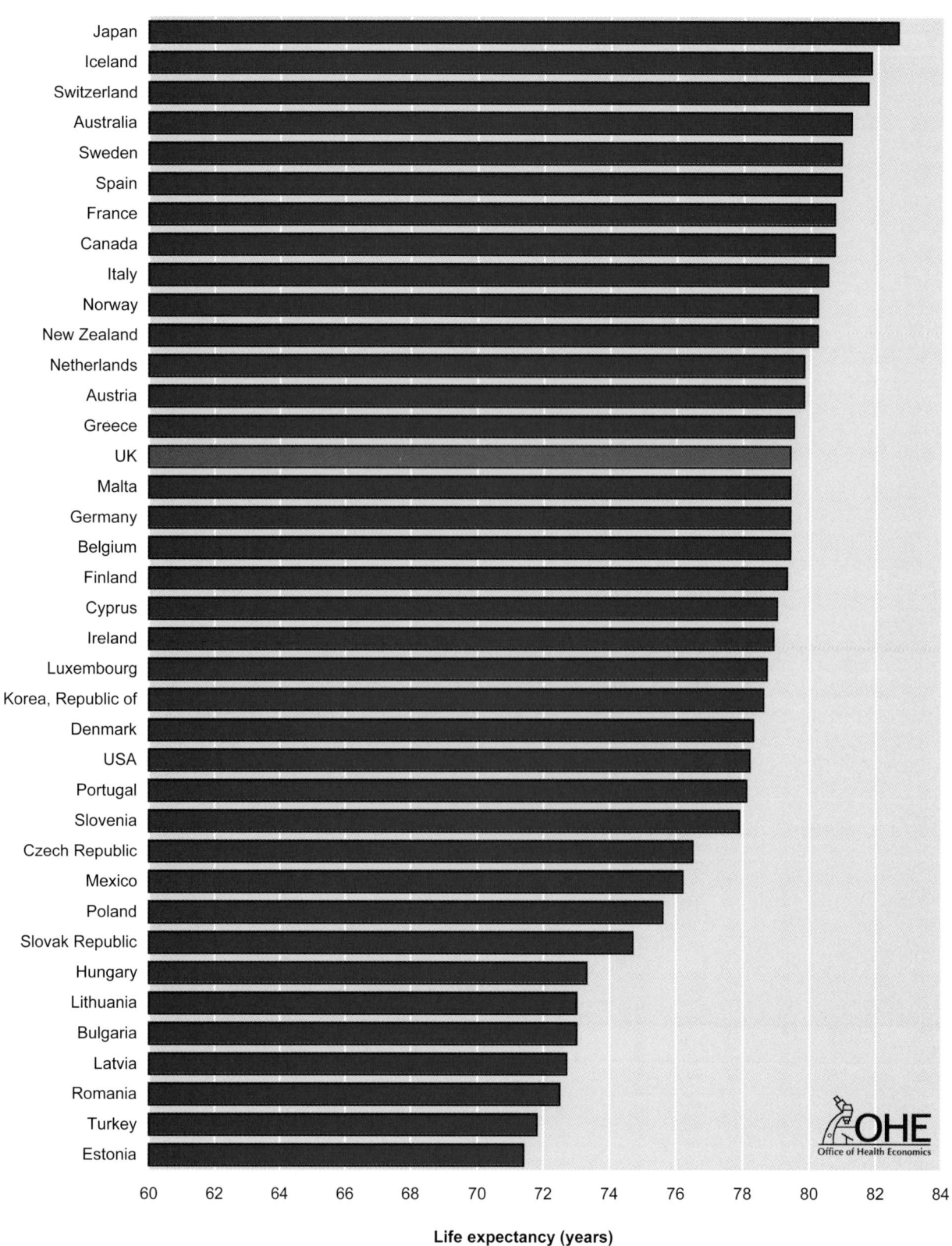

Life expectancy (years)

*Source:*   World Population Prospects (United Nations).

Figure 1.8 **Trends in birth rate, infant[1], childhood and age standardised mortality rates, UK, 1950 - 2005**

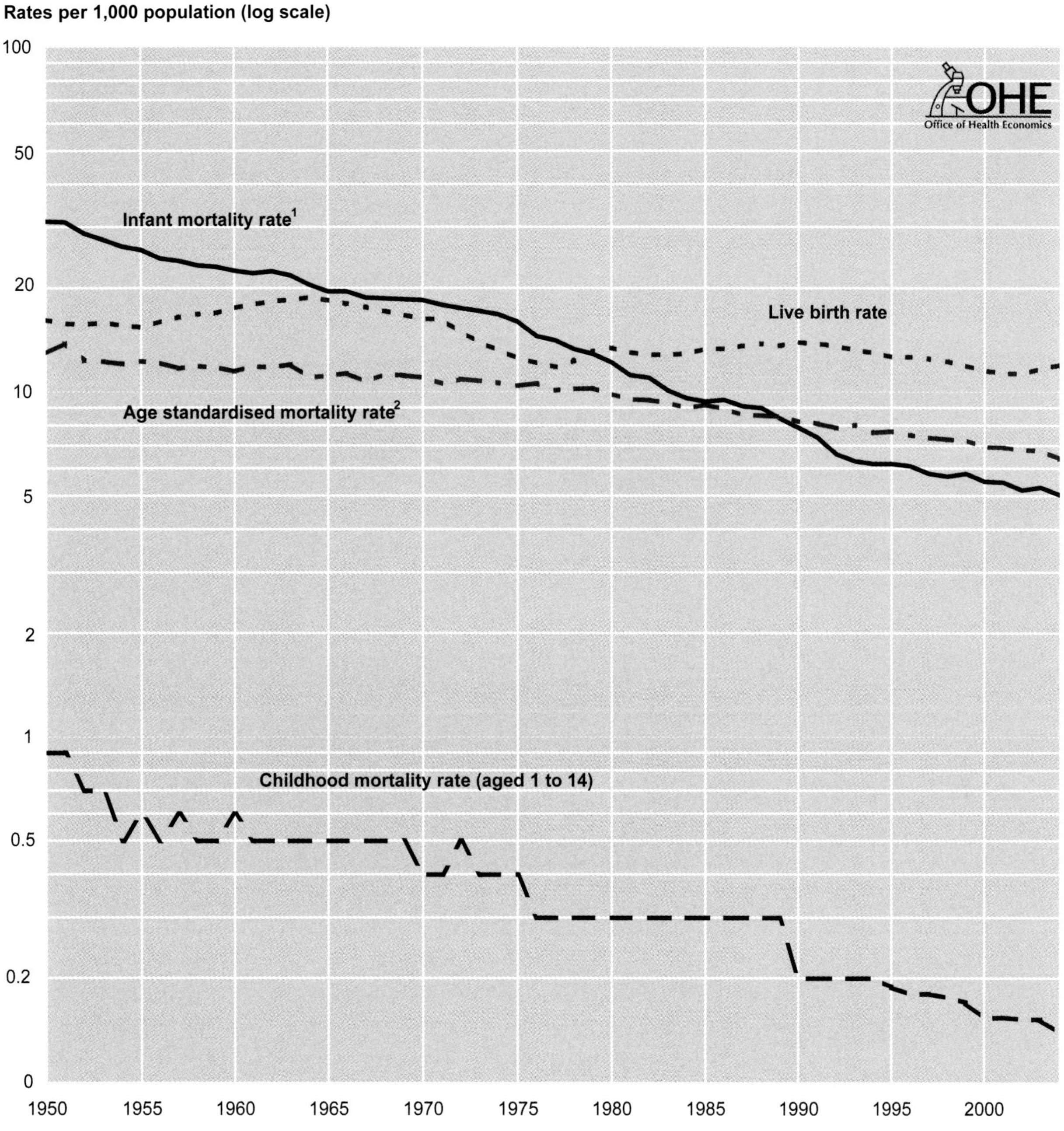

**Rates per 1,000 population (log scale)**

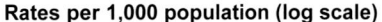

*Infant mortality rate[1]*

*Live birth rate*

*Age standardised mortality rate[2]*

*Childhood mortality rate (aged 1 to 14)*

**Year**

*Notes:*   1 Deaths under 1 year per 1,000 live births.
   2 Standardised via direct age standardisation using European Standard Population.
*Sources:*   Population Trends (ONS).
   Annual Abstract of Statistics (ONS).
   WHO Mortality Database (WHO).

Figure 1.9 **Trends in all causes mortality for males in the countries of the UK, 1950 - 2005**

**Age standardised rate per 100,000 population**

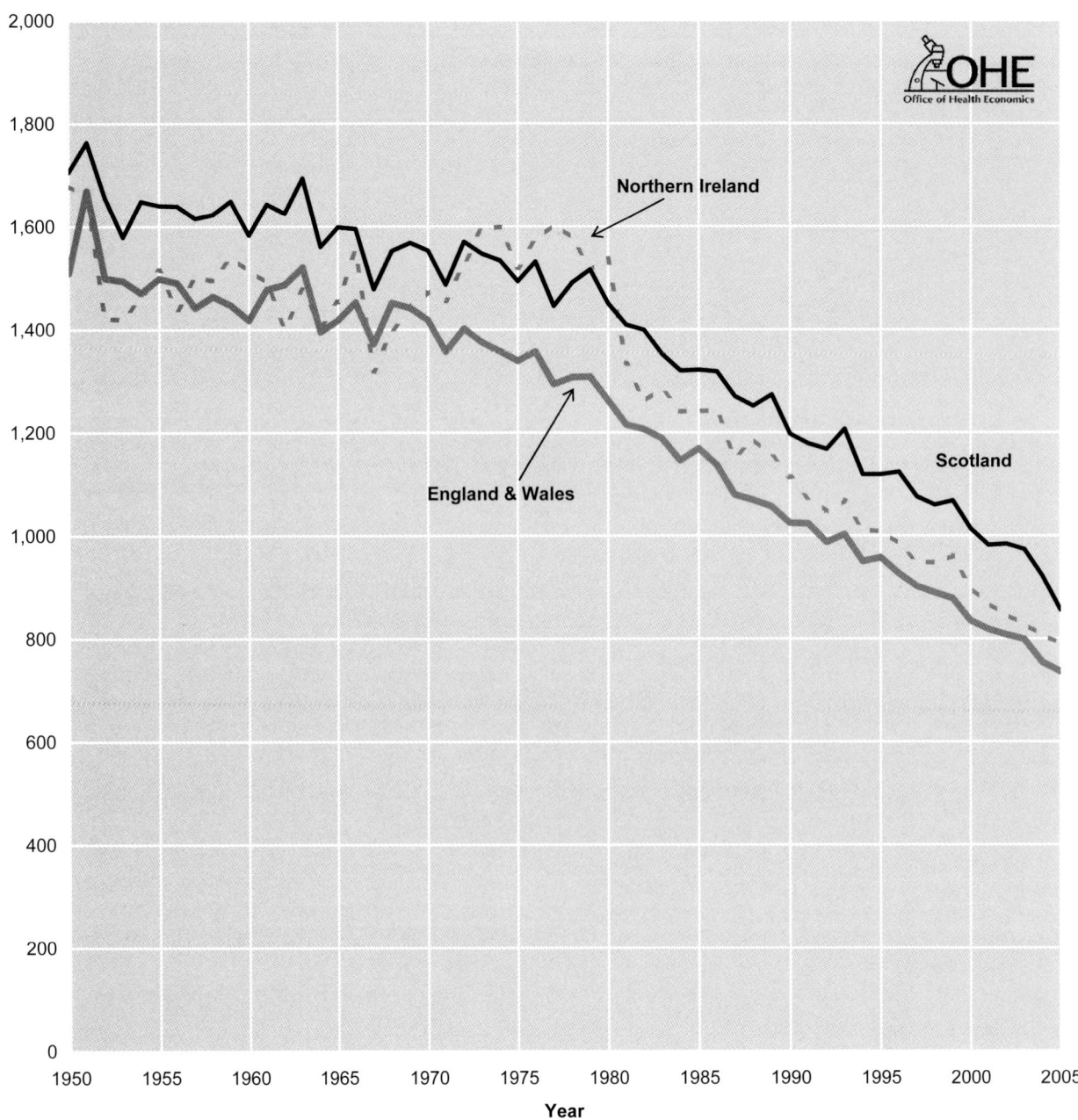

**Year**

*Sources:* OHE calculation based on WHO Mortality Database (WHO).
Mortality Statistics Series DH2 (ONS).
Vital Events Reference Tables (General Register Office of Scotland.
Demographic Statistics (Northern Ireland Statistics and Research Agency).

Figure 1.10 **Trends in all causes mortality for females in the countries of the UK, 1950 - 2005**

**Age standardised rate per 100,000 population**

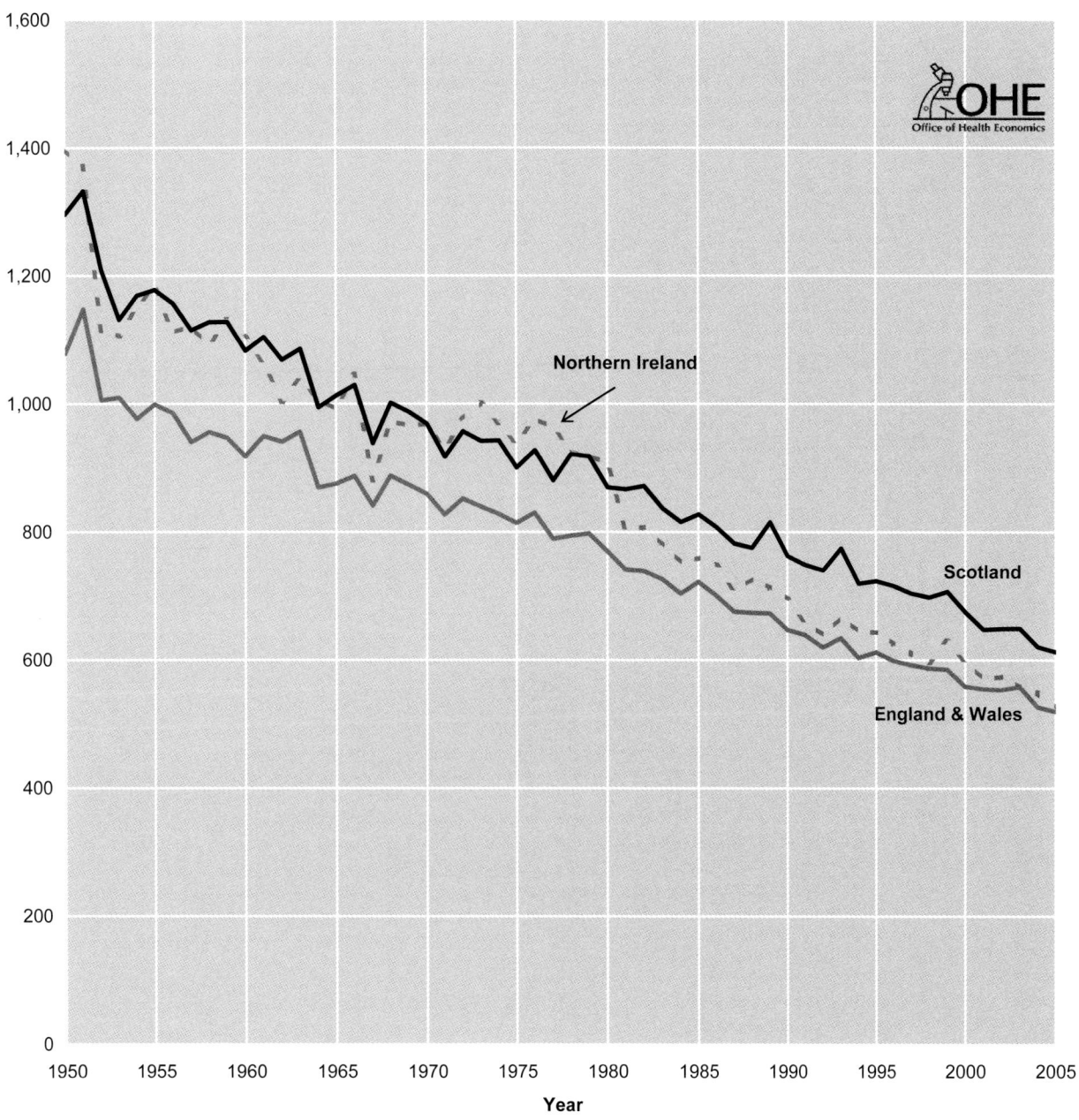

**Year**

*Sources:* OHE calculation based on WHO Mortality Database (WHO).
Mortality Statistics Series DH2 (ONS).
Vital Events Reference Tables (General Register Office of Scotland.
Demographic Statistics (Northern Ireland Statistics and Research Agency).

Table 1.19  **Birth rates, infant and childhood mortality rates, UK, 1870 - 2005**

| Year | Live births '000s | Live births per 1,000 population | Total Fertility Rate (TFR)[1] | Infant deaths '000s | Infant deaths per 1,000 live births | Childhood mortality per 1,000 population | | | |
|---|---|---|---|---|---|---|---|---|---|
| | | | | | | 1 to 4 | 5 to 9 | 10 to 14 | 1 to 14 |
| 1870-2 | 960 | 35.0 | - | 144.0 | 149.7 | 34.60 | 7.90 | 4.50 | 14.90 |
| 1880-2 | 1,043 | 33.6 | - | 143.0 | 137.2 | 30.20 | 6.20 | 3.50 | 12.70 |
| 1890-2 | 1,049 | 30.6 | - | 152.0 | 144.8 | 27.90 | 4.90 | 2.90 | 10.80 |
| 1900-2 | 1,095 | 28.6 | - | 156.0 | 142.5 | 22.50 | 4.20 | 2.50 | 9.00 |
| 1910-2 | 1,037 | 24.6 | - | 114.0 | 109.7 | 16.10 | 3.30 | 2.10 | 6.70 |
| 1920-2 | 1,018 | 23.1 | - | 83.0 | 81.9 | 12.30 | 2.90 | 1.80 | 4.90 |
| 1930-2 | 750 | 16.3 | - | 50.0 | 66.5 | 7.60 | 2.20 | 1.50 | 3.40 |
| 1940 | 702 | 14.6 | 1.75 | 43.0 | 61.0 | 5.20 | 2.00 | 1.40 | 2.70 |
| 1950 | 818 | 16.2 | 2.18 | 26.0 | 31.2 | 1.40 | 0.60 | 0.50 | 0.90 |
| 1955 | 789 | 15.4 | 2.22 | 20.0 | 25.8 | 1.00 | 0.50 | 0.40 | 0.60 |
| 1960 | 918 | 17.5 | 2.68 | 21.0 | 22.5 | 0.90 | 0.50 | 0.40 | 0.60 |
| 1965 | 997 | 18.4 | 2.85 | 20.0 | 19.6 | 0.80 | 0.40 | 0.40 | 0.50 |
| 1966 | 980 | 18.0 | 2.75 | 19.0 | 19.6 | 0.90 | 0.40 | 0.40 | 0.50 |
| 1967 | 962 | 17.6 | 2.65 | 18.0 | 18.8 | 0.80 | 0.40 | 0.40 | 0.50 |
| 1968 | 947 | 17.2 | 2.57 | 18.0 | 18.7 | 0.80 | 0.40 | 0.40 | 0.50 |
| 1969 | 920 | 16.7 | 2.47 | 17.0 | 18.6 | 0.80 | 0.40 | 0.30 | 0.50 |
| 1970 | 904 | 16.3 | 2.40 | 17.0 | 18.5 | 0.70 | 0.40 | 0.30 | 0.40 |
| 1971 | 902 | 16.2 | 2.37 | 16.0 | 17.9 | 0.70 | 0.40 | 0.30 | 0.40 |
| 1972 | 834 | 14.9 | 2.17 | 15.0 | 17.5 | 0.80 | 0.40 | 0.30 | 0.50 |
| 1973 | 780 | 13.9 | 2.00 | 13.0 | 17.2 | 0.70 | 0.40 | 0.30 | 0.40 |
| 1974 | 737 | 13.2 | 1.89 | 12.0 | 16.8 | 0.70 | 0.40 | 0.30 | 0.40 |
| 1975 | 698 | 12.5 | 1.78 | 11.0 | 16.0 | 0.60 | 0.30 | 0.30 | 0.40 |
| 1976 | 676 | 12.1 | 1.71 | 10.0 | 14.5 | 0.60 | 0.30 | 0.30 | 0.30 |
| 1977 | 657 | 11.8 | 1.66 | 9.0 | 14.1 | 0.60 | 0.30 | 0.30 | 0.30 |
| 1978 | 687 | 12.3 | 1.73 | 9.0 | 13.3 | 0.60 | 0.30 | 0.20 | 0.30 |
| 1979 | 735 | 13.1 | 1.84 | 9.0 | 12.9 | 0.50 | 0.30 | 0.30 | 0.30 |
| 1980 | 754 | 13.4 | 1.88 | 9.0 | 12.2 | 0.50 | 0.20 | 0.20 | 0.30 |
| 1981 | 731 | 13.0 | 1.80 | 8.0 | 11.2 | 0.50 | 0.20 | 0.30 | 0.30 |
| 1982 | 719 | 12.8 | 1.76 | 8.0 | 11.0 | 0.50 | 0.30 | 0.30 | 0.30 |
| 1983 | 722 | 12.8 | 1.76 | 7.0 | 10.1 | 0.40 | 0.20 | 0.30 | 0.30 |
| 1984 | 730 | 12.9 | 1.75 | 7.0 | 9.6 | 0.40 | 0.20 | 0.30 | 0.30 |
| 1985 | 751 | 13.3 | 1.78 | 7.0 | 9.4 | 0.50 | 0.20 | 0.30 | 0.30 |
| 1986 | 755 | 13.3 | 1.77 | 7.0 | 9.5 | 0.40 | 0.20 | 0.20 | 0.30 |
| 1987 | 776 | 13.6 | 1.81 | 7.0 | 9.1 | 0.40 | 0.20 | 0.30 | 0.30 |
| 1988 | 788 | 13.8 | 1.82 | 7.0 | 9.0 | 0.40 | 0.20 | 0.30 | 0.30 |
| 1989 | 777 | 13.6 | 1.80 | 7.0 | 8.4 | 0.40 | 0.20 | 0.20 | 0.30 |
| 1990 | 799 | 13.9 | 1.84 | 6.0 | 7.9 | 0.30 | 0.10 | 0.20 | 0.20 |
| 1991 | 793 | 13.7 | 1.82 | 6.0 | 7.4 | 0.30 | 0.10 | 0.20 | 0.20 |
| 1992 | 781 | 13.5 | 1.80 | 5.0 | 6.6 | 0.30 | 0.10 | 0.20 | 0.20 |
| 1993 | 762 | 13.1 | 1.76 | 5.0 | 6.3 | 0.30 | 0.10 | 0.20 | 0.20 |
| 1994 | 751 | 12.9 | 1.75 | 4.6 | 6.2 | 0.20 | 0.10 | 0.20 | 0.20 |
| 1995 | 732 | 12.5 | 1.72 | 4.5 | 6.2 | 0.22 | 0.11 | 0.16 | 0.16 |
| 1996 | 733 | 12.6 | 1.73 | 4.5 | 6.1 | 4.94 | 0.56 | 0.73 | 1.05 |
| 1997 | 727 | 12.5 | 1.73 | 4.3 | 5.8 | 0.29 | 0.13 | 0.13 | 0.17 |
| 1998 | 717 | 12.3 | 1.73 | 4.1 | 5.7 | 0.30 | 0.13 | 0.12 | 0.17 |
| 1999 | 700 | 11.9 | 1.69 | 4.0 | 5.8 | 0.28 | 0.13 | 0.13 | 0.17 |
| 2000 | 679 | 11.5 | 1.64 | 3.8 | 5.5 | 0.23 | 0.13 | 0.13 | 0.15 |
| 2001 | 669 | 11.3 | 1.63 | 3.7 | 5.5 | 0.22 | 0.13 | 0.13 | 0.16 |
| 2002 | 669 | 11.3 | 1.64 | 3.5 | 5.2 | 0.22 | 0.12 | 0.14 | 0.16 |
| 2003 | 696 | 11.7 | 1.72 | 3.7 | 5.3 | 0.23 | 0.11 | 0.14 | 0.16 |
| 2004 | 716 | 12.0 | 1.77 | 3.6 | 5.0 | 0.20 | 0.10 | 0.14 | 0.14 |
| 2005 | 723 | 12.0 | 1.79 | 3.7 | 5.1 | 0.20 | 0.09 | 0.14 | 0.14 |

*Notes:*    Data for childhood mortality and infant deaths prior to 1994 are only accurate to 1 decimal place.
1 Figures prior to 1999 relate to England and Wales only, figures from 1999 onwards are for the UK.

*Sources:*    Annual Abstract of Statistics (ONS).
Population Trends (ONS).
Population Projections Database (GAD).
World Health Organisation (WHO).
StatsWales Birth Statistics (NAW).
General Register Office of Scotland (GROS).
Register General Report for Northern Ireland (NISRA).
Alison Macfarlane et al. Birth Counts: Statistics of Pregnancy and Childbirth, The Stationery Office Books (2000).

# Mortality Statistics

Table 1.20   **Crude mortality rates in OECD and EU countries, 1960 - 2003**

**Crude mortality rates per 1,000 population**

| | Year | | | | | | | | | | | | |
|---|---|---|---|---|---|---|---|---|---|---|---|---|---|
| | 1960 | 1970 | 1980 | 1990 | 1993 | 1995 | 1997 | 1998 | 1999 | 2000 | 2001 | 2002 | 2003[2] |
| **OECD**[1] | **9.7** | **9.8** | **9.4** | **9.4** | **9.5** | **9.4** | **9.2** | **9.2** | **9.3** | **9.1** | **8.8** | **8.8** | **8.8** |
| **EU27**[1] | **9.7** | **9.8** | **9.4** | **9.4** | **10.9** | **10.7** | **10.6** | **10.6** | **10.5** | **10.3** | **10.3** | **10.3** | **10.4** |
| **EU15**[1] | **9.7** | **9.8** | **9.4** | **9.4** | **10.1** | **9.9** | **9.8** | **9.8** | **9.8** | **9.6** | **9.5** | **9.5** | **9.6** |
| Australia | 8.5 | 8.9 | 7.4 | 7.0 | 6.8 | 6.9 | 6.9 | 6.8 | 6.8 | 6.7 | 6.6 | 6.8 | - |
| Austria | 12.7 | 13.2 | 12.2 | 10.7 | 10.3 | 10.1 | 9.8 | 9.7 | 9.7 | 9.5 | 9.2 | 9.5 | 9.5 |
| Belgium | 12.4 | 11.5 | 10.0 | 10.3 | 10.6 | 10.3 | 10.2 | - | - | - | - | 10.0 | - |
| Bulgaria | - | 9.1 | 11.1 | 12.1 | 12.9 | 13.6 | 14.7 | 14.3 | 13.6 | 14.1 | 14.2 | 14.3 | 14.3 |
| Canada | 7.8 | 7.3 | 7.2 | 7.2 | 7.1 | 7.1 | 7.2 | 7.2 | 7.2 | 7.1 | 7.1 | 7.1 | - |
| Cyprus | - | - | - | - | - | - | - | - | - | - | - | 9.4 | - |
| Czech Republic | - | - | - | - | 11.4 | 11.4 | 11.0 | 10.6 | 10.7 | 10.6 | 10.6 | 10.6 | 10.9 |
| Denmark | 9.6 | 9.7 | 10.9 | 11.9 | 11.7 | 11.6 | 11.3 | 11.0 | 11.0 | 10.7 | 10.8 | 10.7 | - |
| Estonia | - | - | - | 12.4 | 14.0 | 14.0 | 12.7 | 13.4 | 12.8 | 13.4 | 13.6 | 13.4 | 13.3 |
| Finland | 9.0 | 9.6 | 9.2 | 10.0 | 10.1 | 9.7 | 9.6 | 9.6 | 9.6 | 9.5 | 9.3 | 9.5 | 9.4 |
| France | 11.3 | 10.6 | 10.1 | 9.4 | 9.2 | 9.1 | 9.0 | 9.1 | 9.2 | 9.0 | 9.0 | 9.0 | - |
| Germany | 11.6 | 12.1 | 11.6 | 11.3 | 11.1 | 10.8 | 10.5 | 10.4 | 10.3 | 10.2 | 10.1 | 10.2 | 10.3 |
| Greece | 7.3 | 8.4 | 9.1 | 9.3 | 9.4 | 9.6 | 9.5 | 9.8 | 9.8 | 9.6 | 9.4 | 9.5 | 9.6 |
| Hungary | - | - | - | - | 14.6 | 14.2 | 13.7 | 13.9 | 14.2 | 13.5 | 13.0 | 13.1 | 13.4 |
| Iceland | 6.6 | 7.1 | 6.7 | 6.7 | 6.6 | 7.2 | 6.8 | 6.7 | 6.9 | 6.5 | 6.1 | 6.6 | 6.3 |
| Ireland | 11.5 | 11.4 | 9.8 | 9.0 | 9.0 | 9.0 | 8.6 | 8.5 | 8.7 | 8.3 | 7.9 | 7.6 | - |
| Italy | 9.6 | 9.9 | 9.9 | 9.6 | 9.7 | 9.7 | 9.8 | 10.0 | 9.8 | 9.7 | 9.8 | 9.8 | - |
| Japan | 7.6 | 6.9 | 6.2 | 6.7 | 7.1 | 7.4 | 7.3 | 7.5 | 7.8 | 7.7 | 7.7 | 7.8 | 8.0 |
| Korea, Republic of | - | - | - | - | 4.9 | 5.2 | 5.1 | 5.1 | 5.2 | 5.2 | 5.0 | 5.1 | - |
| Latvia | - | - | - | 13.0 | 15.2 | 15.5 | 13.6 | 14.0 | 13.5 | 13.6 | 14.0 | 13.9 | 13.7 |
| Lithuania | - | - | - | 10.7 | 12.4 | 12.2 | 11.1 | 11.0 | 10.8 | 10.5 | 11.6 | 11.8 | 11.1 |
| Luxembourg | 11.8 | 12.4 | 11.2 | 9.9 | 9.8 | 9.0 | 8.9 | 9.0 | 8.5 | 8.5 | 8.3 | 8.3 | 8.9 |
| Malta | 8.6 | 9.4 | 10.4 | 7.7 | 7.4 | 7.3 | 7.7 | 8.1 | 8.2 | 7.7 | 7.5 | 7.7 | 8.3 |
| Mexico | - | - | - | - | - | - | - | - | - | - | 4.8 | 4.6 | - |
| Netherlands | 7.5 | 8.4 | 8.0 | 8.6 | 9.0 | 8.8 | 8.7 | 8.8 | 8.9 | 8.8 | 8.7 | 8.8 | 8.7 |
| New Zealand | 8.7 | 8.8 | 8.5 | 7.9 | 7.6 | 7.6 | 7.3 | 6.9 | 7.3 | 6.9 | 7.2 | 7.1 | 7.0 |
| Norway | 9.2 | 10.0 | 10.1 | 10.9 | 10.8 | 10.4 | 10.1 | 10.0 | 10.1 | 9.8 | 9.7 | 9.8 | 9.3 |
| Poland | - | - | - | - | 10.2 | 10.0 | - | - | 9.9 | 9.5 | 9.4 | 9.4 | 9.6 |
| Portugal | 10.5 | 10.3 | 9.9 | 10.4 | 10.8 | 10.5 | 10.6 | 10.7 | 10.8 | 10.4 | 10.3 | 10.3 | 10.4 |
| Romania | 8.7 | 9.5 | 10.4 | 10.6 | 11.6 | 12.0 | 12.4 | 12.0 | 11.8 | 11.4 | 11.6 | 12.4 | 12.3 |
| Slovak Republic | - | - | - | - | - | - | - | - | 9.7 | 9.8 | 9.7 | 9.6 | - |
| Slovenia | - | - | - | 9.3 | 10.1 | 9.6 | 9.6 | 9.6 | 9.6 | 9.4 | 9.3 | 9.4 | 9.8 |
| Spain | 8.6 | 8.4 | 7.7 | 8.5 | 8.7 | 8.8 | 8.9 | 9.2 | 9.4 | 9.0 | 8.9 | 8.9 | 9.2 |
| Sweden | 10.0 | 10.0 | 11.1 | 11.1 | 11.1 | 10.6 | 10.6 | 10.6 | 10.7 | 10.5 | 10.5 | 10.7 | - |
| Switzerland | 9.8 | 9.2 | 9.4 | 9.5 | 9.0 | 9.0 | 8.8 | 8.8 | 8.7 | 8.7 | 8.4 | 8.4 | - |
| Turkey | - | - | - | - | - | - | - | - | - | - | - | 6.2 | - |
| UK | 11.5 | 11.7 | 11.8 | 11.2 | 11.3 | 10.9 | 10.8 | 10.8 | 10.8 | 10.4 | 10.3 | 10.2 | 10.3 |
| USA | 9.5 | 9.5 | 8.8 | 8.6 | 8.8 | 8.8 | 8.6 | 8.6 | 8.8 | 8.5 | 8.5 | 8.5 | - |

*Notes:*   1 Average for countries for which data are available, unless otherwise stated. EU15 as constituted before 1 May 2004. EU27 as constituted since 1 January 2007.
2 OECD includes 2002 figures for Australia, Belgium, Canada, Denmark, France, Ireland, Italy, Mexico, Republic of Korea, Slovak Republic Sweden, Switzerland, Turkey and USA. EU27 figure includes 2002 figures for Belgium, Cyprus, Denmark, France, Ireland, Italy, Slovak Republic and Sweden. EU15 figure includes 2002 figures for Belgium, Denmark, France, Ireland, Italy and Sweden.
- Not available.

*Sources:*   OHE calculation based on data from WHO Mortality Database (WHO).
Population Projections Database (GAD).

Table 1.21    **Infant mortality rates in OECD and EU countries, 1960 - 2005**

**Infant (under 1 year) mortality rates per 1,000 live births**

| | Year | | | | | | | | | | | |
|---|---|---|---|---|---|---|---|---|---|---|---|---|
| | 1960 | 1970 | 1980 | 1990 | 1995 | 1999 | 2000 | 2001 | 2002 | 2003[2] | 2004[2] | 2005[3] |
| **OECD[1]** | **37.4** | **28.7** | **17.9** | **11.0** | **8.4** | **6.9** | **6.7** | **6.4** | **6.1** | **6.0** | **5.7** | **5.4** |
| **EU27[1]** | **35.9** | **25.2** | **15.3** | **10.3** | **8.7** | **6.9** | **6.7** | **6.4** | **6.0** | **5.8** | **5.6** | **5.4** |
| **EU15[1]** | **32.6** | **22.9** | **12.3** | **7.6** | **5.7** | **4.9** | **4.8** | **4.7** | **4.4** | **4.3** | **4.1** | **3.9** |
| Australia | 20.2 | 17.9 | 10.7 | 8.2 | 5.7 | 5.7 | 5.2 | 5.3 | 5.0 | 4.8 | 4.7 | 5.0 |
| Austria | 37.5 | 25.9 | 14.3 | 7.8 | 5.4 | 4.4 | 4.8 | 4.8 | 4.1 | 4.5 | 4.5 | 4.2 |
| Belgium | 23.9 | 21.1 | 12.1 | 6.5 | 5.9 | 4.9 | 4.8 | 4.5 | 4.4 | 4.3 | 4.3 | 3.7 |
| Bulgaria | - | 27.3 | 20.2 | 14.8 | 14.8 | 14.6 | 13.3 | 14.4 | 13.3 | 12.0 | 11.6 | - |
| Canada | 27.3 | 18.8 | 10.4 | 6.8 | 6.1 | 5.3 | 5.3 | 5.2 | 5.4 | 5.3 | 5.3 | - |
| Cyprus | - | - | - | - | - | - | - | - | - | - | 4.5 | - |
| Czech Republic | 20.0 | 20.2 | 16.9 | 10.8 | 7.7 | 4.6 | 4.1 | 4.0 | 4.1 | 3.9 | 3.7 | 3.4 |
| Denmark | 21.5 | 14.2 | 8.4 | 7.5 | 5.1 | 0.0 | 5.3 | 4.9 | 4.4 | 4.4 | 4.4 | - |
| Estonia | - | - | - | 12.3 | 14.8 | 9.5 | 8.4 | 8.8 | 5.7 | 7.0 | 5.7 | - |
| Finland | 21.0 | 13.2 | 7.6 | 5.6 | 3.9 | 3.6 | 3.8 | 3.2 | 3.0 | 3.1 | 3.3 | 3.0 |
| France | 27.7 | 18.2 | 10.0 | 7.3 | 4.9 | 4.3 | 4.4 | 4.5 | 4.1 | 4.0 | 3.9 | 3.6 |
| Germany | 35.0 | 22.5 | 12.4 | 7.0 | 5.3 | 4.5 | 4.4 | 4.3 | 4.2 | 4.2 | 4.1 | 3.9 |
| Greece | 40.1 | 29.6 | 17.9 | 9.7 | 8.1 | 6.2 | 5.4 | 5.1 | 5.1 | 4.0 | 4.1 | 3.8 |
| Hungary | 47.6 | 35.9 | 23.2 | 14.8 | 10.7 | 8.4 | 9.2 | 8.1 | 7.2 | 7.3 | 6.6 | 6.2 |
| Iceland | 13.1 | 13.3 | 7.8 | 5.8 | 6.0 | 2.4 | 3.0 | 2.7 | 2.3 | 2.4 | 2.8 | 2.3 |
| Ireland | 29.3 | 19.5 | 11.1 | 8.2 | 6.4 | 5.9 | 6.2 | 5.7 | 5.0 | 5.3 | 4.6 | 4.0 |
| Italy | 43.3 | 29.0 | 14.6 | 8.2 | 6.2 | 5.1 | 4.5 | 4.6 | 4.3 | 3.9 | 4.1 | 4.7 |
| Japan | 30.7 | 13.1 | 7.5 | 4.6 | 4.3 | 3.4 | 3.2 | 3.1 | 3.0 | 3.0 | 2.8 | 2.8 |
| Korea, Republic of | - | 45.0 | - | - | - | 6.2 | - | - | 5.3 | - | - | - |
| Latvia | - | - | 15.3 | 13.7 | 18.8 | 11.3 | 10.4 | 11.0 | 9.9 | 9.4 | 9.8 | - |
| Lithuania | - | - | - | 10.2 | 12.5 | 8.7 | 8.6 | 7.9 | 7.9 | 6.7 | 7.5 | - |
| Luxembourg | 31.6 | 25.0 | 11.4 | 7.3 | 5.6 | 4.6 | 5.1 | 5.8 | 5.1 | 4.9 | 3.9 | 2.6 |
| Malta | 38.3 | 16.2 | 15.5 | 9.5 | 8.9 | 7.2 | 6.0 | 4.3 | 5.9 | 5.7 | 5.3 | - |
| Mexico | 74.0 | 79.4 | 51.0 | 36.2 | 27.6 | 24.4 | 23.3 | 22.4 | 21.4 | 20.5 | 19.7 | 18.8 |
| Netherlands | 17.9 | 12.7 | 8.6 | 7.1 | 5.5 | 5.2 | 5.1 | 5.4 | 5.0 | 4.8 | 4.4 | 4.9 |
| New Zealand | 22.6 | 16.7 | 13.0 | 8.4 | 6.7 | 5.6 | 6.1 | 5.3 | 5.6 | 4.9 | 5.6 | 5.1 |
| Norway | 18.9 | 12.7 | 8.1 | 6.9 | 4.0 | 3.9 | 3.8 | 3.9 | 3.5 | 3.4 | 3.2 | 3.1 |
| Poland | 54.8 | 36.7 | 25.5 | 19.3 | 13.6 | 8.9 | 8.1 | 7.7 | 7.5 | 7.0 | 6.8 | 6.4 |
| Portugal | 77.5 | 55.5 | 24.2 | 11.0 | 7.5 | 5.8 | 5.5 | 5.0 | 5.0 | 4.1 | 3.8 | 3.5 |
| Romania | 75.7 | 49.4 | 29.3 | 26.9 | 21.2 | 18.6 | 18.6 | 18.4 | 17.3 | 16.7 | 16.8 | - |
| Slovak Republic | 28.6 | 25.7 | 20.9 | 12.0 | 11.0 | 8.3 | 8.6 | 6.2 | 7.6 | 7.9 | 6.8 | 7.2 |
| Slovenia | - | - | - | 8.3 | 5.6 | 4.6 | 4.9 | 4.2 | 3.8 | 4.0 | 4.0 | - |
| Spain | 43.7 | 28.1 | 12.3 | 7.6 | 5.5 | 4.5 | 4.4 | 4.1 | 4.1 | 3.9 | 4.0 | 4.1 |
| Sweden | 16.6 | 11.0 | 6.9 | 6.0 | 4.1 | 3.4 | 3.4 | 3.7 | 3.3 | 3.1 | 3.1 | 2.4 |
| Switzerland | 21.1 | 15.1 | 9.1 | 6.8 | 5.0 | 4.6 | 4.9 | 5.0 | 5.0 | 4.3 | 4.2 | 4.2 |
| Turkey | 189.5 | 145.0 | 117.5 | 55.4 | 43.0 | 33.9 | 28.9 | 27.8 | 26.7 | 28.7 | 24.6 | 23.6 |
| UK | 22.5 | 18.5 | 12.1 | 7.9 | 6.2 | 5.8 | 5.6 | 5.5 | 5.2 | 5.3 | 5.0 | 5.1 |
| USA | 26.0 | 20.0 | 12.6 | 9.2 | 7.6 | 7.1 | 6.9 | 6.8 | 7.0 | 6.9 | 6.8 | - |

*Notes:*    1 Average for countries for which data are available, unless other wise stated. EU15 as constituted before 1 May 2004. EU27 as constituted since 1 January 2007.
2 OECD figure includes 2002 figures for Republic of Korea.
3 OECD figure includes 2002 figures for Republic of Korea and 2004 figures for Canada Denmark and the USA. EU27 figure include 2004 figures for Bulgaria, Cyprus, Denmark, Estonia, Latvia, Lithuania, Malta, Romania and Slovenia. The EU15 figure includes 2004 figures for Denmark.
- Not available.

*Sources:*    OECD Health Database.
OHE calculations based on data from WHO Mortality Database (WHO).
Population Trends (ONS).

Figure 1.11 **Infant mortality rates[1] in selected OECD and EU countries, circa 2005**

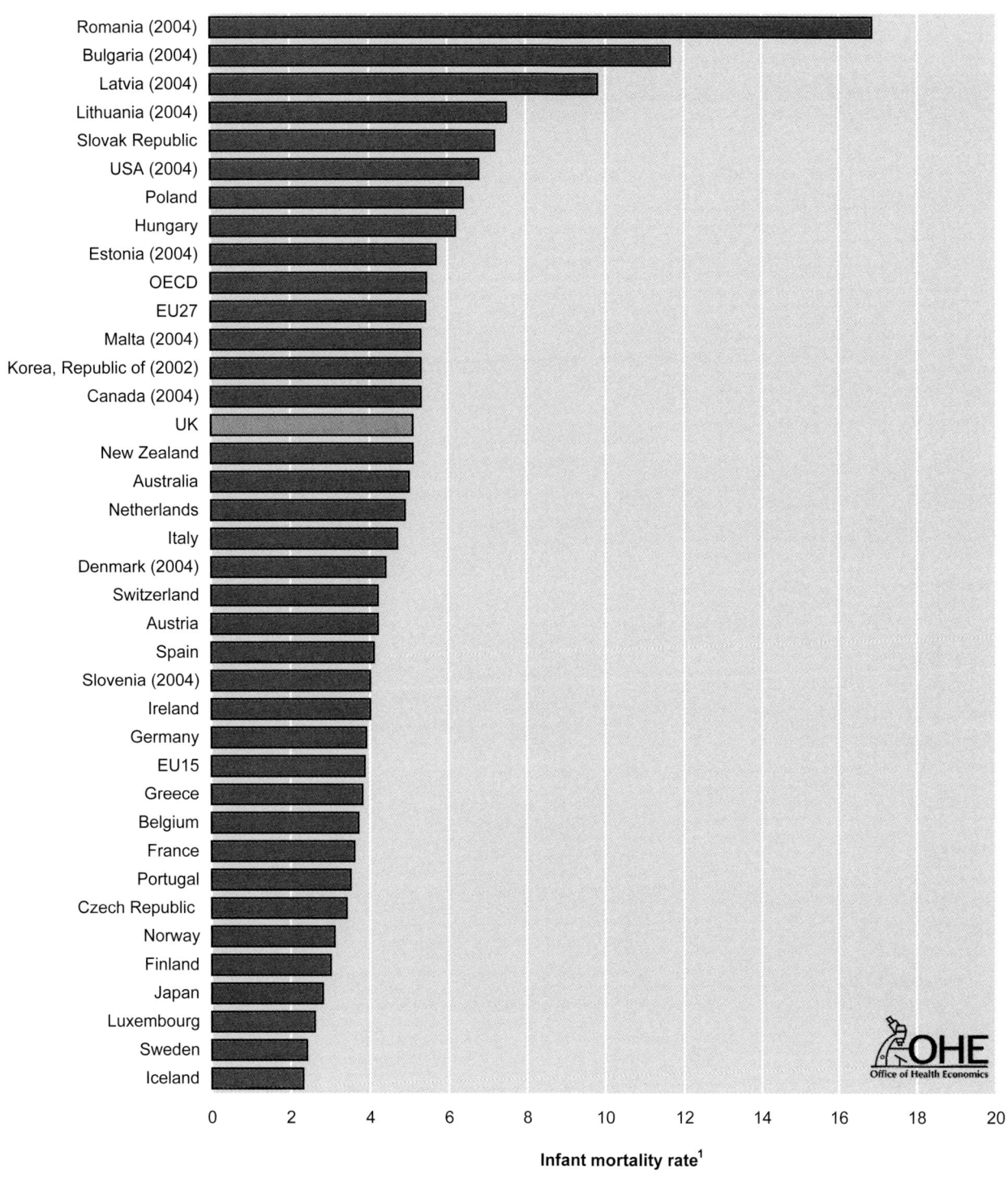

Infant mortality rate[1]

*Notes:*   1 Deaths under 1 year per 1,000 live births.
See Table 1.21 for rates for all available OECD/EU countries.
EU15 as constituted before 1 May 2004.  EU27 as constituted on 1st January 2007.
*Sources:* OHE calculations based on data from WHO Mortality Database (WHO).
OECD Health Database.

Table 1.22    **Infant and neonatal mortality in selected OECD and EU countries, circa 2004**

**Infant deaths[1]**

| | All | | | | Boys | | | | Girls | | | |
|---|---|---|---|---|---|---|---|---|---|---|---|---|
| | Early neonat. | Neo- nat. | Post- neonat. | Infant | Early neonat. | Neo- nat. | Post- neonat | Infant | Early neonat. | Neo- nat. | Post- neonat. | Infant |
| **OECD** | 44,525 | 58,593 | 31,566 | 95,591 | 25,011 | 32,877 | 17,805 | 53,677 | 19,514 | 25,716 | 13,761 | 41,914 |
| **EU27** | 12,357 | 17,078 | 8,874 | 27,070 | 7,025 | 9,653 | 4,971 | 15,220 | 5,332 | 7,425 | 3,903 | 11,850 |
| **EU15** | 8,364 | 11,508 | 5,479 | 18,105 | 4,725 | 6,485 | 3,080 | 10,161 | 3,639 | 5,023 | 2,399 | 7,944 |
| Australia (2002) | 668 | 830 | 396 | 1,226 | 349 | 436 | 227 | 663 | 319 | 394 | 169 | 563 |
| Austria (2004) | 166 | 248 | 105 | 353 | 90 | 135 | 54 | 189 | 76 | 113 | 51 | 164 |
| Bulgaria (2004) | 313 | 459 | 355 | 814 | 184 | 270 | 204 | 474 | 129 | 189 | 151 | 340 |
| Canada (2002) | - | - | - | 1,762 | - | - | - | 980 | - | - | - | 782 |
| Czech Republic (2004) | 130 | 224 | 142 | 366 | 79 | 136 | 74 | 210 | 51 | 88 | 68 | 156 |
| Denmark (2001) | 161 | 214 | 89 | 303 | 75 | 105 | 47 | 152 | 86 | 109 | 42 | 151 |
| Estonia (2003) | 39 | 52 | 39 | 91 | 22 | 30 | 26 | 56 | 17 | 22 | 13 | 35 |
| Finland (2004) | 113 | 142 | 51 | 193 | 63 | 84 | 37 | 121 | 50 | 58 | 14 | 72 |
| France (2002) | 1,399 | 2,018 | 1,096 | 3,114 | 787 | 1,123 | 630 | 1,753 | 612 | 895 | 466 | 1,361 |
| Germany (2004) | 1,446 | 1,892 | 1,026 | 2,918 | 806 | 1,069 | 560 | 1,629 | 640 | 823 | 466 | 1,289 |
| Greece (2003) | 186 | 282 | 138 | 420 | 99 | 158 | 78 | 236 | 87 | 124 | 60 | 184 |
| Hungary (2003) | 336 | 449 | 241 | 690 | 191 | 254 | 135 | 389 | 145 | 195 | 106 | 301 |
| Iceland (2003) | 7 | 1 | 2 | 10 | 3 | 1 | 2 | 6 | 4 | 0 | 0 | 4 |
| Ireland (2002) | 183 | 216 | 89 | 305 | 102 | 125 | 44 | 169 | 81 | 91 | 45 | 136 |
| Italy (2002) | 1,200 | 1,676 | 661 | 2,337 | 697 | 957 | 363 | 1,320 | 503 | 719 | 298 | 1,017 |
| Japan (2003) | 1,303 | 1,879 | 1,485 | 3,364 | 675 | 976 | 811 | 1,787 | 628 | 903 | 674 | 1,577 |
| Korea, Republic of (2002) | - | - | - | 2,545 | - | - | - | 1,416 | - | - | - | 1,129 |
| Latvia (2004) | 77 | 116 | 75 | 191 | 42 | 59 | 36 | 95 | 35 | 57 | 39 | 96 |
| Lithuania (2004) | 104 | 146 | 94 | 240 | 55 | 82 | 50 | 132 | 49 | 64 | 44 | 108 |
| Luxembourg (2004) | 9 | 11 | 8 | 19 | 4 | 5 | 5 | 10 | 5 | 6 | 3 | 9 |
| Malta (2004) | 12 | 17 | 6 | 23 | 9 | 11 | 3 | 14 | 3 | 6 | 3 | 9 |
| Mexico (2001) | 16,727 | 22,348 | 13,419 | 35,767 | 9,548 | 12,754 | 7,535 | 20,289 | 7,179 | 9,594 | 5,884 | 15,478 |
| Netherlands (2004) | 500 | 651 | 201 | 852 | 288 | 373 | 117 | 490 | 212 | 278 | 84 | 362 |
| New Zealand (2000) | 175 | 216 | 143 | 359 | 99 | 118 | 85 | 203 | 76 | 98 | 58 | 156 |
| Norway (2003) | 112 | 140 | 57 | 197 | 65 | 80 | 32 | 112 | 47 | 60 | 25 | 85 |
| Poland (2003) | 1,316 | 1,763 | 708 | 2,471 | 731 | 986 | 398 | 1,384 | 585 | 777 | 310 | 1,087 |
| Portugal (2003) | - | - | - | 471 | - | - | - | 238 | - | - | - | 233 |
| Romania (2004) | 1,464 | 2,065 | 1,576 | 3,641 | 890 | 1,209 | 880 | 2,089 | 574 | 856 | 696 | 1,552 |
| Slovak Republic (2002) | 170 | 238 | 150 | 388 | 79 | 109 | 80 | 189 | 91 | 129 | 70 | 199 |
| Slovenia (2003) | 41 | 52 | 17 | 69 | 22 | 27 | 10 | 37 | 19 | 25 | 7 | 32 |
| Spain (2003) | 690 | 1,106 | 627 | 1,733 | 391 | 625 | 339 | 964 | 299 | 481 | 288 | 769 |
| Sweden (2002) | 161 | 212 | 102 | 314 | 82 | 112 | 61 | 173 | 79 | 100 | 41 | 141 |
| Switzerland (2002) | 222 | 261 | 65 | 326 | 118 | 139 | 42 | 181 | 104 | 122 | 23 | 145 |
| UK (2005) | 2,141 | 2,829 | 1,278 | 4,107 | 1,237 | 1,609 | 740 | 2,349 | 904 | 1,220 | 538 | 1,758 |
| *England and Wales* | *1,919* | *2,528* | *1,155* | *3,683* | *1,109* | *1,438* | *671* | *2,109* | *810* | *1,090* | *484* | *1,574* |
| *Scotland* | *131* | *190* | *94* | *284* | *75* | *107* | *52* | *159* | *56* | *83* | *42* | *125* |
| *Northern Ireland* | *91* | *111* | *29* | *140* | *53* | *64* | *17* | *81* | *38* | *47* | *12* | *59* |
| USA (2002) | 15,004 | 18,747 | 9,287 | 28,034 | 8,353 | 10,408 | 5,309 | 15,717 | 6,651 | 8,339 | 3,978 | 12,317 |

*Notes:*    1 Early neonatal death - death under 1 week; neonatal - under 4 weeks; post neonatal - between 4 weeks and 1 year; infant under 1 year.
EU15 as constituted before 1 May 2004.  EU27 as constituted on 1st January 2007.
For Mexico, figures for boys and girls may not sum to the total due to unknown sex for some deaths.
Recent data were not available for Belgium, Cyprus or Turkey.
- Not available.

*Sources:*    OHE calculation based on WHO Mortality Database (WHO) and Mortality Statistics Series DH3 (ONS).

# Mortality Statistics

Table 1.23    Infant[1] and neonatal mortality rates per 1,000 live births in selected OECD and EU countries, circa 2004

**Infant (under 1 year) mortality rates per 1,000 live births**

| | All | | | | Boys | | | | Girls | | | |
|---|---|---|---|---|---|---|---|---|---|---|---|---|
| | Early neonat. | Neo- nat. | Post- neonat. | Infant | Early neonat. | Neo- nat. | Post- neonat. | Infant | Early neonat. | Neo- nat. | Post- neonat. | Infant |
| OECD[2] | 3.3 | 4.3 | 2.3 | 7.1 | 3.6 | 4.8 | 2.6 | 7.8 | 3.0 | 3.9 | 2.1 | 6.4 |
| EU27[2] | 2.5 | 3.4 | 1.8 | 5.4 | 2.7 | 3.7 | 1.9 | 5.9 | 2.2 | 3.0 | 1.6 | 4.9 |
| EU15[2] | 2.1 | 2.8 | 1.3 | 4.5 | 2.3 | 3.1 | 1.5 | 4.9 | 1.8 | 2.5 | 1.2 | 4.0 |
| | | | | | | | | | | | | |
| Australia (2002) | 2.7 | 3.3 | 1.6 | 4.9 | 2.7 | 3.4 | 1.8 | 5.2 | 2.6 | 3.2 | 1.4 | 4.6 |
| Austria (2004) | 2.1 | 3.1 | 1.3 | 4.5 | 2.2 | 3.3 | 1.3 | 4.7 | 2.0 | 2.9 | 1.3 | 4.3 |
| Bulgaria (2004) | 4.5 | 6.6 | 5.1 | 11.6 | 5.1 | 7.5 | 5.7 | 13.2 | 3.8 | 5.6 | 4.5 | 10.0 |
| Canada (2002) | - | - | - | 5.4 | - | - | - | 5.8 | - | - | - | 4.9 |
| Czech Republic (2004) | 1.3 | 2.3 | 1.5 | 3.7 | 1.6 | 2.7 | 1.5 | 4.2 | 1.1 | 1.9 | 1.4 | 3.3 |
| Denmark (2001) | 2.4 | 3.2 | 1.3 | 4.6 | 2.2 | 3.1 | 1.4 | 4.5 | 2.7 | 3.4 | 1.3 | 4.7 |
| Estonia (2003) | 3.0 | 4.0 | 3.0 | 7.0 | 3.3 | 4.5 | 3.9 | 8.5 | 2.7 | 3.4 | 2.0 | 5.5 |
| Finland (2004) | 2.0 | 2.5 | 0.9 | 3.3 | 2.1 | 2.8 | 1.2 | 4.1 | 1.8 | 2.1 | 0.5 | 2.6 |
| France (2002) | 1.8 | 2.7 | 1.4 | 4.1 | 2.0 | 2.9 | 1.6 | 4.5 | 1.6 | 2.4 | 1.3 | 3.7 |
| Germany (2004) | 2.0 | 2.7 | 1.5 | 4.1 | 2.2 | 3.0 | 1.5 | 4.5 | 1.9 | 2.4 | 1.4 | 3.8 |
| Greece (2003) | 1.8 | 2.7 | 1.3 | 4.0 | 1.8 | 2.9 | 1.5 | 4.4 | 1.7 | 2.4 | 1.2 | 3.6 |
| Hungary (2003) | 3.6 | 4.7 | 2.5 | 7.3 | 3.9 | 5.2 | 2.8 | 8.0 | 3.2 | 4.3 | 2.3 | 6.6 |
| Iceland (2003) | 1.7 | 0.2 | 0.5 | 2.4 | 1.4 | 0.5 | 1.0 | 2.9 | 2.0 | 0.0 | 0.0 | 2.0 |
| Ireland (2002) | 3.0 | 3.6 | 1.5 | 5.0 | 3.3 | 4.0 | 1.4 | 5.4 | 2.7 | 3.1 | 1.5 | 4.6 |
| Italy (2002) | 2.2 | 3.1 | 1.2 | 4.4 | 2.5 | 3.5 | 1.3 | 4.8 | 1.9 | 2.8 | 1.1 | 3.9 |
| Japan (2003) | 1.2 | 1.7 | 1.3 | 3.0 | 1.2 | 1.7 | 1.4 | 3.1 | 1.1 | 1.7 | 1.2 | 2.9 |
| Korea, Republic of (2002) | - | - | - | 4.0 | - | - | - | 4.9 | - | - | - | 4.2 |
| Latvia (2004) | 3.8 | 5.7 | 3.7 | 9.4 | 4.0 | 5.6 | 3.4 | 9.0 | 3.6 | 5.8 | 4.0 | 9.7 |
| Lithuania (2004) | 3.4 | 4.8 | 3.1 | 7.9 | 3.5 | 5.3 | 3.2 | 8.5 | 3.3 | 4.3 | 3.0 | 7.2 |
| Luxembourg (2004) | 1.7 | 2.0 | 1.5 | 3.5 | 1.4 | 1.8 | 1.8 | 3.5 | 1.9 | 2.3 | 1.1 | 3.4 |
| Malta (2004) | 3.1 | 4.4 | 1.5 | 5.9 | 4.5 | 5.5 | 1.5 | 7.0 | 1.6 | 3.2 | 1.6 | 4.8 |
| Mexico (2001) | 7.2 | 9.7 | 5.8 | 15.4 | 8.1 | 10.8 | 6.4 | 17.1 | 6.4 | 8.5 | 5.2 | 13.7 |
| Netherlands (2004) | 2.6 | 3.4 | 1.0 | 4.4 | 2.9 | 3.8 | 1.2 | 4.9 | 2.2 | 2.9 | 0.9 | 3.8 |
| New Zealand (2000) | 3.1 | 3.8 | 2.5 | 6.3 | 3.4 | 4.0 | 2.9 | 7.0 | 2.8 | 3.6 | 2.1 | 5.7 |
| Norway (2003) | 2.0 | 2.5 | 1.0 | 3.5 | 2.2 | 2.8 | 1.1 | 3.9 | 1.7 | 2.2 | 0.9 | 3.1 |
| Poland (2003) | 3.7 | 5.0 | 2.0 | 7.0 | 4.0 | 5.5 | 2.2 | 7.7 | 3.4 | 4.6 | 1.8 | 6.4 |
| Portugal (2003) | - | - | - | 4.2 | - | - | - | 4.1 | - | - | - | 4.3 |
| Romania (2004) | 6.8 | 9.5 | 7.3 | 16.8 | 8.0 | 10.8 | 7.9 | 18.7 | 5.5 | 8.2 | 6.6 | 14.8 |
| Slovak Republic (2002) | 3.3 | 4.7 | 2.9 | 7.6 | 3.0 | 4.1 | 3.0 | 7.1 | 3.7 | 5.2 | 2.8 | 8.1 |
| Slovenia (2003) | 2.4 | 3.0 | 1.0 | 4.0 | 2.5 | 3.0 | 1.1 | 4.1 | 2.3 | 3.0 | 0.8 | 3.8 |
| Spain (2003) | 1.6 | 2.5 | 1.4 | 3.9 | 1.7 | 2.7 | 1.5 | 4.2 | 1.4 | 2.2 | 1.3 | 3.6 |
| Sweden (2002) | 1.7 | 2.2 | 1.1 | 3.3 | 1.7 | 2.3 | 1.2 | 3.5 | 1.7 | 2.1 | 0.9 | 3.0 |
| Switzerland (2002) | 3.1 | 3.6 | 0.9 | 4.5 | 3.2 | 3.7 | 1.1 | 4.9 | 3.0 | 3.5 | 0.7 | 4.1 |
| UK (2005) | 3.0 | 3.9 | 1.8 | 5.7 | 3.3 | 4.3 | 2.0 | 6.3 | 2.6 | 3.5 | 1.5 | 5.0 |
| *England and Wales* | *3.0* | *3.9* | *1.8* | *5.7* | *3.4* | *4.3* | *2.0* | *6.4* | *2.6* | *3.5* | *1.5* | *5.0* |
| *Scotland* | *2.4* | *3.5* | *1.7* | *5.2* | *2.7* | *3.8* | *1.9* | *5.7* | *2.1* | *3.2* | *1.6* | *4.8* |
| *Northern Ireland* | *4.1* | *5.0* | *1.3* | *6.3* | *4.7* | *5.6* | *1.5* | *7.1* | *3.5* | *4.3* | *1.1* | *5.4* |
| USA (2002) | 3.7 | 4.7 | 2.3 | 7.0 | 4.1 | 5.1 | 2.6 | 7.6 | 3.4 | 4.2 | 2.0 | 6.3 |

*Notes:*    1 Early neonatal death - death under 1 week; neonatal - under 4 weeks; post neonatal - between 4 weeks and 1 year; infant under 1 year.
2 Weighted average of countries for which recent data is available.
EU15 as constituted before 1 May 2004.    EU27 as constituted on 1st January 2007.
For Mexico, figures for boys and girls may not sum to the total due to unknown sex for some deaths.
Recent data were not available for Belgium, Cyprus or Turkey.
- Not available.

*Sources:*    OHE calculation based on WHO Mortality Database (WHO) and Mortality Statistics Series DH3 (ONS).

Table 1.24    **Childhood mortality in selected OECD and EU countries, circa 2004**

**Number of deaths**

| | | All | | | Males | | | Females | | |
| | | Age | | | Age | | | Age | | |
| Country | Year | 1-4 | 5-14 | 1-14 | 1-4 | 5-14 | 1-14 | 1-4 | 5-14 | 1-14 |
|---|---|---|---|---|---|---|---|---|---|---|
| Australia | 2002 | 261 | 352 | 613 | 164 | 206 | 370 | 97 | 146 | 243 |
| Austria | 2004 | 50 | 117 | 167 | 30 | 61 | 91 | 20 | 56 | 76 |
| Bulgaria | 2004 | 192 | 211 | 403 | 105 | 125 | 230 | 87 | 86 | 173 |
| Canada | 2002 | 319 | 563 | 882 | 168 | 331 | 499 | 151 | 232 | 383 |
| Czech Republic | 2004 | 76 | 150 | 226 | 41 | 87 | 128 | 35 | 63 | 98 |
| Denmark | 2001 | 67 | 97 | 164 | 33 | 60 | 93 | 34 | 37 | 71 |
| Estonia | 2003 | 26 | 43 | 69 | 14 | 24 | 38 | 12 | 19 | 31 |
| Finland | 2004 | 56 | 104 | 160 | 33 | 57 | 90 | 23 | 47 | 70 |
| France | 2002 | 703 | 987 | 1,690 | 405 | 566 | 971 | 298 | 421 | 719 |
| Germany | 2004 | 619 | 832 | 1,451 | 329 | 488 | 817 | 290 | 344 | 634 |
| Greece | 2003 | 74 | 130 | 204 | 39 | 76 | 115 | 35 | 54 | 89 |
| Hungary | 2003 | 120 | 208 | 328 | 67 | 117 | 184 | 53 | 91 | 144 |
| Iceland | 2003 | 2 | 6 | 8 | 0 | 5 | 5 | 2 | 1 | 3 |
| Ireland | 2002 | 59 | 78 | 137 | 30 | 46 | 76 | 29 | 32 | 61 |
| Italy | 2002 | 437 | 752 | 1,189 | 243 | 477 | 720 | 194 | 275 | 469 |
| Japan | 2003 | 1,154 | 1,325 | 2,479 | 615 | 747 | 1,362 | 539 | 578 | 1,117 |
| Korea, Republic of | 2002 | 1,080 | 1,368 | 2,448 | 608 | 824 | 1,432 | 472 | 544 | 1,016 |
| Latvia | 2004 | 39 | 73 | 112 | 26 | 51 | 77 | 13 | 22 | 35 |
| Lithuania | 2004 | 54 | 98 | 152 | 32 | 61 | 93 | 22 | 37 | 59 |
| Luxembourg | 2004 | 2 | 1 | 3 | 2 | 0 | 2 | 0 | 1 | 1 |
| Malta | 2004 | 8 | 6 | 14 | 3 | 3 | 6 | 5 | 3 | 8 |
| Mexico | 2001 | 6,606 | 7,088 | 13,686 | 3,606 | 4,238 | 7,844 | 2,989 | 2,844 | 5,833 |
| Netherlands | 2004 | 192 | 216 | 408 | 108 | 129 | 237 | 84 | 87 | 171 |
| New Zealand | 2000 | 88 | 114 | 202 | 53 | 69 | 122 | 35 | 45 | 80 |
| Norway | 2003 | 60 | 86 | 146 | 29 | 53 | 82 | 31 | 33 | 64 |
| Poland | 2003 | 391 | 871 | 1,262 | 237 | 532 | 769 | 154 | 339 | 493 |
| Portugal | 2003 | 128 | 228 | 356 | 69 | 130 | 199 | 59 | 98 | 157 |
| Romania | 2004 | 620 | 816 | 1,436 | 357 | 513 | 870 | 263 | 303 | 566 |
| Slovak Republic | 2002 | 74 | 149 | 223 | 38 | 89 | 127 | 36 | 60 | 96 |
| Slovenia | 2003 | 15 | 24 | 39 | 10 | 13 | 23 | 5 | 11 | 16 |
| Spain | 2003 | 442 | 595 | 1,037 | 245 | 355 | 600 | 197 | 240 | 437 |
| Sweden | 2002 | 69 | 103 | 172 | 46 | 57 | 103 | 23 | 46 | 69 |
| Switzerland | 2002 | 75 | 89 | 164 | 44 | 53 | 97 | 31 | 36 | 67 |
| United Kingdom | 2005 | 577 | 823 | 1,400 | 324 | 471 | 795 | 253 | 352 | 605 |
| *England and Wales* | *2005* | *501* | *709* | *1,210* | *282* | *403* | *685* | *219* | *306* | *525* |
| *Scotland* | *2005* | *60* | *78* | *138* | *33* | *49* | *82* | *27* | *29* | *56* |
| *Northern Ireland* | *2005* | *16* | *36* | *52* | *9* | *19* | *28* | *7* | *17* | *24* |
| USA | 2002 | 4,858 | 7,150 | 12,008 | 2,806 | 4,198 | 7,004 | 2,052 | 2,952 | 5,004 |

*Notes:* For Mexico, figures for males and females may not sum to the total due to unknown sex for some deaths.
Recent data were not available for Belgium, Cyprus or Turkey.

*Sources:* OHE calculation based on: WHO Mortality Database (WHO); Mortality Statistics Series DH2 (ONS); Vital Events Reference Tables (General Register Office of Scotland); and Demographic Statistics (Northern Ireland Statistics and Research Agency).

# Mortality Statistics

Table 1.25   **Childhood mortality rates per 100,000 population in selected OECD and EU countries, circa 2004**

**Childhood mortality rates per 100,000 population**

| Country | Year | All Age 1-4 | Age 5-14 | Age 1-14 | Males Age 1-4 | Age 5-14 | Age 1-14 | Females Age 1-4 | Age 5-14 | Age 1-14 |
|---|---|---|---|---|---|---|---|---|---|---|
| OECD[1] | | 35 | 17 | 22 | 38 | 20 | 25 | 32 | 15 | 19 |
| EU27[1,2] | | 26 | 15 | 18 | 29 | 17 | 20 | 23 | 12 | 15 |
| EU15[1,2] | | 23 | 12 | 15 | 25 | 14 | 17 | 20 | 10 | 13 |
| Australia | 2002 | 25 | 13 | 16 | 31 | 15 | 19 | 19 | 11 | 13 |
| Austria | 2004 | 16 | 13 | 13 | 18 | 13 | 14 | 13 | 12 | 12 |
| Bulgaria | 2004 | 72 | 28 | 39 | 76 | 32 | 44 | 67 | 23 | 35 |
| Canada | 2002 | 23 | 14 | 16 | 23 | 16 | 18 | 22 | 12 | 14 |
| Czech Republic | 2004 | 21 | 14 | 16 | 22 | 16 | 17 | 20 | 12 | 14 |
| Denmark | 2001 | 25 | 15 | 18 | 24 | 18 | 19 | 26 | 11 | 16 |
| Estonia | 2003 | 52 | 27 | 33 | 55 | 30 | 36 | 50 | 25 | 31 |
| Finland | 2004 | 25 | 16 | 19 | 28 | 18 | 20 | 21 | 15 | 17 |
| France | 2002 | 24 | 13 | 16 | 27 | 15 | 18 | 20 | 12 | 14 |
| Germany | 2004 | 21 | 10 | 13 | 22 | 11 | 14 | 20 | 8 | 11 |
| Greece | 2003 | 18 | 12 | 14 | 19 | 13 | 15 | 18 | 10 | 12 |
| Hungary | 2003 | 31 | 18 | 21 | 34 | 20 | 24 | 28 | 16 | 19 |
| Iceland | 2003 | 12 | 13 | 13 | 0 | 22 | 16 | 24 | 5 | 10 |
| Ireland | 2002 | 26 | 14 | 18 | 26 | 16 | 19 | 27 | 12 | 16 |
| Italy | 2002 | 21 | 14 | 16 | 23 | 17 | 18 | 19 | 10 | 13 |
| Japan | 2003 | 25 | 11 | 15 | 26 | 12 | 16 | 24 | 10 | 14 |
| Korea, Republic of | 2002 | 43 | 20 | 26 | 46 | 23 | 29 | 39 | 17 | 23 |
| Latvia | 2004 | 49 | 29 | 34 | 64 | 40 | 46 | 33 | 18 | 22 |
| Lithuania | 2004 | 42 | 22 | 27 | 49 | 27 | 32 | 36 | 17 | 21 |
| Luxembourg | 2004 | 9 | 2 | 4 | 17 | 0 | 5 | 0 | 4 | 3 |
| Malta | 2004 | 49 | 12 | 21 | 36 | 11 | 17 | 62 | 12 | 24 |
| Mexico | 2001 | 73 | 32 | 44 | 78 | 37 | 49 | 68 | 26 | 38 |
| Netherlands | 2004 | 23 | 11 | 14 | 26 | 13 | 16 | 21 | 9 | 12 |
| New Zealand | 2000 | 39 | 19 | 25 | 45 | 23 | 29 | 32 | 16 | 20 |
| Norway | 2003 | 25 | 14 | 17 | 24 | 17 | 19 | 27 | 11 | 15 |
| Poland | 2003 | 26 | 18 | 20 | 31 | 21 | 24 | 21 | 14 | 16 |
| Portugal | 2003 | 29 | 21 | 23 | 30 | 23 | 25 | 27 | 18 | 21 |
| Romania | 2004 | 73 | 33 | 44 | 82 | 41 | 52 | 63 | 25 | 35 |
| Slovak Republic | 2002 | 34 | 21 | 24 | 34 | 25 | 27 | 34 | 17 | 21 |
| Slovenia | 2003 | 21 | 12 | 14 | 27 | 12 | 16 | 14 | 11 | 12 |
| Spain | 2003 | 27 | 15 | 18 | 29 | 17 | 21 | 25 | 12 | 16 |
| Sweden | 2002 | 19 | 9 | 11 | 25 | 10 | 13 | 13 | 8 | 9 |
| Switzerland | 2002 | 25 | 10 | 14 | 29 | 12 | 16 | 21 | 9 | 12 |
| United Kingdom | 2005 | 21 | 11 | 14 | 23 | 12 | 15 | 19 | 9 | 12 |
| *England and Wales* | *2005* | *21* | *11* | *14* | *23* | *12* | *15* | *19* | *10* | *12* |
| *Scotland* | *2005* | *28* | *13* | *17* | *31* | *16* | *20* | *26* | *10* | *14* |
| *Northern Ireland* | *2005* | *18* | *15* | *16* | *20* | *15* | *17* | *16* | *14* | *15* |
| USA | 2002 | 31 | 17 | 21 | 35 | 20 | 24 | 27 | 15 | 18 |

*Notes:*   1 Weighted average for countries for which recent data were available.
2 EU15 as constituted before 1 May 2004.  EU27 as constituted on 1st January 2007.
For Mexico, figures for males and females may not sum to the total due to unknown sex for some deaths.
Recent data were not available for Belgium, Cyprus or Turkey.

*Sources:*   OHE calculation based on: WHO Mortality Database (WHO); Mortality Statistics Series DH2 (ONS); Vital Events Reference Tables (General Register Office of Scotland); and Demographic Statistics (Northern Ireland Research and Statistics Agency).

Table 1.26 **Age specific mortality rates per 1,000 population, UK, 1870 - 2005**

| Year | Age Group All ages | <1[2] | 0 - 4 | 5 - 9 | 10 - 14 | 15 - 19 | 20 - 24 | 25 - 34 | 35 - 44 | 45 - 54 | 55 - 64 | 65 - 74 | 75 - 84 | =>85 |
|---|---|---|---|---|---|---|---|---|---|---|---|---|---|---|
| 1870-2[1] | 22.1 | 149.7 | 64.5 | 7.9 | 4.5 | 6.6 | 8.5 | 10.1 | 13.0 | 17.5 | 30.2 | 62.3 | 137.1 | 286.9 |
| 1880-2[1] | 19.7 | 137.2 | 57.0 | 6.3 | 3.5 | 5.0 | 6.4 | 8.1 | 11.8 | 17.0 | 30.6 | 62.0 | 133.6 | 277.6 |
| 1890-2[1] | 19.7 | 144.8 | 57.2 | 4.9 | 2.9 | 4.5 | 5.7 | 7.6 | 11.9 | 18.6 | 34.9 | 71.3 | 148.1 | 297.3 |
| 1900-2[1] | 17.4 | 142.5 | 52.5 | 4.2 | 2.5 | 3.6 | 4.7 | 6.2 | 10.0 | 16.5 | 31.5 | 64.6 | 135.3 | 276.1 |
| 1910-2[1] | 14.1 | 109.7 | 37.3 | 3.3 | 2.1 | 3.0 | 3.7 | 4.7 | 7.4 | 13.2 | 26.5 | 56.4 | 123.8 | 247.8 |
| 1920-2[1] | 12.7 | 81.9 | 30.2 | 2.9 | 1.9 | 2.9 | 3.7 | 4.3 | 6.3 | 10.6 | 22.3 | 51.7 | 121.7 | 245.8 |
| 1930-2[1] | 12.2 | 66.5 | 20.0 | 2.2 | 1.5 | 2.5 | 3.1 | 3.4 | 5.2 | 9.8 | 20.7 | 50.8 | 122.2 | 261.7 |
| 1940 | 14.6 | 61.0 | 16.7 | 2.0 | 1.4 | 2.5 | 3.9 | 3.6 | 5.1 | 10.4 | 23.1 | 53.5 | 134.3 | 284.9 |
| 1945 | 13.0 | 48.8 | 12.7 | 1.2 | 1.0 | 1.7 | 3.4 | 3.1 | 3.7 | 7.7 | 18.0 | 42.9 | 103.6 | 203.9 |
| 1950 | 11.8 | 31.2 | 7.0 | 0.7 | 0.5 | 0.9 | 1.3 | 1.7 | 2.2 | 7.0 | 17.9 | 44.6 | 110.3 | 235.2 |
| 1955 | 11.8 | 25.8 | 6.1 | 0.5 | 0.4 | 0.7 | 0.9 | 1.2 | 2.3 | 6.3 | 17.0 | 43.8 | 110.0 | 243.4 |
| 1960 | 11.5 | 22.5 | 5.7 | 0.5 | 0.4 | 0.7 | 0.8 | 0.9 | 2.2 | 5.9 | 16.3 | 41.6 | 102.8 | 224.0 |
| 1965 | 11.6 | 19.6 | 4.8 | 0.4 | 0.4 | 0.7 | 0.8 | 0.9 | 2.2 | 6.0 | 16.2 | 41.3 | 99.6 | 222.1 |
| 1966 | 11.8 | 19.6 | 4.7 | 0.4 | 0.4 | 0.7 | 0.8 | 0.9 | 2.2 | 6.0 | 16.2 | 41.6 | 101.9 | 233.9 |
| 1967 | 11.2 | 18.8 | 4.4 | 0.4 | 0.4 | 0.7 | 0.7 | 0.8 | 2.1 | 5.7 | 15.5 | 39.7 | 94.8 | 216.5 |
| 1968 | 11.9 | 18.7 | 4.4 | 0.4 | 0.4 | 0.7 | 0.7 | 0.9 | 2.1 | 5.8 | 16.0 | 41.4 | 102.1 | 240.6 |
| 1969 | 11.9 | 18.6 | 4.3 | 0.4 | 0.3 | 0.7 | 0.7 | 0.8 | 2.1 | 6.0 | 16.4 | 42.3 | 99.0 | 226.8 |
| 1970 | 11.8 | 18.5 | 4.2 | 0.3 | 0.3 | 0.7 | 0.7 | 0.8 | 2.0 | 5.9 | 16.0 | 41.2 | 98.0 | 229.2 |
| 1971 | 11.7 | 17.9 | 4.2 | 0.3 | 0.3 | 0.7 | 0.7 | 0.8 | 2.0 | 5.9 | 15.5 | 39.6 | 97.4 | 230.1 |
| 1972 | 12.1 | 17.5 | 4.0 | 0.3 | 0.3 | 0.7 | 0.7 | 0.8 | 2.0 | 6.1 | 15.9 | 40.8 | 99.0 | 222.7 |
| 1973 | 12.0 | 17.2 | 3.7 | 0.3 | 0.3 | 0.7 | 0.8 | 0.8 | 2.0 | 6.0 | 15.7 | 39.5 | 97.0 | 216.7 |
| 1974 | 11.9 | 16.8 | 3.7 | 0.3 | 0.3 | 0.7 | 0.7 | 0.8 | 2.0 | 6.0 | 15.6 | 39.2 | 95.1 | 215.7 |
| 1975 | 11.8 | 16.0 | 3.4 | 0.3 | 0.3 | 0.7 | 0.7 | 0.8 | 1.9 | 5.9 | 15.2 | 38.3 | 94.3 | 212.8 |
| 1976 | 12.1 | 14.5 | 3.1 | 0.3 | 0.3 | 0.6 | 0.7 | 0.8 | 1.9 | 5.8 | 15.3 | 38.8 | 96.4 | 222.0 |
| 1977 | 11.7 | 14.1 | 3.1 | 0.3 | 0.3 | 0.7 | 0.7 | 0.8 | 1.8 | 5.6 | 14.7 | 37.3 | 90.9 | 206.3 |
| 1978 | 11.9 | 13.3 | 3.1 | 0.3 | 0.3 | 0.7 | 0.7 | 0.8 | 1.8 | 5.7 | 14.7 | 37.5 | 91.2 | 208.3 |
| 1979 | 12.0 | 12.9 | 3.3 | 0.3 | 0.3 | 0.6 | 0.7 | 0.8 | 1.8 | 5.6 | 14.7 | 37.2 | 91.4 | 211.6 |
| 1980 | 11.8 | 12.2 | 3.1 | 0.3 | 0.3 | 0.6 | 0.7 | 0.7 | 1.7 | 5.3 | 14.4 | 36.1 | 88.2 | 204.2 |
| 1981 | 12.0 | 11.2 | 2.9 | 0.3 | 0.3 | 0.6 | 0.7 | 0.8 | 1.7 | 5.2 | 14.2 | 36.5 | 90.5 | 215.1 |
| 1982 | 11.8 | 11.0 | 2.6 | 0.3 | 0.3 | 0.6 | 0.7 | 0.7 | 1.5 | 5.0 | 13.9 | 35.6 | 86.6 | 202.2 |
| 1983 | 11.7 | 10.1 | 2.4 | 0.3 | 0.3 | 0.6 | 0.6 | 0.7 | 1.5 | 4.8 | 13.9 | 35.5 | 84.9 | 199.1 |
| 1984 | 11.5 | 9.6 | 2.3 | 0.3 | 0.3 | 0.5 | 0.6 | 0.7 | 1.5 | 4.6 | 13.6 | 34.6 | 81.8 | 191.5 |
| 1985 | 11.9 | 9.4 | 2.3 | 0.2 | 0.3 | 0.5 | 0.6 | 0.7 | 1.5 | 4.5 | 13.7 | 34.9 | 84.8 | 200.9 |
| 1986 | 11.7 | 9.5 | 2.3 | 0.2 | 0.2 | 0.5 | 0.6 | 0.7 | 1.4 | 4.4 | 13.3 | 33.8 | 82.6 | 194.8 |
| 1987 | 11.4 | 9.1 | 2.3 | 0.2 | 0.3 | 0.5 | 0.6 | 0.7 | 1.4 | 4.3 | 12.9 | 32.7 | 79.1 | 177.1 |
| 1988 | 11.4 | 9.0 | 2.2 | 0.2 | 0.3 | 0.5 | 0.6 | 0.7 | 1.5 | 4.2 | 12.6 | 32.2 | 78.5 | 178.1 |
| 1989 | 11.5 | 8.4 | 2.1 | 0.2 | 0.2 | 0.5 | 0.6 | 0.7 | 1.4 | 4.0 | 12.2 | 31.8 | 79.2 | 181.9 |
| 1990 | 11.2 | 7.9 | 2.0 | 0.2 | 0.2 | 0.5 | 0.6 | 0.8 | 1.5 | 3.9 | 11.8 | 31.0 | 76.6 | 172.3 |
| 1991 | 11.2 | 7.4 | 1.8 | 0.2 | 0.2 | 0.5 | 0.6 | 0.8 | 1.5 | 3.9 | 11.3 | 30.9 | 76.8 | 181.8 |
| 1992 | 11.0 | 6.6 | 1.6 | 0.2 | 0.2 | 0.5 | 0.6 | 0.7 | 1.4 | 3.6 | 11.0 | 30.0 | 74.5 | 173.0 |
| 1993 | 11.3 | 6.3 | 1.5 | 0.2 | 0.2 | 0.5 | 0.6 | 0.7 | 1.4 | 3.6 | 10.9 | 30.6 | 77.5 | 181.7 |
| 1994 | 10.8 | 6.2 | 1.4 | 0.1 | 0.2 | 0.4 | 0.6 | 0.7 | 1.4 | 3.4 | 10.1 | 28.5 | 69.7 | 164.9 |
| 1995 | 10.9 | 6.2 | 1.4 | 0.1 | 0.2 | 0.5 | 0.6 | 0.8 | 1.4 | 3.5 | 10.0 | 28.5 | 69.9 | 171.8 |
| 1996 | 10.9 | 6.1 | 1.4 | 0.1 | 0.2 | 0.5 | 0.6 | 0.8 | 1.4 | 3.5 | 9.8 | 27.5 | 67.6 | 169.8 |
| 1997 | 10.8 | 5.8 | 1.4 | 0.1 | 0.2 | 0.4 | 0.6 | 0.7 | 1.4 | 3.4 | 9.4 | 26.6 | 65.9 | 169.9 |
| 1998 | 10.8 | 5.7 | 1.3 | 0.1 | 0.1 | 0.4 | 0.6 | 0.7 | 1.4 | 3.4 | 9.3 | 26.1 | 65.0 | 168.8 |
| 1999 | 10.8 | 5.8 | 1.3 | 0.1 | 0.1 | 0.4 | 0.6 | 0.7 | 1.3 | 3.4 | 9.0 | 25.5 | 64.6 | 172.3 |
| 2000 | 10.3 | 5.6 | 1.3 | 0.1 | 0.1 | 0.4 | 0.6 | 0.7 | 1.3 | 3.3 | 8.6 | 24.0 | 61.5 | 164.6 |
| 2001 | 10.2 | 5.5 | 1.2 | 0.1 | 0.1 | 0.4 | 0.6 | 0.7 | 1.3 | 3.3 | 8.4 | 22.9 | 60.3 | 164.4 |
| 2002 | 10.2 | 5.2 | 1.2 | 0.1 | 0.1 | 0.4 | 0.6 | 0.7 | 1.3 | 3.3 | 8.1 | 22.3 | 60.3 | 168.1 |
| 2003 | 10.3 | 5.3 | 1.3 | 0.1 | 0.1 | 0.4 | 0.5 | 0.7 | 1.3 | 3.2 | 8.0 | 21.8 | 60.6 | 173.6 |
| 2004 | 9.7 | 5.0 | 1.2 | 0.1 | 0.1 | 0.3 | 0.5 | 0.7 | 1.3 | 3.1 | 7.5 | 20.6 | 58.0 | 161.4 |
| 2005 | 9.7 | 5.1 | 1.2 | 0.1 | 0.1 | 0.3 | 0.5 | 0.6 | 1.3 | 3.1 | 7.4 | 20.0 | 56.8 | 159.1 |

*Notes:* 1 Averages for the periods.
2 Death rates per 1,000 live births.
*Sources:* Annual Abstract of Statistics (ONS).
Population Trends (ONS).

Figure 1.12   **Trends in age specific mortality rates, UK, 1948 - 2005**

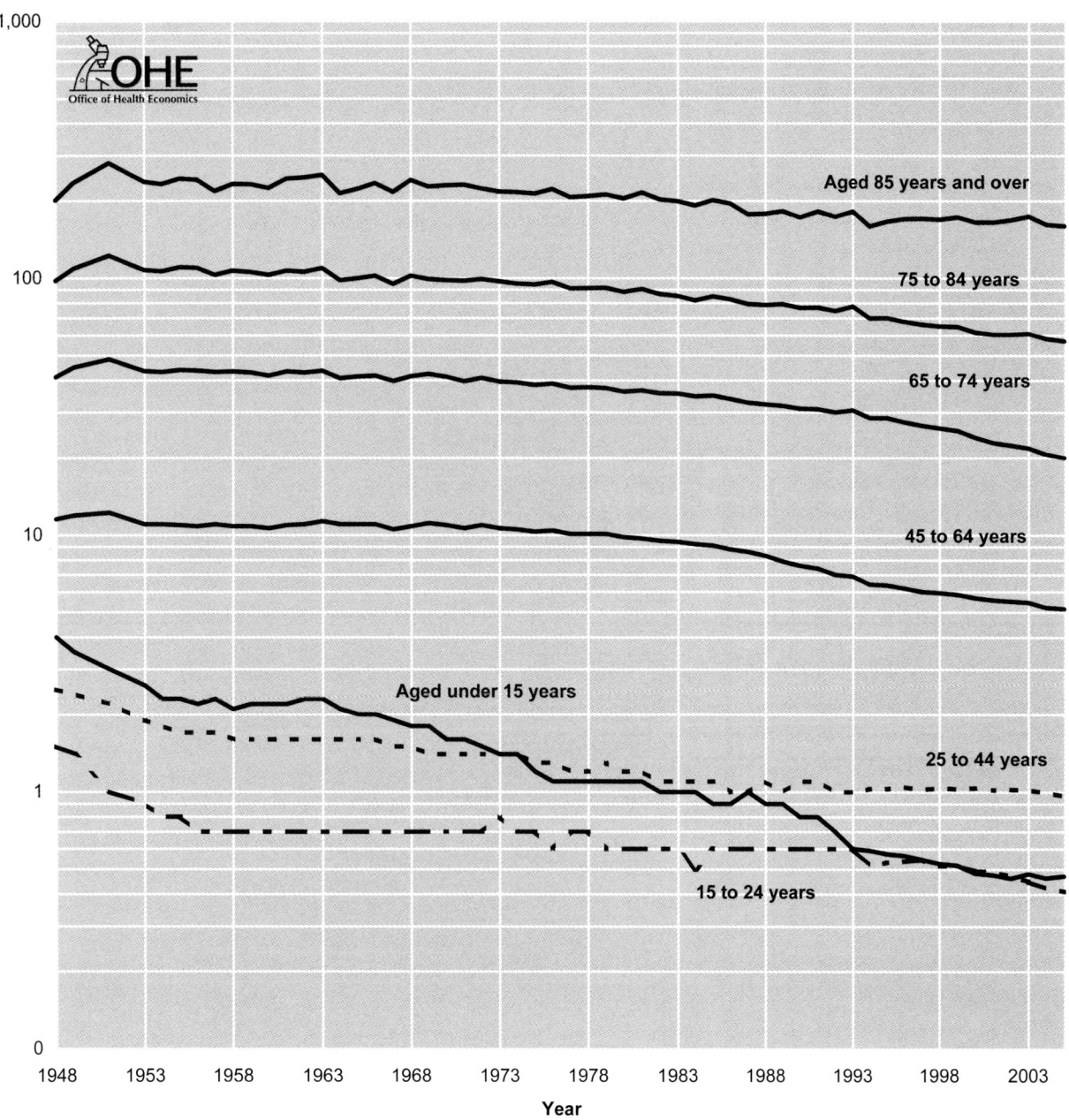

*Sources:*  Annual Abstract of Statistics (ONS).
            Population Projections Database (GAD).
            Population estimates (ONS).

Table 1.27(a) **Deaths and crude death rates by main cause, UK, 1970 - 2005**

**Number of deaths**

| ICD 10 | Causes | 1970 | 1980 | 1990 | 1995 | 2000 | 2002[1] | 2003 | 2004 | 2005 |
|---|---|---|---|---|---|---|---|---|---|---|
| | Total deaths[2] | 655,385 | 661,519 | 641,799 | 635,945 | 608,366 | 606,216 | 611,188 | 583,082 | 582,663 |
| I | Infectious and parasitic diseases | 4,250 | 2,598 | 2,777 | 4,052 | 4,316 | 5,115 | 5,580 | 5,846 | 7,022 |
| II | Neoplasms | 132,653 | 147,497 | 163,239 | 160,344 | 153,695 | 158,991 | 158,654 | 157,233 | 157,688 |
| III | Blood and blood-forming organs | 2,159 | 1,911 | 2,631 | 2,087 | 2,027 | 1,232 | 1,250 | 1,159 | 1,250 |
| IV | Endocrine diseases[3] | 7,697 | 7,392 | 11,060 | 8,707 | 8,197 | 9,037 | 9,220 | 8,739 | 8,723 |
| V | Mental disorders | 1,610 | 3,928 | 14,439 | 10,810 | 13,382 | 15,610 | 17,824 | 17,339 | 17,425 |
| VI-VIII | Nervous system and sense organs | 7,133 | 7,367 | 12,711 | 10,780 | 11,192 | 16,644 | 17,577 | 16,386 | 17,043 |
| IX | Circulatory system | 333,880 | 332,088 | 295,794 | 277,398 | 236,662 | 237,850 | 233,058 | 216,712 | 209,059 |
| X | Respiratory system | 95,484 | 92,448 | 71,030 | 101,622 | 99,950 | 78,589 | 84,674 | 77,906 | 81,531 |
| XI | Digestive system | 15,267 | 18,699 | 20,856 | 22,167 | 25,587 | 27,858 | 28,750 | 28,668 | 29,018 |
| XII | Skin and subcutaneous tissue | 393 | 531 | 923 | 1,205 | 1,376 | 1,609 | 1,807 | 1,820 | 1,935 |
| XIII | Musculo-skeletal system | 2,733 | 3,369 | 5,646 | 3,989 | 3,852 | 5,121 | 5,096 | 4,809 | 4,799 |
| XIV | Genito-urinary system | 8,758 | 8,819 | 8,385 | 8,297 | 8,406 | 9,798 | 10,503 | 10,726 | 11,645 |
| XV | Pregnancy, childbirth etc[3] | 163 | 82 | 61 | 51 | 46 | 40 | 55 | 53 | 41 |
| XVI | Conditions of the perinatal period[3] | 7,787 | 3,647 | 523 | 389 | 315 | 425 | 418 | 428 | 450 |
| XVII | Congenital abnormalities | 5,255 | 3,907 | 1,912 | 1,557 | 1,376 | 1,454 | 1,540 | 1,469 | 1,533 |
| XVIII | Ill-defined conditions[3] | 3,842 | 2,751 | 5,309 | 10,203 | 14,158 | 13,496 | 13,364 | 12,012 | 11,890 |
| XIX | Injury and poisoning | 26,321 | 24,489 | 21,282 | 19,107 | 19,516 | 19,190 | 19,554 | 19,568 | 19,384 |
| | All accidents | 20,130 | 17,115 | 14,817 | 11,986 | 12,476 | 12,121 | 12,669 | 12,573 | 12,829 |
| | Suicide and self-inflicted injury | 4,397 | 4,917 | 4,643 | 4,315 | 4,290 | 4,067 | 3,962 | 4,040 | 3,905 |

Table 1.27(b) **Crude death rates by main cause, rates per 100,000 population, UK, 1970 - 2005**

| ICD 10 | Causes | 1970 | 1980 | 1990 | 1995 | 2000 | 2002[1] | 2003 | 2004 | 2005 |
|---|---|---|---|---|---|---|---|---|---|---|
| | Total deaths[2] | 1,178 | 1,174 | 1,118 | 1,096 | 1,033 | 1,022 | 1,026 | 974 | 967 |
| I | Infectious and parasitic diseases | 8 | 5 | 5 | 7 | 7 | 9 | 9 | 10 | 12 |
| II | Neoplasms | 238 | 262 | 286 | 276 | 261 | 268 | 266 | 263 | 262 |
| III | Blood and blood-forming organs | 4 | 3 | 5 | 4 | 3 | 2 | 2 | 2 | 2 |
| IV | Endocrine diseases[3] | 14 | 13 | 19 | 15 | 14 | 15 | 15 | 15 | 14 |
| V | Mental disorders | 3 | 7 | 25 | 19 | 23 | 26 | 30 | 29 | 29 |
| VI-VIII | Nervous system and sense organs | 13 | 13 | 22 | 19 | 19 | 28 | 30 | 27 | 28 |
| IX | Circulatory system | 600 | 590 | 515 | 478 | 402 | 401 | 391 | 362 | 347 |
| X | Respiratory system | 172 | 164 | 124 | 175 | 170 | 132 | 142 | 130 | 135 |
| XI | Digestive system | 27 | 33 | 36 | 38 | 43 | 47 | 48 | 48 | 48 |
| XII | Skin and subcutaneous tissue | 1 | 1 | 2 | 2 | 2 | 3 | 3 | 3 | 3 |
| XIII | Musculo-skeletal system | 5 | 6 | 10 | 7 | 7 | 9 | 9 | 8 | 8 |
| XIV | Genito-urinary system | 16 | 16 | 15 | 14 | 14 | 17 | 18 | 18 | 19 |
| XV | Pregnancy, childbirth etc[3,4] | 0 | 0 | 0 | 0 | 0 | 0 | 0 | 0 | 0 |
| XVI | Conditions of the perinatal period[3] | 14 | 6 | 1 | 1 | 1 | 1 | 1 | 1 | 1 |
| XVII | Congenital abnormalities | 9 | 7 | 3 | 3 | 2 | 2 | 3 | 2 | 3 |
| XVIII | Ill-defined conditions[3] | 7 | 5 | 9 | 18 | 24 | 23 | 22 | 20 | 20 |
| XIX | Injury and poisoning | 47 | 43 | 37 | 33 | 33 | 32 | 33 | 33 | 32 |
| | All accidents | 36 | 30 | 26 | 21 | 21 | 20 | 21 | 21 | 21 |
| | Suicide and self-inflicted injury | 8 | 9 | 8 | 7 | 7 | 7 | 7 | 7 | 6 |

*Notes:* 1 Since 2001, and in Scotland since 2000, cause of death information is based on ICD10, the 10th version of the International Statistical
Classification of Disease and Health Problems. As a result these figures, in particular for respiratory system, are not strictly compatible with
earlier years.
2 From 1986, a new certificate for deaths within the first 28 days of life was introduced. It is not possible to assign any one underlying
cause of death from this certificate. The 'cause' figures in this table for 1986 onwards exclude all deaths at ages under 28 days.
3 Headings have been abbreviated.
4 Crude death rates of 0 correspond to a rate of less than 5 per million population.

*Source:* Annual Abstract of Statistics (ONS).

Table 1.28 **Number of deaths and age standardised mortality rates by main cause, sex and country, UK, 2005**

**Males**

| Cause | Number of deaths | | | | Age standardised mortality rates[1] | | | |
|---|---|---|---|---|---|---|---|---|
| | United Kingdom | England and Wales | Scotland | Northern Ireland | United Kingdom | England and Wales | Scotland | Northern Ireland |
| All causes | 276,803 | 243,324 | 26,522 | 6,957 | 751 | 736 | 891 | 791 |
| Infectious and parasitic diseases | 3,062 | 2,664 | 318 | 80 | 8 | 8 | 11 | 9 |
| All cancers[2] | 79,958 | 70,394 | 7,664 | 1,900 | 217 | 214 | 253 | 214 |
| Stomach cancer | 3,517 | 3,084 | 342 | 91 | 9 | 9 | 11 | 10 |
| Colorectal cancer | 8,666 | 7,583 | 860 | 223 | 23 | 23 | 28 | 25 |
| Lung cancer | 19,552 | 16,852 | 2,195 | 505 | 53 | 51 | 72 | 57 |
| Breast cancer[3] | - | - | - | - | - | - | - | - |
| Prostate cancer | 10,029 | 9,042 | 765 | 222 | 26 | 26 | 24 | 25 |
| Diabetes Mellitus | 3,104 | 2,660 | 347 | 97 | 8 | 8 | 11 | 11 |
| Circulatory system | 100,156 | 88,292 | 9,434 | 2,430 | 265 | 261 | 310 | 272 |
| Hypertensive disease | 1,769 | 1,590 | 151 | 28 | 5 | 5 | 5 | 3 |
| Coronary heart disease | 56,449 | 49,317 | 5,629 | 1,503 | 151 | 147 | 185 | 169 |
| Cerebrovascular disease | 21,966 | 19,333 | 2,134 | 499 | 57 | 56 | 69 | 55 |
| Respiratory system | 36,745 | 32,689 | 3,190 | 866 | 95 | 94 | 104 | 98 |
| Pneumonia | 13,531 | 12,164 | 1,026 | 341 | 35 | 35 | 34 | 39 |
| BEA and COPD[4] | 14,938 | 13,243 | 1,369 | 326 | 38 | 38 | 43 | 36 |
| Digestive system | 13,398 | 11,561 | 1,559 | 278 | 38 | 37 | 55 | 32 |
| Ulcer of stomach and duodenum | 1,680 | 1,546 | 106 | 28 | 5 | 5 | 4 | 3 |
| Chronic liver disease and cirrhosis | 5,282 | 4,351 | 817 | 114 | 17 | 16 | 30 | 14 |
| External causes of injury and poisoning | 11,708 | 9,851 | 1,346 | 511 | 37 | 35 | 51 | 60 |
| Motor vehicle traffic accidents | 2,370 | 2,023 | 216 | 131 | 8 | 7 | 8 | 15 |
| Suicide and self-inflicted injury | 2,985 | 2,436 | 399 | 150 | 10 | 9 | 16 | 18 |

**Females**

| Cause | Number of deaths | | | | Age standardised mortality rates[1] | | | |
|---|---|---|---|---|---|---|---|---|
| | United Kingdom | England and Wales | Scotland | Northern Ireland | United Kingdom | England and Wales | Scotland | Northern Ireland |
| All causes | 305,860 | 269,368 | 29,225 | 7,267 | 528 | 519 | 613 | 526 |
| Infectious and parasitic diseases | 3,960 | 3,477 | 401 | 82 | 7 | 7 | 9 | 6 |
| All cancers[2] | 74,164 | 64,858 | 7,471 | 1,835 | 156 | 154 | 181 | 153 |
| Stomach cancer | 2,161 | 1,843 | 248 | 70 | 4 | 4 | 6 | 5 |
| Colorectal cancer | 7,490 | 6,563 | 715 | 212 | 14 | 14 | 16 | 17 |
| Lung cancer | 14,073 | 11,940 | 1,814 | 319 | 30 | 29 | 44 | 28 |
| Breast cancer | 12,488 | 11,040 | 1,144 | 304 | 28 | 28 | 30 | 27 |
| Prostate cancer | - | - | - | - | - | - | - | - |
| Diabetes Mellitus | 3,542 | 3,017 | 398 | 127 | 6 | 6 | 9 | 9 |
| Circulatory system | 108,903 | 95,705 | 10,626 | 2,572 | 167 | 164 | 199 | 169 |
| Hypertensive disease | 2,420 | 2,156 | 219 | 45 | 4 | 4 | 4 | 3 |
| Coronary heart disease | 44,861 | 38,954 | 4,702 | 1,205 | 71 | 68 | 91 | 81 |
| Cerebrovascular disease | 35,902 | 31,439 | 3,655 | 808 | 53 | 52 | 66 | 51 |
| Respiratory system | 44,786 | 39,828 | 3,903 | 1,055 | 69 | 68 | 74 | 69 |
| Pneumonia | 21,290 | 19,279 | 1,457 | 554 | 29 | 30 | 25 | 34 |
| BEA and COPD[4] | 13,998 | 12,123 | 1,575 | 300 | 25 | 24 | 33 | 22 |
| Digestive system | 15,620 | 13,652 | 1,662 | 306 | 29 | 28 | 39 | 24 |
| Ulcer of stomach and duodenum | 1,876 | 1,720 | 124 | 32 | 3 | 3 | 3 | 2 |
| Chronic liver disease and cirrhosis | 3,107 | 2,538 | 496 | 73 | 9 | 8 | 16 | 8 |
| External causes of injury and poisoning | 7,676 | 6,560 | 866 | 250 | 16 | 15 | 22 | 23 |
| Motor vehicle traffic accidents | 795 | 674 | 77 | 44 | 2 | 2 | 3 | 5 |
| Suicide and self-inflicted injury | 933 | 741 | 156 | 36 | 3 | 2 | 6 | 4 |

Notes:   1 Per 100,000 population.
   2 All cancers relate to ICD code C00-C97. Figures differ from Tables 1.27 and 1.30 which relate to all Neoplasms ICD codes C00-D48.
   3 Although deaths from breast cancer do occur in males, they are very rare.
   4 Bronchitis, emphysema and other chronic obstructive pulmonary disease.

Sources:  Mortality Statistics Series DH2 (ONS).
   Vital Events Reference Tables (General Register Office of Scotland).
   Demographic Statistics (Northern Ireland Statistics and Research Agency).
   Population Projections Database (GAD).

Table 1.29  **Years of potential working life lost[1] due to premature deaths by selected causes, England and Wales, 1980 - 2005**

| | Year | | | | | | | |
|---|---|---|---|---|---|---|---|---|
| | 1980 | 1990 | 2000 | 2001 | 2002 | 2003 | 2004 | 2005 |
| **Males** | | | | | | | | |
| | | | | Years (Thousands) | | | | |
| **All causes** | 1,043 | 995 | 827 | 817 | 811 | 802 | 773 | 764 |
| | | | | As % of total years of potential working life lost | | | | |
| **All malignant neoplasms** | 18 | 18 | 19 | 20 | 20 | 20 | 20 | 20 |
| *-digestive organs and peritoneum* | 5 | 5 | 5 | 5 | 5 | 6 | 5 | 6 |
| *-trachea, bronchus and lungs* | 5 | 4 | 4 | 4 | 4 | 3 | 4 | 4 |
| *-genito-urinary organs* | 2 | 2 | 2 | 2 | 2 | 2 | 2 | 2 |
| *-leukaemia* | 1 | 1 | 1 | 1 | 1 | 1 | 1 | 1 |
| **Circulatory diseases** | 27 | 22 | 20 | 20 | 20 | 20 | 19 | 19 |
| *-ischaemic heart disease* | 20 | 16 | 12 | 12 | 12 | 12 | 11 | 11 |
| *-other heart and hypertension* | 2 | 2 | 3 | 3 | 3 | 3 | 3 | 4 |
| *-cerebrovascular disease* | 3 | 3 | 3 | 3 | 3 | 3 | 3 | 3 |
| **Respiratory system** | 7 | 4 | 5 | 4 | 4 | 4 | 4 | 4 |
| *-bronchitis, emphysema and asthma[2]* | 5 | 4 | 4 | 4 | 4 | 3 | 4 | 4 |
| **All accidental deaths** | 15 | 16 | 14 | 13 | 12 | 12 | 12 | 12 |
| *-motor vehicle traffic accidents* | 10 | 10 | 7 | 7 | 7 | 8 | 7 | 7 |
| **Suicide[3]** | 5 | 10 | 11 | 10 | 10 | 10 | 10 | 9 |
| **Females** | | | | | | | | |
| | | | | Years (Thousands) | | | | |
| **All causes** | 735 | 636 | 511 | 505 | 497 | 487 | 499 | 480 |
| | | | | As % of total years of potential working life lost | | | | |
| **All malignant neoplasms** | 30 | 34 | 35 | 35 | 35 | 34 | 35 | 35 |
| *-digestive organs and peritoneum* | 5 | 5 | 5 | 5 | 5 | 5 | 5 | 5 |
| *-trachea, bronchus and lungs* | 3 | 4 | 4 | 4 | 4 | 4 | 4 | 4 |
| *-female breast* | 9 | 10 | 10 | 10 | 10 | 9 | 9 | 10 |
| *-genito-urinary organs* | 6 | 6 | 6 | 6 | 6 | 5 | 6 | 5 |
| *-leukaemia* | 2 | 2 | 1 | 2 | 2 | 1 | 1 | 2 |
| **Circulatory diseases** | 16 | 14 | 13 | 13 | 14 | 13 | 12 | 12 |
| *-ischaemic heart disease* | 7 | 6 | 5 | 5 | 5 | 4 | 4 | 4 |
| *-other heart and hypertension* | 2 | 2 | 3 | 3 | 3 | 3 | 3 | 3 |
| *-cerebrovascular disease* | 5 | 4 | 4 | 4 | 4 | 4 | 4 | 4 |
| **Respiratory system** | 8 | 5 | 6 | 5 | 5 | 5 | 5 | 5 |
| *-bronchitis, emphysema and asthma[2]* | 2 | 1 | 1 | 1 | 1 | 1 | 1 | 1 |
| **All accidental deaths** | 8 | 8 | 6 | 6 | 6 | 6 | 6 | 6 |
| *-motor vehicle traffic accidents* | 4 | 4 | 3 | 3 | 3 | 3 | 3 | 3 |
| **Suicide[3]** | 4 | 5 | 5 | 5 | 5 | 5 | 5 | 5 |

*Notes:*   1 Years of potential working life lost relate to all ages ≤ 64 years.
2 Including chronic obstructive pulmonary disease.
3 Including events of undetermined intent.

*Source:*   OHE calculation based on data from Mortality Statistics Series DH2 (ONS).

Table 1.30  **Deaths by main cause in selected OECD and EU countries, circa 2004**

**Number of deaths**

| Country | Year | All causes | Neoplasms | Circulatory system | Respiratory system | Digestive system | External causes |
|---|---|---|---|---|---|---|---|
| OECD[1] | | 8,393,678 | 2,208,582 | 3,168,028 | 770,115 | 354,182 | 511,764 |
| EU27[1] | | 4,683,399 | 1,199,205 | 1,986,605 | 353,255 | 219,463 | 243,429 |
| EU15[1] | | 3,540,487 | 950,206 | 1,369,566 | 301,129 | 165,140 | 170,023 |
| Australia | 2002 | 132,982 | 38,258 | 49,957 | 11,634 | 4,479 | 7,785 |
| Austria | 2004 | 74,292 | 19,755 | 32,486 | 4,490 | 3,336 | 4,166 |
| Bulgaria | 2004 | 110,110 | 16,266 | 74,064 | 3,192 | 2,905 | 3,880 |
| Canada | 2002 | 223,600 | 66,590 | 74,626 | 17,761 | 8,454 | 13,834 |
| Czech Republic | 2004 | 107,177 | 29,304 | 55,042 | 4,755 | 4,537 | 6,991 |
| Denmark | 2001 | 57,632 | 15,971 | 20,873 | 5,339 | 2,800 | 3,078 |
| Estonia | 2003 | 18,110 | 3,375 | 9,945 | 615 | 642 | 1,816 |
| Finland | 2004 | 47,757 | 10,768 | 19,758 | 2,971 | 2,331 | 4,353 |
| France | 2002 | 535,140 | 152,738 | 158,095 | 33,607 | 24,087 | 40,888 |
| Germany | 2004 | 818,271 | 214,863 | 368,472 | 52,500 | 42,213 | 33,309 |
| Greece | 2003 | 105,529 | 24,799 | 52,763 | 7,430 | 2,470 | 4,041 |
| Hungary | 2003 | 135,812 | 34,062 | 69,049 | 5,439 | 9,445 | 9,427 |
| Iceland | 2003 | 1,826 | 502 | 731 | 146 | 64 | 102 |
| Ireland | 2002 | 29,683 | 7,621 | 11,652 | 4,344 | 1,025 | 1,603 |
| Italy | 2002 | 560,390 | 163,070 | 237,198 | 35,941 | 24,719 | 26,693 |
| Japan | 2003 | 1,014,249 | 319,157 | 312,304 | 147,832 | 39,242 | 75,225 |
| Korea, Republic of | 2002 | 246,493 | 63,485 | 61,517 | 16,621 | 14,130 | 28,833 |
| Latvia | 2004 | 32,039 | 5,812 | 17,896 | 801 | 1,038 | 3,179 |
| Lithuania | 2004 | 41,338 | 8,074 | 22,531 | 1,630 | 1,632 | 5,076 |
| Luxembourg | 2004 | 3,530 | 931 | 1,373 | 287 | 182 | 230 |
| Malta | 2004 | 2,999 | 724 | 1,255 | 323 | 129 | 125 |
| Mexico | 2001 | 438,550 | 58,578 | 98,827 | 37,116 | 42,437 | 50,497 |
| Netherlands | 2004 | 136,553 | 40,300 | 44,638 | 12,755 | 5,604 | 5,226 |
| New Zealand | 2000 | 26,718 | 7,771 | 10,920 | 2,053 | 721 | 1,614 |
| Norway | 2003 | 42,550 | 10,723 | 16,623 | 3,941 | 1,304 | 2,462 |
| Poland | 2003 | 365,230 | 90,641 | 172,292 | 17,330 | 14,923 | 24,811 |
| Portugal | 2003 | 109,148 | 23,257 | 41,035 | 9,553 | 4,612 | 5,630 |
| Romania | 2004 | 258,890 | 43,985 | 159,253 | 13,678 | 15,119 | 13,462 |
| Slovak Republic | 2002 | 51,756 | 11,609 | 28,375 | 2,793 | 2,686 | 3,042 |
| Slovenia | 2003 | 19,451 | 5,147 | 7,337 | 1,570 | 1,267 | 1,597 |
| Spain | 2003 | 384,828 | 99,826 | 129,783 | 43,803 | 19,576 | 16,697 |
| Sweden | 2002 | 95,071 | 22,185 | 42,381 | 6,578 | 3,167 | 4,725 |
| Switzerland | 2002 | 61,768 | 15,711 | 23,738 | 4,062 | 2,354 | 3,653 |
| United Kingdom | 2005 | 582,663 | 157,688 | 209,059 | 81,531 | 29,018 | 19,384 |
| England and Wales | 2005 | 512,692 | 138,454 | 183,997 | 72,517 | 25,213 | 16,411 |
| Scotland | 2005 | 55,747 | 15,408 | 20,060 | 7,093 | 3,221 | 2,212 |
| Northern Ireland | 2005 | 14,224 | 3,826 | 5,002 | 1,921 | 584 | 761 |
| USA | 2002 | 2,443,030 | 570,563 | 923,288 | 234,619 | 86,703 | 163,962 |

*Notes:*  1 Including all constituent countries for which recent data are available.
EU15 as constituted before 1 May 2004 and EU27 as constituted since 1 January 2007.
Recent data were not available for Belgium, Cyprus, Mexico and Turkey.
OHE calculation based on WHO Mortality Database (WHO).

*Sources:*  Mortality Statistics Series DH2 (ONS).
Vital Events Reference Tables (General Register Office of Scotland).
Demographic Statistics (Northern Ireland Statistics and Research Agency).

Table 1.31  **Age standardised mortality rates for all persons by main cause in selected OECD and EU countries, circa 2004**

All persons age standardised mortality rates per 100,000 population

| Country | Year | All causes | Neoplasms | Circulatory system | Respiratory system | Digestive system | External causes |
|---|---|---|---|---|---|---|---|
| **OECD[1]** | | **636** | **178** | **225** | **54** | **28** | **47** |
| **EU27[1]** | | **685** | **186** | **271** | **48** | **34** | **43** |
| **EU15[1]** | | **617** | **179** | **220** | **48** | **31** | **37** |
| Australia | 2002 | 551 | 169 | 195 | 46 | 19 | 37 |
| Austria | 2004 | 620 | 175 | 248 | 35 | 31 | 42 |
| Bulgaria | 2004 | 1056 | 157 | 685 | 33 | 29 | 45 |
| Canada | 2002 | 588 | 185 | 186 | 44 | 23 | 40 |
| Czech Republic | 2004 | 852 | 231 | 431 | 37 | 37 | 61 |
| Denmark | 2001 | 749 | 225 | 250 | 66 | 38 | 46 |
| Estonia | 2003 | 1064 | 196 | 551 | 37 | 40 | 128 |
| Finland | 2004 | 637 | 147 | 248 | 37 | 34 | 72 |
| France | 2002 | 606 | 191 | 161 | 33 | 29 | 54 |
| Germany | 2004 | 628 | 174 | 263 | 38 | 35 | 32 |
| Greece | 2003 | 674 | 161 | 326 | 46 | 16 | 33 |
| Hungary | 2003 | 1048 | 268 | 508 | 41 | 80 | 80 |
| Iceland | 2003 | 547 | 163 | 208 | 42 | 19 | 35 |
| Ireland | 2002 | 721 | 194 | 278 | 101 | 25 | 39 |
| Italy | 2002 | 571 | 182 | 220 | 33 | 26 | 34 |
| Japan | 2003 | 475 | 156 | 137 | 60 | 19 | 46 |
| Korea, Republic of | 2002 | 745 | 180 | 192 | 56 | 38 | 71 |
| Latvia | 2004 | 1091 | 195 | 578 | 28 | 37 | 129 |
| Lithuania | 2004 | 1017 | 198 | 529 | 39 | 42 | 143 |
| Luxembourg | 2004 | 615 | 168 | 230 | 48 | 32 | 44 |
| Malta | 2004 | 628 | 155 | 255 | 67 | 27 | 28 |
| Netherlands | 2004 | 630 | 198 | 197 | 55 | 25 | 27 |
| New Zealand | 2000 | 627 | 193 | 245 | 47 | 16 | 41 |
| Norway | 2003 | 608 | 173 | 215 | 51 | 19 | 44 |
| Poland | 2003 | 895 | 220 | 417 | 41 | 36 | 62 |
| Portugal | 2003 | 727 | 164 | 256 | 60 | 33 | 46 |
| Romania | 2004 | 1076 | 178 | 649 | 60 | 63 | 60 |
| Slovak Republic | 2002 | 981 | 217 | 539 | 53 | 51 | 56 |
| Slovenia | 2003 | 795 | 207 | 295 | 62 | 53 | 70 |
| Spain | 2003 | 600 | 172 | 187 | 62 | 32 | 34 |
| Sweden | 2002 | 599 | 160 | 243 | 38 | 20 | 40 |
| Switzerland | 2002 | 546 | 155 | 189 | 32 | 22 | 40 |
| United Kingdom | 2005 | 627 | 181 | 211 | 79 | 34 | 26 |
| *England and Wales* | *2005* | *616* | *178* | *208* | *79* | *33* | *25* |
| *Scotland* | *2005* | *739* | *210* | *250* | *86* | *47* | *36* |
| *Northern Ireland* | *2005* | *641* | *178* | *214* | *80* | *28* | *41* |
| USA | 2002 | 703 | 178 | 250 | 64 | 26 | 54 |

*Notes:*  1 Including all constituent countries for which recent data are available.
EU15 as constituted before 1 May 2004 and EU27 as constituted since 1 January 2007.
Recent data were not available for Belgium, Cyprus, Mexico and Turkey.

*Sources:*  OHE calculation based on WHO Mortality Database (WHO).
Mortality Statistics Series DH2 (ONS).
Vital Events Reference Tables (General Register Office of Scotland).
Demographic Statistics (Northern Ireland Statistics and Research Agency).
Population Projections Database (GAD).

Table 1.32  **Age standardised mortality rates for males by main cause in selected OECD and EU countries, circa 2004**

**Male age standardised mortality rates per 100,000 population**

| Country | Year | All causes | Neoplasms | Circulatory system | Respiratory system | Digestive system | External causes |
|---|---|---|---|---|---|---|---|
| OECD[1] | | 812 | 235 | 278 | 75 | 37 | 69 |
| EU27[1] | | 880 | 249 | 335 | 69 | 45 | 65 |
| EU15[1] | | 787 | 238 | 272 | 68 | 39 | 53 |
| | | | | | | | |
| Australia | 2002 | 684 | 213 | 237 | 61 | 22 | 53 |
| Austria | 2004 | 792 | 228 | 298 | 52 | 41 | 66 |
| Bulgaria | 2004 | 1345 | 210 | 841 | 48 | 45 | 73 |
| Canada | 2002 | 728 | 226 | 236 | 59 | 27 | 57 |
| Czech Republic | 2004 | 1107 | 315 | 531 | 55 | 50 | 89 |
| Denmark | 2001 | 910 | 261 | 321 | 80 | 45 | 63 |
| Estonia | 2003 | 1544 | 298 | 752 | 69 | 56 | 224 |
| Finland | 2004 | 850 | 193 | 335 | 60 | 46 | 108 |
| France | 2002 | 812 | 273 | 210 | 50 | 39 | 78 |
| Germany | 2004 | 790 | 224 | 315 | 56 | 44 | 47 |
| Greece | 2003 | 796 | 218 | 355 | 54 | 21 | 52 |
| Hungary | 2003 | 1410 | 375 | 648 | 65 | 117 | 121 |
| Iceland | 2003 | 632 | 169 | 264 | 49 | 20 | 46 |
| Ireland | 2002 | 907 | 241 | 354 | 130 | 28 | 58 |
| Italy | 2002 | 745 | 248 | 274 | 52 | 34 | 50 |
| Japan | 2003 | 657 | 221 | 178 | 95 | 27 | 68 |
| Korea, Republic of | 2002 | 1007 | 283 | 235 | 90 | 62 | 103 |
| Latvia | 2004 | 1559 | 298 | 792 | 54 | 52 | 214 |
| Lithuania | 2004 | 1463 | 295 | 693 | 78 | 59 | 248 |
| Luxembourg | 2004 | 825 | 238 | 291 | 79 | 45 | 64 |
| Malta | 2004 | 753 | 194 | 294 | 98 | 30 | 33 |
| Netherlands | 2004 | 787 | 252 | 253 | 80 | 29 | 37 |
| New Zealand | 2000 | 782 | 237 | 305 | 62 | 18 | 61 |
| Norway | 2003 | 761 | 214 | 273 | 66 | 21 | 63 |
| Poland | 2003 | 1217 | 309 | 536 | 67 | 50 | 102 |
| Portugal | 2003 | 932 | 228 | 299 | 87 | 47 | 73 |
| Romania | 2004 | 1357 | 239 | 762 | 87 | 88 | 97 |
| Slovak Republic | 2002 | 1302 | 311 | 660 | 80 | 77 | 95 |
| Slovenia | 2003 | 1094 | 294 | 376 | 102 | 77 | 109 |
| Spain | 2003 | 792 | 251 | 227 | 96 | 43 | 52 |
| Sweden | 2002 | 734 | 188 | 308 | 49 | 25 | 59 |
| Switzerland | 2002 | 692 | 202 | 235 | 47 | 28 | 56 |
| United Kingdom | 2005 | 750 | 217 | 265 | 95 | 38 | 37 |
| *England and Wales* | *2005* | *734* | *213* | *260* | *94* | *37* | *35* |
| *Scotland* | *2005* | *909* | *256* | *317* | *107* | *55* | *51* |
| *Northern Ireland* | *2005* | *790* | *214* | *272* | *98* | *32* | *60* |
| USA | 2002 | 855 | 216 | 306 | 78 | 32 | 79 |

*Notes:*  1 Including all constituent countries for which recent data are available.
EU15 as constituted before 1 May 2004 and EU27 as constituted since 1 January 2007.
Recent data were not available for Belgium, Cyprus, Mexico and Turkey.

*Sources:*  OHE calculation based on WHO Mortality Database (WHO).
Mortality Statistics Series DH2 (ONS).
Vital Events Reference Tables (General Register Office of Scotland).
Demographic Statistics (Northern Ireland Statistics and Research Agency).
Population Projections Database (GAD).

Table 1.33   **Age standardised mortality rates for females by main cause in selected OECD and EU countries, circa 2004**

**Female age standardised mortality rates per 100,000 population**

| Country | Year | All causes | Neoplasms | Circulatory system | Respiratory system | Digestive system | External causes |
|---|---|---|---|---|---|---|---|
| **OECD[1]** | | **499** | **138** | **182** | **41** | **21** | **26** |
| **EU27[1]** | | **532** | **141** | **221** | **35** | **25** | **23** |
| **EU15[1]** | | **484** | **137** | **179** | **35** | **23** | **21** |
| | | | | | | | |
| Australia | 2002 | 443 | 137 | 158 | 36 | 15 | 21 |
| Austria | 2004 | 491 | 139 | 210 | 25 | 21 | 22 |
| Bulgaria | 2004 | 820 | 116 | 560 | 21 | 15 | 20 |
| Canada | 2002 | 478 | 157 | 146 | 34 | 18 | 24 |
| Czech Republic | 2004 | 662 | 173 | 357 | 26 | 26 | 34 |
| Denmark | 2001 | 627 | 203 | 195 | 59 | 32 | 29 |
| Estonia | 2003 | 748 | 139 | 427 | 18 | 29 | 49 |
| Finland | 2004 | 476 | 120 | 182 | 24 | 22 | 38 |
| France | 2002 | 445 | 130 | 123 | 23 | 21 | 34 |
| Germany | 2004 | 501 | 139 | 219 | 27 | 26 | 18 |
| Greece | 2003 | 563 | 113 | 297 | 39 | 12 | 14 |
| Hungary | 2003 | 784 | 195 | 410 | 27 | 50 | 44 |
| Iceland | 2003 | 476 | 161 | 161 | 37 | 17 | 23 |
| Ireland | 2002 | 575 | 161 | 213 | 83 | 22 | 21 |
| Italy | 2002 | 442 | 134 | 179 | 21 | 20 | 19 |
| Japan | 2003 | 339 | 108 | 105 | 40 | 12 | 25 |
| Korea, Republic of | 2002 | 561 | 111 | 162 | 38 | 19 | 43 |
| Latvia | 2004 | 785 | 139 | 444 | 12 | 26 | 58 |
| Lithuania | 2004 | 705 | 141 | 417 | 17 | 29 | 54 |
| Luxembourg | 2004 | 467 | 117 | 189 | 32 | 22 | 27 |
| Malta | 2004 | 531 | 128 | 222 | 47 | 24 | 22 |
| Netherlands | 2004 | 517 | 162 | 156 | 41 | 22 | 19 |
| New Zealand | 2000 | 507 | 162 | 197 | 37 | 15 | 22 |
| Norway | 2003 | 491 | 147 | 169 | 42 | 17 | 26 |
| Poland | 2003 | 659 | 162 | 331 | 27 | 25 | 27 |
| Portugal | 2003 | 564 | 117 | 221 | 41 | 22 | 22 |
| Romania | 2004 | 846 | 131 | 558 | 40 | 42 | 26 |
| Slovak Republic | 2002 | 744 | 153 | 450 | 36 | 31 | 21 |
| Slovenia | 2003 | 587 | 154 | 236 | 42 | 34 | 35 |
| Spain | 2003 | 446 | 112 | 153 | 39 | 22 | 16 |
| Sweden | 2002 | 493 | 142 | 192 | 31 | 16 | 23 |
| Switzerland | 2002 | 435 | 124 | 152 | 23 | 16 | 25 |
| United Kingdom | 2005 | 528 | 156 | 167 | 69 | 29 | 16 |
| *England and Wales* | *2005* | *519* | *154* | *164* | *68* | *28* | *15* |
| *Scotland* | *2005* | *613* | *181* | *199* | *74* | *39* | *22* |
| *Northern Ireland* | *2005* | *525* | *153* | *169* | *69* | *24* | *23* |
| USA | 2002 | 581 | 151 | 205 | 55 | 21 | 30 |

*Notes:*   1 Including all constituent countries for which recent data are available.
EU15 as constituted before 1 May 2004 and EU27 as constituted since 1 January 2007.
Recent data were not available for Belgium, Cyprus, Mexico and Turkey.

*Sources:*   OHE calculation based on WHO Mortality Database (WHO).
Mortality Statistics Series DH2 (ONS).
Vital Events Reference Tables (General Register Office of Scotland).
Demographic Statistics (Northern Ireland Statistics and Research Agency).
Population Projections Database (GAD).

Table 1.34  **Crude death rates per 100,000 population for leading causes of death, UK, 1970 - 2005**

| | Year | | | | | | | | | |
|---|---|---|---|---|---|---|---|---|---|---|
| | 1970 | 1980 | 1990 | 1995 | 2000 | 2001 | 2002 | 2003 | 2004 | 2005 |
| **All deaths** | **1,178.0** | **1,174.0** | **1,118.0** | **1,112.4** | **1,033.1** | **1,018.8** | **1,021.9** | **1,026.2** | **974.3** | **967.3** |
| From natural causes | 1,131.0 | 1,131.0 | 1,075.0 | 1,074.2 | 996.0 | 982.2 | 985.9 | 989.6 | 937.9 | 931.4 |
| Coronary heart disease | 290.0 | 314.0 | 295.0 | 260.9 | 207.6 | 204.8 | 198.3 | 191.5 | 177.3 | 168.2 |
| Cerebrovascular disease | 165.0 | 147.0 | 133.0 | 118.4 | 101.7 | 112.9 | 113.7 | 110.5 | 101.1 | 96.1 |
| Pneumonia[1] | 84.0 | 104.0 | 57.0 | 104.3 | 101.5 | 59.3 | 60.9 | 64.3 | 56.7 | 57.8 |
| Malignant neoplasm of trachea[2] | 62.0 | 71.0 | 68.0 | 62.5 | 56.5 | 56.6 | 56.8 | 56.2 | 55.3 | 55.8 |
| Bronchitis, emphysema and COPD[4] | - | - | - | - | - | 45.9 | 47.0 | 49.4 | 44.4 | 46.0 |
| Diseases of pulmonary circulation[3] | 57.0 | 69.0 | 40.0 | 51.0 | 46.0 | 46.0 | 46.6 | 47.7 | 44.6 | 44.7 |
| Malignant neoplasm of breast[6] | - | - | - | 47.5 | 42.4 | 43.3 | 42.7 | 41.8 | 40.7 | 40.9 |
| Chronic liver disease and cirrhosis | 3.0 | 5.0 | 6.0 | 7.3 | 9.8 | 10.9 | 11.3 | 12.0 | 11.8 | 11.9 |
| Diabetes mellitus | 10.0 | 10.0 | 15.0 | 11.5 | 10.8 | 11.8 | 11.9 | 12.1 | 11.3 | 11.0 |
| Malignant neoplasm of stomach | 26.0 | 22.0 | 17.0 | 13.7 | 11.1 | 10.9 | 10.8 | 10.1 | 9.8 | 9.4 |
| Leukaemia | 6.0 | 7.0 | 7.0 | 6.7 | 6.7 | 7.1 | 7.3 | 7.3 | 7.1 | 7.2 |
| Hypertensive disease | 20.0 | 11.0 | 6.0 | 5.6 | 5.5 | 6.0 | 4.3 | 6.9 | 6.5 | 7.0 |
| Suicide and self-inflicted injury | 8.0 | 9.0 | 8.0 | 7.4 | 7.2 | 6.8 | 6.9 | 6.7 | 6.8 | 6.5 |
| Benign and unspecified neoplasms | 3.0 | 2.0 | 3.0 | 3.3 | 3.0 | 6.0 | 6.3 | 6.4 | 6.0 | 5.9 |
| Ulcer of stomach and duodenum | 8.0 | 9.0 | 8.0 | 7.6 | 7.4 | 7.2 | 6.9 | 6.8 | 6.5 | 5.9 |
| Malignant neoplasm of uterus[6] | 8.0 | 7.0 | 6.0 | 4.9 | 4.9 | 5.0 | 5.0 | 5.2 | 5.4 | 5.3 |
| Motor vehicle accidents | 14.0 | 12.0 | 10.0 | 6.3 | 5.6 | 5.9 | 5.7 | 5.7 | 5.3 | 5.3 |
| Malignant neoplasm of cervix[6] | - | - | - | 5.0 | 4.1 | 3.9 | 3.7 | 3.6 | 3.6 | 3.4 |
| Asthma | 3.0 | 3.0 | 4.0 | 2.8 | 2.4 | 2.4 | 2.4 | 2.4 | 2.3 | 2.2 |
| Chronic rheumatic heart disease | 15.0 | 6.0 | 4.0 | 3.3 | 2.7 | 3.0 | 2.2 | 2.2 | 2.2 | 2.2 |
| Hernia of abdominal cavity[4] | 5.0 | 4.0 | 4.0 | 3.7 | 3.6 | 4.0 | 4.0 | 1.4 | 1.4 | 1.5 |
| Anaemias | 3.0 | 2.0 | 2.0 | 1.3 | 0.9 | 0.0 | 0.0 | 1.1 | 0.9 | 1.0 |
| Tuberculosis[5] | 2.0 | 1.0 | 1.0 | 0.7 | 0.5 | 0.9 | 0.9 | 0.9 | 0.8 | 0.8 |
| Hyperplasia of prostrate | 3.0 | 1.0 | 1.0 | 0.5 | 0.3 | 0.0 | 0.0 | 0.3 | 0.6 | 0.6 |
| Meningitis | 1.0 | 1.0 | 0.0 | 0.4 | 0.4 | 0.4 | 0.3 | 0.4 | 0.3 | 0.3 |
| Appendicitis | 1.0 | 0.0 | 0.0 | 0.2 | 0.2 | 0.0 | 0.0 | 0.3 | 0.3 | 0.2 |
| Other tuberculosis[5] | 1.0 | 1.0 | 1.0 | 0.3 | 0.0 | 0.0 | 0.0 | 0.2 | 0.2 | 0.2 |
| Meningococcal infection | 0.0 | 0.0 | 0.0 | 0.4 | 0.4 | 0.4 | 0.2 | 0.2 | 0.1 | 0.2 |
| Nutritional deficiencies | 0.0 | 0.0 | 0.0 | 0.2 | 0.1 | 0.0 | 0.0 | 0.2 | 0.2 | 0.1 |
| Influenza | 15.0 | 1.0 | 2.0 | 0.5 | 1.1 | 0.1 | 0.1 | 0.2 | 0.0 | 0.1 |
| Whooping cough | - | - | - | 0.0 | 0.0 | 0.0 | 0.0 | 0.0 | 0.0 | 0.0 |
| Abortion | 0.0 | 0.0 | 0.0 | 0.0 | 0.0 | 0.0 | 0.0 | 0.0 | 0.0 | 0.0 |
| Syphilis | 0.0 | 0.0 | 0.0 | 0.0 | 0.0 | 0.0 | 0.0 | 0.0 | 0.0 | 0.0 |
| Measles | 0.0 | 0.0 | 0.0 | 0.0 | 0.0 | 0.0 | 0.0 | 0.0 | 0.0 | 0.0 |
| Malaria | 0.0 | 0.0 | 0.0 | 0.0 | 0.0 | 0.0 | 0.0 | 0.0 | 0.0 | 0.0 |
| Nephritis, nephrotic syndrome[3] | 5.0 | 9.0 | 8.0 | 6.9 | 5.2 | 5.0 | 5.0 | 0.0 | 0.0 | 0.0 |
| Birth trauma, hypoxia, birth asphyxia[6] | 7.0 | 4.0 | 0.0 | 0.4 | 0.0 | 0.0 | 0.0 | 0.0 | 0.0 | 0.0 |

*Notes:* - Not available.

0.0: <5 deaths per million population.

Prior to 1995, data is accurate to 0 decimal places.

1 From 2001, and in Scotland from 2000, cause of death information is based on ICD10, the 10th version of the International Statistical Classification of Disease and Health Problems. As a result these figures are not strictly compatible with earlier years.

2 Including bronchus and lung.

3 Including other forms of heart disease.

4 COPD - chronic obstructive pulmonary disease.

5 Respiratory and other tuberculosis including late effects.

6 Per female population.

*Sources:* Annual Abstract of Statistics (ONS).

Mortality Statistics Series DH2 (ONS).

Vital Events Reference Tables (General Register Office of Scotland).

Demographic Statistics (Northern Ireland Research and Statistics Agency).

Population Projections Database (GAD).

Table 1.35 **Age standardised mortality rates from coronary heart disease, cerebrovascular disease, lung cancer and breast cancer, men and women aged 15 - 74, in selected OECD and EU countries, circa 2004**

**Age standardised mortality rate per 100,000 population**

| Country | Year | Coronary heart disease | | Cerebrovascular disease | | Lung cancer | | Breast cancer |
|---|---|---|---|---|---|---|---|---|
| | | Males | Females | Males | Females | Males | Females | Females |
| OECD[1] | | 89 | 31 | 36 | 23 | 57 | 22 | 23 |
| EU27 | | - | - | - | - | - | - | - |
| EU15[1] | | 76 | 22 | 26 | 16 | 57 | 17 | 26 |
| Australia | 2002 | 79 | 26 | 19 | 12 | 41 | 21 | 25 |
| Austria | 2004 | 80 | 26 | 21 | 12 | 51 | 18 | 24 |
| Bulgaria | 2004 | 171 | 62 | 141 | 81 | 68 | 10 | 23 |
| Canada | 2002 | 88 | 29 | 17 | 12 | 59 | 38 | 26 |
| Czech Republic | 2004 | 143 | 49 | 58 | 31 | 85 | 19 | 26 |
| Denmark | 2001 | 88 | 31 | 33 | 23 | 59 | 44 | 37 |
| Estonia | 2003 | 311 | 89 | 125 | 59 | 93 | 10 | 27 |
| Finland | 2004 | 132 | 29 | 34 | 20 | 39 | 11 | 22 |
| France | 2002 | 45 | 10 | 22 | 11 | 67 | 13 | 27 |
| Germany | 2004 | 89 | 27 | 24 | 15 | 54 | 18 | 27 |
| Greece | 2003 | 104 | 28 | 42 | 27 | 69 | 10 | 20 |
| Hungary | 2003 | 222 | 81 | 112 | 55 | 126 | 36 | 32 |
| Iceland | 2003 | 82 | 25 | 17 | 13 | 32 | 40 | 23 |
| Ireland | 2002 | 136 | 41 | 25 | 17 | 50 | 25 | 30 |
| Italy | 2002 | 62 | 17 | 25 | 15 | 64 | 13 | 26 |
| Japan | 2003 | 33 | 10 | 41 | 19 | 34 | 9 | 14 |
| Korea, Republic of | 2002 | 36 | 15 | 92 | 54 | 59 | 13 | 7 |
| Latvia | 2004 | 332 | 97 | 147 | 82 | 85 | 9 | 29 |
| Lithuania | 2004 | 306 | 89 | 88 | 47 | 82 | 8 | 28 |
| Luxembourg | 2004 | 74 | 30 | 25 | 20 | 56 | 15 | 18 |
| Malta | 2004 | 107 | 37 | 36 | 24 | 48 | 6 | 22 |
| Netherlands | 2004 | 60 | 21 | 23 | 16 | 64 | 31 | 31 |
| New Zealand | 2000 | 118 | 43 | 25 | 21 | 44 | 25 | 32 |
| Norway | 2003 | 78 | 23 | 22 | 15 | 44 | 26 | 23 |
| Poland | 2003 | 142 | 42 | 74 | 41 | 102 | 22 | 23 |
| Portugal | 2003 | 61 | 21 | 60 | 34 | 45 | 8 | 22 |
| Romania | 2004 | 198 | 83 | 156 | 102 | 78 | 12 | 25 |
| Slovak Republic | 2002 | 221 | 87 | 66 | 31 | 81 | 11 | 26 |
| Slovenia | 2003 | 92 | 23 | 51 | 24 | 75 | 19 | 28 |
| Spain | 2003 | 63 | 16 | 26 | 14 | 67 | 8 | 21 |
| Sweden | 2002 | 94 | 31 | 27 | 18 | 29 | 22 | 22 |
| Switzerland | 2002 | 61 | 16 | 15 | 9 | 44 | 17 | 26 |
| United Kingdom | 2005 | 102 | 33 | 24 | 19 | 45 | 28 | 28 |
| *England and Wales* | *2005* | *98* | *31* | *24* | *18* | *43* | *27* | *28* |
| *Scotland* | *2005* | *133* | *47* | *30* | *24* | *62* | *41* | *30* |
| *Northern Ireland* | *2005* | *109* | *37* | *24* | *16* | *48* | *26* | *26* |
| United States of America | 2002 | 124 | 51 | 23 | 19 | 63 | 38 | 25 |

*Notes:* 1 Including all constituent countries for which recent data are available.
EU15 as constituted before 1 May 2004 and EU27 as constituted since 1 January 2007.
Recent data were not available for Belgium, Cyprus, Mexico and Turkey.

*Sources:* OHE calculation based on WHO Mortality Database (WHO).
Mortality Statistics Series DH2 (ONS).
Vital Events Reference Tables (General Register Office of Scotland).
Demographic Statistics (Northern Ireland Statistics and Research Agency).

Figure 1.13 **Age standardised mortality rates from coronary heart disease, men and women aged 15 - 74, in selected OECD and EU countries, circa 2004**

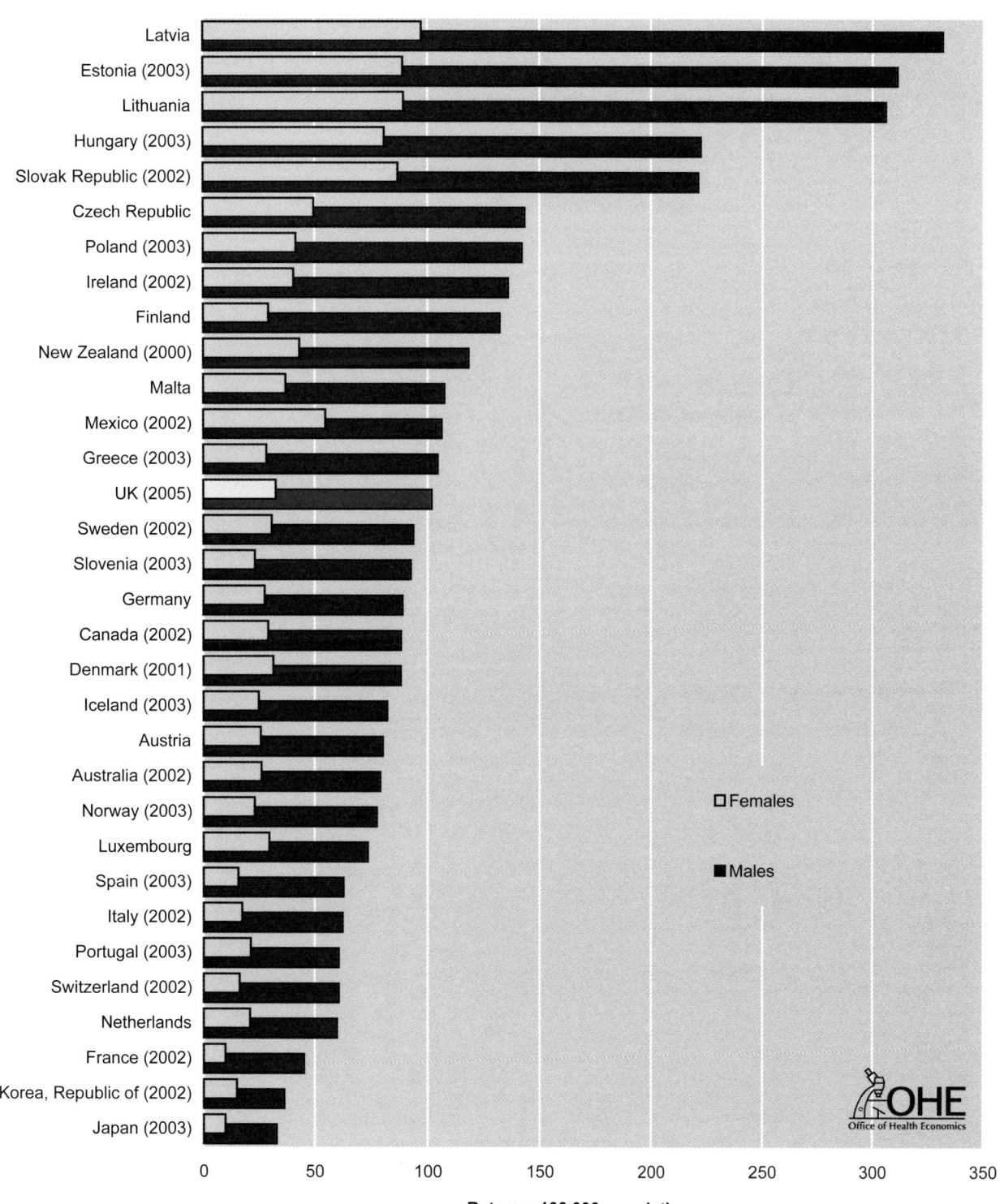

**Rate per 100,000 population**

*Note:* Year is 2004 unless stated otherwise.
*Sources:* OHE calculations based on WHO Mortality Database (WHO).
Mortality Statistics Series DH2 (ONS).
Vital Events Reference Tables (General Register Office of Scotland).
Demographic Statistics (Northern Ireland Statistics and Research Agency).

Figure 1.14 **Age standardised mortality rates from cerebrovascular disease, men and women aged 15 - 74, in selected OECD and EU countries, circa 2004**

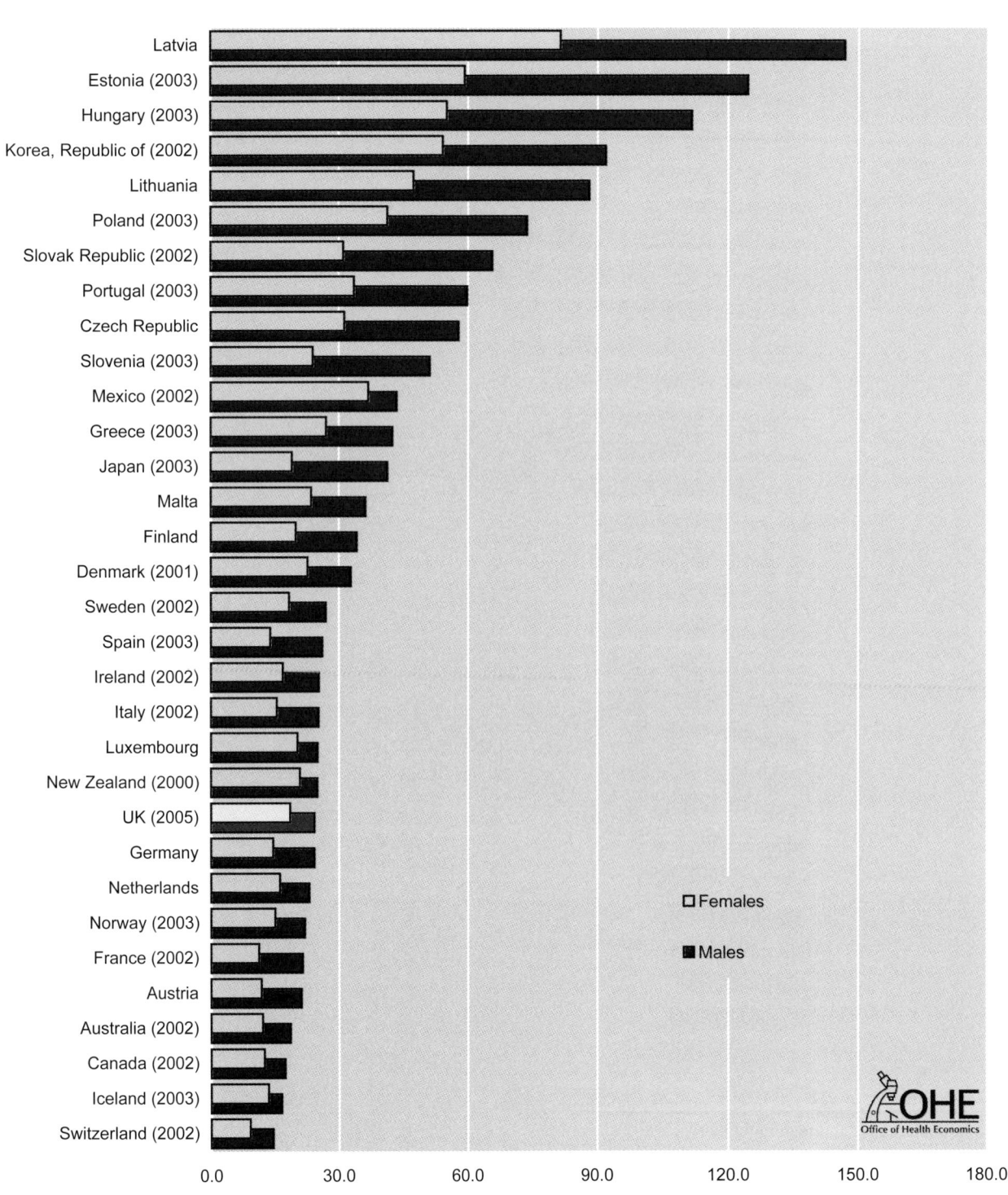

**Rate per 100,000 population**

*Note:*    Year is 2004 unless stated otherwise.
*Sources:* OHE calculations based on WHO Mortality Database (WHO).
           Mortality Statistics Series DH2 (ONS).
           Vital Events Reference Tables (General Register Office of Scotland).
           Demographic Statistics (Northern Ireland Statistics and Research Agency).

Figure 1.15 **Age standardised mortality rates from lung cancer, men and women aged 15 - 74, in selected OECD and EU countries, circa 2004**

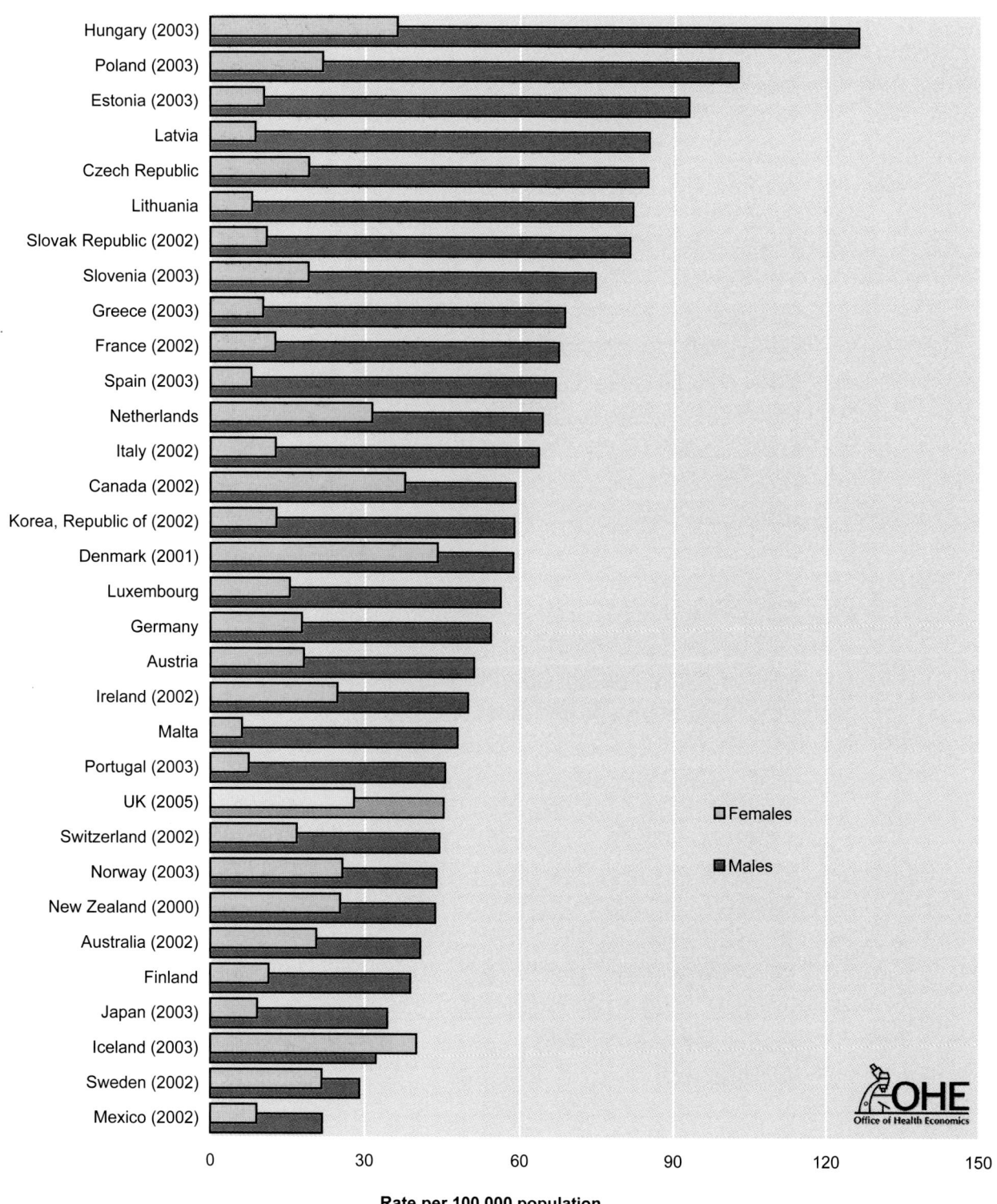

**Rate per 100,000 population**

*Note:*     Year is 2004 unless stated otherwise.
*Sources:* OHE calculations based on WHO Mortality Database (WHO).
          Mortality Statistics Series DH2 (ONS).
          Vital Events Reference Tables (General Register Office of Scotland).
          Demographic Statistics (Northern Ireland Statistics and Research Agency).

# Mortality Statistics

Figure 1.16 **Age standardised mortality rates from breast cancer, women aged 15 - 74, in selected OECD and EU countries, circa 2004**

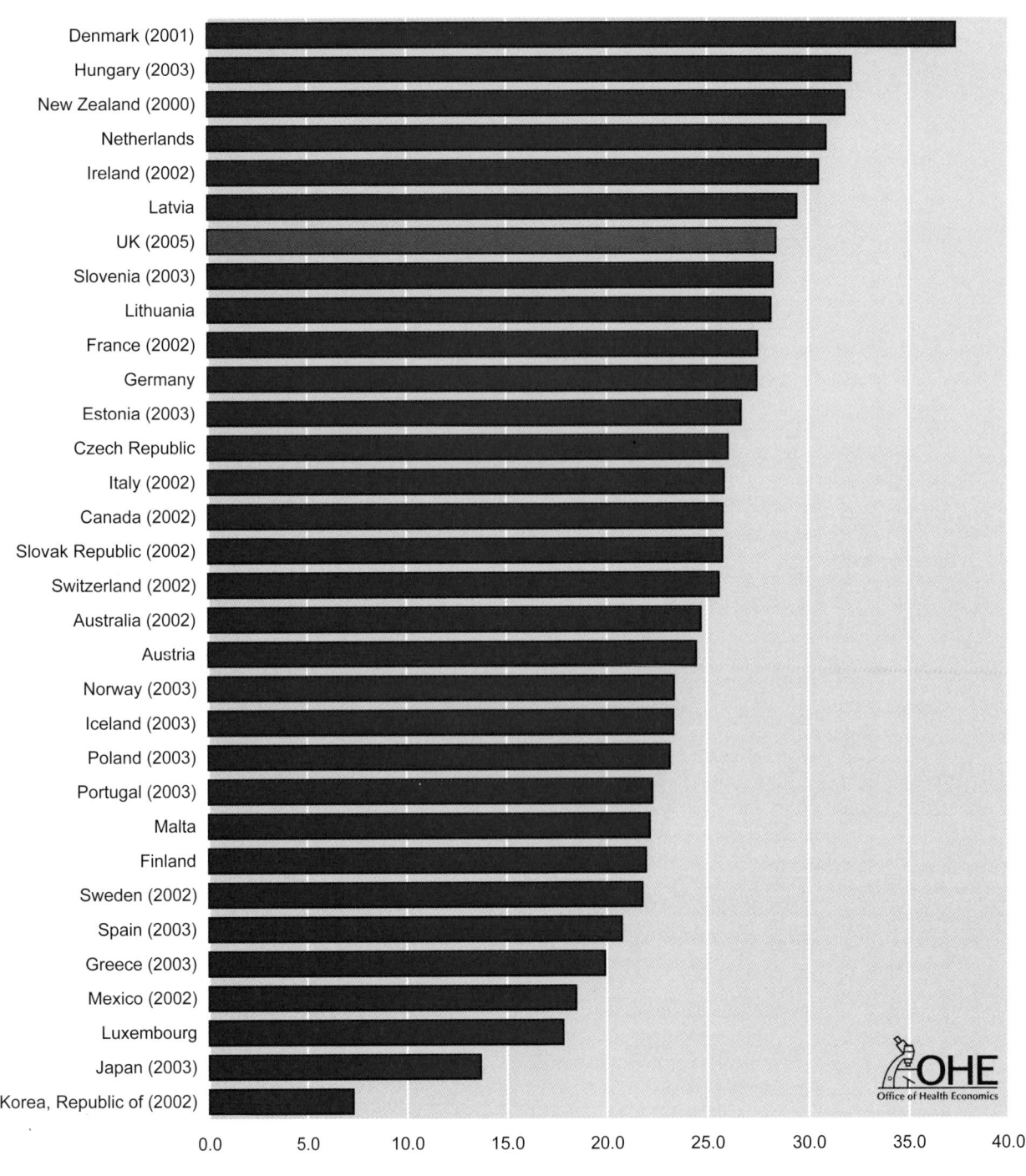

**Rate per 100,000 population**

*Note:* Year is 2004 unless stated otherwise.

*Sources:* OHE calculations based on WHO Mortality Database (WHO).
Mortality Statistics Series DH2 (ONS).
Vital Events Reference Tables (General Register Office of Scotland).
Demographic Statistics (Northern Ireland Statistics and Research Agency).

Table 1.36 **Registrations of newly diagnosed cases of cancer, selected sites, by sex and country, UK, 2004**

| ICD 10 | Description | Numbers | | | | |
|---|---|---|---|---|---|---|
| | | UK | England | Wales | Scotland | Northern Ireland |
| **Males** | | | | | | |
| C00-C99 xC44 | All malignant neoplasms excluding NMSC[1] | 143,136 | 117,805 | 8,740 | 13,164 | 3,427 |
| C00-C14 | All lip and mouth | 3,608 | 2,829 | 213 | 461 | 105 |
| C15 | Oesophagus | 4,943 | 4,047 | 254 | 536 | 106 |
| C16 | Stomach | 5,157 | 4,210 | 309 | 515 | 123 |
| C18-C21 | Colorectal | 19,632 | 16,103 | 1,108 | 1,914 | 507 |
| C25 | Pancreas | 3,605 | 3,039 | 209 | 286 | 71 |
| C33,C34 | Trachea, bronchus & lung | 22,495 | 18,105 | 1,313 | 2,506 | 571 |
| C43 | Melanoma of skin | 4,015 | 3,307 | 207 | 389 | 112 |
| C50 | Breast | 323 | 272 | 18 | 31 | 2 |
| C53 | Cervix | - | - | - | - | - |
| C54 | Uterus | - | - | - | - | - |
| C56 | Ovary | - | - | - | - | - |
| C61 | Prostate | 34,987 | 29,406 | 2,274 | 2,550 | 757 |
| C62 | Testis | 1,959 | 1,616 | 95 | 178 | 70 |
| C64-C66, C68 | Kidney | 4,303 | 3,567 | 268 | 360 | 108 |
| C67 | Bladder | 7,171 | 5,800 | 664 | 559 | 148 |
| C71 | Brain | 2,488 | 2,086 | 138 | 220 | 44 |
| C81-C96 | Lymphomas and leukaemias | 12,386 | 10,234 | 770 | 1,079 | 303 |
| C81 | Hodgkin's disease | 844 | 697 | 45 | 79 | 23 |
| C82-C85, C96 | Non-Hodgkin's lymphoma | 5,290 | 4,419 | 283 | 453 | 135 |
| C88, C90 | Multiple myeloma[2] | 2,202 | 1,814 | 156 | 174 | 58 |
| C91-C95 | All leukaemias | 4,036 | 3,306 | 286 | 357 | 87 |
| **Females** | | | | | | |
| C00-C99 xC44 | All malignant neoplasms excluding NMSC[1] | 141,433 | 115,816 | 8,073 | 13,949 | 3,595 |
| C00-C14 | All lip and mouth | 1,924 | 1,559 | 96 | 221 | 48 |
| C15 | Oesophagus | 2,710 | 2,171 | 154 | 336 | 49 |
| C16 | Stomach | 3,022 | 2,395 | 217 | 330 | 80 |
| C18-C21 | Colorectal | 16,429 | 13,448 | 894 | 1,640 | 447 |
| C25 | Pancreas | 3,797 | 3,181 | 230 | 304 | 82 |
| C33,C34 | Trachea, bronchus & lung | 15,817 | 12,354 | 942 | 2,160 | 361 |
| C43 | Melanoma of skin | 4,924 | 4,056 | 242 | 478 | 148 |
| C50 | Breast | 44,333 | 36,939 | 2,360 | 3,917 | 1,117 |
| C53 | Cervix | 2,726 | 2,221 | 156 | 282 | 67 |
| C54 | Uterus | 6,099 | 5,029 | 389 | 525 | 156 |
| C56 | Ovary | 6,478 | 5,293 | 361 | 619 | 205 |
| C61 | Prostate | - | - | - | - | - |
| C62 | Testis | - | - | - | - | - |
| C64-C66, C68 | Kidney | 2,655 | 2,178 | 168 | 230 | 79 |
| C67 | Bladder | 2,924 | 2,337 | 252 | 273 | 62 |
| C71 | Brain | 1,717 | 1,425 | 86 | 161 | 45 |
| C81-C96 | Lymphomas and leukaemias | 10,154 | 8,329 | 611 | 946 | 268 |
| C81 | Hodgkin's disease | 675 | 560 | 27 | 71 | 17 |
| C82-C85, C96 | Non-Hodgkin's lymphoma | 4,700 | 3,885 | 241 | 427 | 147 |
| C88, C90 | Multiple myeloma[2] | 1,788 | 1,456 | 129 | 159 | 44 |
| C91-C95 | All leukaemias | 2,964 | 2,414 | 214 | 278 | 58 |

*Notes:* 1 NMSC: non-melanoma skin cancer.
2 Figures for Northern Ireland for Multiple myeloma relate to ICD codes C90.
xC44: excluding C44.
- Not applicable.

*Sources:* Cancer Registration Statistics (ONS), Cancer Statistics (ISD), Welsh Cancer Intelligence and Surveillance Unit (WCISU), Northern Ireland Cancer Registry (NICR). Population estimates and projections (ONS).

Table 1.37 **Age standardised registration rates of newly diagnosed cases of cancer, selected sites, by sex and country, UK, 2004**

| | | Rates[1] per 100,000 population | | | | |
|---|---|---|---|---|---|---|
| ICD 10 | Description | UK[2] | England[2] | Wales | Scotland[2] | Northern Ireland[3] |
| **Males** | | | | | | |
| C00-C99 xC44 | All malignant neoplasms excluding NMSC[4] | 408.7 | 400.7 | 465.2 | 451.0 | 401.2 |
| C00-C14 | All lip and mouth | 11.2 | 10.5 | 12.9 | 16.6 | 12.9 |
| C15 | Oesophagus | 14.2 | 13.8 | 13.4 | 18.4 | 12.6 |
| C16 | Stomach | 14.3 | 13.9 | 16.2 | 17.2 | 14.2 |
| C18-C21 | Colorectal | 55.4 | 54.1 | 57.3 | 64.9 | 59.5 |
| C25 | Pancreas | 10.2 | 10.3 | 11.0 | 9.6 | 8.5 |
| C33,C34 | Trachea, bronchus & lung | 63.0 | 60.4 | 68.4 | 84.1 | 65.6 |
| C43 | Melanoma of skin | 12.3 | 12.1 | 12.3 | 14.3 | 13.3 |
| C50 | Breast | 0.9 | 0.9 | 0.9 | 1.1 | 0.2 |
| C53 | Cervix | - | - | - | - | - |
| C54 | Uterus | - | - | - | - | - |
| C56 | Ovary | - | - | - | - | - |
| C61 | Prostate | 98.0 | 98.3 | 115.8 | 85.9 | 88.6 |
| C62 | Testis | 6.6 | 6.5 | 7.0 | 7.1 | 8.1 |
| C64-C66, C68 | Kidney | 14.1 | 12.5 | 14.9 | 32.1 | 12.6 |
| C67 | Bladder | 19.6 | 18.8 | 34.6 | 18.5 | 16.7 |
| C71 | Brain | 7.6 | 7.6 | 8.3 | 7.9 | 5.3 |
| C81-C96 | Lymphomas and leukaemias | 36.4 | 35.8 | 42.2 | 38.3 | *36.0* |
| C81 | Hodgkin's disease | 2.8 | 2.7 | 2.9 | 3.2 | 2.7 |
| C82-C85, C96 | Non-Hodgkin's lymphoma | 15.7 | 15.6 | 16.0 | 16.0 | 16.0 |
| C88, C90 | Multiple myeloma[5] | 6.2 | 6.1 | 8.2 | 6.5 | 6.7 |
| C91-C95 | All leukaemias | 11.6 | 11.4 | 15.5 | 12.6 | 10.2 |
| | | | | | | |
| **Females** | | | | | | |
| C00-C99 xC44 | All malignant neoplasms excluding NMSC[4] | 347.3 | 341.5 | 372.4 | 387.1 | 351.8 |
| C00-C14 | All lip and mouth | 5.0 | 4.9 | 4.9 | 6.6 | 4.8 |
| C15 | Oesophagus | 5.5 | 5.3 | 5.9 | 7.9 | 3.7 |
| C16 | Stomach | 6.1 | 5.8 | 7.8 | 7.6 | 6.4 |
| C18-C21 | Colorectal | 35.4 | 34.7 | 36.2 | 40.3 | 40.4 |
| C25 | Pancreas | 7.9 | 8.0 | 9.0 | 7.5 | 7.1 |
| C33,C34 | Trachea, bronchus & lung | 35.9 | 33.6 | 40.5 | 55.3 | 32.9 |
| C43 | Melanoma of skin | 13.8 | 13.6 | 13.0 | 15.7 | 15.8 |
| C50 | Breast | 120.5 | 120.7 | 120.8 | 120.0 | 117.7 |
| C53 | Cervix | 8.0 | 7.8 | 9.3 | 9.6 | 7.2 |
| C54 | Uterus | 16.0 | 15.8 | 19.2 | 15.7 | 16.0 |
| C56 | Ovary | 16.9 | 16.6 | 17.7 | 17.8 | 21.0 |
| C61 | Prostate | - | - | - | - | - |
| C62 | Testis | - | - | - | - | - |
| C64-C66, C68 | Kidney | 6.9 | 6.2 | 7.8 | 12.4 | 7.6 |
| C67 | Bladder | 5.8 | 5.5 | 10.0 | 6.5 | 5.8 |
| C71 | Brain | 4.6 | 4.6 | 4.6 | 4.9 | 4.9 |
| C81-C96 | Lymphomas and leukaemias | 24.4 | 23.9 | 27.2 | 26.2 | *25.2* |
| C81 | Hodgkin's disease | 2.1 | 2.1 | 1.8 | 2.6 | 1.9 |
| C82-C85, C96 | Non-Hodgkin's lymphoma | 11.4 | 11.3 | 10.6 | 11.7 | 13.4 |
| C88, C90 | Multiple myeloma[5] | 3.9 | 3.8 | 5.4 | 4.0 | 4.2 |
| C91-C95 | All leukaemias | 6.9 | 6.6 | 9.7 | 7.9 | 5.8 |

*Notes:* 1 Age standardised using the European Standard population.
2 Figures are OHE estimates using published registration statistics for 2004, 2006-based population estimates for 2004, standardised using the European Standard Population. The Northern Ireland component of the UK figures are based on aggregated data covering the period 2002-2005.
3 Figures in italics for Northern Ireland are OHE estimates based on aggregated data covering the period 2002-2005.
4 NMSC: non-melanoma skin cancer.
5 Figures for Northern Ireland for Multiple myeloma relate to ICD codes C90.
xC44: excluding C44.
- Not applicable.

*Sources:* Cancer Registration Statistics (ONS), Cancer Statistics (ISD), Welsh Cancer Intelligence and Surveillance Unit (WCISU), Northern Ireland Cancer Registry (NICR). Population estimates and projections (ONS).

## Morbidity Statistics

Table 1.38(a)    **Prevalence of longstanding illness by age and sex, Great Britain, 1975 - 2005**

**Per cent of population reporting longstanding illness**

| Year | 1975 | 1980 | 1985 | 1990/91 | 1995/96 | 2000/01 | 2001/02 | 2002/03 | 2003/04 | 2004/05 | 2005 |
|---|---|---|---|---|---|---|---|---|---|---|---|
| **Males** | **23** | **29** | **29** | **33** | **31** | **33** | **32** | **34** | **31** | **31** | **32** |
| 0-4 | 8 | 8 | 11 | 14 | 14 | 14 | 17 | 17 | 14 | 15 | 14 |
| 5-15[1] | 12 | 16 | 18 | 20 | 20 | 23 | 20 | 21 | 18 | 19 | 19 |
| 16-44[1] | 17 | 23 | 21 | 25 | 23 | 23 | 22 | 23 | 20 | 20 | 22 |
| 45-64 | 35 | 43 | 42 | 46 | 43 | 45 | 44 | 46 | 41 | 43 | 44 |
| 65-74 | 50 | 54 | 55 | 58 | 55 | 61 | 58 | 65 | 62 | 57 | 58 |
| over 75 | 63 | 59 | 58 | 66 | 56 | 63 | 64 | 71 | 61 | 63 | 65 |
| **Females** | **25** | **31** | **31** | **35** | **31** | **32** | **31** | **35** | **32** | **32** | **33** |
| 0-4 | 6 | 8 | 9 | 12 | 11 | 13 | 12 | 12 | 10 | 11 | 10 |
| 5-15[1] | 9 | 11 | 13 | 17 | 17 | 18 | 16 | 19 | 17 | 15 | 16 |
| 16-44[1] | 16 | 23 | 22 | 25 | 22 | 22 | 21 | 25 | 22 | 22 | 24 |
| 45-64 | 33 | 42 | 43 | 47 | 39 | 42 | 42 | 44 | 41 | 42 | 43 |
| 65-74 | 54 | 60 | 56 | 61 | 54 | 54 | 56 | 61 | 59 | 55 | 61 |
| over 75 | 61 | 66 | 65 | 70 | 66 | 64 | 63 | 72 | 65 | 63 | 64 |
| **All** | **24** | **30** | **30** | **34** | **31** | **32** | **32** | **35** | **31** | **31** | **33** |
| 0-4 | 7 | 8 | 10 | 13 | 13 | 14 | 14 | 15 | 12 | 13 | 12 |
| 5-15[1] | 10 | 14 | 16 | 19 | 19 | 20 | 18 | 20 | 18 | 17 | 18 |
| 16-44[1] | 16 | 23 | 22 | 25 | 23 | 22 | 22 | 24 | 21 | 21 | 23 |
| 45-64 | 34 | 42 | 43 | 46 | 41 | 44 | 43 | 45 | 41 | 43 | 43 |
| 65-74 | 52 | 57 | 56 | 60 | 55 | 57 | 57 | 63 | 60 | 56 | 60 |
| over 75 | 62 | 64 | 63 | 69 | 63 | 64 | 63 | 72 | 64 | 63 | 64 |

Table 1.38(b)    **Prevalence of limiting longstanding illness by age and sex, Great Britain, 1975 - 2005**

**Per cent of population reporting limiting longstanding illness**

| Year | 1975 | 1980 | 1985 | 1990/91 | 1995/96 | 2000/01 | 2001/02 | 2002/03 | 2003/04 | 2004/05 | 2005 |
|---|---|---|---|---|---|---|---|---|---|---|---|
| **Males** | **14** | **18** | **16** | **19** | **18** | **18** | **18** | **20** | **17** | **17** | **18** |
| 0-4 | 3 | 3 | 4 | 5 | 5 | 4 | 5 | 5 | 4 | 4 | 5 |
| 5-15[1] | 6 | 8 | 8 | 9 | 8 | 9 | 9 | 8 | 7 | 8 | 7 |
| 16-44[1] | 9 | 12 | 10 | 13 | 12 | 11 | 10 | 12 | 10 | 10 | 11 |
| 45-64 | 27 | 28 | 27 | 29 | 28 | 27 | 28 | 28 | 24 | 26 | 26 |
| 65-74 | 36 | 39 | 38 | 38 | 37 | 38 | 36 | 43 | 37 | 33 | 36 |
| over 75 | 46 | 45 | 43 | 47 | 41 | 44 | 47 | 52 | 41 | 43 | 44 |
| **Females** | **16** | **20** | **18** | **22** | **20** | **19** | **19** | **22** | **19** | **19** | **20** |
| 0-4 | 2 | 3 | 3 | 3 | 3 | 4 | 4 | 3 | 4 | 4 | 3 |
| 5-15[1] | 4 | 5 | 6 | 7 | 8 | 8 | 8 | 9 | 7 | 7 | 7 |
| 16-44[1] | 9 | 12 | 11 | 14 | 13 | 11 | 12 | 14 | 11 | 12 | 13 |
| 45-64 | 22 | 26 | 26 | 30 | 26 | 27 | 26 | 28 | 25 | 24 | 26 |
| 65-74 | 39 | 42 | 38 | 42 | 37 | 35 | 37 | 39 | 37 | 33 | 39 |
| over 75 | 49 | 54 | 51 | 53 | 52 | 48 | 45 | 53 | 46 | 48 | 48 |
| **All** | **15** | **19** | **17** | **21** | **19** | **19** | **19** | **21** | **18** | **18** | **19** |
| 0-4 | 3 | 3 | 3 | 4 | 4 | 4 | 4 | 4 | 4 | 4 | 4 |
| 5-15[1] | 5 | 7 | 7 | 8 | 8 | 8 | 8 | 8 | 7 | 8 | 7 |
| 16-44[1] | 9 | 12 | 10 | 14 | 12 | 11 | 11 | 13 | 11 | 11 | 12 |
| 45-64 | 24 | 27 | 26 | 29 | 27 | 27 | 27 | 28 | 24 | 25 | 26 |
| 65-74 | 38 | 41 | 38 | 40 | 37 | 37 | 36 | 41 | 37 | 33 | 37 |
| over 75 | 48 | 51 | 48 | 51 | 48 | 47 | 46 | 53 | 44 | 46 | 47 |

*Notes:*    Longstanding illness refers to an illness, disability or infirmity that has occurred or is likely to occur over a period of time.  Limiting
requires a longstanding illness that is limiting of activity.
Data shown for 2000 onwards are based on data weighted to compensate for differential non-response.
From 1988 to 2004 the General Household Survey was on a financial year basis with interviews taking place from April to the following March.
1 In 1975, figures relate to age groups 5-14 and 15-44, respectively.

*Source:*    Living in Britain: Results from the General Household Survey (ONS).

Figure 1.17   **Trends in prevalence of longstanding illness by age group, Great Britain, 1972 - 2005**

**Per cent reporting illness**

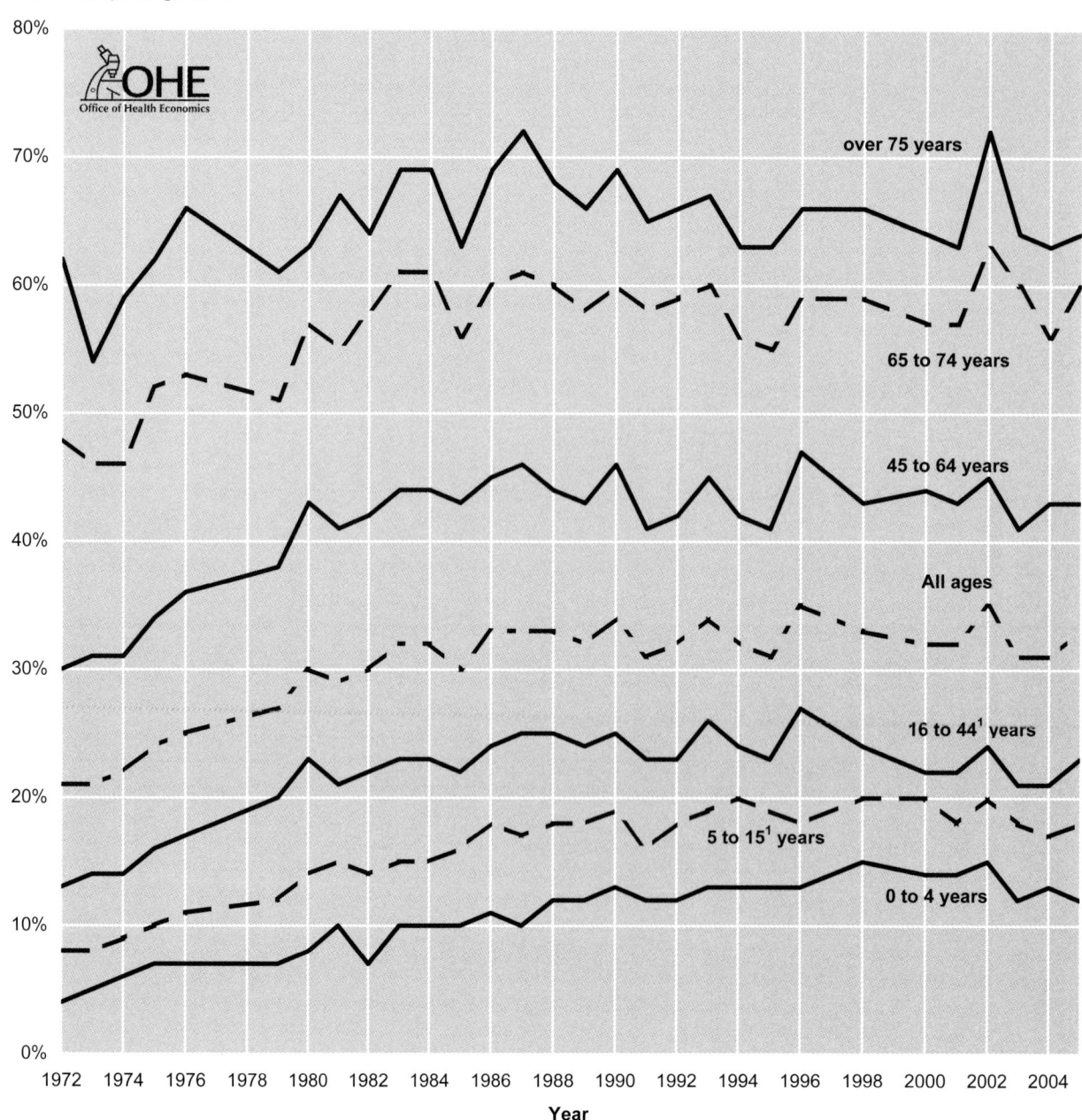

Year

*Notes:*   Interpolated figures for 1977, 1978, 1997 and 1999.
All figures are subject to sampling error.  Trends should be interpreted with caution.
From 1988 to 2004 the General Household Survey was on a financial year basis with interviews taking place from April to the following March.
1 From 1972 to 1978, figures relate to age groups 5-14 and 15-44.
Data shown for 1998 onwards are based on data weighted to compensate for differential non-response.
*Source:*   Living in Britain: Results from the General Household Survey (ONS).

Figure 1.18  **Prevalence of longstanding illness by socio-economic classification, Great Britain, 2005**

**Per cent reporting illness**

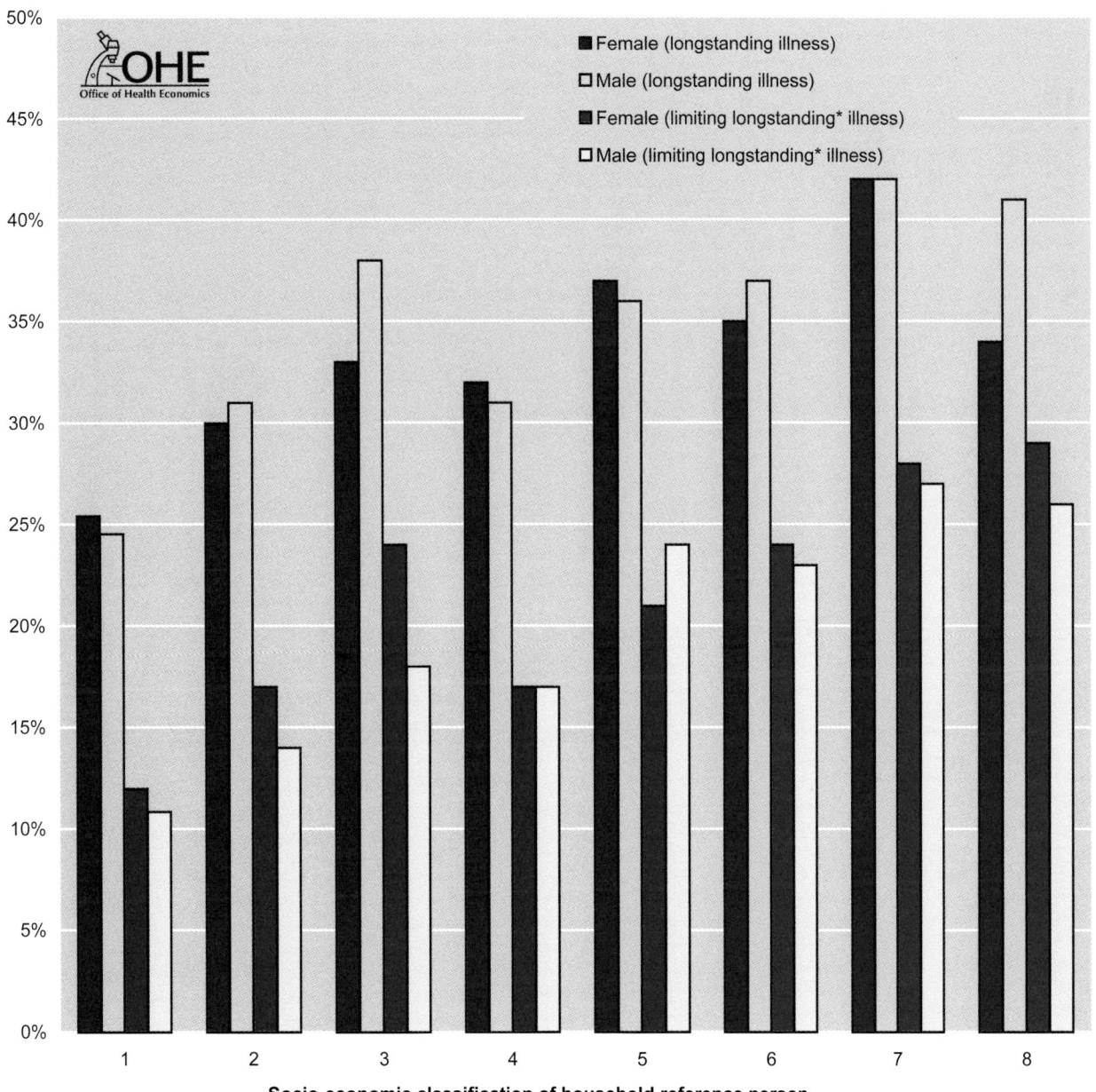

**Socio-economic classification of household reference person**

*Notes:*    * Figures for limiting longstanding illness refer to the proportion of the sample who reported that their usual level of activity had been restricted by illness or injury in the 14 days before the interview. These figures are subject to sampling error and should be interpreted with caution.

1: Large employers and higher managerial and higher professional occupations
2: Lower managerial and professional occupations
3: Intermediate occupations
4: Small employers and own account workers
5: Lower supervisory and technical occupations
6: Semi-routine occupations
7: Routine occupations
8: Never worked and long-term unemployed

*Source:*    Living in Britain: Results from the General Household Survey (ONS).

Table 1.39(a)   **Percentage of population consulting a NHS GP in a two-week period, Great Britain, 1975 - 2005**

**Per cent of population**

| | Year | | | | | | | | | | |
|---|---|---|---|---|---|---|---|---|---|---|---|
| | 1975 | 1980 | 1985 | 1990/91 | 1995/96 | 2000/01 | 2001/02 | 2002/03 | 2003/04 | 2004/05 | 2005 |
| **Males** | **9** | **11** | **11** | **13** | **13** | **12** | **11** | **13** | **11** | **11** | **11** |
| 0-4 | 13 | 19 | 22 | 26 | 22 | 18 | 18 | 19 | 17 | 15 | 15 |
| 5-15[1] | 7 | 10 | 9 | 10 | 9 | 8 | 7 | 8 | 7 | 7 | 7 |
| 16-44[1] | 8 | 9 | 7 | 10 | 10 | 8 | 8 | 9 | 8 | 8 | 8 |
| 45-64 | 11 | 12 | 12 | 14 | 14 | 15 | 13 | 15 | 12 | 14 | 13 |
| 65-74 | 12 | 17 | 15 | 17 | 17 | 20 | 18 | 22 | 18 | 17 | 17 |
| over 75 | 20 | 21 | 19 | 24 | 22 | 20 | 22 | 21 | 21 | 21 | 21 |
| **Females** | **12** | **15** | **16** | **19** | **18** | **16** | **16** | **17** | **16** | **16** | **16** |
| 0-4 | 13 | 17 | 21 | 22 | 21 | 14 | 18 | 14 | 14 | 17 | 15 |
| 5-15[1] | 7 | 10 | 11 | 13 | 13 | 9 | 9 | 8 | 7 | 7 | 6 |
| 16-44[1] | 13 | 17 | 17 | 19 | 18 | 16 | 15 | 18 | 15 | 16 | 17 |
| 45-64 | 12 | 14 | 15 | 19 | 17 | 17 | 18 | 17 | 17 | 17 | 17 |
| 65-74 | 16 | 17 | 17 | 19 | 23 | 22 | 18 | 21 | 22 | 21 | 21 |
| over 75 | 17 | 20 | 20 | 22 | 23 | 22 | 20 | 27 | 20 | 22 | 21 |
| **All** | **11** | **13** | **14** | **16** | **16** | **14** | **13** | **15** | **13** | **14** | **14** |
| 0-4 | 13 | 18 | 21 | 24 | 21 | 16 | 18 | 17 | 16 | 16 | 15 |
| 5-15[1] | 7 | 10 | 10 | 12 | 11 | 8 | 8 | 8 | 7 | 7 | 7 |
| 16-44[1] | 10 | 13 | 12 | 14 | 14 | 12 | 11 | 14 | 12 | 12 | 12 |
| 45-64 | 11 | 13 | 14 | 16 | 16 | 16 | 16 | 16 | 15 | 15 | 15 |
| 65-74 | 14 | 17 | 16 | 18 | 20 | 21 | 18 | 22 | 20 | 19 | 19 |
| over 75 | 18 | 20 | 20 | 23 | 23 | 21 | 21 | 25 | 20 | 22 | 21 |

Table 1.39(b)  **Average number of NHS GP consultations per person per year, Great Britain, 1975 - 2005**

**Average number**

| | Year | | | | | | | | | | |
|---|---|---|---|---|---|---|---|---|---|---|---|
| | 1975 | 1980 | 1985 | 1990/91 | 1995/96 | 2000/01 | 2001/02 | 2002/03 | 2003/04 | 2004/05 | 2005 |
| **Males** | **3** | **4** | **3** | **4** | **4** | **4** | **4** | **4** | **3** | **3** | **4** |
| 0-4 | 4 | 6 | 7 | 9 | 7 | 6 | 6 | 7 | 6 | 5 | 5 |
| 5-15[1] | 2 | 3 | 3 | 3 | 3 | 2 | 2 | 3 | 2 | 2 | 2 |
| 16-44[1] | 2 | 3 | 2 | 3 | 3 | 3 | 3 | 3 | 3 | 3 | 3 |
| 45-64 | 4 | 4 | 4 | 5 | 4 | 5 | 4 | 5 | 4 | 4 | 4 |
| 65-74 | 4 | 6 | 5 | 5 | 5 | 6 | 5 | 7 | 6 | 5 | 5 |
| over 75 | 7 | 7 | 6 | 7 | 8 | 6 | 7 | 7 | 7 | 7 | 7 |
| **Females** | **4** | **5** | **5** | **6** | **6** | **5** | **5** | **6** | **5** | **5** | **5** |
| 0-4 | 4 | 5 | 7 | 7 | 7 | 4 | 6 | 4 | 5 | 6 | 5 |
| 5-15[1] | 2 | 3 | 3 | 4 | 4 | 3 | 3 | 2 | 2 | 2 | 2 |
| 16-44[1] | 4 | 5 | 5 | 6 | 6 | 5 | 5 | 6 | 5 | 5 | 6 |
| 45-64 | 4 | 4 | 5 | 6 | 5 | 5 | 6 | 5 | 5 | 6 | 5 |
| 65-74 | 5 | 6 | 5 | 6 | 7 | 7 | 5 | 7 | 7 | 7 | 7 |
| over 75 | 6 | 6 | 7 | 7 | 7 | 7 | 6 | 9 | 6 | 7 | 7 |
| **All** | **3** | **4** | **4** | **5** | **5** | **4** | **4** | **5** | **4** | **4** | **4** |
| 0-4 | 4 | 6 | 7 | 8 | 7 | 5 | 6 | 5 | 5 | 5 | 5 |
| 5-15[1] | 2 | 3 | 3 | 4 | 3 | 2 | 3 | 2 | 2 | 2 | 2 |
| 16-44[1] | 3 | 4 | 4 | 5 | 4 | 4 | 4 | 4 | 4 | 4 | 4 |
| 45-64 | 4 | 4 | 4 | 5 | 5 | 5 | 5 | 5 | 5 | 5 | 5 |
| 65-74 | 4 | 6 | 5 | 6 | 6 | 6 | 5 | 7 | 6 | 6 | 6 |
| over 75 | 6 | 7 | 6 | 7 | 7 | 7 | 6 | 8 | 7 | 7 | 7 |

*Notes:*   All figures relate to 14 days before survey interview.
1 In 1975, figures relate to age groups 5-14 and 15-44, respectively.
From 1988 to 2004 the General Household Survey was on a financial year basis with interviews taking place from April to the following March.
Alternative estimates from 1995 to 2006 based on different methodology are available from the Information Centre (IC)

*Source:*   Living in Britain: Results from the General Household Survey (ONS).

Table 1.40 **Longstanding chronic sickness rates by age and condition groups, Great Britain, 2005**

*Rate per 1,000 population*

| ICD[2] | | Total[1] | 16-44 | 45-64 | 65-74 | >= 75 |
|---|---|---|---|---|---|---|
| XIII | Musculoskeletal system | 143 | 64 | 188 | 296 | 308 |
| | *Arthritis and rheumatism* | *71* | *14* | *91* | *179* | *183* |
| | *Back problems* | *38* | *28* | *53* | *40* | *31* |
| | *Other bone and joint problems* | *40* | *21* | *43* | *77* | *96* |
| VII | Heart and circulatory system | 104 | 17 | 145 | 274 | 320 |
| | *Hypertension* | *46* | *7* | *68* | *116* | *99* |
| | *Heart attack* | *19* | *1* | *22* | *55* | *68* |
| | *Stroke* | *7* | *1* | *7* | *16* | *32* |
| | *Other heart complaints* | *30* | *6* | *36* | *70* | *100* |
| | *Other blood vessel/embolic disorders* | *8* | *2* | *10* | *16* | *19* |
| VIII | Respiratory system | 62 | 53 | 60 | 96 | 87 |
| | *Asthma* | *43* | *43* | *42* | *52* | *40* |
| | *Bronchitis and emphysema* | *7* | *0* | *8* | *21* | *20* |
| | *Hay fever* | *3* | *5* | *1* | *2* | *0* |
| | *Other respiratory complaints* | *9* | *4* | *10* | *20* | *27* |
| III | Endocrine and metabolic | 49 | 18 | 71 | 115 | 96 |
| V | Mental disorders | 30 | 33 | 33 | 17 | 15 |
| VI | Nervous system | 29 | 22 | 37 | 36 | 33 |
| IX | Digestive system | 27 | 15 | 34 | 50 | 47 |
| VI | Eye complaints | 14 | 5 | 15 | 24 | 66 |
| X | Genito-urinary system | 15 | 11 | 15 | 23 | 36 |
| VI | Ear complaints | 13 | 6 | 13 | 27 | 46 |
| II | Neoplasms and benign growths | 13 | 4 | 19 | 32 | 33 |
| XII | Skin complaints | 8 | 8 | 8 | 8 | 9 |
| IV | Blood and related organs | 5 | 3 | 5 | 6 | 17 |
| | Other complaints[3] | 3 | 2 | 4 | 2 | 7 |
| I | Infectious diseases | 2 | 1 | 3 | 4 | 2 |

*Notes:* 1 Ages 16 and over.

2 Longstanding Illness has been categorised into broad groups based on symptoms, which only approximately correspond to ICD.

3 Including general complaints and non-specific conditions.

Individuals may have more than one condition.

0: less than 5 per 10,000 population.

*Sources:* OHE calculations based on General Household Survey England.

Government Actuary's Department (GAD).

Table 1.41 **Estimated days off work due to self-reported illness caused or made worse by work, by complaint type, Great Britain, 2001/02 - 2005/06**

Millions of days - Estimate (95% Confidence Interval)

| Complaint | Year | | | |
|---|---|---|---|---|
| | 2001/02 | 2003/04 | 2004/05 | 2005/06 |
| | **Males** | | | |
| **Total** | **18.2 (16.1, 20.2)** | **17.1 (14.9, 19.2)** | **15.9 (13.7, 18)** | **13.5 (11.6, 15.5)** |
| Bone, joint or muscle problem | 8 (6.6, 9.3) | 7.3 (5.9, 8.7) | 7.3 (5.8, 8.8) | 6.6 (5.2, 7.9) |
| *mainly affects upper limbs or neck* | *2.5 (1.8, 3.2)* | *2.4 (1.6, 3.1)* | *2.8 (1.8, 3.8)* | *2.3 (1.5, 3.1)* |
| *mainly affects the lower limbs* | *1.8 (1.1, 2.5)* | *1.6 (0.9, 2.3)* | *1.5 (0.8, 2.2)* | *1.7 (1, 2.4)* |
| *mainly affects the back* | *3.7 (2.7, 4.6)* | *3.3 (2.4, 4.3)* | *3 (2.1, 3.9)* | *2.5 (1.7, 3.4)* |
| Breathing or lung problem | 0.9 (0.5, 1.4) | 0.5 (0.2, 0.8) | 0.6 (0.2, 0.9) | 0.5 (0.2, 0.8) |
| Skin problem | - | - | - | - |
| Hearing problem | - | - | - | - |
| Stress, depression or anxiety | 5.9 (4.7, 7.1) | 6.4 (5, 7.8) | 6.2 (4.9, 7.5) | 4.7 (3.5, 5.8) |
| Headache and/or eyestrain | 0.1 (0, 0.2) | - | - | - |
| Heart disease/attack, other circulatory system | - | - | - | - |
| Infectious disease | 0.1 (0, 0.2) | 0.1 (0, 0.2) | - | - |
| Other | 1.4 (0.9, 2) | 1.6 (1, 2.3) | 0.9 (0.5, 1.3) | 1.1 (0.4, 1.7) |
| | **Females** | | | |
| **Total** | **18.2 (16.1, 20.2)** | **17.1 (14.9, 19.2)** | **12.5 (10.9, 14.1)** | **10.8 (9.3, 12.3)** |
| Bone, joint or muscle problem | 3.8 (3, 4.6) | 4.6 (3.6, 5.5) | 4.3 (3.3, 5.3) | 2.9 (2.1, 3.6) |
| *mainly affects upper limbs or neck* | *1.5 (1, 1.9)* | *2.4 (1.6, 3.1)* | *1.9 (1.2, 2.6)* | *1.3 (0.8, 1.9)* |
| *mainly affects the lower limbs* | *0.6 (0.2, 0.9)* | *0.6 (0.3, 0.9)* | *0.9 (0.5, 1.3)* | *0.3 (0.1, 0.6)* |
| *mainly affects the back* | *1.8 (1.3, 2.3)* | *1.6 (1.1, 2.1)* | *1.5 (0.9, 2.1)* | *1.2 (0.7, 1.7)* |
| Breathing or lung problem | 0.2 (0.1, 0.3) | 0.3 (0.1, 0.5) | 0.2 (0.1, 0.4) | - |
| Skin problem | - | - | - | - |
| Hearing problem | - | - | - | - |
| Stress, depression or anxiety | 7.1 (5.9, 8.2) | 6.4 (5.3, 7.5) | 6.6 (5.5, 7.7) | 5.9 (4.7, 7) |
| Headache and/or eyestrain | 0.1 (0, 0.1) | 0.1 (0, 0.2) | - | - |
| Heart disease/attack, other circulatory system | - | - | - | - |
| Infectious disease | 0.3 (0.1, 0.6) | 0.2 (0, 0.3) | 0.1 (0, 0.1) | - |
| Other | 1.6 (0.9, 2.2) | 1 (0.6, 1.5) | 0.8 (0.4, 1.2) | 1 (0.5, 1.4) |

*Notes:* Data should be interpreted with caution due to the small sample numbers in some groups, and are presented with 95% confidence intervals. 95% confidence intervals correspond to the range of values which we are 95% confident contains the true value. This reflects the potential error that results from surveying a sample rather obtaining information on the entire population.
Estimated days (full-day equivalent) off work due to self-reported work-related illness.
Work-related injuries are not included, they represented approximately 6 million additional working days lost in 2005/06.

*Source:* Labour Force Survey (HSE).

Table 1.42  **Prevalence of cigarette smoking by sex and age, Great Britain, 1974- 2005**

| | Percentage smoking cigarettes | | | | | | |
|---|---|---|---|---|---|---|---|
| | **Males** | | | | | | |
| Year | All aged 16 and over | 16-19 | 20-24 | 25-34 | 35-49 | 50-59 | 60 and over |
| 1974 | 51 | 42 | 52 | 56 | 55 | 53 | 44 |
| 1978 | 45 | 35 | 45 | 48 | 48 | 48 | 38 |
| 1982 | 38 | 31 | 41 | 40 | 40 | 42 | 33 |
| 1986 | 35 | 30 | 41 | 37 | 37 | 35 | 29 |
| 1990/91 | 31 | 28 | 38 | 36 | 34 | 28 | 24 |
| 1994/95 | 28 | 28 | 40 | 34 | 31 | 27 | 18 |
| 1998/99[1] | 30 | 30 | 41 | 38 | 33 | 28 | 16 |
| 2000/01 | 29 | 30 | 35 | 39 | 31 | 27 | 16 |
| 2001/02 | 28 | 25 | 40 | 38 | 31 | 26 | 16 |
| 2002/03 | 27 | 22 | 37 | 36 | 29 | 27 | 17 |
| 2003/04 | 28 | 27 | 38 | 38 | 32 | 26 | 16 |
| 2004/05 | 26 | 23 | 36 | 35 | 31 | 26 | 15 |
| 2005 | 25 | 23 | 34 | 34 | 29 | 25 | 14 |
| | **Females** | | | | | | |
| | All aged 16 and over | 16-19 | 20-24 | 25-34 | 35-49 | 50-59 | 60 and over |
| 1974 | 41 | 38 | 44 | 46 | 49 | 48 | 26 |
| 1978 | 37 | 33 | 43 | 42 | 43 | 42 | 24 |
| 1982 | 33 | 30 | 40 | 37 | 38 | 40 | 23 |
| 1986 | 31 | 30 | 38 | 35 | 34 | 35 | 22 |
| 1990/91 | 29 | 32 | 39 | 34 | 33 | 29 | 20 |
| 1994/95 | 26 | 27 | 38 | 30 | 28 | 26 | 17 |
| 1998/99[1] | 26 | 32 | 39 | 33 | 29 | 27 | 16 |
| 2000/01 | 25 | 28 | 35 | 32 | 27 | 28 | 15 |
| 2001/02 | 26 | 31 | 35 | 31 | 28 | 25 | 17 |
| 2002/03 | 25 | 29 | 38 | 33 | 27 | 24 | 14 |
| 2003/04 | 24 | 25 | 34 | 31 | 28 | 23 | 14 |
| 2004/05 | 23 | 25 | 29 | 28 | 28 | 22 | 14 |
| 2005 | 23 | 26 | 30 | 29 | 26 | 23 | 13 |
| | **All persons** | | | | | | |
| | All aged 16 and over | 16-19 | 20-24 | 25-34 | 35-49 | 50-59 | 60 and over |
| 1974 | 45 | 40 | 48 | 51 | 52 | 51 | 34 |
| 1978 | 40 | 34 | 44 | 45 | 45 | 45 | 30 |
| 1982 | 35 | 30 | 40 | 38 | 39 | 41 | 27 |
| 1986 | 33 | 30 | 39 | 36 | 36 | 35 | 25 |
| 1990/91 | 30 | 30 | 38 | 35 | 34 | 29 | 21 |
| 1994/95 | 27 | 27 | 39 | 32 | 30 | 27 | 17 |
| 1998/99[1] | 28 | 31 | 40 | 35 | 31 | 28 | 16 |
| 2000/01 | 27 | 29 | 35 | 35 | 29 | 27 | 16 |
| 2001/02 | 27 | 28 | 37 | 34 | 29 | 26 | 17 |
| 2002/03 | 26 | 25 | 38 | 34 | 28 | 26 | 15 |
| 2003/04 | 26 | 26 | 36 | 34 | 30 | 25 | 15 |
| 2004/05 | 25 | 24 | 32 | 31 | 29 | 24 | 14 |
| 2005 | 24 | 24 | 32 | 31 | 27 | 24 | 14 |

Notes:    1 Data from 1998 onwards are weighted.
Data on the prevelence of cigarette smoking was only available in the General Household Survey for the years shown.
From 1988 to 2004 the General Household Survey was on a financial year basis with interviews taking place from April to the following March.

Source:    Living in Britain: Results from the General Household Survey (ONS).

Figure 1.19   **Prevalence of cigarette smoking by country, 1978 - 2005**

**Percentage smoking cigarettes**

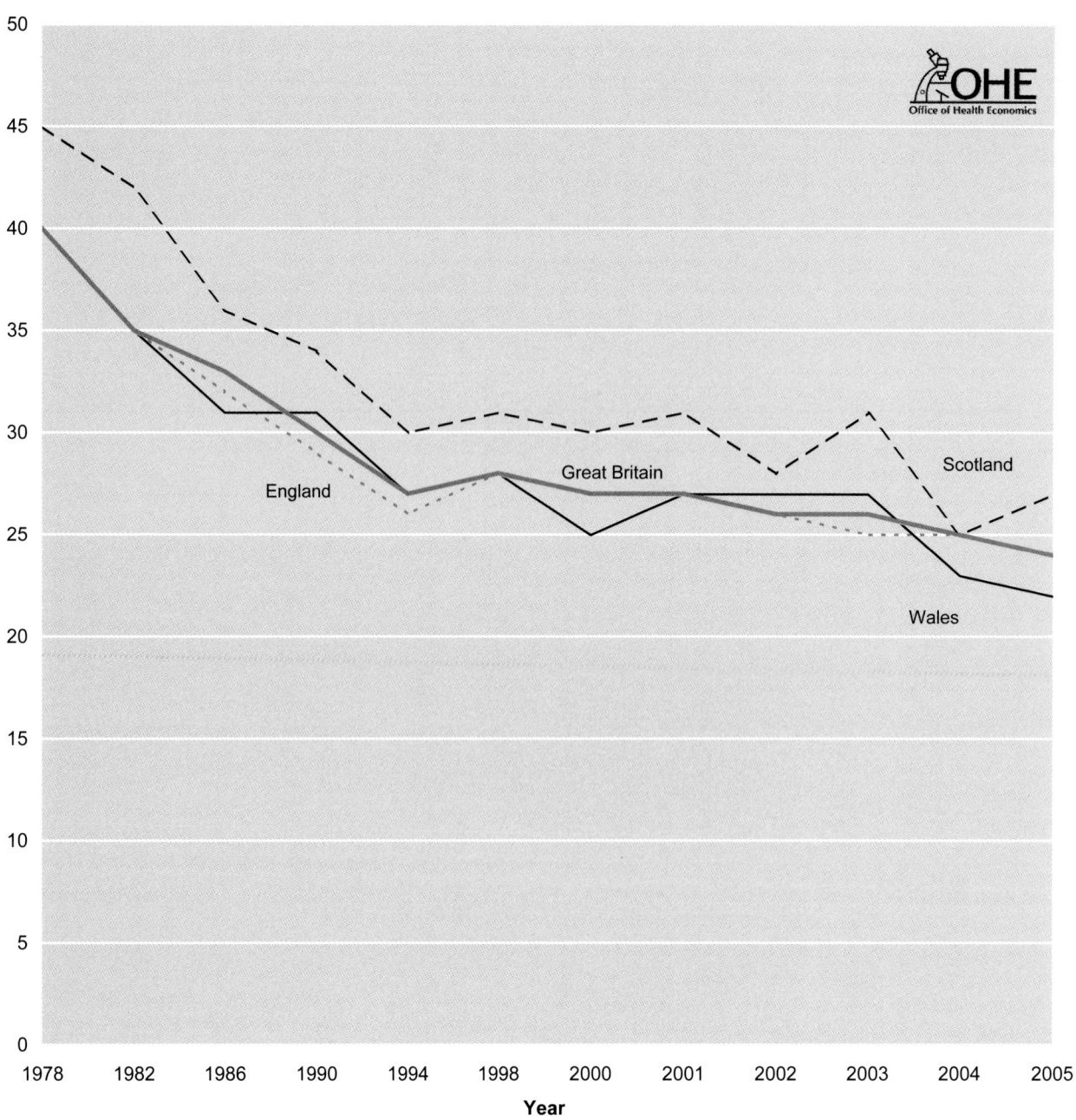

Year

*Notes:*   Data from 1998 onwards are weighted.
          From 1988 to 2004 the General Household Survey was on a financial year basis with interviews taking place from April to the following March.
*Source:* Living in Britain: Results from the General Household Survey (ONS).

Figure 1.20  **Prevalence of smoking among males and females aged 15[1] and over in selected OECD and EU countries, circa 2005**

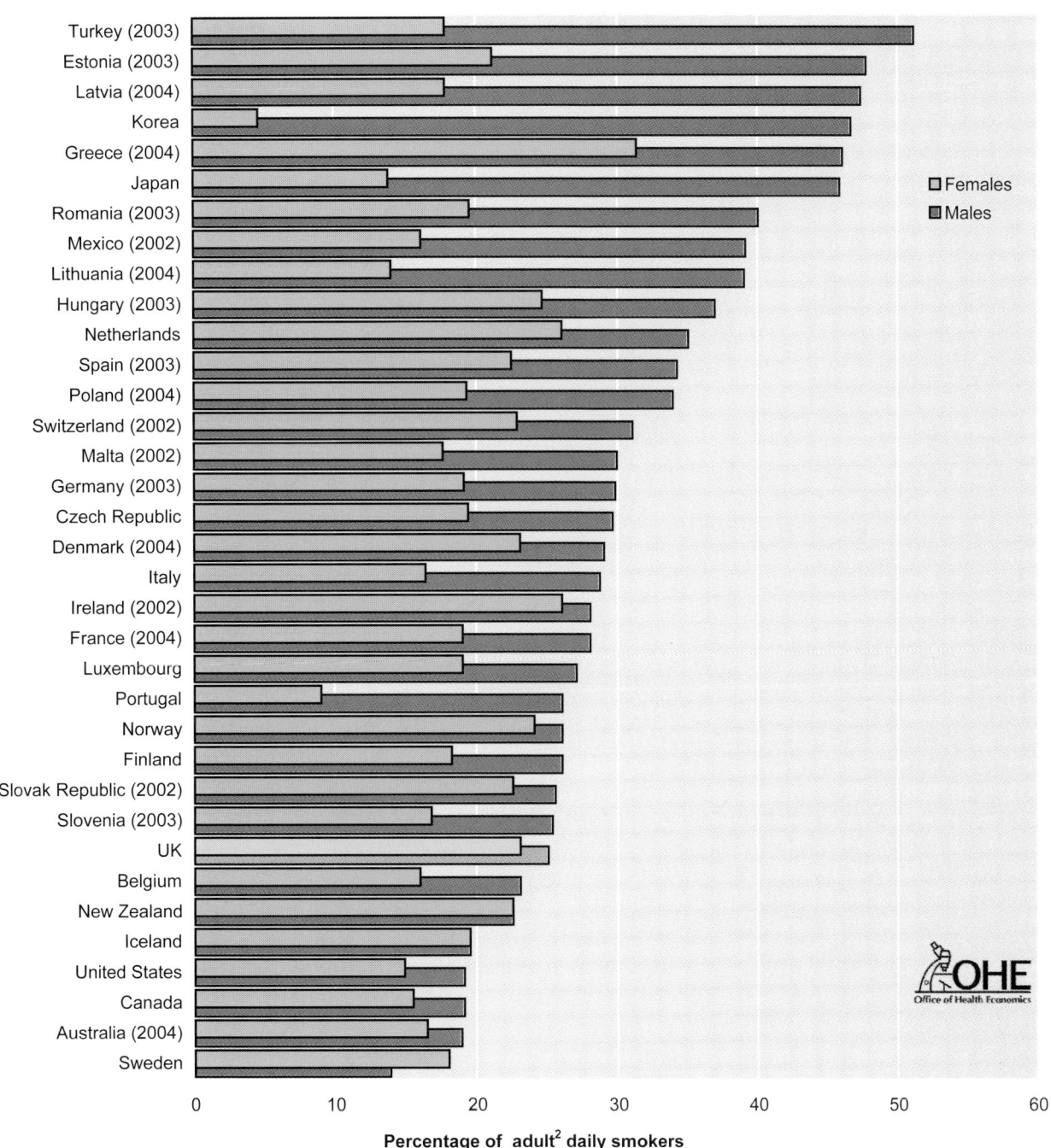

**Percentage of adult[2] daily smokers**

Notes:    Data relates to daily smokers.

      1 Data for Estonia relates to age group 16-64, Latvia to age group 15-64, Lithuania to age group 20-64, Malta to age group 15-98, Romania to age group 14-60 and Slovenia to age group 18+.

      2 Data relates to those aged 15 and over who are daily smokers.

Sources: OECD Health Database (OECD).

      WHO InfoBase (WHO).

Table 1.43 **Weekly consumption of alcohol (in units) by sex and age, Great Britain, 1988/89 - 2005**

| | **Weekly consumption of alcohol** | | | | | | | | | |
|---|---|---|---|---|---|---|---|---|---|---|
| | **Males** | | | | | **Females** | | | | |
| | Total | 16-24 | 25-44 | 45-64 | **65 and** over | Total | 16-24 | 25-44 | 45-64 | **65 and** over |
| **Year** | percentage drinking over 21 units | | | | | percentage drinking over 14 units | | | | |
| 1988/89 | 26 | 31 | 34 | 24 | 13 | 10 | 15 | 14 | 9 | 4 |
| 1990/91 | 27 | 31 | 34 | 24 | 13 | 11 | 16 | 13 | 10 | 5 |
| 1992/93 | 26 | 32 | 31 | 25 | 15 | 11 | 17 | 14 | 11 | 5 |
| 1994/95 | 27 | 29 | 30 | 27 | 17 | 13 | 19 | 15 | 12 | 7 |
| 1996/97 | 27 | 35 | 30 | 26 | 18 | 14 | 22 | 16 | 13 | 7 |
| 1998/99[1] | 28 | 38 | 28 | 30 | 16 | 15 | 25 | 16 | 15 | 6 |
| 2000/01 | 29 | 41 | 30 | 28 | 17 | 17 | 33 | 19 | 14 | 7 |
| 2001/02 | 28 | 40 | 30 | 26 | 15 | 15 | 32 | 17 | 14 | 6 |
| 2002/03 | 27 | 37 | 29 | 28 | 15 | 17 | 33 | 19 | 14 | 7 |
| 2005 | 24 | 27 | 26 | 25 | 14 | 13 | 24 | 14 | 13 | 5 |
| | Total | 16-24 | 25-44 | 45-64 | **65 and** over | Total | 16-24 | 25-44 | 45-64 | **65 and** over |
| | percentage drinking over 50 units | | | | | percentage drinking over 35 units | | | | |
| 1988/89 | 7 | 10 | 9 | 6 | 2 | 2 | 3 | 2 | 1 | 0 |
| 1990/91 | 7 | 11 | 9 | 6 | 2 | 2 | 3 | 2 | 1 | 1 |
| 1992/93 | 6 | 9 | 8 | 6 | 2 | 2 | 4 | 2 | 1 | 0 |
| 1994/95 | 6 | 9 | 7 | 6 | 3 | 2 | 4 | 2 | 2 | 1 |
| 1996/97 | 6 | 10 | 6 | 5 | 3 | 2 | 5 | 2 | 2 | 1 |
| 1998/99[1] | 7 | 14 | 6 | 7 | 3 | 2 | 7 | 2 | 2 | 1 |
| 2000/01 | 7 | 14 | 7 | 6 | 3 | 3 | 9 | 3 | 2 | 1 |
| 2001/02 | 7 | 15 | 7 | 5 | 2 | 3 | 10 | 3 | 2 | 1 |
| 2002/03 | 7 | 12 | 8 | 6 | 3 | 3 | 10 | 3 | 2 | 1 |
| 2005 | 6 | 9 | 5 | 6 | 3 | 2 | 6 | 2 | 2 | 1 |

*Notes:*    1 Data from 1998 onwards are weighted.
From 1988 to 2004 the General Household Survey was on a financial year basis with interviews taking place from April to the following March.
Data for 2003 and 2004 are not available.

*Source:*    Living in Britain: Results from the General Household Survey (ONS).

Figure 1.21   **Percentage who drank more than 3 or 4 units on a least one day in the last week by sex and country, 1998 - 2005**

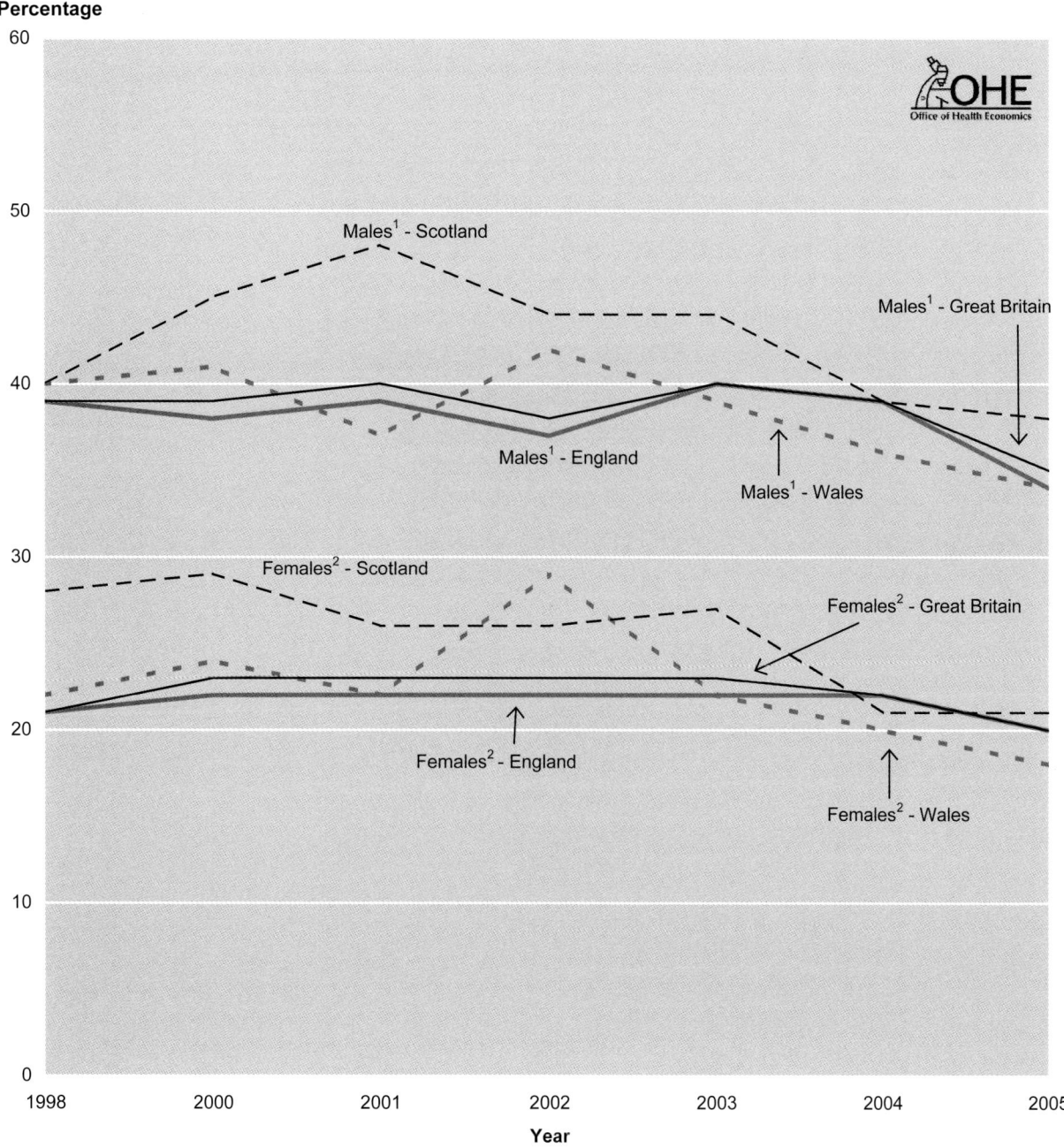

**Percentage**

*Notes:*    1 Percentage who drank more than 4 units on at least one day in the week preceding the survey.
            2 Percentage who drank more than 3 units on at least one day in the week preceding the survey.
*Source:*   Health Survey for England (Information Centre (IC)).

Figure 1.22   Annual consumption of pure alcohol (in litres) per person aged 15 and over in selected OECD and EU countries, circa 2005

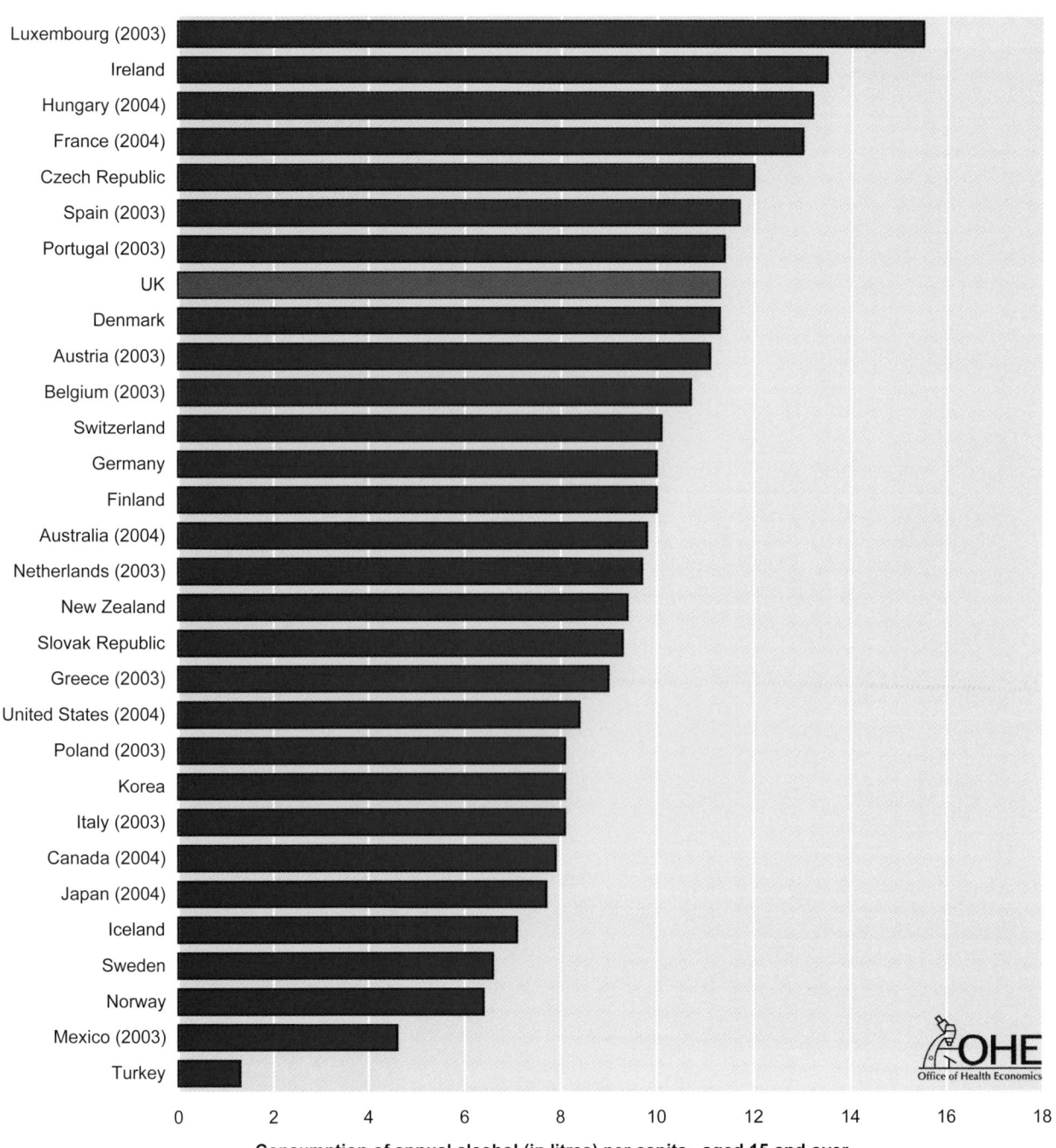

**Consumption of annual alcohol (in litres) per capita,  aged 15 and over**

*Notes:*   Data relates to annual consumption of pure alcohol in litres per person aged 15 and over.
Methodology to convert alcoholic drinks to pure alcohol may differ across countries.
*Source:*   OECD Health Database (OECD).

Table 1.44(a)  **Percentage of men, women and children who are overweight, 1995 - 2005**

| | 1995 | 1996 | 1997 | 1998 | 1999 | 2000 | 2001 | 2002 | 2003[1] | 2004 | 2005 |
|---|---|---|---|---|---|---|---|---|---|---|---|
| Age group | | | | | **Males overweight[2]** | | | | | | |
| 2 - 10 | 22.5 | 24.8 | 24.3 | 26.0 | 30.2 | 25.8 | 29.1 | 28.5 | 29.7 | 30.5 | 33.0 |
| 11 - 15 | 26.9 | 28.6 | 28.3 | 30.9 | 31.8 | 28.9 | 32.9 | 34.2 | 34.5 | 37.0 | 35.3 |
| 16 and over | 59.3 | 61.0 | 62.2 | 62.8 | 62.6 | 65.5 | 67.5 | 65.5 | 65.4 | 66.6 | 64.7 |
| | | | | | **Females overweight[2]** | | | | | | |
| 2 - 10 | 22.9 | 21.2 | 22.6 | 24.3 | 36.5 | 23.3 | 26.7 | 28.9 | 25.8 | 27.7 | 29.0 |
| 11 - 15 | 29.3 | 28.5 | 31.6 | 33.2 | 28.9 | 32.6 | 35.2 | 34.3 | 38.5 | 46.0 | 34.9 |
| 16 and over | 50.4 | 52.0 | 52.5 | 53.3 | 53.9 | 55.2 | 56.4 | 56.5 | 55.6 | 57.1 | 56.4 |

Table 1.44(b)  **Percentage of men, women and children who are obese, 1995 - 2005**

| | 1995 | 1996 | 1997 | 1998 | 1999 | 2000 | 2001 | 2002 | 2003[1] | 2004 | 2005 |
|---|---|---|---|---|---|---|---|---|---|---|---|
| Age group | | | | | **Males obese[3]** | | | | | | |
| 2 - 10 | 9.6 | 11.0 | 11.1 | 11.4 | 16.1 | 12.2 | 13.5 | 15.2 | 15.1 | 15.9 | 16.9 |
| 11 - 15 | 13.5 | 13.8 | 15.6 | 16.3 | 16.9 | 18.8 | 18.8 | 19.8 | 20.0 | 24.2 | 20.4 |
| 16 and over | 15.3 | 16.4 | 17.0 | 17.3 | 18.7 | 21.0 | 21.0 | 22.1 | 22.2 | 22.7 | 22.1 |
| | | | | | **Females obese[3]** | | | | | | |
| 2 - 10 | 10.3 | 10.2 | 10.7 | 11.8 | 13.0 | 11.8 | 12.7 | 15.8 | 12.4 | 12.8 | 16.8 |
| 11 - 15 | 15.4 | 15.0 | 16.2 | 17.5 | 15.2 | 18.1 | 17.7 | 19.2 | 22.1 | 26.7 | 20.8 |
| 16 and over | 17.5 | 18.4 | 19.7 | 21.2 | 21.1 | 21.4 | 23.5 | 22.8 | 23.0 | 23.2 | 24.3 |

*Notes:*   BMI = Body Mass index.  A measure that takes weight in kilogrammes divided by height in metres squared.
1 Data from 2003 onwards are weighted.
2 BMI over 25 (i.e. overweight including obese).
3 BMI over 30
*Source:*   Health Survey for England (Information Centre).

Figure 1.23 **Percentage of population who are overweight or obese by sex by country, 2004**

**Percentage**

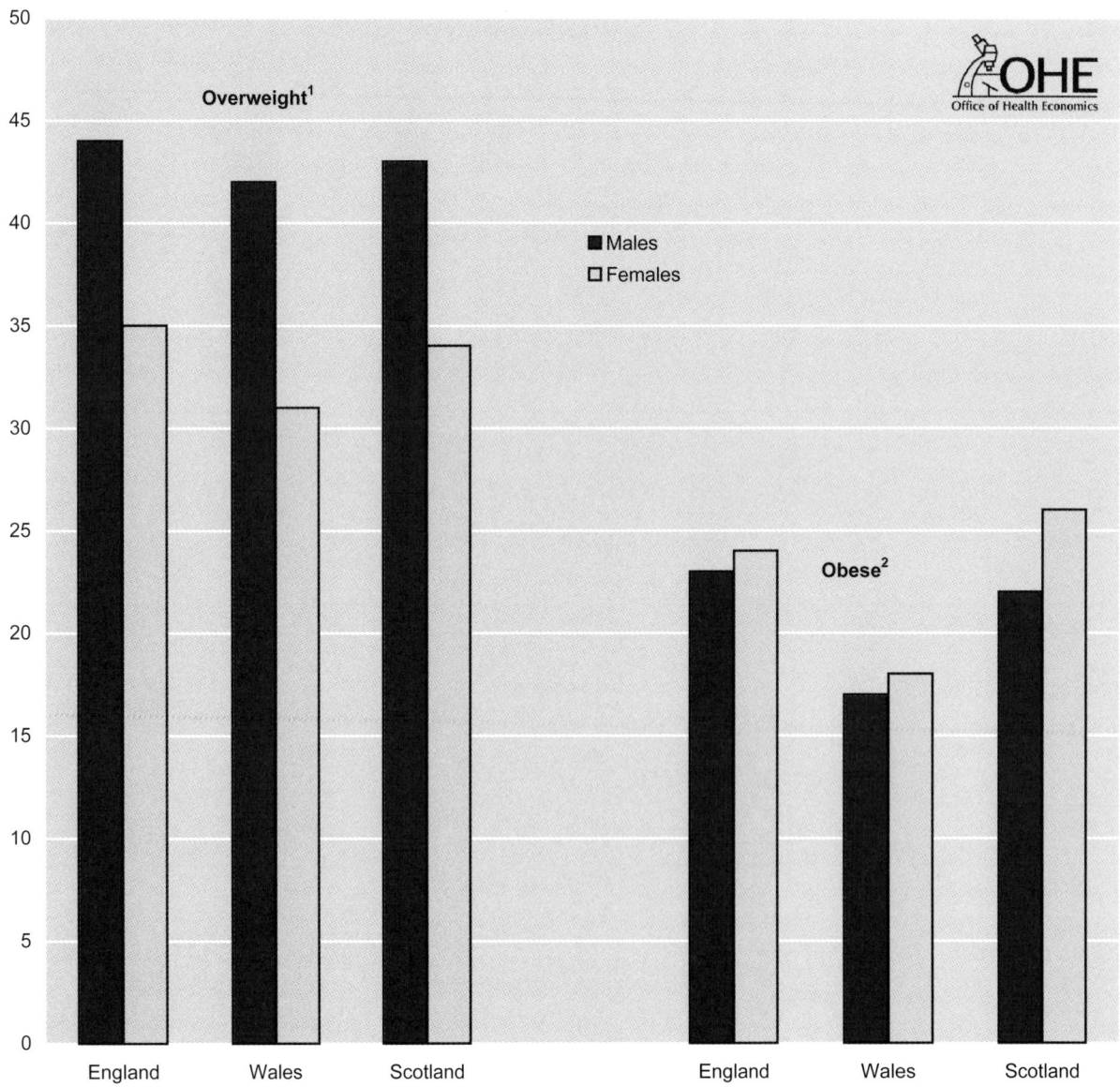

*Notes:* 1 Overweight is defined as BMI over 25 (i.e. overweight including obese).
2 Obese is defined as BMI over 30.

*Source:* Diet, physical activity and obesity statistics 2006, British Heart Foundation and Department of Public Health, University of Oxford.

Figure 1.24  **Prevalence of obesity, males and females in OECD and EU countries, 2005[1]**

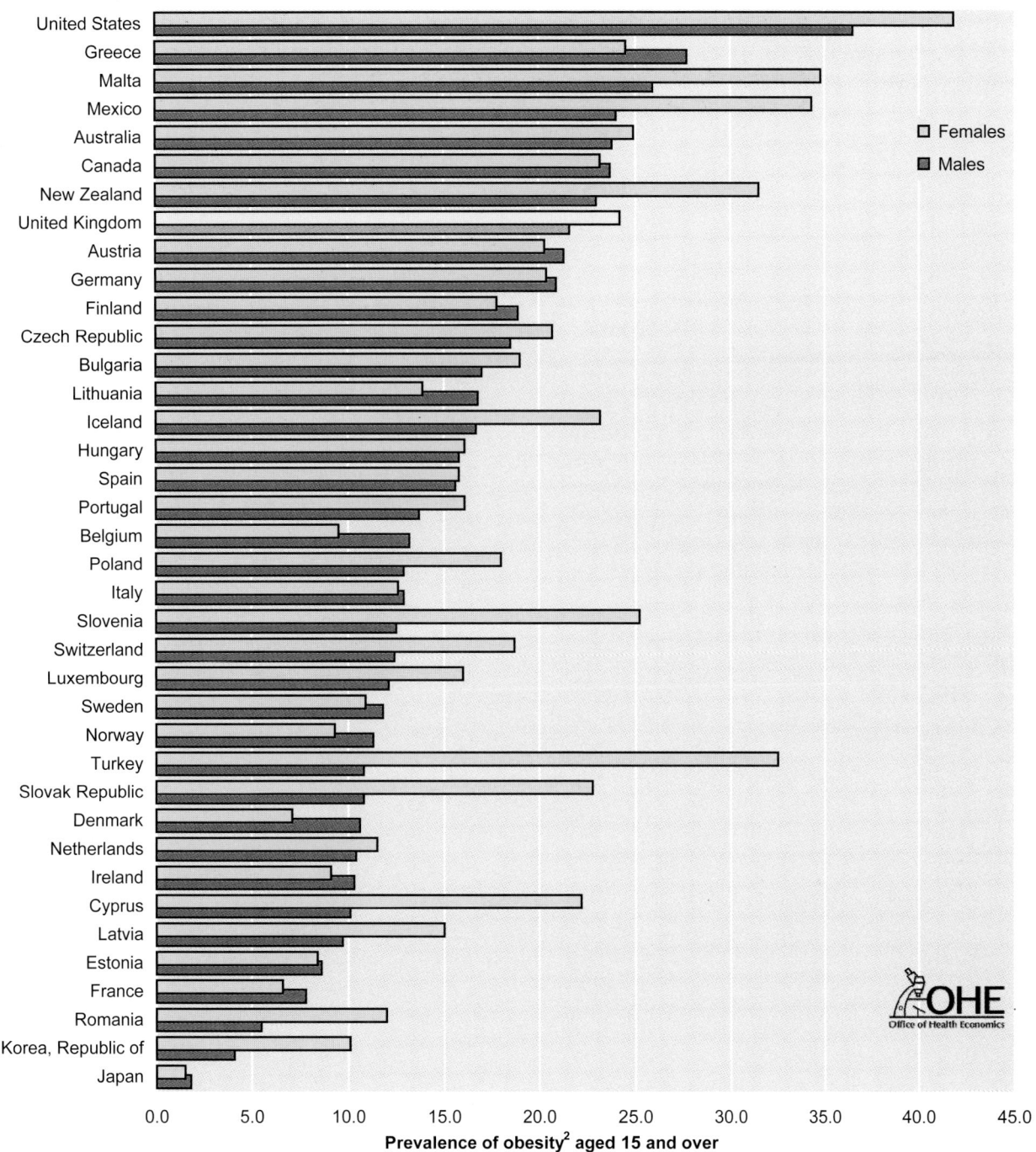

Prevalence of obesity[2] aged 15 and over

*Notes:*  1 Data are WHO estimates, adjusted to be representative of the national population where possible, age standardised and projected using available trend data to a standard reporting year - 2005.
2 Obesity is defined as BMI => 30.
*Source:*  WHO Global InfoBase (WHO).

# Total Health Care Expenditure in the UK

## *Main Points*

- Total health care expenditure in the UK rose to an estimated £121 billion in 2006/07, representing 9.1% of GDP, up from 6.6% in 1996/97.

- The gross cost of the NHS rose to an estimated £104 billion in 2006/07, (7.9% of GDP)

- Relative to England, NET per capita spend on the NHS in 2005/06 was 5.5% lower in Wales, 4.4% higher in Northern Ireland and 14% higher in Scotland.

- The number of people covered by private medical insurance was 6.5 million in 2005, equivalent to 10.9% of the UK population, compared with a peak of 6.9 million in 2000 (11.7% of the population).

### UK total health care expenditure

The total UK healthcare market in the public and private sectors in 2006/07 was estimated to be worth £121 billion, with expenditure rising by an estimated 7.2% between 2005/06 and 2006/07 (**Table 2.1**). Between 1999/2000 and 2006/07 total health care spending increased by 62% in real terms, continuing the marked increase that had begun in 1999 (**Figure 2.1** and **Box 1**).

| Box 1 **Percentage change in real[1] GDP and total real[1] UK health spending in five year periods** | | |
|---|---|---|
| Year | GDP | Total health spending |
| 1981/82 - 1986/87 | 17 | 15 |
| 1986/87 - 1991/92 | 11 | 27 |
| 1991/92 - 1996/97 | 14 | 20 |
| 1996/97 - 2001/02 | 16 | 33 |
| 2001/02 - 2006/07 | 14 | 37 |

*Note:* 1 As adjusted by the GDP deflator.
*Sources:* Economic Trends (ONS).
The Government's Expenditure Plans (DH).

UK health care expenditure per capita is now around the EU15 level. Recent increases have resulted in a per capita spend of £1,830 in the UK in 2005 (**Table 2.3**). However, several countries still spend considerably more per capita, with the USA, Switzerland and Luxembourg all having expenditures greater than £3,000 per person.

In 2006/07 total health care spending as a proportion of Gross Domestic Product (GDP) at market prices rose to an estimated 9.1% in the UK, up from the 6.6% observed a decade earlier (**Table 2.1** and **Figure 2.1**). All countries within the EU and OECD have increased expenditure in relation to GDP over the last few years (**Table 2.4**). However, the increase observed in the UK since 2000 is one of the highest (**Table 2.5**).

The proportion of total health care financed publicly in the UK was approximately 86% in 2006/07 (**Table 2.1**), higher than in most other EU and OECD countries (**Table 2.8**, **Figure 2.7**). In 2005 the highest percentage of public spending on total health care recorded was in Czech Republic, 89%. In contrast, only 45% of total health care spending was financed publicly in the USA.

**Figure 2.3** indicates the consistently faster growth in NHS pay rates and prices compared to the general rate of inflation in the UK economy. Once the relative increase in NHS pay and prices is taken into account, the volume of NHS resources increased by approximately 80% between 1975/76 and 2005/06, compared to an increase in GDP deflated terms of over 200% over the same period (**Figure 2.4**).

In parallel with the increased spending on health care there has been an improvement in key indicators of health, such as infant mortality and life expectancy. **Tables 2.10** and **2.11** and **Figure 2.10** indicate the relationship between health care expenditure and both infant mortality and life expectancy, with those countries spending particularly low amounts on health care per capita tending to have higher infant mortality rates and lower life expectancy. The levels achieved for these key health indicators in the UK are in the middle of the range of those observed across OECD countries.

*Note:*
1. Figures published by the OECD may differ from those taken from other sources due to differences in the definitions used in compiling data and in the exact timing.

# Total Health Care Expenditure in the UK

Table 2.1  **Total health care expenditure, UK, 1972/73 - 2007/08**

| Calendar year | UK health care expenditure | | | | Health care expenditure per capita | | UK health care expenditure as % of GDP[5] | | |
|---|---|---|---|---|---|---|---|---|---|
| | NHS[1] £m | Private health care[2] £m | Other medical products[3] £m | Total £m | £ Cash | Constant prices[4] 1972/73=100 | NHS | Private & other | Total |
| 1972/73 | 2,684 | 26 | 52 | 2,761 | 49 | 100 | 4.0 | 0.1 | 4.1 |
| 1975/76 | 5,358 | 142 | 285 | 5,785 | 103 | 130 | 4.8 | 0.4 | 5.2 |
| 1980/81 | 11,677 | 382 | 634 | 12,692 | 225 | 145 | 4.9 | 0.4 | 5.4 |
| 1981/82 | 13,229 | 496 | 714 | 14,438 | 256 | 150 | 5.1 | 0.5 | 5.6 |
| 1982/83 | 14,363 | 613 | 816 | 15,792 | 281 | 153 | 5.1 | 0.5 | 5.6 |
| 1983/84 | 15,371 | 660 | 948 | 16,978 | 301 | 158 | 5.0 | 0.5 | 5.5 |
| 1984/85 | 16,349 | 652 | 1,108 | 18,108 | 321 | 160 | 4.9 | 0.5 | 5.5 |
| 1985/86 | 17,514 | 765 | 1,234 | 19,513 | 345 | 163 | 4.8 | 0.5 | 5.4 |
| 1986/87 | 19,048 | 901 | 1,381 | 21,330 | 376 | 173 | 4.9 | 0.6 | 5.5 |
| 1987/88 | 21,829 | 1,111 | 1,474 | 24,414 | 430 | 187 | 5.0 | 0.6 | 5.6 |
| 1988/89 | 24,252 | 1,273 | 1,643 | 27,168 | 477 | 195 | 5.0 | 0.6 | 5.6 |
| 1989/90 | 26,169 | 1,421 | 1,819 | 29,409 | 515 | 197 | 5.0 | 0.6 | 5.6 |
| 1990/91 | 29,178 | 1,710 | 2,014 | 32,902 | 574 | 204 | 5.1 | 0.7 | 5.8 |
| 1991/92 | 33,044 | 1,981 | 2,407 | 37,432 | 651 | 219 | 5.5 | 0.7 | 6.3 |
| 1992/93 | 36,233 | 2,046 | 2,787 | 41,066 | 713 | 233 | 5.8 | 0.8 | 6.6 |
| 1993/94 | 37,563 | 2,201 | 3,164 | 42,928 | 743 | 237 | 5.7 | 0.8 | 6.5 |
| 1994/95 | 40,432 | 2,426 | 3,825 | 46,684 | 806 | 254 | 5.8 | 0.9 | 6.7 |
| 1995/96 | 42,326 | 2,681 | 3,989 | 48,996 | 844 | 259 | 5.8 | 0.9 | 6.7 |
| 1996/97 | 43,921 | 3,211 | 4,244 | 51,375 | 883 | 262 | 5.6 | 1.0 | 6.6 |
| 1997/98 | 46,240 | 3,722 | 4,456 | 54,417 | 933 | 270 | 5.6 | 1.0 | 6.6 |
| 1998/99 | 48,770 | 4,126 | 4,767 | 57,663 | 985 | 279 | 5.6 | 1.0 | 6.6 |
| 1999/00 | 53,429 | 4,465 | 5,060 | 62,954 | 1,072 | 299 | 5.8 | 1.0 | 6.8 |
| 2000/01 | 58,279 | 5,310 | 5,379 | 68,969 | 1,170 | 322 | 6.0 | 1.1 | 7.1 |
| 2001/02 | 64,430 | 5,961 | 5,858 | 76,249 | 1,289 | 348 | 6.4 | 1.2 | 7.5 |
| 2002/03 | 71,657 | 6,872 | 6,335 | 84,864 | 1,429 | 376 | 6.7 | 1.2 | 7.9 |
| 2003/04 | 81,259 | 7,550 | 6,594 | 95,403 | 1,600 | 411 | 7.2 | 1.2 | 8.4 |
| 2004/05 | 88,141 | 8,215 | 6,694 | 103,050 | 1,719 | 432 | 7.4 | 1.2 | 8.6 |
| 2005/06 | 97,230 | *8,958* | 6,653 | 112,841 | 1,871 | 463 | 7.8 | *1.2* | 9.0 |
| *2006/07e* | *104,099* | *9,680* | *7,149* | *120,928* | *1,993* | *483* | *7.9* | *1.3* | *9.1* |
| *2007/08e* | *114,350* | *10,402* | *7,557* | *132,309* | *2,166* | *514* | *8.1* | *1.3* | *9.4* |

*Notes:*  e = OHE estimates based, see notes below for further information.

1 Including charges paid by patients. Figures in italics are OHE estimates based on published data.

2 Consumer expenditure on private medical insurance (PMI) and private medical treatment. Figures in italics are OHE estimates based on trend.

3 Figures relate to consumer expenditure on medical goods including medicines not purchased on NHS prescription, and expenditure on therapeutic equipment such as spectacles, contact lenses and hearing aids. Figures in italics are OHE estimates based on trend over previous 10 years.

4 Figures have been adjusted by the GDP deflator at market prices and hence may include relative price effects.

5 Gross Domestic Product (GDP) at market prices.

*Sources:*  Consumer Trends (ONS).
Annual Abstract of Statistics (ONS).
Economic Trends (ONS).
The Government's Expenditure Plans (DH).
Department of Health Departmental Report (DH).
Health Statistics Wales (NAW).
NHS Board Operating Costs and Capital Expenditure, ISD Scotland (ISD).
Public Expenditure Statistical Analyses (HM Treasury).
Laing's Healthcare Market Review (Laing and Buisson).
Population Projections Database (GAD).
UK dentistry market research report (MBD).

Figure 2.1 **Total health care expenditure, UK, 1972/73 - 2007/08**

**Total health care expenditure (£ billion)**

**Per cent**

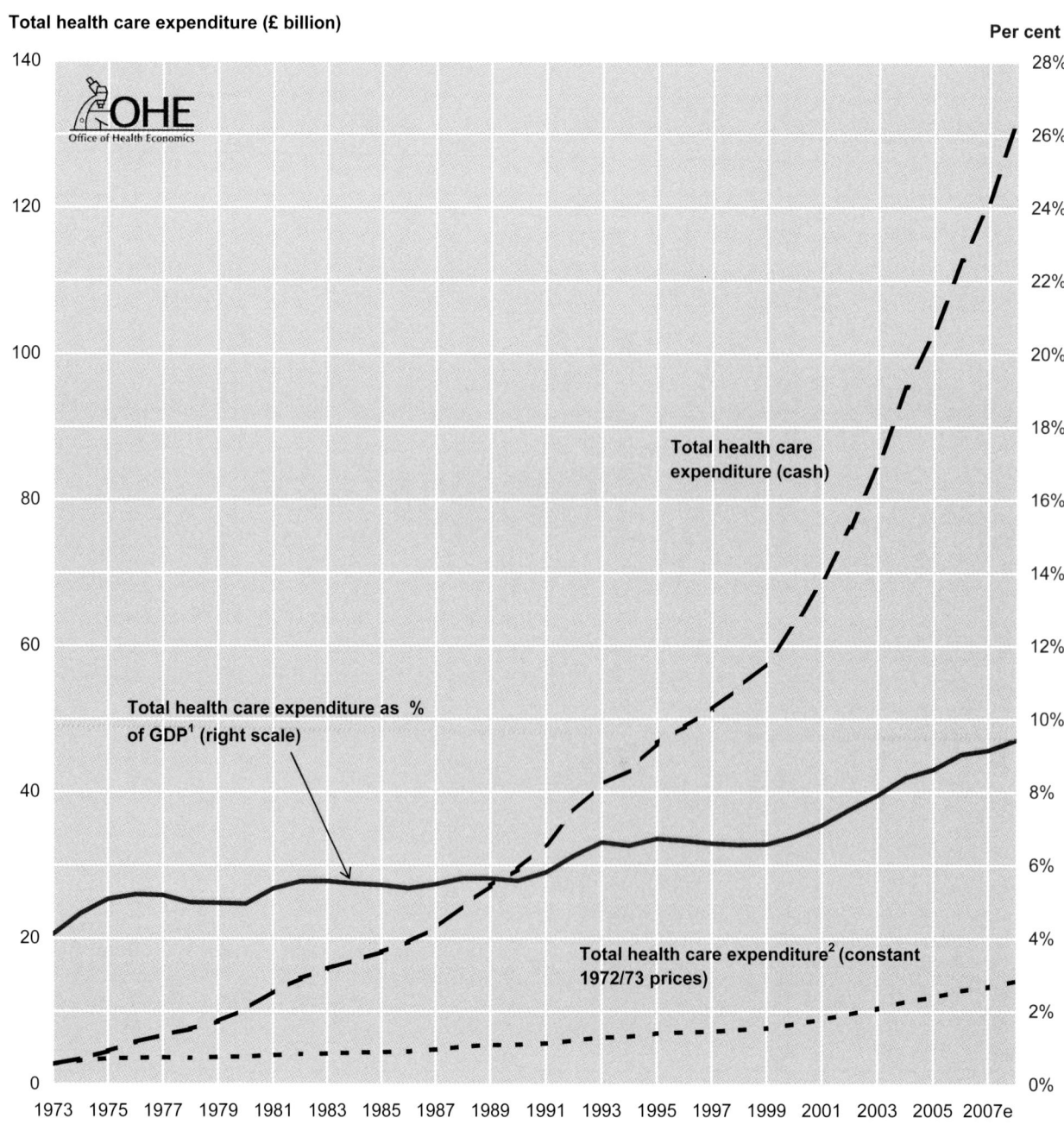

**Financial year ending**

*Notes:*    1 GDP = Gross Domestic Product at market prices.

        2 As adjusted by the GDP deflator at 1972/73 prices.

        Figures are for financial year ending 31 March (e.g. 2007 = 2006/07).

        e = OHE estimates.

*Sources:*   Consumer Trends (ONS).

        Annual Abstract of Statistics (ONS).

        Economic Trends (ONS).

        The Government's Expenditure Plans (DH).

        Department of Health Departmental Report (DH).

        Health Statistics Wales (NAW).

        NHS Board Operating Costs and Capital Expenditure, ISD Scotland (ISD).

        Public Expenditure Statistical Analyses (HM Treasury).

        Laing's Healthcare Market Review (Laing and Buisson).

        Population Projections Database (GAD).

# Total Health Care Expenditure in the UK

Figure 2.2 **Relationship between total UK health care expenditure and GDP[1], 1972/73 - 2007/08**

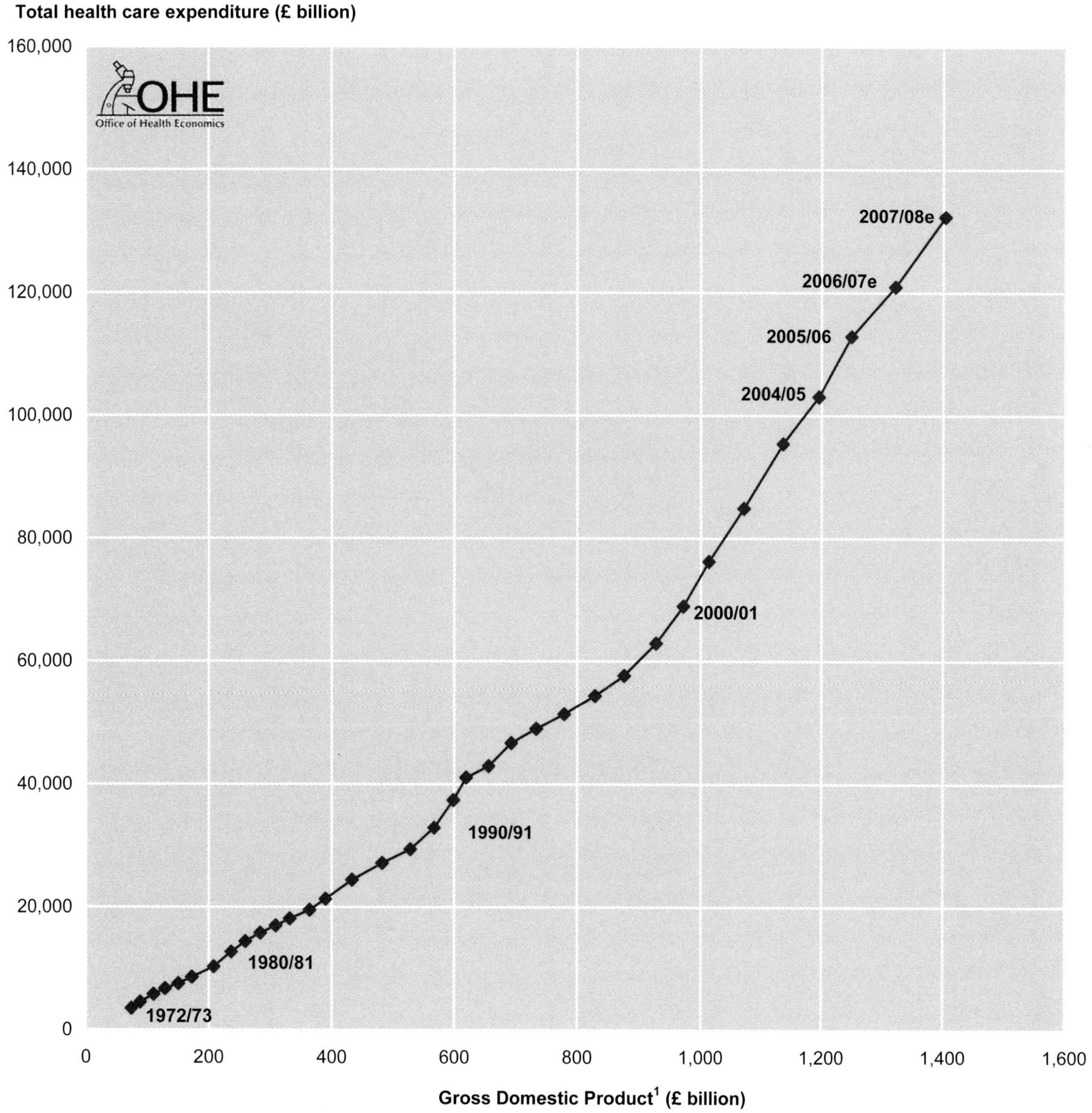

**Total health care expenditure (£ billion)**

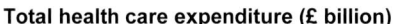

*Notes:* Total health care expenditure includes both the NHS and the private sector (see also Table 2.1).
1 GDP = Gross Domestic Product at market prices.
e = OHE estimates.

*Sources:* Consumer Trends (ONS).
Annual Abstract of Statistics (ONS).
Economic Trends (ONS).
The Government's Expenditure Plans (DH).
Department of Health Departmental Report (DH).
Health Statistics Wales (NAW).
NHS Board Operating Costs and Capital Expenditure, ISD Scotland (ISD).
Public Expenditure Statistical Analyses (HM Treasury).
Laing's Healthcare Market Review (Laing and Buisson).
Population Projections Database (GAD).

# Total Health Care Expenditure in the UK

Figure 2.3  **NHS pay and prices index and GDP[1] deflator index, 1975/76 - 2005/06**

**Index (1975/76 = 100)**

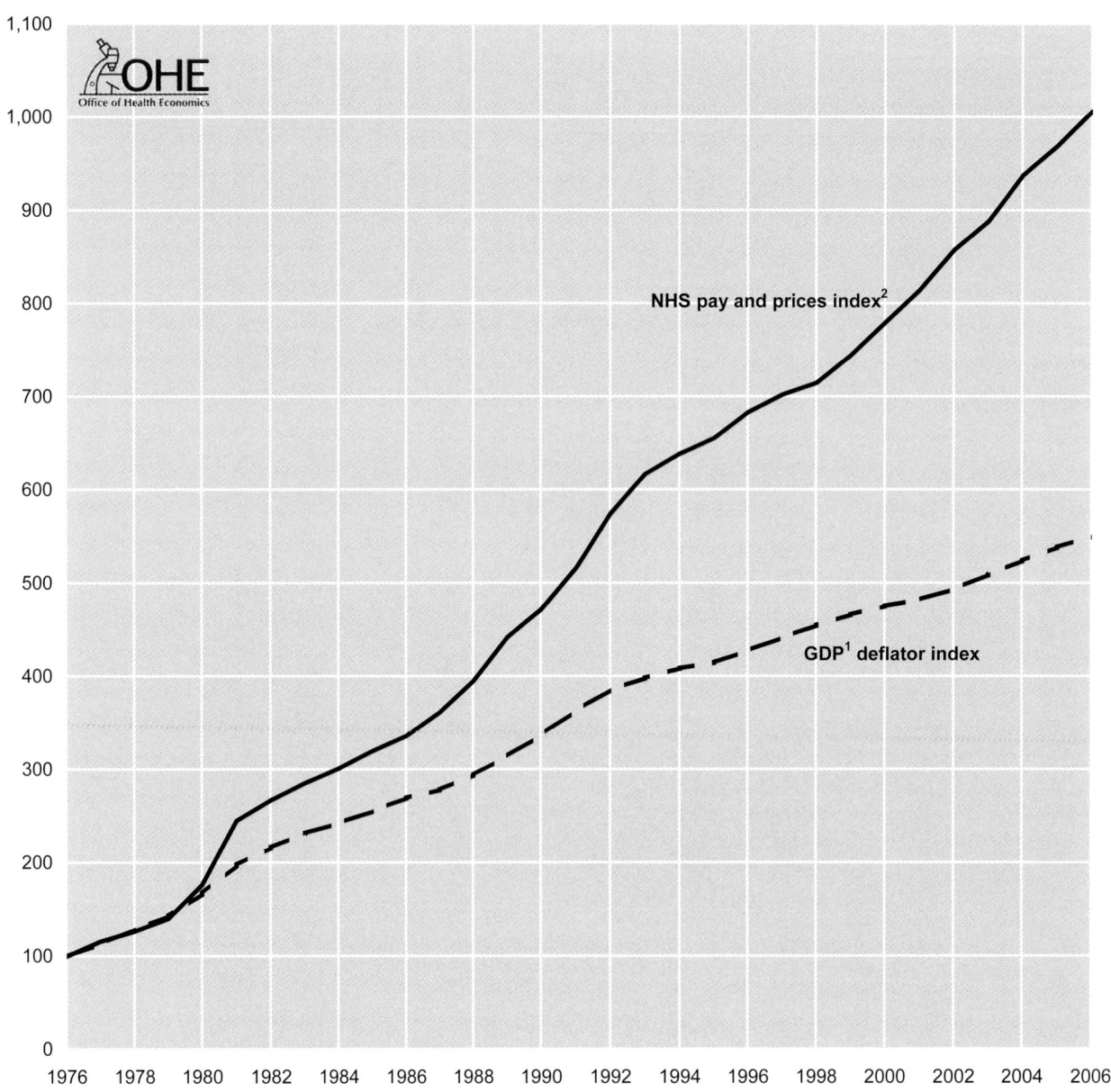

**Financial year ending**

*Notes:*  Data shown reflect data for the financial year ending 31 March e.g.2000 = 1999/2000..
        Figures are for financial year ending 31 March (e.g. 2007 = 2006/07).
        1 UK Gross Domestic Product (GDP) at market prices.
        2 Figures relate to Hospital and Community Health Services in England.
*Sources:*  Public Expenditure Team, Finance Directorate (Department of Health).
        Economic Data (HM Treasury).

## Total Health Care Expenditure in the UK

Figure 2.4  **Indices of total UK NHS expenditure at constant prices, 1975/76 - 2005/06**

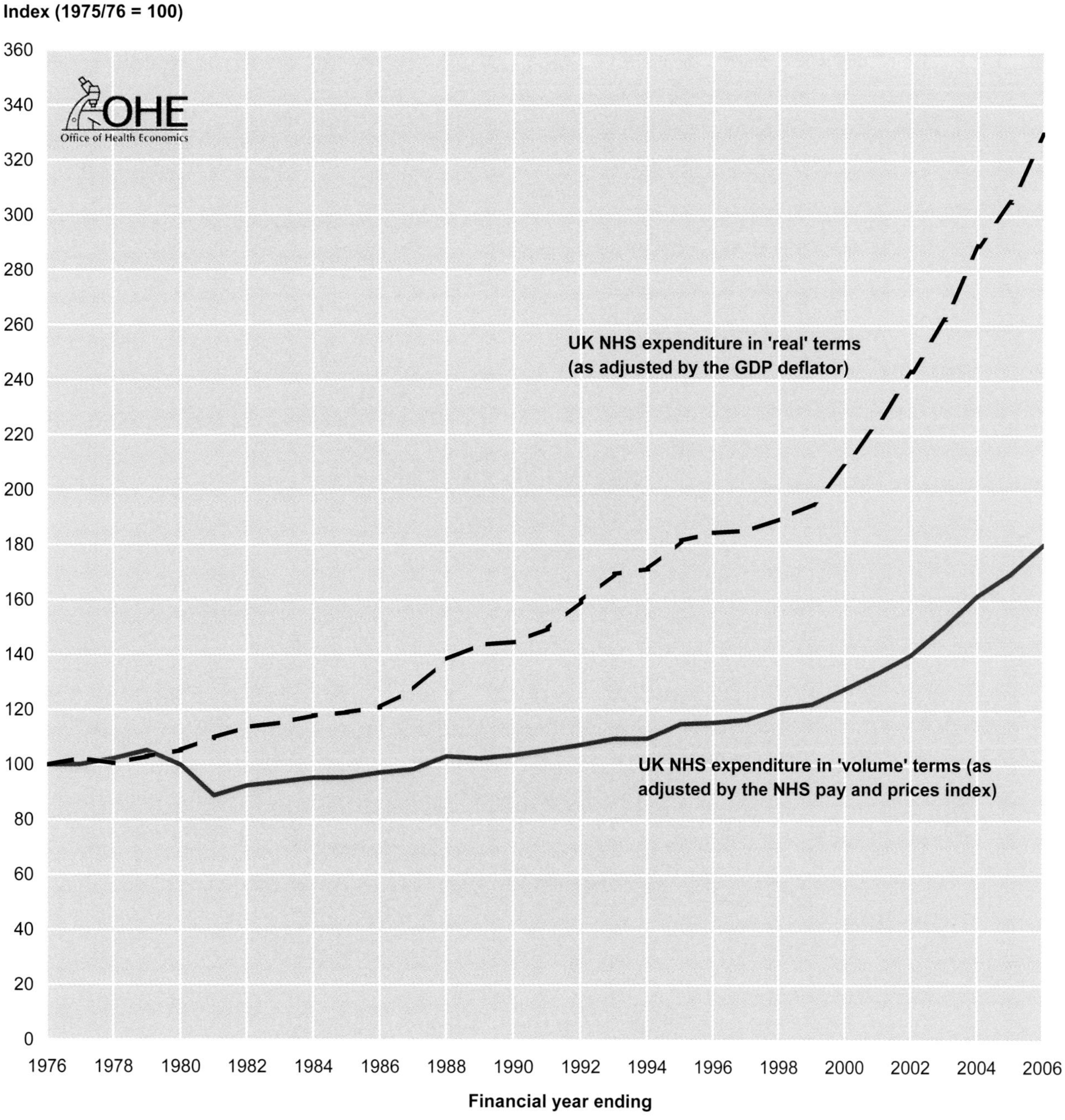

**Index (1975/76 = 100)**

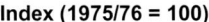

UK NHS expenditure in 'real' terms (as adjusted by the GDP deflator)

UK NHS expenditure in 'volume' terms (as adjusted by the NHS pay and prices index)

**Financial year ending**

Notes:    Data shown reflect data for the financial year ending 31 March e.g. 2000 = 1999/2000.
          GDP = Gross Domestic Product.
Sources:  Consumer Trends (ONS).
          Annual Abstract of Statistics (ONS).
          The Government's Expenditure Plans (DH).
          Department of Health Departmental Report (DH).
          Health Statistics Wales (NAW).
          NHS Board Operating Costs and Capital Expenditure, ISD Scotland (ISD).
          Public Expenditure Statistical Analyses (HM Treasury).
          Public Expenditure Team, Finance Directorate (DH).
          Economic Data (HM Treasury).
          Laing's Healthcare Market Review (Laing and Buisson).
          Population Projections Database (GAD).

# Total Health Care Expenditure in the UK

Figure 2.5 **Indices of UK spending on public and private health care at constant prices [1], 1973/74 - 2006/07**

**Index (1973/74 = 100)**

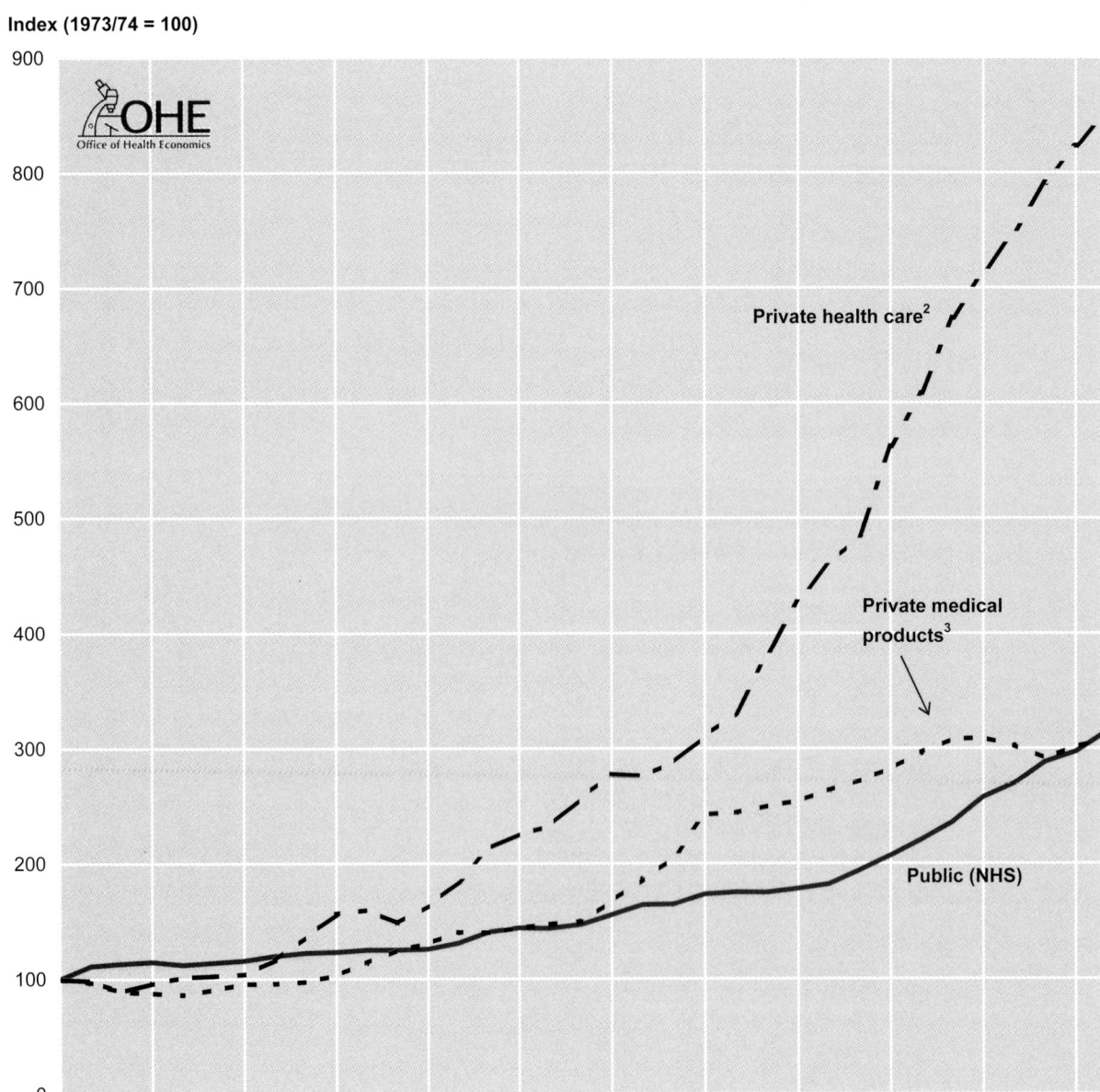

**Financial year ending**

*Notes:* 1 As adjusted by the Gross Domestic Product (GDP) deflator at market prices.
2 Consumer expenditure on private medical insurance (PMSI) and private medical treatment.
3 Figures relate to consumer expenditure on medical goods including medicines not purchased on NHS prescription and expenditure on therapeutic equipment such as spectacles, contact lenses and hearing aids.
2007 = OHE estimate.
Figures relate to financial year ending 31 March (e.g. 2000 = 1999/2000).

*Sources:* Consumer Trends (ONS).
Annual Abstract of Statistics (ONS).
The Government's Expenditure Plans (DH).
Department of Health Departmental Report (DH).
Health Statistics Wales (NAW).
NHS Board Operating Costs and Capital Expenditure, ISD Scotland (ISD).
Public Expenditure Statistical analyses (HM Treasury).
Laing's Healthcare Market Review (Laing and Buisson).
Population Projections Database (GAD).
Economic Data (HM Treasury)

# Total Health Care Expenditure in the UK

Table 2.2   Total[1] health care expenditure (£ billion) in OECD and EU countries, 1960 - 2005

**Total health care expenditure (£ billion)**

| | Year | | | | | | | | | | |
|---|---|---|---|---|---|---|---|---|---|---|---|
| | 1960 | 1970 | 1980 | 1990 | 1995 | 2000 | 2001 | 2002 | 2003 | 2004 | 2005[3] |
| **OECD** | 15.7 | 55.3 | 261.4 | 855.1 | 1,450.1 | 1,699.4 | 1,865.8 | 1,941.4 | 2,042.2 | 2,020.1 | 2,161.9 |
| **EU27[2]** | - | - | - | - | - | 475.2 | 517.3 | 558.0 | 648.4 | 671.2 | 717.4 |
| **EU15[2]** | 4.5 | 17.0 | 106.4 | 290.6 | 484.9 | 459.1 | 498.1 | 536.1 | 624.1 | 645.2 | 687.8 |
| Australia | 0.3 | 0.8 | 5.0 | 13.5 | 19.5 | 23.2 | 23.6 | 25.9 | 30.7 | 34.3 | - |
| Austria | 0.1 | 0.3 | 2.6 | 6.4 | 14.9 | 12.7 | 13.4 | 14.0 | 15.9 | 16.3 | 17.2 |
| Belgium | 0.1 | 0.4 | 3.4 | 8.2 | 14.8 | 13.2 | 14.0 | 15.1 | 19.0 | 20.0 | 21.0 |
| Bulgaria | - | - | - | - | - | 0.5 | 0.7 | 0.8 | 1.0 | 1.1 | 1.2 |
| Canada | 0.8 | 2.5 | 8.1 | 28.8 | 33.9 | 42.1 | 46.1 | 46.9 | 51.7 | 52.9 | 60.8 |
| Cyprus | - | - | - | - | - | 0.4 | 0.4 | 0.4 | 0.5 | 0.5 | - |
| Czech Republic | - | - | - | 0.8 | 2.5 | 2.5 | 2.9 | 3.5 | 4.2 | 4.3 | 4.9 |
| Denmark | 0.1 | 0.4 | 2.7 | 6.3 | 9.4 | 8.7 | 9.5 | 10.1 | 11.8 | 12.3 | 13.0 |
| Estonia | - | - | - | - | 0.2 | 0.2 | 0.2 | 0.2 | 0.3 | 0.3 | - |
| Finland | 0.1 | 0.3 | 1.4 | 6.0 | 6.2 | 5.3 | 5.8 | 6.4 | 7.3 | 7.6 | 8.1 |
| France | 0.8 | 3.3 | 21.0 | 58.3 | 98.1 | 83.7 | 90.2 | 97.3 | 119.4 | 123.2 | 131.2 |
| Germany | 1.2 | 4.8 | 30.7 | 73.0 | 161.9 | 128.6 | 136.8 | 143.2 | 160.7 | 157.5 | 164.4 |
| Greece | - | 0.3 | 1.3 | 3.4 | 7.2 | 9.0 | 10.2 | 11.1 | 13.6 | 13.8 | 15.8 |
| Hungary | - | - | - | 1.2 | 2.1 | 2.2 | 2.7 | 3.4 | 4.3 | 4.5 | - |
| Iceland | 0.0 | 0.0 | 0.1 | 0.3 | 0.4 | 0.5 | 0.5 | 0.6 | 0.7 | 0.7 | 0.8 |
| Ireland | 0.0 | 0.1 | 0.7 | 1.6 | 2.9 | 4.0 | 5.0 | 5.8 | 7.0 | 7.4 | 8.3 |
| Italy | 0.5 | 2.3 | 13.5 | 48.8 | 51.9 | 58.2 | 63.6 | 67.8 | 76.6 | 81.3 | 87.1 |
| Japan | 0.5 | 3.9 | 29.7 | 101.0 | 228.7 | 236.9 | 226.1 | 207.8 | 209.2 | 202.2 | - |
| Korea, Republic of | - | 0.1 | 1.0 | 6.4 | 13.6 | 16.1 | 18.1 | 19.3 | 20.2 | 20.4 | 25.8 |
| Latvia | - | - | - | - | 0.2 | 0.3 | 0.4 | 0.4 | 0.4 | 0.5 | - |
| Lithuania | - | - | - | - | 0.2 | 0.5 | 0.5 | 0.6 | 0.7 | 0.8 | - |
| Luxembourg | - | 0.0 | 0.1 | 0.4 | 0.7 | 0.8 | 0.9 | 1.0 | 1.4 | 1.5 | - |
| Malta | - | - | - | - | 0.2 | 0.2 | 0.2 | 0.2 | 0.3 | 0.3 | - |
| Mexico | - | - | - | 7.1 | 10.2 | 21.3 | 25.8 | 26.6 | 24.8 | 24.1 | 27.0 |
| Netherlands | 0.2 | 0.8 | 5.8 | 13.2 | 22.1 | 20.1 | 23.0 | 25.9 | 30.0 | 30.4 | - |
| New Zealand | 0.1 | 0.1 | 0.6 | 1.7 | 2.8 | 2.7 | 2.8 | 3.3 | 4.0 | 4.6 | 5.4 |
| Norway | 0.1 | 0.2 | 1.9 | 5.0 | 7.4 | 9.4 | 10.4 | 12.5 | 13.8 | 13.6 | 15.0 |
| Poland | - | - | - | 1.7 | 4.8 | 6.2 | 7.8 | 8.4 | 8.3 | 8.6 | 10.4 |
| Portugal | - | 0.1 | 0.7 | 2.5 | 5.6 | 6.5 | 7.1 | 7.6 | 9.2 | 9.5 | 10.4 |
| Romania | - | - | - | - | - | 1.3 | 1.5 | 1.8 | 1.8 | 2.0 | 2.8 |
| Slovak Republic | - | - | - | - | - | 0.7 | 0.8 | 0.9 | 1.2 | 1.7 | 1.9 |
| Slovenia | - | - | - | - | 1.1 | 1.1 | 1.2 | 1.3 | 1.5 | 1.5 | - |
| Spain | 0.1 | 0.6 | 5.2 | 19.1 | 28.1 | 27.5 | 30.6 | 33.2 | 42.2 | 45.7 | 51.2 |
| Sweden | 0.2 | 1.0 | 5.1 | 11.3 | 12.8 | 13.4 | 13.4 | 14.8 | 17.3 | 17.3 | 17.9 |
| Switzerland | 0.2 | 0.5 | 3.5 | 10.9 | 19.4 | 16.9 | 19.0 | 20.5 | 22.6 | 22.7 | 23.3 |
| Turkey | - | 0.2 | 1.0 | 3.3 | 3.3 | 8.6 | 7.5 | 9.0 | 11.1 | 12.7 | 15.2 |
| UK | 1.0 | 2.3 | 12.2 | 32.0 | 48.3 | 67.4 | 74.4 | 82.8 | 92.7 | 101.2 | 110.3 |
| USA | 9.4 | 30.0 | 104.2 | 382.7 | 616.7 | 851.0 | 973.6 | 1,016.9 | 1,011.5 | 967.7 | 1,042.6 |

Notes:   Figures are dependent on exchange rates between national currencies and £ sterling over time.
Trends over time should be interpreted with caution as there are several breaks in series (see OECD Health Database for further information).
2005 figures for Belgium, Cyprus, Denmark, Estonia, Japan, Latvia, Lithuania, Malta, Slovak Republic and Slovenia are WHO provisional estimates.
1 Public and private spending.
2 EU15 as constituted before 1 May 2004 and EU27 as constituted since 1 January 2007.
3 OECD figure includes 2004 data for Australia, Hungary, Japan, Luxembourg and the Netherlands.  EU27 figure includes 2004 data for Cyprus, Estonia, Hungary, Latvia, Lithuania, Luxembourg, Malta, the Netherlands and Slovenia.  EU15 figure includes 2004 data for Luxembourg and the Netherlands.
- Not available. Expenditure less than £500 million is displayed as 0.0.
Sources:   OECD Health Database (OECD).
World Development Indicators (World Bank).
World Health Report: Core Health Indicators (WHO).
World Health Organisation National Health Accounts Series (WHO).
For sources of UK data refer to Table 2.1.

# Total Health Care Expenditure in the UK

Table 2.3   Total[1] health care expenditure per capita (£ cash) in OECD and EU countries, 1960 - 2005

**Total health care expenditure per capita (£ cash)**

| | Year | | | | | | | | | | |
|---|---|---|---|---|---|---|---|---|---|---|---|
| | 1960 | 1970 | 1980 | 1990 | 1995 | 2000 | 2001 | 2002 | 2003 | 2004 | 2005[3] |
| OECD[2] | 26 | 74 | 320 | 839 | 1,339 | 1,506 | 1,641 | 1,696 | 1,772 | 1,741 | 1,849 |
| EU27[2] | - | - | - | - | - | 987 | 1,072 | 1,152 | 1,335 | 1,377 | 1,465 |
| EU15[2] | 16 | 53 | 315 | 835 | 1,307 | 1,219 | 1,317 | 1,410 | 1,634 | 1,682 | 1,782 |
| | | | | | | | | | | | |
| Australia | 26 | 61 | 337 | 790 | 1,076 | 1,209 | 1,218 | 1,317 | 1,546 | 1,706 | - |
| Austria | 14 | 44 | 345 | 829 | 1,855 | 1,564 | 1,650 | 1,727 | 1,953 | 1,999 | 2,092 |
| Belgium | 15 | 44 | 344 | 823 | 1,465 | 1,284 | 1,364 | 1,459 | 1,832 | 1,917 | 2,009 |
| Bulgaria | - | - | - | - | - | 64 | 86 | 98 | 123 | 137 | 158 |
| Canada | 44 | 116 | 331 | 1,041 | 1,155 | 1,370 | 1,488 | 1,494 | 1,634 | 1,653 | 1,885 |
| Cyprus | - | - | - | - | 532 | 586 | 488 | 527 | 632 | 632 | - |
| Czech Republic | - | - | - | 80 | 237 | 239 | 281 | 348 | 408 | 421 | 478 |
| Denmark | 17 | 81 | 523 | 1,234 | 1,791 | 1,636 | 1,781 | 1,888 | 2,196 | 2,275 | 2,392 |
| Estonia | - | - | - | - | 131 | 144 | 155 | 172 | 220 | 250 | - |
| Finland | 16 | 56 | 299 | 1,212 | 1,215 | 1,018 | 1,124 | 1,221 | 1,408 | 1,446 | 1,552 |
| France | 18 | 65 | 390 | 1,028 | 1,696 | 1,419 | 1,519 | 1,628 | 1,985 | 2,036 | 2,155 |
| Germany | 22 | 80 | 498 | 1,155 | 1,983 | 1,566 | 1,663 | 1,737 | 1,947 | 1,910 | 1,994 |
| Greece | - | 32 | 138 | 342 | 674 | 823 | 935 | 1,006 | 1,229 | 1,249 | 1,422 |
| Hungary | - | - | - | 118 | 205 | 215 | 260 | 330 | 421 | 446 | - |
| Iceland | 16 | 51 | 394 | 1,091 | 1,367 | 1,886 | 1,754 | 2,029 | 2,356 | 2,433 | 2,839 |
| Ireland | 9 | 31 | 220 | 463 | 794 | 1,052 | 1,311 | 1,490 | 1,755 | 1,838 | 2,009 |
| Italy | 10 | 44 | 243 | 860 | 914 | 1,017 | 1,109 | 1,180 | 1,333 | 1,413 | 1,499 |
| Japan | 5 | 37 | 253 | 817 | 1,821 | 1,866 | 1,776 | 1,630 | 1,639 | 1,584 | - |
| Korea, Republic of | - | 3 | 26 | 149 | 301 | 343 | 382 | 405 | 423 | 424 | 535 |
| Latvia | - | - | - | - | 73 | 115 | 150 | 165 | 186 | 205 | - |
| Lithuania | - | - | - | - | 53 | 185 | 152 | 175 | 215 | 230 | - |
| Luxembourg | - | 55 | 368 | 987 | 1,767 | 1,786 | 2,016 | 2,295 | 3,036 | 3,315 | - |
| Malta | - | - | - | - | 452 | 533 | 529 | 614 | 677 | 666 | - |
| Mexico | - | - | - | 87 | 112 | 216 | 258 | 262 | 241 | 232 | 255 |
| Netherlands | 14 | 64 | 408 | 881 | 1,427 | 1,265 | 1,436 | 1,604 | 1,846 | 1,869 | - |
| New Zealand | 26 | 50 | 183 | 503 | 759 | 696 | 733 | 835 | 990 | 1,143 | 1,328 |
| Norway | 15 | 60 | 466 | 1,186 | 1,704 | 2,083 | 2,315 | 2,757 | 3,021 | 2,967 | 3,249 |
| Poland | - | - | - | 46 | 125 | 163 | 203 | 219 | 217 | 224 | 272 |
| Portugal | - | 10 | 73 | 251 | 567 | 640 | 686 | 737 | 883 | 903 | 984 |
| Romania | - | - | - | - | - | 58 | 69 | 81 | 81 | 94 | 128 |
| Slovak Republic | - | - | - | - | - | 137 | 150 | 170 | 220 | 308 | 344 |
| Slovenia | - | - | - | - | 540 | 520 | 615 | 657 | 749 | 765 | - |
| Spain | 2 | 17 | 137 | 492 | 714 | 683 | 750 | 804 | 1,006 | 1,070 | 1,179 |
| Sweden | 31 | 125 | 608 | 1,318 | 1,451 | 1,505 | 1,510 | 1,659 | 1,930 | 1,927 | 1,977 |
| Switzerland | 30 | 83 | 551 | 1,627 | 2,758 | 2,357 | 2,623 | 2,810 | 3,080 | 3,076 | 3,129 |
| Turkey | - | 5 | 22 | 59 | 54 | 128 | 110 | 131 | 158 | 178 | 211 |
| UK | 19 | 41 | 217 | 559 | 832 | 1,145 | 1,259 | 1,395 | 1,557 | 1,691 | 1,830 |
| USA | 52 | 146 | 459 | 1,533 | 2,316 | 3,016 | 3,415 | 3,531 | 3,478 | 3,295 | 3,517 |

*Notes:*   Figures are dependent on exchange rates between national currencies and £ sterling over time.
Trends over time should be interpreted with caution as there are several breaks in series (see OECD Health Database for further information).
2005 figures for Belgium, Cyprus, Denmark, Estonia, Japan, Latvia, Lithuania, Malta, Slovak Republic and Slovenia are WHO provisional estimates.
1 Public and private spending.
2 Weighted average. EU15 as constituted before 1 May 2004 and EU27 as constituted since 1 January 2007.
3 OECD figure includes data for 2004 for Australia, Hungary, Japan, Luxembourg and the Netherlands.  EU27 figure includes 2004 data for Cyprus, Estonia, Hungary, Latvia, Lithuania, Luxembourg, Malta, the Netherlands and Slovenia.  EU15 includes 2004 data for Luxembourg and the Netherlands.
- Not available.

*Sources:*   OECD Health Database (OECD).
World Development Indicators (World Bank).
World Health Report: Core Health Indicators (WHO).
World Health Organisation National Health Accounts Series (WHO).
For sources of UK data refer to Table 2.1.

# Total Health Care Expenditure in the UK

Figure 2.6 **Total[1] annual health care expenditure per capita in OECD and EU countries, circa 2005**

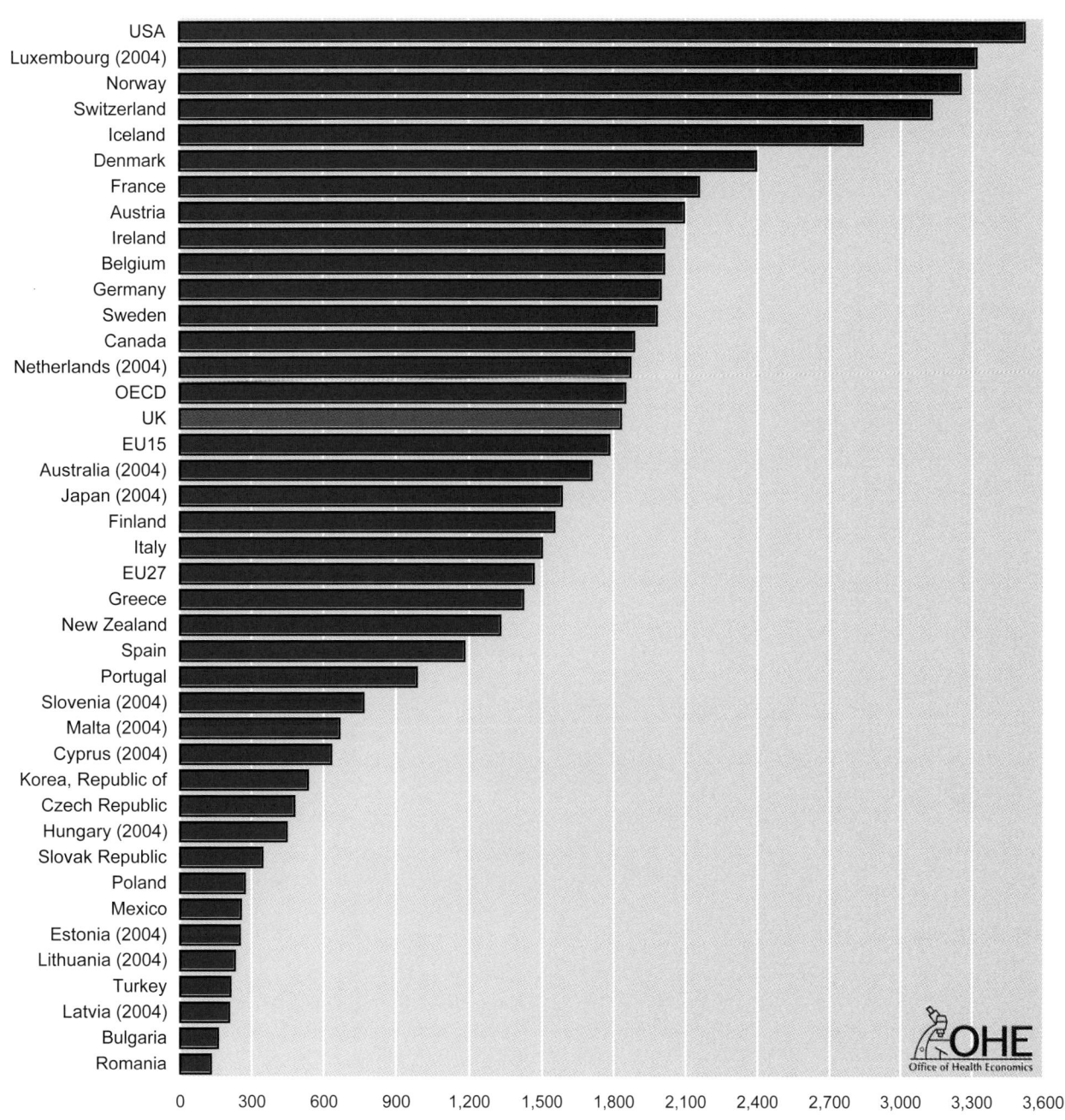

**Total[1] annual health care expenditure per capita (£ cash)**

*Notes:* 1 Public and private spending.

2005 figures for Belgium, Cyprus, Denmark, Estonia, Japan, Latvia, Lithuania, Malta, Slovak Republic and Slovenia are WHO provisional estimates.

Figures are dependent on exchange rates between national currencies and £ sterling over time.

Figures for OECD, EU27 and EU15 are weighted averages.

*Sources:* OECD Health Database (OECD).

World Development Indicators (World Bank).

World Health Report: Core Health Indicators (WHO).

World Health Organisation National Health Accounts Series (WHO).

For sources of UK data refer to Table 2.1.

# Total Health Care Expenditure in the UK

Table 2.4 **Total health care expenditure as per cent of GDP in OECD and EU countries, 1960 - 2005**

**Total health care expenditure as per cent of GDP**

| | Year | | | | | | | | | | |
|---|---|---|---|---|---|---|---|---|---|---|---|
| | 1960 | 1970 | 1980 | 1990 | 1995 | 2000 | 2001 | 2002 | 2003 | 2004 | 2005[2] |
| **OECD**[1] | **4.6** | **6.0** | **7.5** | **8.6** | **9.5** | **10.0** | **10.6** | **10.9** | **11.2** | **11.1** | **11.3** |
| **EU27**[1] | - | - | - | - | - | **8.5** | **8.7** | **9.0** | **9.3** | **9.4** | **9.5** |
| **EU15**[1] | **3.9** | **5.2** | **7.0** | **7.5** | **8.7** | **8.7** | **8.9** | **9.1** | **9.5** | **9.5** | **9.7** |
| Australia | 3.9 | 4.1 | 6.8 | 7.5 | 8.0 | 8.8 | 8.9 | 9.1 | 9.2 | 9.5 | - |
| Austria | 4.3 | 5.2 | 7.5 | 7.0 | 9.8 | 10.0 | 10.0 | 10.1 | 10.2 | 10.3 | 10.2 |
| Belgium | 3.4 | 3.9 | 6.3 | 7.2 | 8.2 | 8.6 | 8.7 | 9.0 | 10.1 | 10.2 | 10.3 |
| Bulgaria | - | - | - | - | - | 6.2 | 7.2 | 7.5 | 7.9 | 8.0 | 8.3 |
| Canada | 5.4 | 6.9 | 7.0 | 8.9 | 9.0 | 8.8 | 9.3 | 9.6 | 9.8 | 9.8 | 9.8 |
| Cyprus | - | - | - | - | - | - | 5.9 | 6.1 | 6.4 | 6.2 | - |
| Czech Republic | - | - | - | 4.7 | 7.0 | 6.5 | 6.7 | 7.1 | 7.4 | 7.3 | 7.2 |
| Denmark | 3.6 | 5.8 | 8.9 | 8.3 | 8.1 | 8.3 | 8.6 | 8.8 | 9.1 | 9.2 | 9.1 |
| Estonia | - | - | - | - | 8.6 | 6.1 | 5.1 | 5.0 | 5.3 | 5.5 | - |
| Finland | 3.8 | 5.5 | 6.3 | 7.7 | 7.5 | 6.6 | 6.7 | 7.0 | 7.3 | 7.4 | 7.5 |
| France | 3.8 | 5.4 | 7.0 | 8.4 | 9.9 | 9.6 | 9.7 | 10.0 | 10.9 | 11.0 | 11.1 |
| Germany | 4.7 | 6.0 | 8.4 | 8.3 | 10.1 | 10.3 | 10.4 | 10.6 | 10.8 | 10.6 | 10.7 |
| Greece | - | 4.7 | 5.1 | 5.8 | 7.5 | 9.3 | 9.8 | 9.7 | 10.0 | 9.6 | 10.1 |
| Hungary | - | - | - | 6.1 | 7.3 | 6.9 | 7.2 | 7.6 | 8.3 | 8.1 | - |
| Iceland | 3.0 | 4.8 | 6.3 | 7.8 | 8.2 | 9.3 | 9.2 | 10.0 | 10.3 | 10.0 | 9.5 |
| Ireland | 3.7 | 5.1 | 8.3 | 6.1 | 6.7 | 6.3 | 7.0 | 7.2 | 7.3 | 7.5 | 7.5 |
| Italy | 3.6 | 5.0 | 6.8 | 7.7 | 7.3 | 8.1 | 8.2 | 8.3 | 8.3 | 8.7 | 8.9 |
| Japan | 3.0 | 4.6 | 6.5 | 6.0 | 6.9 | 7.7 | 7.9 | 8.0 | 8.1 | 8.0 | - |
| Korea, Republic of | - | 2.3 | 3.7 | 4.3 | 4.1 | 4.8 | 5.4 | 5.3 | 5.4 | 5.5 | 6.0 |
| Latvia | - | - | - | - | 6.5 | 5.9 | 6.2 | 6.3 | 6.4 | 6.4 | - |
| Lithuania | - | - | - | - | 5.2 | 6.0 | 6.3 | 6.5 | 6.6 | 6.5 | - |
| Luxembourg | - | 3.1 | 5.2 | 5.4 | 5.6 | 5.8 | 6.4 | 6.8 | 7.8 | 8.3 | - |
| Malta | - | - | - | - | 8.3 | 8.8 | 8.0 | 9.1 | 9.3 | 9.2 | - |
| Mexico | - | - | - | 4.8 | 5.6 | 5.6 | 6.0 | 6.2 | 6.3 | 6.5 | 6.4 |
| Netherlands | 3.7 | 5.6 | 7.5 | 8.0 | 8.3 | 8.0 | 8.3 | 8.9 | 9.1 | 9.2 | - |
| New Zealand | 4.3 | 5.1 | 5.9 | 6.9 | 7.2 | 7.7 | 7.8 | 8.2 | 8.0 | 8.6 | 9.0 |
| Norway | 2.9 | 4.4 | 7.0 | 7.6 | 7.9 | 8.4 | 8.8 | 9.8 | 10.0 | 9.7 | 9.1 |
| Poland | - | - | - | 4.8 | 5.5 | 5.5 | 5.9 | 6.3 | 6.2 | 6.2 | 6.2 |
| Portugal | - | 2.5 | 5.3 | 5.9 | 7.8 | 8.8 | 8.8 | 9.0 | 9.7 | 9.8 | 10.2 |
| Romania | - | - | - | - | - | 5.1 | 5.2 | 5.6 | 4.9 | 4.9 | 5.1 |
| Slovak Republic | - | - | - | - | - | 5.5 | 5.5 | 5.6 | 5.9 | 7.2 | 7.1 |
| Slovenia | - | - | - | - | 9.1 | 8.6 | 9.0 | 8.9 | 8.8 | 8.7 | - |
| Spain | 1.5 | 3.5 | 5.3 | 6.5 | 7.4 | 7.2 | 7.2 | 7.3 | 7.9 | 8.1 | 8.2 |
| Sweden | 4.4 | 6.8 | 9.0 | 8.3 | 8.1 | 8.4 | 8.7 | 9.1 | 9.3 | 9.1 | 9.1 |
| Switzerland | 4.9 | 5.5 | 7.4 | 8.3 | 9.7 | 10.4 | 10.9 | 11.1 | 11.5 | 11.5 | 11.6 |
| Turkey | - | 2.4 | 3.3 | 4.0 | 3.4 | 6.6 | 7.5 | 7.4 | 7.6 | 7.7 | 7.6 |
| UK | 3.9 | 4.5 | 5.3 | 5.7 | 6.7 | 7.1 | 7.5 | 7.9 | 8.3 | 8.5 | 8.9 |
| USA | 5.1 | 7.0 | 8.8 | 11.9 | 13.3 | 13.2 | 13.9 | 14.7 | 15.2 | 15.2 | 15.3 |

*Notes:* 1 Weighted average. EU15 as constituted before 1 May 2004 and EU27 as constituted since 1 January 2007.
2 OECD figure includes 2004 data for Australia, Hungary, Japan, Luxembourg and the Netherlands. EU27 figure includes 2004 data for Cyprus, Estonia, Hungary, Latvia, Lithuania, Luxembourg, Malta, the Netherlands and Slovenia. EU15 figure includes 2004 data for Luxembourg and the Netherlands.
2005 figures for Belgium, Cyprus, Denmark, Estonia, Japan, Latvia, Lithuania, Malta, Slovak Republic and Slovenia are WHO provisional estimates.
GDP = Gross Domestic Product.
- Not available.

*Sources:* OECD Health Database (OECD).
World Development Indicators (World Bank).
World Health Report: Core Health Indicators (WHO).
World Health Organisation National Health Accounts Series (WHO).
For sources of UK data refer to Table 2.1.

# Total Health Care Expenditure in the UK

Table 2.5   Index (2000=100) of total health care expenditure as per cent of GDP in OECD and EU countries, 1960 - 2005

**Index of health care expenditure as per cent of GDP (2000=100)**

| | Year | | | | | | | | | | |
|---|---|---|---|---|---|---|---|---|---|---|---|
| | 1960 | 1970 | 1980 | 1990 | 1995 | 2000 | 2001 | 2002 | 2003 | 2004 | 2005[2] |
| **OECD** | **46** | **60** | **75** | **86** | **95** | **100** | **105** | **109** | **111** | **111** | **118** |
| **EU27[1]** | - | - | - | - | - | **100** | **102** | **105** | **109** | **110** | **112** |
| **EU15[1]** | **45** | **60** | **81** | **87** | **100** | **100** | **102** | **105** | **109** | **110** | **112** |
| Australia | 45 | 47 | 78 | 86 | 91 | 100 | 102 | 105 | 105 | 109 | - |
| Austria | 43 | 52 | 75 | 70 | 98 | 100 | 101 | 101 | 102 | 103 | 103 |
| Belgium | 39 | 45 | 73 | 84 | 95 | 100 | 101 | 104 | 117 | 119 | 119 |
| Bulgaria | - | - | - | - | - | 100 | 117 | 121 | 128 | 131 | 135 |
| Canada | 61 | 78 | 80 | 101 | 102 | 100 | 105 | 109 | 111 | 111 | 111 |
| Cyprus | - | - | - | - | - | 100 | 102 | 105 | 110 | 107 | - |
| Czech Republic | - | - | - | 72 | 107 | 100 | 102 | 108 | 114 | 111 | 109 |
| Denmark | 43 | 70 | 108 | 101 | 98 | 100 | 104 | 106 | 110 | 112 | 110 |
| Estonia | - | - | - | - | - | 100 | 93 | 91 | 96 | 100 | - |
| Finland | 58 | 84 | 95 | 117 | 113 | 100 | 102 | 107 | 111 | 112 | 115 |
| France | 39 | 56 | 73 | 87 | 103 | 100 | 101 | 104 | 114 | 115 | 116 |
| Germany | 46 | 58 | 82 | 80 | 98 | 100 | 101 | 103 | 105 | 103 | 104 |
| Greece | - | 51 | 55 | 62 | 80 | 100 | 106 | 104 | 108 | 104 | 108 |
| Hungary | - | - | - | 88 | 105 | 100 | 103 | 109 | 119 | 117 | - |
| Iceland | 32 | 52 | 68 | 84 | 88 | 100 | 99 | 108 | 111 | 108 | 102 |
| Ireland | 58 | 81 | 132 | 96 | 106 | 100 | 111 | 114 | 116 | 119 | 119 |
| Italy | 44 | 62 | 85 | 96 | 90 | 100 | 102 | 103 | 104 | 108 | 111 |
| Japan | 38 | 59 | 85 | 78 | 89 | 100 | 103 | 104 | 105 | 105 | - |
| Korea, Republic of | - | 49 | 77 | 91 | 87 | 100 | 113 | 111 | 114 | 115 | 125 |
| Latvia | - | - | - | - | - | 100 | 103 | 105 | 107 | 107 | - |
| Lithuania | - | - | - | - | - | 100 | 97 | 100 | 102 | 100 | - |
| Luxembourg | - | 53 | 89 | 92 | 95 | 100 | 109 | 116 | 133 | 141 | - |
| Malta | - | - | - | - | - | 100 | 100 | 114 | 116 | 115 | - |
| Mexico | - | - | - | 87 | 102 | 100 | 107 | 111 | 114 | 116 | 115 |
| Netherlands | 46 | 71 | 94 | 101 | 105 | 100 | 104 | 111 | 115 | 116 | - |
| New Zealand | 55 | 66 | 76 | 89 | 93 | 100 | 101 | 106 | 104 | 112 | 117 |
| Norway | 34 | 52 | 83 | 91 | 94 | 100 | 105 | 116 | 119 | 115 | 108 |
| Poland | - | - | - | 87 | 99 | 100 | 106 | 115 | 113 | 113 | 113 |
| Portugal | - | 28 | 60 | 66 | 88 | 100 | 100 | 102 | 110 | 110 | 115 |
| Romania | - | - | - | - | - | 100 | 103 | 110 | 96 | 97 | 101 |
| Slovak Republic | - | - | - | - | - | 100 | 100 | 102 | 107 | 132 | 130 |
| Slovenia | - | - | - | - | - | 100 | 105 | 103 | 102 | 101 | - |
| Spain | 21 | 49 | 74 | 91 | 103 | 100 | 100 | 101 | 109 | 112 | 114 |
| Sweden | 53 | 82 | 108 | 100 | 96 | 100 | 104 | 109 | 111 | 109 | 109 |
| Switzerland | 47 | 53 | 71 | 79 | 93 | 100 | 105 | 107 | 110 | 111 | 111 |
| Turkey | - | 37 | 50 | 60 | 51 | 100 | 113 | 112 | 114 | 117 | 115 |
| United Kingdom | 55 | 63 | 75 | 81 | 95 | 100 | 106 | 111 | 117 | 120 | 126 |
| United States | 39 | 53 | 66 | 90 | 100 | 100 | 105 | 111 | 115 | 115 | 116 |

*Notes:*   Trends over time should be interpreted with caution as there are several breaks in series (see OECD Health Database for further information).
1 EU15 as constituted before 1 May 2004 and EU27 as constituted since 1 January 2007.
2 OECD figure includes 2004 data for Australia, Hungary, Japan, Luxembourg and the Netherlands. EU27 figure includes 2004 data for Cyprus, Estonia, Hungary, Latvia, Lithuania, Luxembourg, Malta, the Netherlands and Slovenia. EU15 figure includes 2004 data for Luxembourg and the Netherlands.
2005 figures for Belgium, Cyprus, Denmark, Estonia, Japan, Latvia, Lithuania, Malta, Slovak Republic and Slovenia are WHO provisional estimates.
GDP = Gross Domestic Product.
- Not available.

*Sources:*   OECD Health Database (OECD).
World Development Indicators (World Bank).
World Health Report: Core Health Indicators (WHO).
World Health Organisation National Health Accounts Series (WHO).
For sources of UK data refer to Table 2.1.

# Total Health Care Expenditure in the UK

Table 2.6   **GDP per capita in OECD and EU countries (£ cash), 1960 - 2005**

| | Year | | | | | | | | | | |
|---|---|---|---|---|---|---|---|---|---|---|---|
| | 1960 | 1970 | 1980 | 1990 | 1995 | 2000 | 2001 | 2002 | 2003 | 2004 | 2005[2] |
| **OECD**[1] | **548** | **1,235** | **4,060** | **9,760** | **14,054** | **15,003** | **15,532** | **15,486** | **15,844** | **15,611** | **16,461** |
| **EU27**[1] | **391** | **1,011** | **4,484** | **9,662** | **13,211** | **11,576** | **12,291** | **12,862** | **14,286** | **14,646** | **15,414** |
| **EU15**[1] | **391** | **1,011** | **4,484** | **11,084** | **15,067** | **14,085** | **14,872** | **15,521** | **17,231** | **17,605** | **18,396** |
| | | | | | | | | | | | |
| Australia | 671 | 1,484 | 4,969 | 10,477 | 13,456 | 13,810 | 13,636 | 14,395 | 16,797 | 17,910 | 19,933 |
| Austria | 327 | 852 | 4,620 | 11,913 | 18,932 | 15,709 | 16,460 | 17,152 | 19,157 | 19,439 | 20,450 |
| Belgium | 441 | 1,139 | 5,492 | 11,362 | 17,790 | 14,870 | 15,604 | 16,263 | 18,195 | 18,722 | 19,570 |
| Bulgaria | - | - | - | - | - | 1,042 | 1,192 | 1,312 | 1,559 | 1,700 | 1,900 |
| Canada | 810 | 1,683 | 4,708 | 11,745 | 12,791 | 15,539 | 16,003 | 15,577 | 16,743 | 16,951 | 19,301 |
| Cyprus | - | - | - | - | - | 7,678 | 8,278 | 8,635 | 9,870 | 10,190 | - |
| Czech Republic | - | - | - | 1,698 | 3,389 | 3,644 | 4,200 | 4,911 | 5,478 | 5,787 | 6,665 |
| Denmark | 473 | 1,405 | 5,841 | 14,788 | 22,043 | 19,794 | 20,802 | 21,546 | 24,138 | 24,623 | 26,245 |
| Estonia | - | - | - | - | - | 2,638 | 3,042 | 3,450 | 4,154 | 4,548 | - |
| Finland | 415 | 1,013 | 4,754 | 15,744 | 16,298 | 15,474 | 16,716 | 17,380 | 19,243 | 19,637 | 20,579 |
| France | 490 | 1,204 | 5,546 | 12,286 | 17,217 | 14,790 | 15,630 | 16,264 | 18,224 | 18,486 | 19,386 |
| Germany | 470 | 1,327 | 5,915 | 13,932 | 19,646 | 15,201 | 15,925 | 16,319 | 18,009 | 18,031 | 18,667 |
| Greece | 200 | 674 | 2,691 | 5,938 | 9,007 | 8,844 | 9,513 | 10,342 | 12,259 | 12,960 | 14,114 |
| Hungary | - | - | - | 1,930 | 2,815 | 3,100 | 3,634 | 4,370 | 5,098 | 5,517 | 6,013 |
| Iceland | 540 | 1,057 | 6,273 | 13,988 | 16,661 | 20,296 | 19,120 | 20,287 | 22,921 | 24,293 | 29,839 |
| Ireland | 243 | 603 | 2,657 | 7,624 | 11,837 | 16,704 | 18,818 | 20,829 | 24,002 | 24,591 | 26,799 |
| Italy | 292 | 872 | 3,567 | 11,161 | 12,592 | 12,611 | 13,500 | 14,149 | 15,970 | 16,282 | 16,815 |
| Japan | 170 | 809 | 3,872 | 13,669 | 26,478 | 24,270 | 22,343 | 20,463 | 20,274 | 19,690 | 19,568 |
| Korea, Republic of | - | 115 | 719 | 3,444 | 7,266 | 7,184 | 7,067 | 7,644 | 7,775 | 7,725 | 8,962 |
| Latvia | - | - | - | - | - | 2,150 | 2,424 | 2,620 | 2,908 | 3,203 | 3,764 |
| Lithuania | - | - | - | - | - | 2,147 | 2,413 | 2,697 | 3,252 | 3,537 | - |
| Luxembourg | 677 | 1,774 | 7,071 | 18,435 | 31,755 | 30,555 | 31,665 | 33,899 | 39,114 | 40,159 | 44,380 |
| Malta | - | - | - | - | - | 6,442 | 6,618 | 6,744 | 7,275 | 7,236 | - |
| Mexico | - | - | 1,531 | 1,812 | 1,987 | 3,884 | 4,317 | 4,255 | 3,805 | 3,584 | 3,973 |
| Netherlands | 381 | 1,139 | 5,442 | 10,991 | 17,139 | 15,891 | 17,301 | 18,087 | 20,207 | 20,274 | 21,283 |
| New Zealand | 615 | 979 | 3,133 | 7,291 | 10,598 | 9,016 | 9,371 | 10,222 | 12,327 | 13,217 | 14,718 |
| Norway | 528 | 1,370 | 6,697 | 15,525 | 21,630 | 24,738 | 26,300 | 28,160 | 30,175 | 30,741 | 35,862 |
| Poland | - | - | - | 948 | 2,288 | 2,953 | 3,459 | 3,447 | 3,467 | 3,606 | 4,359 |
| Portugal | 119 | 383 | 1,375 | 4,275 | 7,304 | 7,238 | 7,780 | 8,192 | 9,117 | 9,252 | 9,691 |
| Romania | - | - | - | - | - | 1,147 | 1,315 | 1,443 | 1,665 | 1,891 | 2,495 |
| Slovak Republic | - | - | - | - | 2,329 | 2,499 | 2,725 | 3,034 | 3,751 | 4,261 | 4,838 |
| Slovenia | - | - | - | - | - | 6,327 | 6,839 | 7,383 | 8,506 | 8,796 | - |
| Spain | 139 | 491 | 2,592 | 7,538 | 9,592 | 9,478 | 10,364 | 11,082 | 12,806 | 13,261 | 14,332 |
| Sweden | 712 | 1,821 | 6,759 | 15,836 | 17,999 | 18,008 | 17,293 | 18,156 | 20,762 | 21,180 | 21,757 |
| Switzerland | 604 | 1,506 | 7,408 | 19,655 | 28,388 | 22,590 | 24,022 | 25,212 | 26,845 | 26,641 | 26,932 |
| Turkey | 178 | 212 | 665 | 1,502 | 1,593 | 1,936 | 1,473 | 1,765 | 2,089 | 2,310 | 2,773 |
| UK | 490 | 926 | 4,095 | 9,737 | 12,381 | 16,194 | 16,862 | 17,679 | 18,642 | 19,659 | 20,352 |
| USA | 1,025 | 2,086 | 5,234 | 12,911 | 17,471 | 22,839 | 24,542 | 24,074 | 22,944 | 21,669 | 22,986 |

*Notes:*    1 Weighted average. EU15 as constituted before 1 May 2004 and EU27 as constituted since 1 January 2007.
    2 OECD figure include s2004 data for Australia, Hungary, Japan, Luxembourg and the Netherlands. EU27 figure includes 2004 data for Cyprus, Estonia, Hungary, Latvia, Lithuania, Luxembourg, Malta, the Netherlands and Slovenia. EU15 figure includes 2004 data for Luxembourg and the Netherlands.
    GDP = Gross Domestic Product.
    Figures are dependent on exchange rates between national currencies and £ sterling over time.
    Trends over time should be interpreted with caution as there are several breaks in series (see OECD Health Database for further information).
    - Not available.

*Sources:*   OECD Health Database (OECD).
    World Development Indicators (World Bank).
    World Health Report: Core Health Indicators (WHO).
    World Health Organisation National Health Accounts Series (WHO).
    Economic Trends (ONS).

# Total Health Care Expenditure in the UK

Table 2.7   Index of GDP per capita at £ cash prices (2000=100) in OECD and EU countries, 1960 - 2005

**Index of GDP per capita at cash price (2000=100)**

| | Year | | | | | | | | | | |
|---|---|---|---|---|---|---|---|---|---|---|---|
| | 1960 | 1970 | 1980 | 1990 | 1995 | 2000 | 2001 | 2002 | 2003 | 2004 | 2005[2] |
| OECD[1] | 4 | 8 | 27 | 65 | 94 | 100 | 104 | 103 | 106 | 104 | 110 |
| EU27[1] | 3 | 9 | 39 | 83 | 114 | 100 | 106 | 111 | 123 | 127 | 133 |
| EU15[1] | 3 | 7 | 32 | 79 | 107 | 100 | 106 | 110 | 122 | 125 | 131 |
| Australia | 5 | 11 | 36 | 76 | 97 | 100 | 99 | 104 | 122 | 130 | 144 |
| Austria | 2 | 5 | 29 | 76 | 121 | 100 | 105 | 109 | 122 | 124 | 130 |
| Belgium | 3 | 8 | 37 | 76 | 120 | 100 | 105 | 109 | 122 | 126 | 132 |
| Bulgaria | - | - | - | - | - | 100 | 114 | 126 | 150 | 163 | 182 |
| Canada | 5 | 11 | 30 | 76 | 82 | 100 | 103 | 100 | 108 | 109 | 124 |
| Cyprus | - | - | - | - | - | 100 | 108 | 112 | 129 | 133 | - |
| Czech Republic | - | - | - | 47 | 93 | 100 | 115 | 135 | 150 | 159 | 183 |
| Denmark | 2 | 7 | 30 | 75 | 111 | 100 | 105 | 109 | 122 | 124 | 133 |
| Estonia | - | - | - | - | - | 100 | 115 | 131 | 157 | 172 | - |
| Finland | 3 | 7 | 31 | 102 | 105 | 100 | 108 | 112 | 124 | 127 | 133 |
| France | 3 | 8 | 37 | 83 | 116 | 100 | 106 | 110 | 123 | 125 | 131 |
| Germany | 3 | 9 | 39 | 92 | 129 | 100 | 105 | 107 | 118 | 119 | 123 |
| Greece | 2 | 8 | 30 | 67 | 102 | 100 | 108 | 117 | 139 | 147 | 160 |
| Hungary | - | - | - | 62 | 91 | 100 | 117 | 141 | 164 | 178 | 194 |
| Iceland | 3 | 5 | 31 | 69 | 82 | 100 | 94 | 100 | 113 | 120 | 147 |
| Ireland | 1 | 4 | 16 | 46 | 71 | 100 | 113 | 125 | 144 | 147 | 160 |
| Italy | 2 | 7 | 28 | 89 | 100 | 100 | 107 | 112 | 127 | 129 | 133 |
| Japan | 1 | 3 | 16 | 56 | 109 | 100 | 92 | 84 | 84 | 81 | 81 |
| Korea, Republic of | - | 2 | 10 | 48 | 101 | 100 | 98 | 106 | 108 | 108 | 125 |
| Latvia | - | - | - | - | - | 100 | 113 | 122 | 135 | 149 | 175 |
| Lithuania | - | - | - | - | - | 100 | 112 | 126 | 151 | 165 | - |
| Luxembourg | 2 | 6 | 23 | 60 | 104 | 100 | 104 | 111 | 128 | 131 | 145 |
| Malta | - | - | - | - | - | 100 | 103 | 105 | 113 | 112 | - |
| Mexico | - | - | 39 | 47 | 51 | 100 | 111 | 110 | 98 | 92 | 102 |
| Netherlands | 2 | 7 | 34 | 69 | 108 | 100 | 109 | 114 | 127 | 128 | 134 |
| New Zealand | 7 | 11 | 35 | 81 | 118 | 100 | 104 | 113 | 137 | 147 | 163 |
| Norway | 2 | 6 | 27 | 63 | 87 | 100 | 106 | 114 | 122 | 124 | 145 |
| Poland | - | - | - | 32 | 77 | 100 | 117 | 117 | 117 | 122 | 148 |
| Portugal | 2 | 5 | 19 | 59 | 101 | 100 | 107 | 113 | 126 | 128 | 134 |
| Romania | - | - | - | - | - | 100 | 115 | 126 | 145 | 165 | 218 |
| Slovak Republic | - | - | - | - | 93 | 100 | 109 | 121 | 150 | 171 | 194 |
| Slovenia | - | - | - | - | - | 100 | 108 | 117 | 134 | 139 | - |
| Spain | 1 | 5 | 27 | 80 | 101 | 100 | 109 | 117 | 135 | 140 | 151 |
| Sweden | 4 | 10 | 38 | 88 | 100 | 100 | 96 | 101 | 115 | 118 | 121 |
| Switzerland | 3 | 7 | 33 | 87 | 126 | 100 | 106 | 112 | 119 | 118 | 119 |
| Turkey | 9 | 11 | 34 | 78 | 82 | 100 | 76 | 91 | 108 | 119 | 143 |
| UK | 3 | 6 | 25 | 60 | 76 | 100 | 104 | 109 | 115 | 121 | 126 |
| USA | 4 | 9 | 23 | 57 | 76 | 100 | 107 | 105 | 100 | 95 | 101 |

*Notes:*   1 Weighted average. EU15 as constituted before 1 May 2004 and EU27 as constituted since 1 January 2007.
2 OECD figure includes 2004 data for Australia, Hungary, Japan, Luxembourg and the Netherlands.  EU27 figure includes 2004 data for Cyprus, Estonia, Hungary, Latvia, Lithuania, Luxembourg, Malta, the Netherlands and Slovenia.  EU15 figure includes 2004 data for Luxembourg and the Netherlands.
Figures are dependent on exchange rates between national currencies and £ sterling over time.
Trends over time should be interpreted with caution as there are several breaks in series (see OECD Health Database for further information).
GDP = Gross Domestic Product.
- Not available.

*Sources:*   OECD Health Database (OECD).
World Development Indicators (World Bank).
World Health Report: Core Health Indicators (WHO).
World Health Organisation National Health Accounts Series (WHO).
Economic Trends (ONS).

# Total Health Care Expenditure in the UK

Table 2.8   **Public health spending as a percentage of total health care expenditure in OECD and EU countries, 1960 - 2005**

**Public health spending as % of total health care expenditure**

| | Year | | | | | | | | | | |
|---|---|---|---|---|---|---|---|---|---|---|---|
| | 1960 | 1970 | 1980 | 1990 | 1995 | 2000 | 2001 | 2002 | 2003 | 2004 | 2005[2] |
| OECD[1] | 40 | 54 | 63 | 60 | 64 | 60 | 60 | 59 | 60 | 61 | 61 |
| EU27[1] | - | - | - | - | - | 77 | 77 | 77 | 77 | 77 | 77 |
| EU15[1] | 72 | 78 | 81 | 79 | 78 | 77 | 77 | 77 | 77 | 77 | 77 |
| | | | | | | | | | | | |
| Australia | 50 | 69 | 63 | 67 | 67 | 68 | 67 | 68 | 67 | 67 | - |
| Austria | 69 | 63 | 69 | 74 | 71 | 76 | 76 | 75 | 75 | 76 | 76 |
| Belgium | 62 | 87 | 83 | 89 | 79 | 76 | 77 | 75 | 72 | 73 | 72 |
| Bulgaria | - | - | - | - | - | 59 | 56 | 60 | 62 | 58 | 58 |
| Canada | 43 | 70 | 76 | 75 | 71 | 70 | 70 | 70 | 70 | 70 | 70 |
| Cyprus | - | - | - | - | - | 42 | 42 | 45 | 49 | 48 | - |
| Czech Republic | - | - | - | 97 | 91 | 90 | 90 | 90 | 90 | 89 | 89 |
| Denmark | 89 | 86 | 88 | 83 | 83 | 82 | 83 | 83 | 84 | 84 | 84 |
| Estonia | - | - | - | - | - | 78 | 79 | 77 | 77 | 76 | - |
| Finland | 54 | 74 | 79 | 81 | 76 | 75 | 76 | 76 | 76 | 77 | 78 |
| France | 62 | 75 | 80 | 77 | 79 | 78 | 78 | 79 | 79 | 79 | 80 |
| Germany | 66 | 73 | 79 | 76 | 82 | 80 | 79 | 79 | 79 | 77 | 77 |
| Greece | - | 43 | 56 | 54 | 52 | 44 | 47 | 47 | 46 | 45 | 43 |
| Hungary | - | - | - | - | 84 | 71 | 69 | 70 | 71 | 71 | - |
| Iceland | 63 | 64 | 88 | 87 | 84 | 82 | 82 | 83 | 82 | 82 | 83 |
| Ireland | 76 | 81 | 82 | 72 | 72 | 73 | 74 | 76 | 77 | 78 | 78 |
| Italy | 83 | 87 | 80 | 80 | 71 | 73 | 75 | 75 | 75 | 76 | 77 |
| Japan | 60 | 70 | 71 | 78 | 83 | 81 | 82 | 81 | 81 | 82 | - |
| Korea, Republic of | - | - | - | 37 | 36 | 47 | 53 | 52 | 52 | 53 | 53 |
| Latvia | - | - | - | - | - | 55 | 51 | 52 | 51 | 52 | - |
| Lithuania | - | - | - | - | - | 70 | 73 | 75 | 76 | 75 | - |
| Luxembourg | - | 89 | 93 | 93 | 92 | 89 | 88 | 90 | 91 | 91 | - |
| Malta | - | - | - | - | - | 77 | 78 | 80 | 80 | 78 | - |
| Mexico | - | - | - | 40 | 42 | 47 | 45 | 44 | 44 | 46 | 45 |
| Netherlands | 33 | 84 | 69 | 67 | 71 | 63 | 63 | 62 | 63 | 62 | - |
| New Zealand | 81 | 80 | 88 | 82 | 77 | 78 | 76 | 78 | 78 | 78 | 78 |
| Norway | 78 | 92 | 85 | 83 | 84 | 82 | 84 | 83 | 84 | 84 | 84 |
| Poland | - | - | - | 92 | 73 | 70 | 72 | 71 | 70 | 69 | 69 |
| Portugal | - | 59 | 64 | 66 | 63 | 73 | 72 | 72 | 73 | 72 | 73 |
| Romania | - | - | - | - | - | 67 | 66 | 65 | 79 | 72 | 75 |
| Slovak Republic | - | - | - | - | - | 89 | 89 | 89 | 88 | 74 | 74 |
| Slovenia | - | - | - | - | - | 78 | 77 | 77 | 76 | 77 | - |
| Spain | 59 | 65 | 80 | 79 | 72 | 72 | 71 | 71 | 70 | 71 | 71 |
| Sweden | 73 | 86 | 93 | 90 | 87 | 85 | 85 | 85 | 85 | 85 | 85 |
| Switzerland | 49 | 60 | 63 | 52 | 54 | 56 | 57 | 58 | 58 | 59 | 60 |
| Turkey | - | 89 | 64 | 92 | 70 | 63 | 68 | 70 | 72 | 72 | 71 |
| UK | 87 | 86 | 92 | 89 | 87 | 85 | 85 | 85 | 86 | 86 | 87 |
| USA | 23 | 36 | 41 | 39 | 45 | 44 | 45 | 45 | 44 | 45 | 45 |

*Notes:*   1 Weighted average. EU15 as constituted before 1 May 2004 and EU27 as constituted since 1 January 2007.

2 OECD figure include s2004 data for Australia, Hungary, Japan, Luxembourg and the Netherlands. EU27 figure includes 2004 data for Cyprus, Estonia, Hungary, Latvia, Lithuania, Luxembourg, Malta, the Netherlands and Slovenia. EU15 figure include s2004 data for Luxembourg and the Netherlands.

2005 figures for Belgium, Cyprus, Denmark, Estonia, Japan, Latvia, Lithuania, Malta, Slovak Republic and Slovenia are WHO provisional estimates.

- Not available.

*Sources:*   OECD Health Database (OECD).

World Development Indicators (World Bank).

World Health Report: Core Health Indicators (WHO).

World Health Organisation National Health Accounts Series (WHO).

For sources of UK data refer to Table 2.1.

# Total Health Care Expenditure in the UK

Table 2.9 **Private health spending as a percentage of total health care expenditure in OECD and EU countries, 1960 - 2005**

**Private health spending as % of total health care expenditure**

| | Year | | | | | | | | | | |
|---|---|---|---|---|---|---|---|---|---|---|---|
| | 1960 | 1970 | 1980 | 1990 | 1995 | 2000 | 2001 | 2002 | 2003 | 2004 | 2005[2] |
| OECD[1] | 60 | 46 | 37 | 40 | 36 | 40 | 40 | 41 | 40 | 39 | 39 |
| EU27[1] | - | - | - | - | - | 23 | 23 | 23 | 23 | 23 | 23 |
| EU15[1] | 28 | 22 | 19 | 21 | 22 | 23 | 23 | 23 | 23 | 23 | 23 |
| Australia | 50 | 31 | 37 | 33 | 33 | 32 | 33 | 32 | 33 | 33 | - |
| Austria | 31 | 37 | 31 | 26 | 29 | 24 | 24 | 25 | 25 | 24 | 24 |
| Belgium | 38 | 13 | 17 | 11 | 21 | 24 | 23 | 25 | 28 | 27 | 28 |
| Bulgaria | - | - | - | - | - | 41 | 44 | 40 | 38 | 42 | 42 |
| Canada | 57 | 30 | 24 | 25 | 29 | 30 | 30 | 30 | 30 | 30 | 30 |
| Cyprus | - | - | - | - | - | 58 | 58 | 55 | 51 | 52 | 52 |
| Czech Republic | - | - | - | 3 | 9 | 10 | 10 | 10 | 10 | 11 | 11 |
| Denmark | 11 | 14 | 12 | 17 | 17 | 18 | 17 | 17 | 16 | 16 | 16 |
| Estonia | - | - | - | - | - | 23 | 21 | 23 | 23 | 24 | - |
| Finland | 46 | 26 | 21 | 19 | 24 | 25 | 24 | 24 | 24 | 23 | 22 |
| France | 38 | 25 | 20 | 23 | 21 | 22 | 22 | 21 | 21 | 21 | 20 |
| Germany | 34 | 27 | 21 | 24 | 18 | 20 | 21 | 21 | 21 | 23 | 23 |
| Greece | - | 57 | 44 | 46 | 48 | 56 | 53 | 53 | 54 | 55 | 57 |
| Hungary | - | - | - | - | 16 | 29 | 31 | 30 | 29 | 29 | - |
| Iceland | 38 | 36 | 12 | 13 | 16 | 18 | 18 | 17 | 18 | 18 | 17 |
| Ireland | 24 | 19 | 18 | 28 | 28 | 27 | 26 | 24 | 23 | 22 | 22 |
| Italy | 17 | 13 | 20 | 20 | 29 | 27 | 25 | 25 | 25 | 24 | 23 |
| Japan | 40 | 30 | 29 | 22 | 17 | 19 | 18 | 19 | 19 | 18 | - |
| Korea, Republic of | - | - | - | 63 | 64 | 53 | 47 | 48 | 48 | 47 | 47 |
| Latvia | - | - | - | - | - | 45 | 49 | 48 | 49 | 48 | - |
| Lithuania | - | - | - | - | - | 30 | 27 | 25 | 24 | 25 | - |
| Luxembourg | - | 11 | 7 | 7 | 8 | 11 | 12 | 10 | 9 | 9 | - |
| Malta | - | - | - | - | - | 24 | 22 | 20 | 20 | 22 | - |
| Mexico | - | - | - | 60 | 58 | 53 | 55 | 56 | 56 | 54 | 55 |
| Netherlands | 67 | 16 | 31 | 33 | 29 | 37 | 37 | 38 | 37 | 38 | - |
| New Zealand | 19 | 20 | 12 | 18 | 23 | 22 | 24 | 22 | 22 | 22 | 22 |
| Norway | 22 | 8 | 15 | 17 | 16 | 18 | 16 | 17 | 16 | 16 | 16 |
| Poland | - | - | - | 8 | 27 | 30 | 28 | 29 | 30 | 31 | 31 |
| Portugal | - | 41 | 36 | 34 | 37 | 27 | 28 | 28 | 27 | 28 | 27 |
| Romania | - | - | - | - | - | 33 | 34 | 35 | 21 | 28 | 25 |
| Slovak Republic | - | - | - | - | - | 11 | 11 | 11 | 12 | 26 | 26 |
| Slovenia | - | - | - | - | - | 22 | 23 | 24 | 24 | 23 | - |
| Spain | 41 | 35 | 20 | 21 | 28 | 28 | 29 | 29 | 30 | 29 | 29 |
| Sweden | 27 | 14 | 7 | 10 | 13 | 15 | 15 | 15 | 15 | 15 | 15 |
| Switzerland | 51 | 40 | 37 | 48 | 46 | 44 | 43 | 42 | 42 | 41 | 40 |
| Turkey | - | 11 | 36 | 8 | 30 | 37 | 32 | 30 | 28 | 28 | 29 |
| UK | 13 | 14 | 8 | 11 | 13 | 15 | 15 | 15 | 14 | 14 | 13 |
| USA | 77 | 64 | 59 | 61 | 55 | 56 | 55 | 55 | 56 | 55 | 55 |

*Notes:* 1 Weighted average. EU15 as constituted before 1 May 2004 and EU27 as constituted since 1 January 2007.
2 OECD figure includes 2004 data for Australia, Hungary, Japan, Luxembourg and the Netherlands. EU27 figure includes 2004 data for Cyprus, Estonia, Hungary, Latvia, Lithuania, Luxembourg, Malta, the Netherlands and Slovenia. EU15 figure includes 2004 data for Luxembourg and the Netherlands.
2005 figures for Belgium, Cyprus, Denmark, Estonia, Japan, Latvia, Lithuania, Malta, Slovak Republic and Slovenia are WHO provisional estimates.
- Not available.

*Sources:* OECD Health Database (OECD).
World Development Indicators (World Bank).
World Health Report: Core Health Indicators (WHO).
World Health Organisation National Health Accounts Series (WHO).
For sources of UK data refer to Table 2.1.

Figure 2.7 **Public and private health spending as a percentage of total health care expenditure, OECD and EU countries, circa 2005**

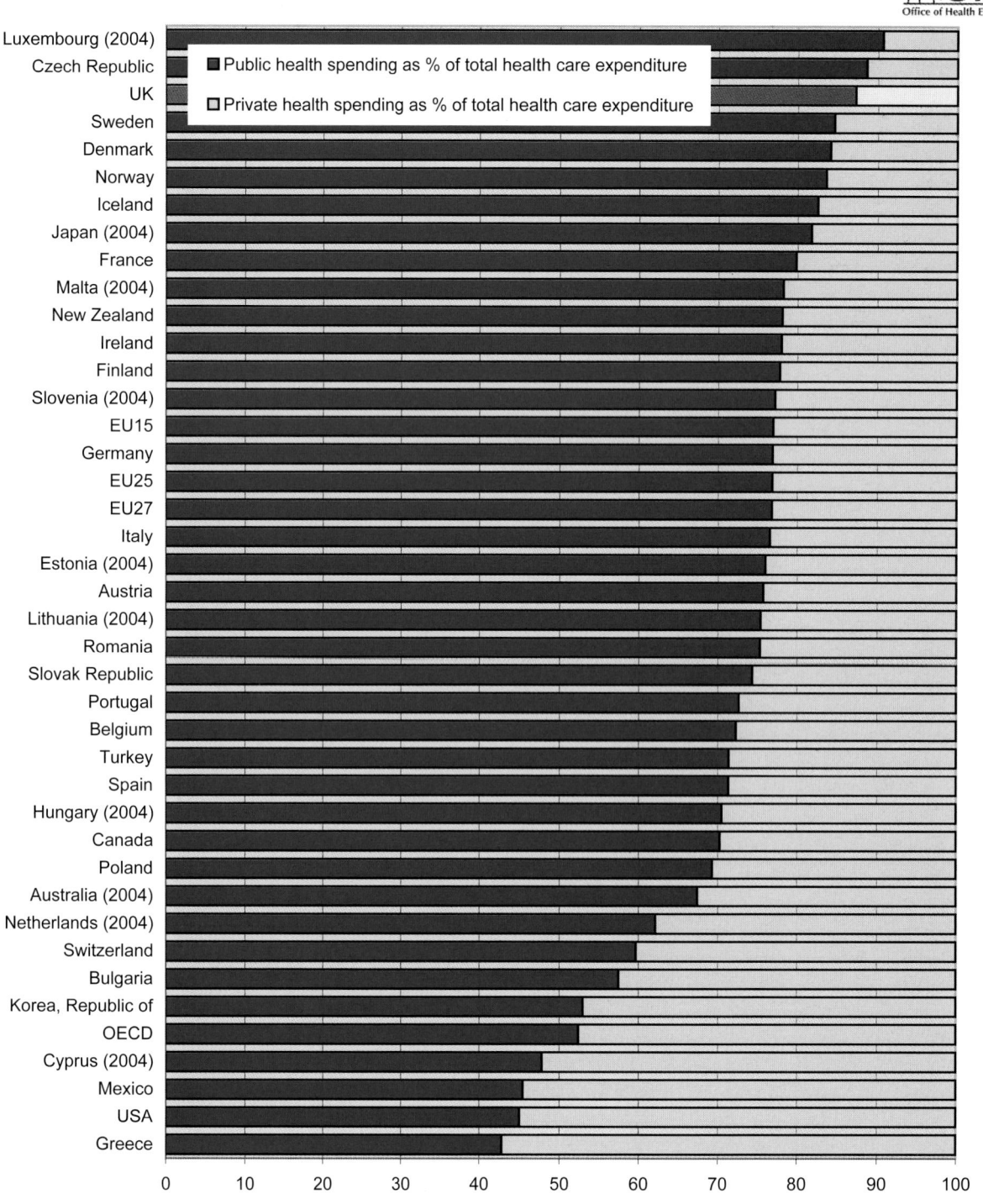

**Public and private health spending as % total health care expenditure**

*Notes:* 2005 figures for Belgium, Cyprus, Denmark, Estonia, Japan, Latvia, Lithuania, Malta, Slovak Republic and Slovenia are WHO provisional estimates,

Figures for OECD, EU27 and EU15 are weighted averages.

EU15 as constituted before 1 May 2004 and EU27 as constituted since 1 January 2007.

*Sources:* OECD Health Database (OECD).

World Development Indicators (World Bank).

World Health Report: Core Health Indicators (WHO).

World Health Organisation National Health Accounts Series (WHO).

For sources of UK data refer to Table 2.1.

Figure 2.8 **Total, public and private health care expenditure as a percentage of GDP\* in OECD and EU countries, circa 2005**

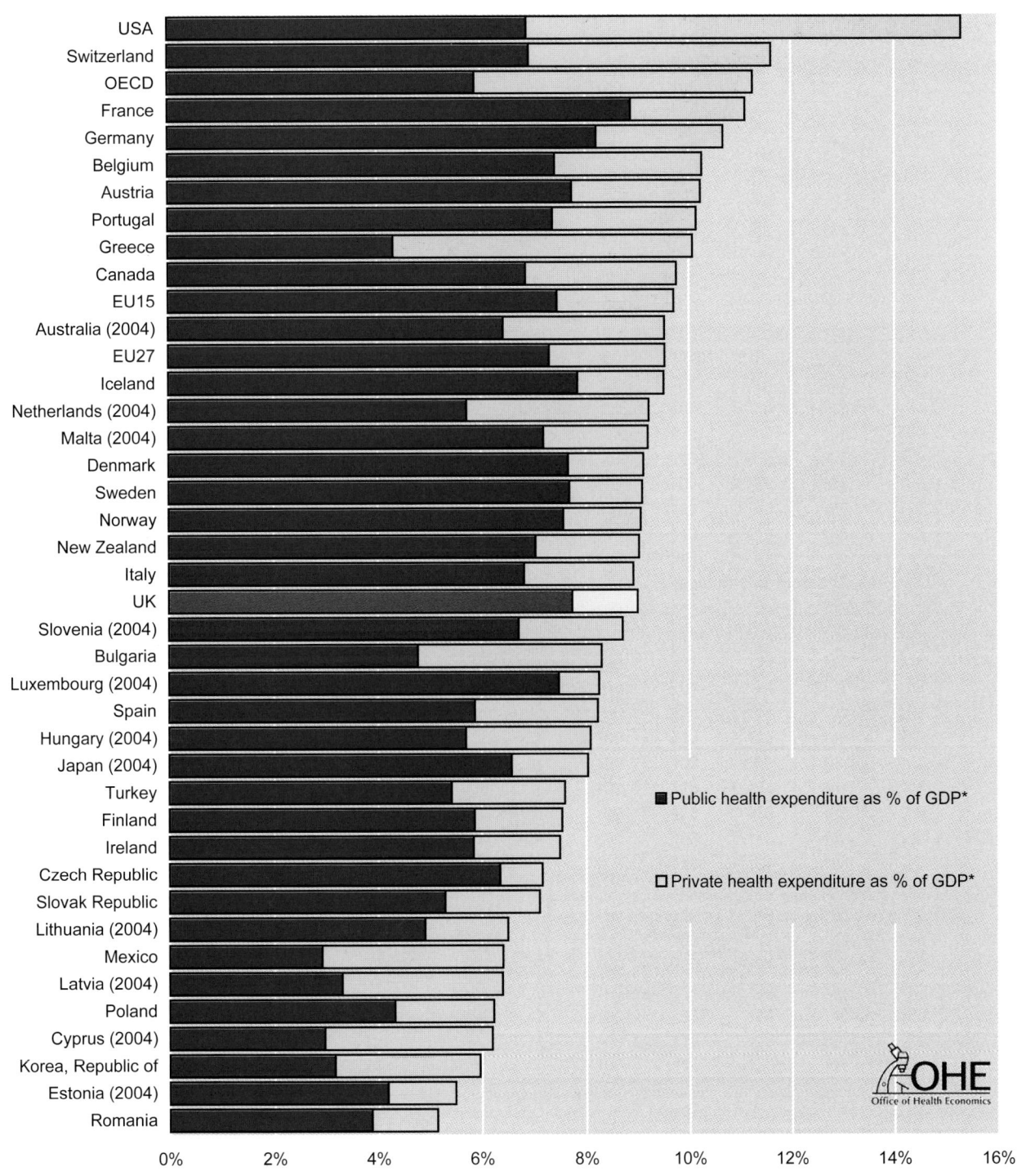

**Total health care expenditure as per cent of GDP\***

*Notes:*    \* GDP = Gross Domestic Product at market prices.

2005 figures for Belgium, Cyprus, Denmark, Estonia, Japan, Latvia, Lithuania, Malta, Slovak Republic and Slovenia are WHO provisional estimates.

Figures for OECD, EU27 and EU15 are weighted averages.

Year is 2005 unless otherwise stated.

*Sources:*   OECD Health Database (OECD).

World Development Indicators (World Bank).

World Health Report: Core Health Indicators (WHO).

World Health Organisation National Health Accounts Series (WHO).

For sources of UK data refer to Table 2.1.

Figure 2.9 **Relationship between total health care spending per capita and GDP[1] per capita in OECD and EU countries, circa 2005**

**Total health care spending per capita (£ cash)**

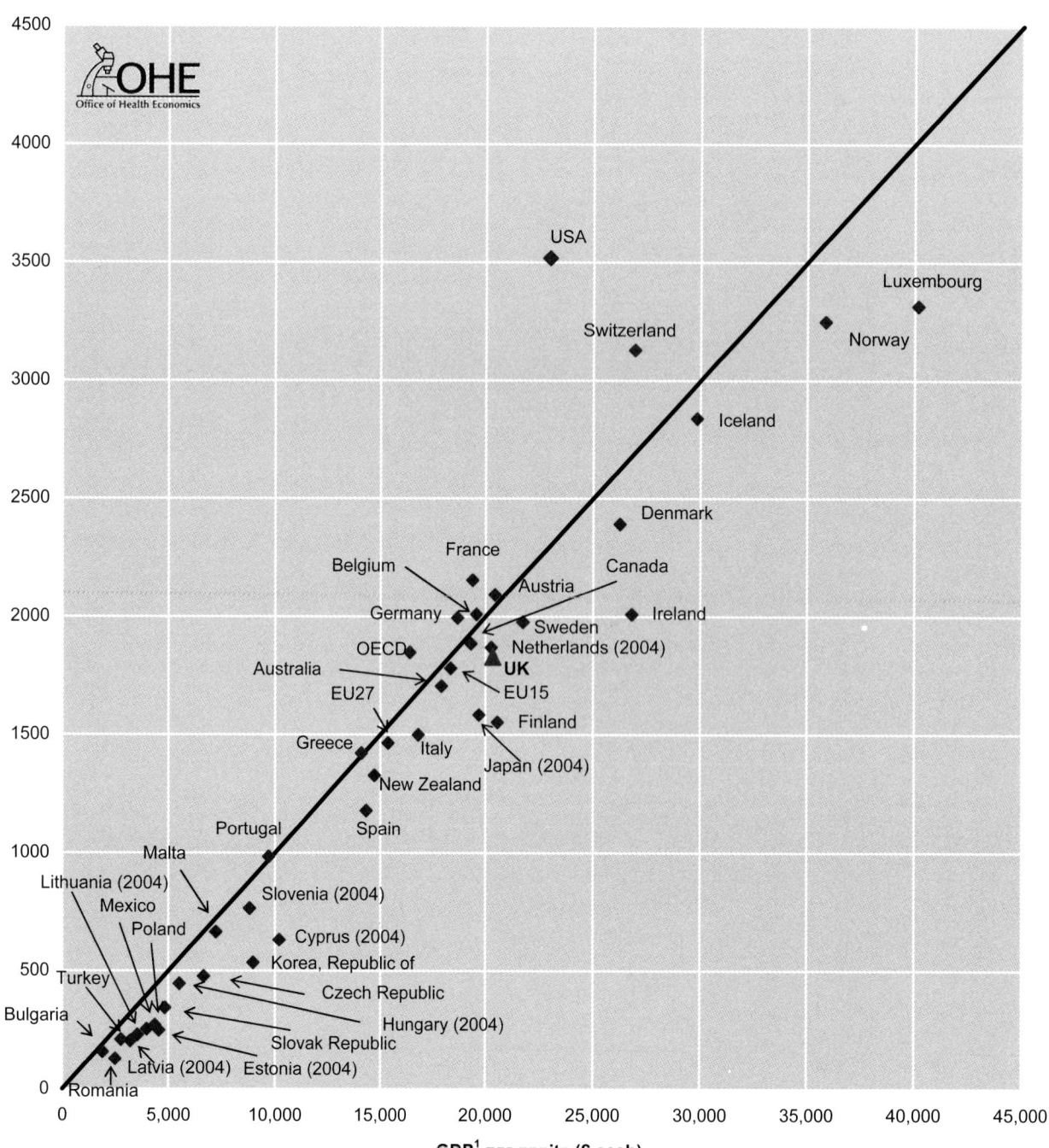

**GDP[1] per capita (£ cash)**

*Notes:* 1 GDP = Gross Domestic Product at market prices.

Figures are dependant on exchange rates between national currencies, US dollars and £ sterling over time.

The solid line is a reference line. Countries on the line have total health spending equal to 10 per cent of GDP. Countries above the line spend more, those below it spend less.

See Table 2.3.

*Sources:* OECD Health Database (OECD).

World Development Indicators (World Bank).

World Health Report: Core Health Indicators (WHO).

World Health Organisation National Health Accounts Series (WHO).

For sources of UK data refer to Table 2.1 and Table 1.20.

Economic Trends (ONS).

# Total Health Care Expenditure in the UK

Table 2.10 **Total health care expenditure, infant mortality and life expectancy in OECD and EU countries, 1960 and 2005**

| | Health care expenditure as % of GDP[1] | | Health care expenditure per capita £ cash[1] | | Infant mortality rate[2] | | Male life expectancy[3] | |
|---|---|---|---|---|---|---|---|---|
| | 1960 | 2005 | 1960 | 2005 | 1960 | 2005 | 1960 | 2005 |
| **OECD** | **4.5** | **11.3** | **22** | **1,741** | **38.3** | **6.0** | **66** | **76** |
| **EU27** | **-** | **9.5** | **-** | **1,377** | **35.4** | **5.4** | **67** | **74** |
| **EU15** | **3.8** | **9.7** | **15** | **1,682** | **32.6** | **3.9** | **68** | **77** |
| Australia | 3.9 | 9.5 | 26 | 1,706 | 20.2 | 5.0 | 68 | 79 |
| Austria | 4.3 | 10.2 | 14 | 2,092 | 37.5 | 4.2 | 65 | 77 |
| Belgium | 3.4 | 10.3 | 15 | 2,009 | 23.9 | 3.7 | 68 | 76 |
| Bulgaria | - | 8.3 | - | 158 | 24.9 | 11.6 | - | 69 |
| Canada | 5.4 | 9.8 | 44 | 1,885 | 27.3 | 5.3 | 71 | 78 |
| Cyprus | - | 6.2 | - | 632 | - | 4.5 | - | 77 |
| Czech Republic | - | 7.2 | - | 478 | 20.0 | 3.4 | 68 | 73 |
| Denmark | 3.6 | 9.1 | 17 | 2,392 | 21.5 | 4.4 | 70 | 76 |
| Estonia | - | 5.5 | - | 250 | - | 5.7 | - | 66 |
| Finland | 3.8 | 7.5 | 16 | 1,552 | 21.0 | 3.0 | 66 | 76 |
| France | 3.8 | 11.1 | 18 | 2,155 | 27.5 | 3.6 | 67 | 77 |
| Germany | 4.7 | 10.7 | 22 | 1,994 | 35.0 | 3.9 | 67 | 76 |
| Greece | - | 10.1 | - | 1,422 | 40.1 | 3.8 | 67 | 77 |
| Hungary | - | 8.1 | - | 446 | 47.6 | 6.2 | 66 | 69 |
| Iceland | 3.0 | 9.5 | 16 | 2,839 | 13.0 | 2.3 | 71 | 79 |
| Ireland | 3.7 | 7.5 | 9 | 2,009 | 29.3 | 4.0 | 68 | 77 |
| Italy | 3.6 | 8.9 | 10 | 1,499 | 43.9 | 4.7 | 70 | 78 |
| Japan | 3.0 | 8.0 | 5 | 1,584 | 30.7 | 2.8 | 65 | 79 |
| Korea, Republic of | - | 6.0 | - | 535 | - | 5.3 | 51 | 75 |
| Latvia | - | 6.4 | - | 205 | - | 9.8 | - | 66 |
| Lithuania | - | 6.5 | - | 230 | - | 7.5 | - | 66 |
| Luxembourg | - | 8.3 | - | 3,315 | 31.5 | 2.6 | 67 | 76 |
| Malta | - | 9.2 | - | 666 | - | 5.3 | - | 76 |
| Mexico | - | 6.4 | - | 255 | 74.0 | 18.8 | 56 | 73 |
| Netherlands | 3.7 | 9.2 | 14 | 1,869 | 17.9 | 4.9 | 72 | 77 |
| New Zealand | 4.3 | 9.0 | 26 | 1,328 | 22.6 | 5.1 | 69 | 78 |
| Norway | 2.9 | 9.1 | 15 | 3,249 | 18.9 | 3.1 | 71 | 78 |
| Poland | - | 6.2 | - | 272 | 54.8 | 6.4 | 65 | 71 |
| Portugal | - | 10.2 | - | 984 | 77.5 | 3.5 | 61 | 75 |
| Romania | - | 5.1 | - | 128 | 78.5 | 16.8 | - | 68 |
| Slovak Republic | - | 7.1 | - | 344 | 28.6 | 7.2 | 68 | 70 |
| Slovenia | - | 8.7 | - | 765 | - | 4.0 | - | 73 |
| Spain | 1.5 | 8.2 | 2 | 1,179 | 43.7 | 4.1 | 67 | 77 |
| Sweden | 4.4 | 9.1 | 31 | 1,977 | 16.6 | 2.4 | 71 | 78 |
| Switzerland | 4.9 | 11.6 | 30 | 3,129 | 21.1 | 4.2 | 69 | 79 |
| Turkey | - | 7.6 | - | 211 | 189.5 | 23.6 | 46 | 69 |
| UK | 3.9 | 9.0 | 19 | 1,830 | 22.5 | 5.1 | 68 | 77 |
| USA | 5.1 | 15.3 | 52 | 3,517 | 26.0 | 6.8 | 67 | 75 |

*Notes:* EU15 as constituted before 1 May 2004 and EU27 as constituted since 1 January 2007.

Figures are for 2005 unless specified otherwise.

1 Figures relate to public and private health expenditure as a percentage of GDP and per capita and figures for the OECD, EU27 and EU15 are weighted averages. 2005 figures for Belgium, Cyprus, Denmark, Estonia, Japan, Latvia, Lithuania, Malta, Slovak Republic and Slovenia are WHO provisional estimates. Figures in italics are for 2004.

2 Infant deaths per 1,000 live births. Figures for the OECD, EU27 and EU15 are unweighted averages.

Figures in italics are for 2004 except for Korea which relate to 2002.

3 Figures for the OECD, EU27 and EU15 are unweighted averages. Figures in italics are for 2004.

GDP = Gross Domestic Product.

- Not available.

*Sources:* See Table 2.9.

For sources of UK data refer to Table 2.1 and Table 1.20.

Life Tables (GAD).

# Total Health Care Expenditure in the UK

Table 2.11   Relative indices (UK=100) for total health care expenditure, infant mortality and life expectancy in OECD and EU countries, 1960 and 2005

| | Health care expenditure as % of GDP[1] | | Health care expenditure per capita £ cash[1] | | Infant mortality rate[2] | | Male life expectancy[3] | |
|---|---|---|---|---|---|---|---|---|
| | 1960 | 2005 | 1960 | 2055 | 1960 | 2005 | 1960 | 2005 |
| **OECD** | **115** | **125** | **115** | **95** | **170** | **118** | **97** | **98** |
| **EU27** | **-** | **106** | **-** | **75** | **157** | **106** | **99** | **96** |
| **EU15** | **98** | **108** | **78** | **92** | **145** | **76** | **99** | **100** |
| Australia | 101 | *106* | 139 | *93* | 90 | 98 | 99 | 102 |
| Austria | 110 | 114 | 73 | 114 | 167 | 82 | 96 | 100 |
| Belgium | 87 | 114 | 78 | 110 | 106 | 73 | 99 | 99 |
| Bulgaria | - | 92 | - | 9 | 111 | *228* | - | 90 |
| Canada | 139 | 109 | 230 | 103 | 121 | *104* | 105 | *101* |
| Cyprus | - | 69 | - | 35 | - | 88 | - | *100* |
| Czech Republic | - | 80 | - | 26 | 89 | 67 | 99 | 95 |
| Denmark | 91 | 101 | 88 | 131 | 96 | *86* | 103 | 98 |
| Estonia | - | *61* | - | *14* | - | 112 | - | *86* |
| Finland | 99 | 84 | 83 | 85 | 93 | 59 | 96 | 98 |
| France | 97 | 124 | 97 | 118 | 122 | 71 | 98 | 100 |
| Germany | 121 | 119 | 116 | 109 | 156 | 76 | 98 | 99 |
| Greece | - | 112 | - | 78 | 178 | 75 | 99 | 100 |
| Hungary | - | 90 | - | 24 | 212 | 122 | 96 | 89 |
| Iceland | 77 | 106 | 85 | 155 | 58 | 45 | 104 | 103 |
| Ireland | 94 | 83 | 47 | 110 | 130 | 78 | 100 | 100 |
| Italy | 92 | 99 | 55 | 82 | 195 | 92 | 102 | 101 |
| Japan | 76 | *89* | 26 | *87* | 136 | 55 | 96 | 102 |
| Korea, Republic of | - | 66 | - | 29 | - | *104* | 75 | 98 |
| Latvia | - | *71* | - | *11* | - | 192 | - | *86* |
| Lithuania | - | *72* | - | *13* | - | 147 | - | *86* |
| Luxembourg | - | 92 | - | *181* | 140 | 51 | 97 | 99 |
| Malta | - | *102* | - | *36* | - | *104* | - | 99 |
| Mexico (1997) | - | 71 | - | 14 | 329 | 369 | 82 | 95 |
| Netherlands | 95 | *103* | 74 | *102* | 80 | 96 | 105 | 100 |
| New Zealand | 110 | 100 | 137 | 73 | 100 | 100 | 101 | 101 |
| Norway | 74 | 101 | 80 | 178 | 84 | 61 | 104 | 101 |
| Poland | - | 69 | - | 15 | 244 | 125 | 95 | 92 |
| Portugal | - | 113 | - | 54 | 344 | 69 | 90 | 97 |
| Romania | - | 57 | - | 7 | 349 | *330* | - | 88 |
| Slovak Republic | - | 79 | - | *19* | 127 | 141 | 100 | 91 |
| Slovenia | - | 97 | - | *42* | - | 78 | - | *95* |
| Spain | 38 | 92 | 11 | 64 | 194 | 80 | 99 | 101 |
| Sweden | 113 | 101 | 164 | 108 | 74 | 47 | 104 | 102 |
| Switzerland | 126 | 129 | 155 | 171 | 94 | 82 | 101 | 102 |
| Turkey | - | 84 | - | 12 | 842 | 463 | 68 | 90 |
| UK | 100 | 100 | 100 | 100 | 100 | 100 | 100 | 100 |
| USA | 131 | 170 | 274 | 192 | 116 | *133* | 98 | *98* |

Notes:    EU15 as constituted before 1 May 2004 and EU27 as constituted since 1 January 2007.
Figures are for 2005 unless specified otherwise.
1 Figures relate to public and private health expenditure as a percentage of GDP and per capita and figures for the OECD, EU27 and EU15 are weighted averages.  2005 figures for Belgium, Cyprus, Denmark, Estonia, Japan, Latvia, Lithuania, Malta, Slovak Republic and Slovenia are WHO provisional estimates.  Figures in italics are for 2004.
2 Infant deaths per 1,000 live births.  Figures for the OECD, EU27 and EU15 are unweighted averages.
Figures in italics are for 2004 except  for Korea which relate to 2002.
3 Figures for the OECD, EU27 and EU15 are unweighted averages. Figures in italics are for 2004.
GDP = Gross Domestic Product.
- Not available.
Sources:  See Table 2.9.
For sources of UK data refer to Table 2.1 and Table 1.20.
Life Tables (GAD).

**Figure 2.10** **Relationship between total health care expenditure per capita[1] and infant mortality rate[2] in OECD and EU countries, circa 2005**

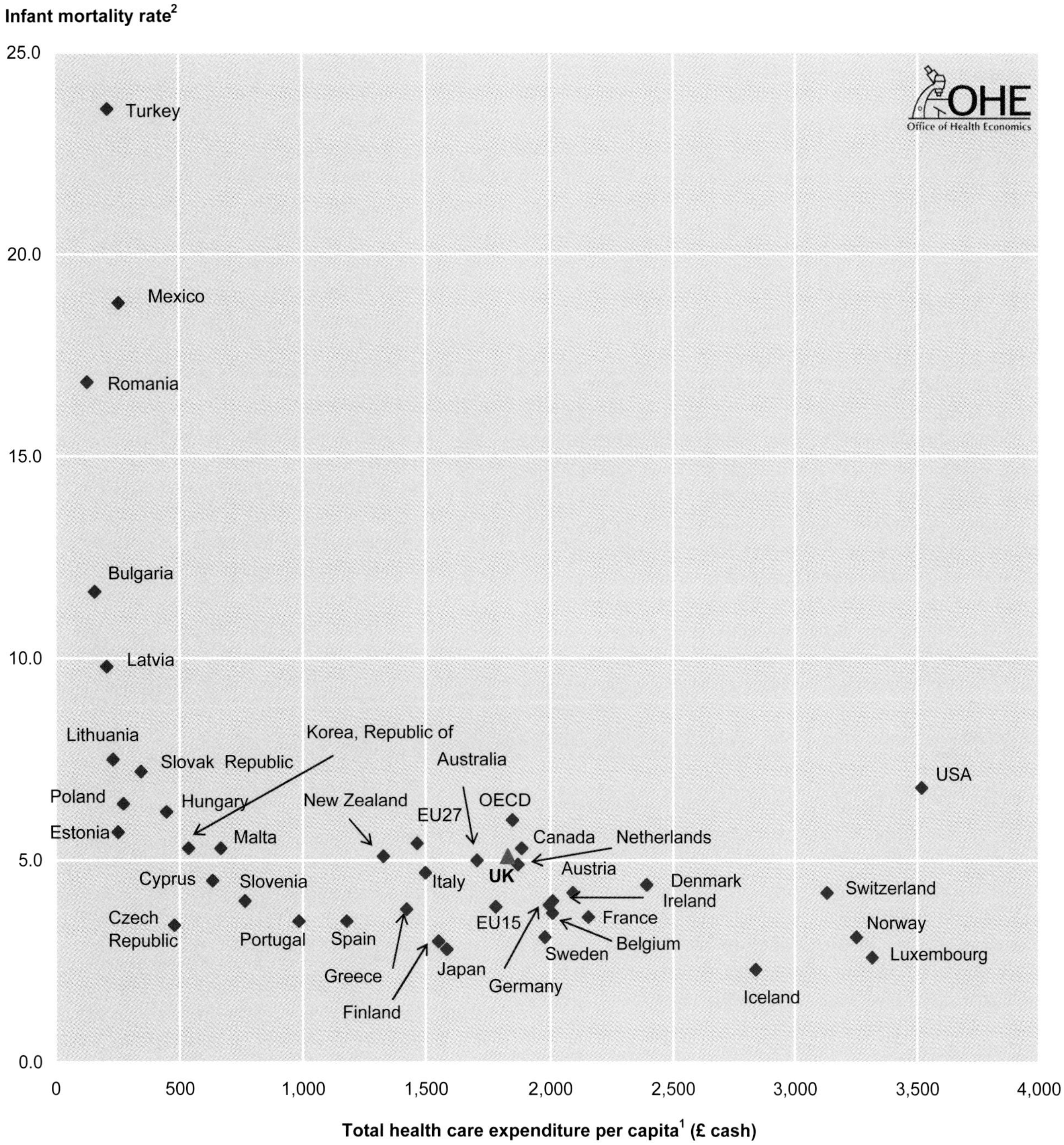

**Infant mortality rate[2]**

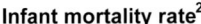

*Figure showing scatter plot of infant mortality rate versus total health care expenditure per capita (£ cash) for OECD and EU countries. Countries plotted include Turkey, Mexico, Romania, Bulgaria, Latvia, Lithuania, Slovak Republic, Poland, Hungary, Estonia, Malta, Cyprus, Slovenia, Czech Republic, Portugal, Spain, Greece, Finland, Japan, Germany, Korea Republic of, New Zealand, Australia, OECD, EU27, Italy, UK, EU15, Canada, Netherlands, Austria, France, Belgium, Sweden, Denmark, Ireland, Iceland, Switzerland, Norway, Luxembourg, USA.*

**Total health care expenditure per capita[1] (£ cash)**

*Notes:* 1 Public and private spending. 2005 figures for Belgium, Cyprus, Denmark, Estonia, Japan, Latvia, Lithuania, Malta, Slovak Republic and Slovenia are WHO provisional estimates.
 Infant deaths (aged under 1 year) per 1,000 live births.
 See Table 2.10 for years of data related to each country.
*Sources:* OECD Health Database (OECD).
 World Development Indicators (World Bank).
 World Health Reports: Core Indicators (WHO).
 World Health Organisation National Health Accounts Series (WHO).
 For sources of UK data refer to Table 2.1 and Table 1.20.

# Cost of the NHS

## The National Health Service (NHS)

The UK health care market is dominated by the National Health Service (NHS), which, according to the World Health Organisation (WHO), is amongst the largest public health care services in the world. The UK NHS was established on 5 July 1948, with the aim of providing a comprehensive range of health services to all UK citizens, financed by general taxation and free at the point of use.

The responsibility for the provision and development of health services lies ultimately with the Secretary of State for Health in England, the Minister for Health and Community Care for Scotland, the Minister for Health and Social Services for Wales and the Minister for Health, Social Services and Public Safety for Northern Ireland. They are supported by the Department of Health (DH) in England, the Scottish Executive Department of Health in Scotland, the NHS Directorate in Wales, and the Department of Health, Social Services and Public Safety (DHSSPS) in Northern Ireland. Devolution has created a Parliament for Scotland which took on its full powers on 1 July 1999. These include competence over matters such as health, education and housing. In Wales, the National Assembly (NAW) was set up at the same time with powers to shape delivery of health services there. However, unlike the Scottish Parliament, the Welsh Assembly does not have law-making power over the running of the NHS. The Northern Ireland Assembly is takes an active role in shaping health services in the Province.

## NHS expenditure

In 2006/07, total expenditure on the main healthcare services of the NHS was estimated at £104 billion, (**Table 2.1**). This represents a 137% increase in cash terms on expenditure compared to just 10 years earlier. Since 1999 there has been a particularly steep increase in expenditure on the NHS (**Figure 2.11**). **Box 2** indicates the considerably higher rate of rise between 2001/02 and 2006/07, compared to earlier years.

NHS gross cost in the UK was estimated to be £1,715 per person and £4,033 per household in 2006/07 (**Table 2.13**). This represents approximately eight times the per capita cost of the NHS when it was first established, after allowing for inflation. NHS net expenditure per capita has been consistently highest in Scotland and lowest in England (**Table 2.22**). In 2005/06 NHS expenditure was £1,745 per capita in Scotland, compared to £1,569 in Northern Ireland, £1,422 in Wales, and £1,500 in England. Public expenditure on health in the UK was above the average observed across both EU and OECD countries in 2005 (**Table**

2.16). The strong positive relationship between public health spending per capita and GDP at market prices per capita across EU and OECD countries can be seen in **Figure 2.15**.

| Box 2 | **Change (per cent) in UK real NHS cost[1] and GDP in five year periods** | | | |
|---|---|---|---|---|
| Year | Total NHS[1] | NHS per capita[1] | Real GDP[1] | NHS as a % of GDP |
| 1981/82 - 1986/87 | 12 | 11 | 17 | -4 |
| 1986/87 - 1991/92 | 25 | 24 | 11 | 13 |
| 1991/92 - 1996/97 | 16 | 15 | 14 | 2 |
| 1996/97 - 2001/02 | 31 | 29 | 16 | 13 |
| 2001/02 - 2006/07 | 41 | 38 | 14 | 24 |

Notes: All figures include charges paid by patients.
1 At constant prices, as adjusted by the GDP deflator.
Sources: Annual Abstract of Statistics (ONS).
The Governments' Expenditure Plans (DH).

In 1949/50 expenditure on the NHS was 3.5% of GDP. This figure had reached an estimated 7.9% of GDP by 2006/07 (**Table 2.12** and **Figure 2.11**). Over the past 50 years the variation of health care expenditure as a fraction of GDP with GDP itself has shown marked cyclical fluctuations, but has been on a steadily upward path since 1998/90 (**Figure 2.13**).

Public expenditure on health care in the UK as a share of GDP is now slightly above average compared to the EU15 countries, reversing the pattern seen in the 1970s, 1980s and 1990s, where expenditure as a percentage of GDP was below average the EU15 average in the UK (**Table 2.14**). The increase in public health care spend as a share of national income seen in the UK since 2000 is amongst the highest observed across the EU and OECD, with only Bulgaria, Turkey and Luxembourg having greater increases (**Table 2.15**). Despite this substantial increase the UK is still below Germany and France with regards to the proportion of GDP spent on public health care (**Table 2.14**).

The pay bill is the single largest component of the NHS budget. Expenditure on salaries and wages accounts for 60% of total Hospital and Community Health Services expenditure in England (**Figure 2.17** and **Table 2.20**). Although NHS Foundation Trusts remain part of the NHS, the purchase of services from Foundation Trusts is not broken down into the constituent elements of salaries and wages, capital charges, etc. As the number of Foundation Trusts increases over time this element of expenditure can be expected to increase (**Table 2.20**).

# Cost of the NHS

## NHS workforce

According to the Office of National Statistics, those employed in the NHS increased to 1.5 million in 2007, more than double the number employed in 1970 (**Table 2.21**). **Figure 2.18** shows the particularly steep increase in the number of employees in the NHS since 2000, and the high proportion of public sector staff who were employed in the NHS.

## NHS expenditure by sector

Since the foundation of the NHS, the largest portion of its expenditure has been absorbed by hospital services, but this proportion is now down from nearly two thirds at its peak in the 1970s to 46% (**Table 2.24**). The share of General Medical Services is now at its highest for 40 years. Pharmaceutical services have grown as a share of total NHS spend since the early 1980s but peaked in 1999/00 and have since fallen back to 10.7 per cent.

NHS expenditures on Hospital, Community and Family Health Services (except for ophthalmic services) in the UK have all increased over the past 30 years after adjusting for inflation (**Table 2.23** and **Box 3**).

HCHS per capita expenditure across age groups in England has not been produced since 2003/04, at that time those aged over 84 had the greatest per capita spend, an estimated £3,136, (**Figure 2.16**). The lowest per capita spend on HCHS was for those in the age group 5 to 15, at an estimated £203. Of the total HCHS gross expenditure, 4% was spent on births, 10% on children under 16, 39% on those aged 16-64 and another 47% on those aged 65 and above (**Table 2.19**).

The NHS reforms of 1991 led to new accounting methods, resulting in difficulty in distinguishing between the costs of hospital services and community health services. The HCHS budget now aggregates expenditure on hospital, community health and various minor services formerly classified under 'other' services, plus the cash limited expenditure of family health and related services (FHS). Only the FHS Pharmaceutical, Dental and Ophthalmic Services were unaffected by these changes.

## Sources of NHS finance

In 2006, 80.3% of NHS funding came from taxes and 18.4% from NHS contributions paid by employers and employees via the National Insurance Scheme. Contributions from patient payments reached £1.3 billion in 2006 but remain a small proportion of NHS funding at just 1.0%. **Table 2.26** shows the amount of patient charges for hospital services, prescriptions and dental care across the UK for over 50 years, and indicates that dental charges have been the largest category of patient charges for the last decade. Since 1999/00 the NHS has been the fastest growing area of UK public expenditure (**Figure 2.19**), reaching an estimated 18.1% of all public expenditure in 2006/07 (**Table 2.27**).

| Box 3 | NHS per capita gross expenditure (£) by sector, at 2005/06 prices[1] | | | |
|---|---|---|---|---|
| Year | HCHS[2] | Ratio of HCHS to FHS | FHS[3] | All NHS |
| 1995/96 | 636 | 2.8 | 228 | 938 |
| 1996/97 | 595 | 2.5 | 235 | 939 |
| 1998/99 | 622 | 2.5 | 246 | 983 |
| 1999/00 | 660 | 2.5 | 262 | 1052 |
| 2000/01 | 709 | 2.6 | 275 | 1127 |
| 2001/02 | 738 | 2.6 | 287 | 1212 |
| 2002/03 | 781 | 2.6 | 298 | 1303 |
| 2003/04 | 832 | 2.6 | 315 | 1430 |
| 2004/05 | 892 | 2.5 | 359 | 1501 |
| 2005/06 | 950 | 2.5 | 371 | 1612 |

Notes: All figures include charges paid by patients.
1 As adjusted by the GDP deflator, at market prices.
2 Hospital and Community Health Services.
3 Family Health Services, including Pharmaceutical, Medical, Dental and Ophthalmic Services.

Sources: NHS Summarised Accounts (House of Commons).
The Government's Expenditure Plans (DH).
Annual Abstract of Statistics (ONS).

Table 2.12 **GDP and NHS expenditure, UK, 1949/50 - 2006/07**

| Year | GDP at market prices (£ billion) | NHS expenditure | | | Total NHS as % of GDP | Total NHS cost per head £ cash | Total NHS cost | |
|---|---|---|---|---|---|---|---|---|
| | | Public[1] £m | Patients[2] £m | Total £m | | | At 1949 prices[3] £m | Index[3] 1949=100 |
| 1949/50 | 12.75 | 447 | - | 447 | 3.50 | 9 | 447 | 100 |
| 1950/51 | 13.54 | 474 | 8 | 482 | 3.56 | 10 | 471 | 105 |
| 1954/55 | 18.31 | 522 | 27 | 550 | 3.00 | 11 | 438 | 98 |
| 1955/56 | 19.62 | 567 | 29 | 596 | 3.03 | 12 | 464 | 104 |
| 1959/60 | 24.45 | 773 | 37 | 811 | 3.31 | 16 | 529 | 118 |
| 1960/61 | 26.05 | 839 | 45 | 883 | 3.39 | 17 | 568 | 127 |
| 1964/65 | 33.94 | 1,123 | 48 | 1,171 | 3.45 | 22 | 680 | 152 |
| 1965/66 | 36.37 | 1,273 | 33 | 1,306 | 3.59 | 24 | 723 | 162 |
| 1969/70 | 47.61 | 1,738 | 56 | 1,795 | 3.77 | 32 | 839 | 188 |
| 1970/71 | 52.93 | 1,983 | 64 | 2,046 | 3.87 | 37 | 882 | 197 |
| 1972/73 | 67.18 | 2,594 | 90 | 2,684 | 3.99 | 48 | 979 | 219 |
| 1973/74 | 74.80 | 3,075 | 100 | 3,176 | 4.25 | 56 | 1,083 | 242 |
| 1974/75 | 89.27 | 4,048 | 109 | 4,158 | 4.66 | 74 | 1,185 | 265 |
| 1975/76 | 111.30 | 5,244 | 115 | 5,358 | 4.81 | 95 | 1,218 | 272 |
| 1976/77 | 129.93 | 6,093 | 131 | 6,224 | 4.79 | 111 | 1,246 | 279 |
| 1977/78 | 151.17 | 6,804 | 147 | 6,951 | 4.60 | 124 | 1,225 | 274 |
| 1978/79 | 172.96 | 7,750 | 164 | 7,914 | 4.58 | 141 | 1,255 | 281 |
| 1979/80 | 208.06 | 9,246 | 209 | 9,456 | 4.54 | 168 | 1,283 | 287 |
| 1980/81 | 237.00 | 11,396 | 281 | 11,677 | 4.93 | 207 | 1,341 | 300 |
| 1981/82 | 260.08 | 12,883 | 346 | 13,229 | 5.09 | 235 | 1,387 | 310 |
| 1982/83 | 284.12 | 13,962 | 401 | 14,363 | 5.06 | 255 | 1,406 | 315 |
| 1983/84 | 309.17 | 14,926 | 444 | 15,371 | 4.97 | 273 | 1,438 | 322 |
| 1984/85 | 331.80 | 15,872 | 476 | 16,349 | 4.93 | 290 | 1,453 | 325 |
| 1985/86 | 363.99 | 17,012 | 502 | 17,514 | 4.81 | 310 | 1,476 | 330 |
| 1986/87 | 389.76 | 18,481 | 567 | 19,048 | 4.89 | 336 | 1,555 | 348 |
| 1987/88 | 433.26 | 21,176 | 653 | 21,829 | 5.04 | 384 | 1,687 | 377 |
| 1988/89 | 482.43 | 23,421 | 831 | 24,252 | 5.03 | 426 | 1,752 | 392 |
| 1989/90 | 528.22 | 25,180 | 989 | 26,169 | 4.95 | 458 | 1,764 | 395 |
| 1990/91 | 567.39 | 27,980 | 1,198 | 29,178 | 5.14 | 509 | 1,824 | 408 |
| 1991/92 | 598.71 | 31,757 | 1,287 | 33,044 | 5.52 | 575 | 1,947 | 436 |
| 1992/93 | 619.52 | 34,961 | 1,272 | 36,233 | 5.85 | 629 | 2,068 | 463 |
| 1993/94 | 656.35 | 36,431 | 1,132 | 37,563 | 5.72 | 650 | 2,089 | 467 |
| 1994/95 | 693.61 | 39,515 | 917 | 40,432 | 5.83 | 698 | 2,215 | 496 |
| 1995/96 | 734.28 | 41,407 | 919 | 42,326 | 5.76 | 729 | 2,251 | 503 |
| 1996/97 | 778.72 | 43,056 | 865 | 43,921 | 5.64 | 755 | 2,259 | 505 |
| 1997/98 | 829.02 | 45,321 | 919 | 46,240 | 5.58 | 792 | 2,311 | 517 |
| 1998/99 | 876.27 | 47,825 | 945 | 48,770 | 5.57 | 833 | 2,377 | 532 |
| 1999/00 | 927.33 | 52,403 | 1,026 | 53,429 | 5.76 | 910 | 2,553 | 571 |
| 2000/01 | 971.32 | 57,210 | 1,069 | 58,279 | 6.00 | 989 | 2,745 | 614 |
| 2001/02 | 1,013.37 | 63,232 | 1,198 | 64,430 | 6.36 | 1,089 | 2,964 | 663 |
| 2002/03 | 1,071.47 | 70,373 | 1,284 | 71,657 | 6.69 | 1,207 | 3,197 | 715 |
| 2003/04 | 1,136.19 | 79,888 | 1,371 | 81,259 | 7.15 | 1,363 | 3,523 | 788 |
| 2004/05 | 1,195.52 | 86,864 | 1,277 | 88,141 | 7.37 | 1,470 | 3,719 | 832 |
| 2005/06 | 1,249.28 | 95,987 | 1,243 | 97,230 | 7.78 | 1,612 | 4,018 | 899 |
| 2006/07e | 1,322.58 | 102,784 | 1,315 | 104,099 | 7.87 | 1,715 | 4,185 | 936 |

*Notes:* 1 Excluding patient charges.
2 Figures relate to NHS charges paid by patients for prescription medicines etc (see also Table 2.19). Data on patient charges from 2004/05 onwards is not strictly comparable with previous uears, see Table 2.26 for further information.
3 Figures have been adjusted by the GDP deflator at market prices.
e = OHE estimates, based on published data shown in italics.
GDP = Gross Domestic Product.

*Sources:* Consumer Trends (ONS).
Annual Abstract of Statistics (ONS).
Economic Trends (ONS).
The Government's Expenditure Plans (DH).
Department of Health Departmental Report (DH).
Health Statistics Wales (NAW).
NHS Board Operating Costs and Capital Expenditure, ISD Scotland (ISD).
Public Expenditure Statistical Analyses (HM Treasury).
Laing's Healthcare Market Review (Laing and Buisson).
Population Projections Database (GAD).

# Cost of the NHS

Table 2.13 **GDP[1] and NHS expenditure per capita, UK, 1949/50 - 2006/07**

| Year | GDP[1] per capita £ cash | NHS gross cost per: Person £ cash | NHS gross cost per: Household £ cash | GDP[1] per capita Real index[2] | NHS gross cost per: Person Real index[2] | NHS gross cost per: Household Real index[2] |
|---|---|---|---|---|---|---|
| 1949/50 | 253 | 9 | 32 | 100 | 100 | 100 |
| 1950/51 | 268 | 10 | 33 | 103 | 105 | 104 |
| 1954/55 | 360 | 11 | 35 | 114 | 97 | 88 |
| 1955/56 | 385 | 12 | 37 | 118 | 103 | 91 |
| 1958/59 | 446 | 14 | 45 | 120 | 110 | 96 |
| 1959/60 | 470 | 16 | 47 | 121 | 115 | 97 |
| 1960/61 | 496 | 17 | 51 | 126 | 122 | 104 |
| 1964/65 | 628 | 22 | 64 | 144 | 142 | 119 |
| 1965/66 | 668 | 24 | 73 | 146 | 150 | 128 |
| 1966/67 | 705 | 26 | 79 | 148 | 157 | 132 |
| 1967/68 | 743 | 28 | 84 | 151 | 165 | 138 |
| 1968/69 | 803 | 30 | 91 | 156 | 168 | 142 |
| 1969/70 | 858 | 32 | 96 | 158 | 170 | 142 |
| 1970/71 | 950 | 37 | 108 | 162 | 179 | 148 |
| 1971/72 | 1,057 | 42 | 121 | 165 | 186 | 152 |
| 1972/73 | 1,197 | 48 | 138 | 173 | 197 | 160 |
| 1973/74 | 1,330 | 56 | 160 | 179 | 217 | 173 |
| 1974/75 | 1,588 | 74 | 213 | 179 | 238 | 193 |
| 1975/76 | 1,980 | 95 | 272 | 178 | 244 | 196 |
| 1976/77 | 2,312 | 111 | 313 | 183 | 250 | 199 |
| 1977/78 | 2,690 | 124 | 347 | 187 | 246 | 194 |
| 1978/79 | 3,078 | 141 | 393 | 193 | 252 | 198 |
| 1979/80 | 3,698 | 168 | 466 | 198 | 257 | 201 |
| 1980/81 | 4,207 | 207 | 570 | 191 | 268 | 208 |
| 1981/82 | 4,617 | 235 | 637 | 191 | 277 | 212 |
| 1982/83 | 5,047 | 255 | 687 | 195 | 282 | 213 |
| 1983/84 | 5,488 | 273 | 729 | 203 | 288 | 216 |
| 1984/85 | 5,878 | 290 | 768 | 206 | 290 | 217 |
| 1985/86 | 6,432 | 310 | 814 | 214 | 294 | 218 |
| 1986/87 | 6,872 | 336 | 876 | 222 | 309 | 227 |
| 1987/88 | 7,624 | 384 | 993 | 233 | 335 | 244 |
| 1988/89 | 8,470 | 426 | 1,090 | 242 | 347 | 250 |
| 1989/90 | 9,248 | 458 | 1,163 | 246 | 348 | 249 |
| 1990/91 | 9,904 | 509 | 1,284 | 245 | 359 | 255 |
| 1991/92 | 10,417 | 575 | 1,441 | 242 | 382 | 269 |
| 1992/93 | 10,752 | 629 | 1,569 | 242 | 404 | 284 |
| 1993/94 | 11,365 | 650 | 1,617 | 250 | 408 | 285 |
| 1994/95 | 11,979 | 698 | 1,729 | 259 | 431 | 301 |
| 1995/96 | 12,647 | 729 | 1,799 | 266 | 437 | 304 |
| 1996/97 | 13,380 | 755 | 1,857 | 272 | 438 | 303 |
| 1997/98 | 14,207 | 792 | 1,947 | 280 | 446 | 309 |
| 1998/99 | 14,972 | 833 | 2,041 | 288 | 458 | 316 |
| 1999/00 | 15,788 | 910 | 2,220 | 298 | 490 | 337 |
| 2000/01 | 16,479 | 989 | 2,398 | 307 | 525 | 359 |
| 2001/02 | 17,128 | 1,089 | 2,618 | 311 | 565 | 382 |
| 2002/03[3] | 18,044 | 1,207 | 2,884 | 318 | 607 | 408 |
| 2003/04[3] | 19,054 | 1,363 | 3,242 | 326 | 666 | 446 |
| 2004/05[3] | 19,944 | 1,470 | 3,487 | 332 | 699 | 467 |
| 2005/06[3] | 20,709 | 1,612 | 3,806 | 338 | 751 | 499 |
| 2006/07e[3] | 21,795 | 1,715 | 4,033 | 346 | 777 | 515 |

*Notes:*   1 GDP = Gross Domestic Product at market prices.
2 At constant prices, as adjusted by the GDP deflator at market prices.
3 Household numbers are based on OHE estimates.
e = OHE estimates based on published data, shown in italics.  2006/07 GDP at market prices is an outturn figure, not an OHE estimate.

*Sources:*   Regional Trends (ONS).
Household estimates and projections (DCLG).
Household projections (GROS).
Household data (NISRA).
See also Table 2.1.

Figure 2.11  **Gross cost of NHS, in cash and real terms and NHS cost as a per cent of GDP, UK, 1949/50 - 2006/07**

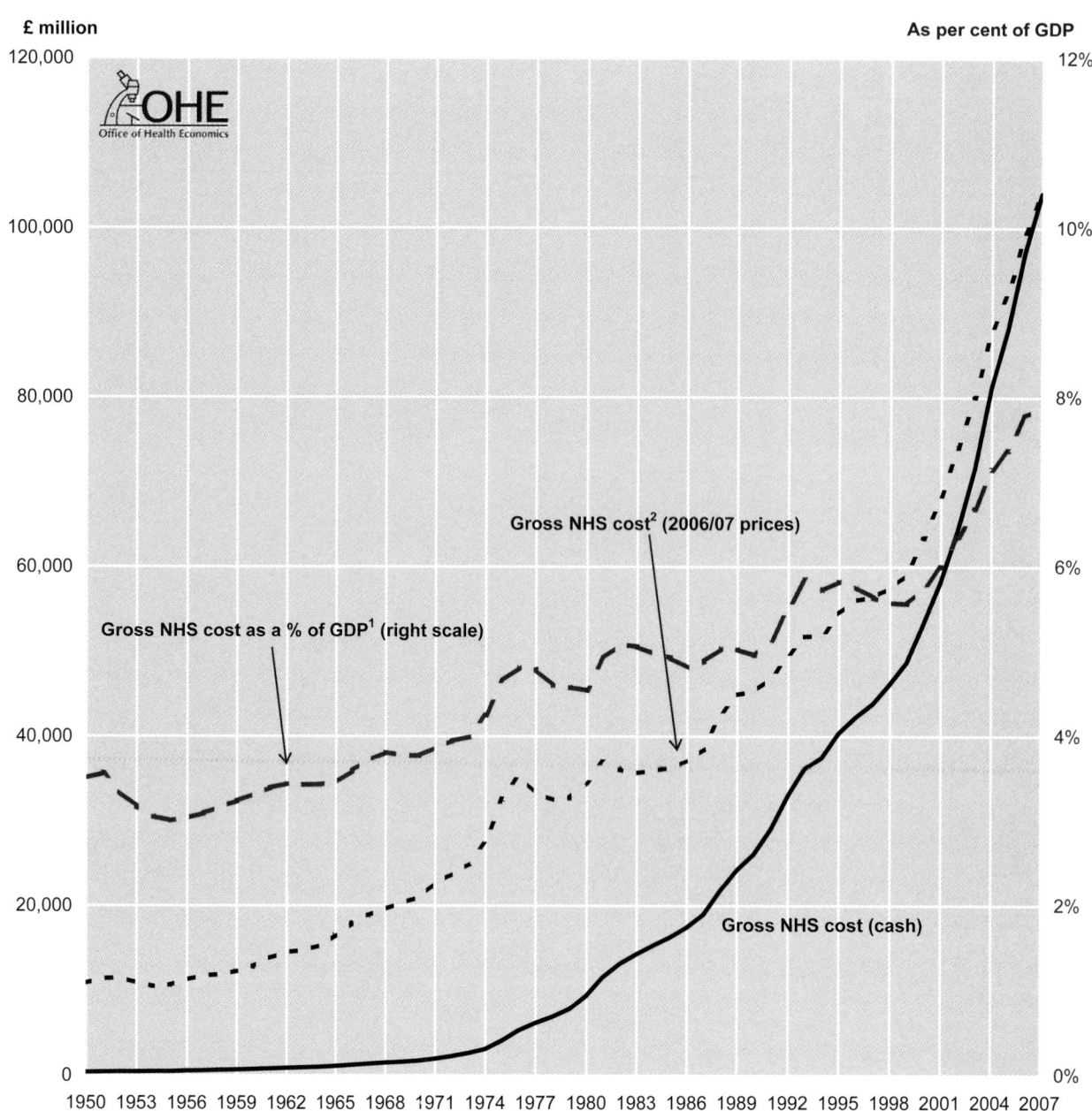

**£ million**

**As per cent of GDP**

Gross NHS cost[2] (2006/07 prices)

Gross NHS cost as a % of GDP[1] (right scale)

Gross NHS cost (cash)

**Financial year ending**

*Notes:*   All figures include charges paid by patients.
Figures are for financial year ending 31 March (e.g. 2007 = 2006/07).
1 GDP = Gross Domestic Product at market prices.
2 As adjusted by the GDP deflator at market prices.
2006/07 figures are OHE estimates.

*Sources:*   Consumer Trends (ONS).
Annual Abstract of Statistics (ONS).
Economic Trends (ONS).
The Government's Expenditure Plans (DH).
Department of Health Departmental Report (DH).
Health Statistics Wales (NAW).
NHS Board Operating Costs and Capital Expenditure, ISD Scotland (ISD).
Public Expenditure Statistical Analyses (HM Treasury).
Laing's Healthcare Market Review (Laing and Buisson).
Population Projections Database (GAD).

Figure 2.12 **Relationship between gross NHS cost and GDP[1], UK, 1949/50 - 2006/07**

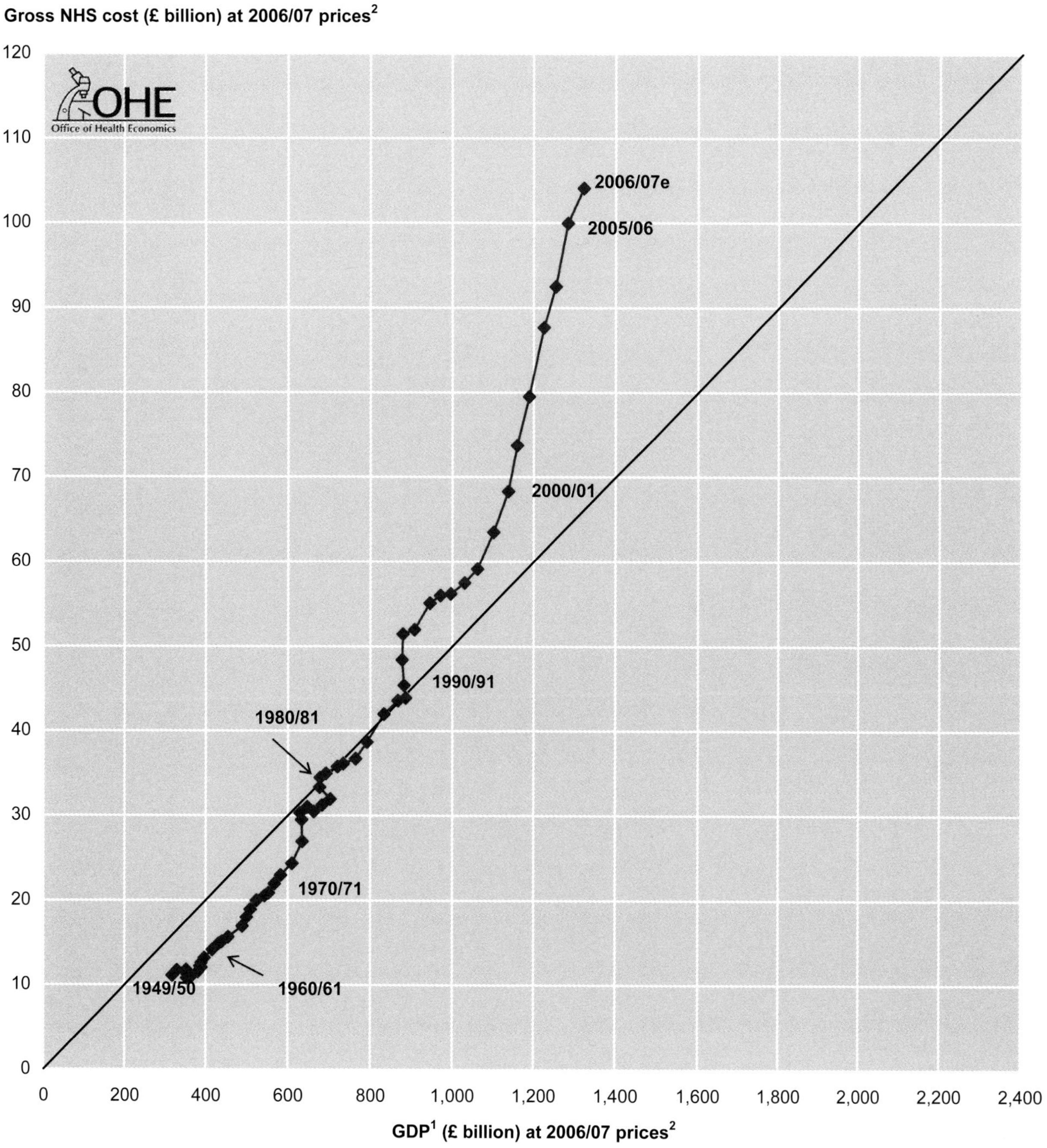

**Gross NHS cost (£ billion) at 2006/07 prices[2]**

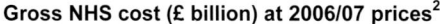

**GDP[1] (£ billion) at 2006/07 prices[2]**

*Notes:* 1 GDP = Gross Domestic Product at market prices.
2 As adjusted by the GDP deflator at market prices.
The solid line shown is a reference line, indicating where points would lie if NHS gross costs were equal to five per cent of GDP.
e = OHE estimate based on published data..

*Sources:* Consumer Trends (ONS).
Annual Abstract of Statistics (ONS).
Economic Trends (ONS).
The Government's Expenditure Plans (DH).
Department of Health Departmental Report (DH).
Health Statistics Wales (NAW).
NHS Board Operating Costs and Capital Expenditure, ISD Scotland (ISD).
Public Expenditure Statistical Analyses (HM Treasury).
Laing's Healthcare Market Review (Laing and Buisson).
Population Projections Database (GAD).

Figure 2.13  **Relationship between NHS cost as a percentage of GDP and GDP [1], UK, 1949/50 - 2006/07**

**NHS gross cost as per cent of GDP at 2006/07 prices [2]**

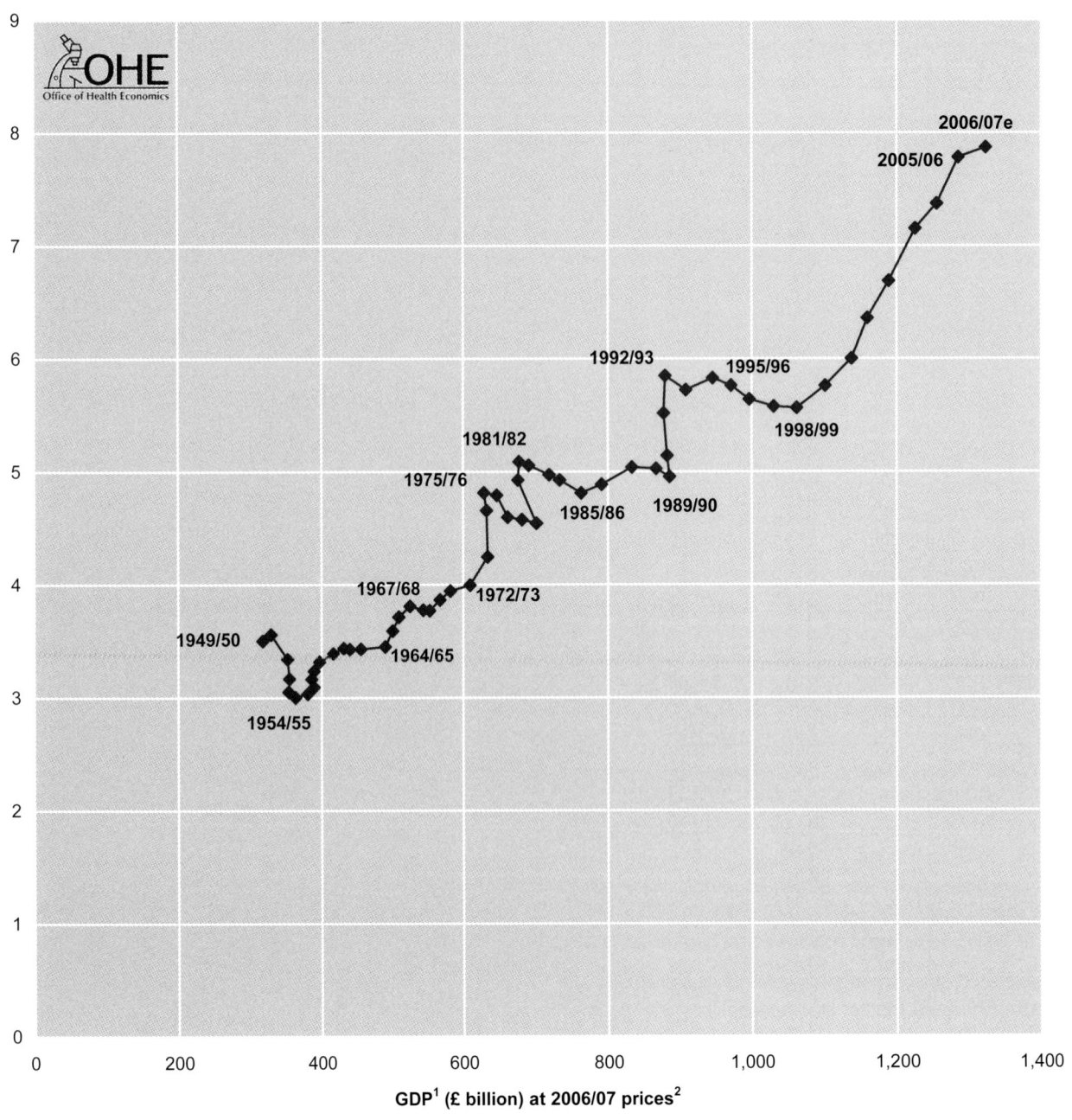

**GDP [1] (£ billion) at 2006/07 prices [2]**

Notes:     1 GDP = Gross Domestic Product at market prices.
           2 As adjusted by the GDP deflator at market prices.
           e = OHE estimate based on published data.

Sources:  Consumer Trends (ONS).
          Annual Abstract of Statistics (ONS).
          Economic Trends (ONS).
          The Government's Expenditure Plans (DH).
          Department of Health Departmental Report (DH).
          Health Statistics Wales (NAW).
          NHS Board Operating Costs and Capital Expenditure, ISD Scotland (ISD).
          Public Expenditure Statistical Analyses (HM Treasury).
          Laing's Healthcare Market Review (Laing and Buisson).
          Population Projections Database (GAD).

Table 2.14    **Public health expenditure[1] as a percentage of GDP at market prices, in OECD and EU countries, 1960 - 2005**

**Public health expenditure as a percentage of GDP**

| | Year | | | | | | | | | | |
|---|---|---|---|---|---|---|---|---|---|---|---|
| | 1960 | 1970 | 1980 | 1990 | 1995 | 2000 | 2001 | 2002 | 2003 | 2004 | 2005[3] |
| OECD[2] | 1.8 | 3.3 | 4.6 | 5.1 | 6.0 | 6.0 | 6.3 | 6.5 | 6.7 | 6.8 | 6.9 |
| EU27[2] | - | - | - | - | - | 6.6 | 6.7 | 6.9 | 7.2 | 7.2 | 7.3 |
| EU15[2] | 2.7 | 4.1 | 5.7 | 5.9 | 6.8 | 6.7 | 6.8 | 7.0 | 7.3 | 7.3 | 7.5 |
| Australia | 2.0 | 2.9 | 4.3 | 5.1 | 5.3 | 6.0 | 6.0 | 6.2 | 6.2 | 6.4 | - |
| Austria | 3.0 | 3.3 | 5.1 | 5.1 | 7.0 | 7.6 | 7.6 | 7.6 | 7.7 | 7.8 | 7.7 |
| Belgium | 2.1 | 3.4 | 5.2 | 6.4 | 6.5 | 6.6 | 6.7 | 6.7 | 7.2 | 7.5 | 7.4 |
| Bulgaria | - | - | - | - | - | 3.7 | 4.0 | 4.5 | 4.9 | 4.6 | 4.8 |
| Canada | 2.3 | 4.8 | 5.3 | 6.6 | 6.4 | 6.2 | 6.5 | 6.7 | 6.8 | 6.8 | 6.9 |
| Cyprus | - | - | - | - | - | 2.4 | 2.5 | 2.7 | 3.1 | 3.0 | - |
| Czech Republic | - | - | - | 4.6 | 6.4 | 5.9 | 6.0 | 6.4 | 6.7 | 6.5 | 6.4 |
| Denmark | 3.2 | 5.0 | 7.9 | 6.9 | 6.7 | 6.8 | 7.1 | 7.3 | 7.7 | 7.8 | 7.7 |
| Estonia | - | - | - | - | - | 4.3 | 4.0 | 3.9 | 4.1 | 4.2 | - |
| Finland | 2.1 | 4.1 | 5.0 | 6.2 | 5.6 | 4.9 | 5.1 | 5.4 | 5.6 | 5.7 | 5.9 |
| France | 2.4 | 4.1 | 5.6 | 6.4 | 7.7 | 7.5 | 7.6 | 7.9 | 8.6 | 8.7 | 8.9 |
| Germany | 3.1 | 4.4 | 6.6 | 6.3 | 8.2 | 8.2 | 8.3 | 8.4 | 8.5 | 8.1 | 8.2 |
| Greece | 1.4 | 2.0 | 2.8 | 3.1 | 3.9 | 4.1 | 4.7 | 4.6 | 4.7 | 4.3 | 4.3 |
| Hungary | - | - | - | - | 6.1 | 4.9 | 4.9 | 5.3 | 5.9 | 5.7 | - |
| Iceland | 1.9 | 3.1 | 5.5 | 6.8 | 6.9 | 7.6 | 7.5 | 8.3 | 8.5 | 8.3 | 7.9 |
| Ireland | 2.8 | 4.1 | 6.8 | 4.4 | 4.8 | 4.6 | 5.1 | 5.4 | 5.6 | 5.8 | 5.8 |
| Italy | 3.0 | 4.4 | 5.5 | 6.1 | 5.1 | 5.8 | 6.1 | 6.2 | 6.2 | 6.6 | 6.8 |
| Japan | 1.8 | 3.2 | 4.7 | 4.6 | 5.7 | 6.2 | 6.5 | 6.5 | 6.6 | 6.6 | - |
| Korea, Republic of | - | - | - | 1.6 | 1.5 | 2.2 | 2.9 | 2.7 | 2.8 | 2.9 | 3.2 |
| Latvia | - | - | - | - | - | 3.3 | 3.2 | 3.3 | 3.3 | 3.3 | - |
| Lithuania | - | - | - | - | - | 4.5 | 4.6 | 4.9 | 5.0 | 4.9 | - |
| Luxembourg | - | 2.8 | 4.8 | 5.0 | 5.1 | 5.2 | 5.6 | 6.1 | 7.0 | 7.5 | - |
| Malta | - | - | - | - | - | 6.1 | 6.2 | 7.3 | 7.4 | 7.2 | - |
| Mexico | - | - | - | 2.0 | 2.4 | 2.6 | 2.7 | 2.7 | 2.8 | 3.0 | 2.9 |
| Netherlands | 1.2 | 4.7 | 5.2 | 5.4 | 5.9 | 5.0 | 5.2 | 5.5 | 5.8 | 5.7 | - |
| New Zealand | 3.4 | 4.1 | 5.1 | 5.7 | 5.5 | 6.0 | 6.0 | 6.4 | 6.3 | 6.7 | 7.0 |
| Norway | 2.2 | 4.0 | 5.9 | 6.3 | 6.6 | 6.9 | 7.4 | 8.2 | 8.4 | 8.1 | 7.6 |
| Poland | - | - | - | 4.4 | 4.0 | 3.9 | 4.2 | 4.5 | 4.4 | 4.3 | 4.3 |
| Portugal | - | 1.5 | 3.4 | 3.8 | 4.9 | 6.4 | 6.3 | 6.5 | 7.1 | 7.0 | 7.4 |
| Romania | - | - | - | - | - | 3.4 | 3.5 | 3.6 | 3.9 | 3.5 | 3.9 |
| Slovak Republic | - | - | - | - | - | 4.9 | 4.9 | 5.0 | 5.2 | 5.3 | 5.3 |
| Slovenia | - | - | - | - | - | 6.7 | 6.9 | 6.8 | 6.7 | 6.7 | - |
| Spain | 0.9 | 2.3 | 4.2 | 5.1 | 5.4 | 5.2 | 5.2 | 5.2 | 5.5 | 5.7 | 5.9 |
| Sweden | 3.2 | 5.9 | 8.3 | 7.5 | 7.0 | 7.1 | 7.4 | 7.8 | 7.9 | 7.7 | 7.7 |
| Switzerland | 2.4 | 3.3 | 4.7 | 4.3 | 5.2 | 5.8 | 6.2 | 6.5 | 6.7 | 6.8 | 6.9 |
| Turkey | - | 2.2 | 2.1 | 3.6 | 2.4 | 4.2 | 5.1 | 5.2 | 5.4 | 5.6 | 5.4 |
| UK | 3.4 | 3.8 | 4.9 | 5.1 | 5.8 | 6.0 | 6.3 | 6.7 | 7.1 | 7.3 | 7.7 |
| USA | 1.2 | 2.5 | 3.6 | 4.7 | 6.0 | 5.8 | 6.2 | 6.6 | 6.7 | 6.8 | 6.9 |

*Notes:*    Trends over time should be interpreted with caution as there are several breaks in series (see OECD Health Database for further information).
1 Including patient payments (e.g. prescription charges).
2 Weighted average. EU15 as constituted before 1 May 2004 and EU27 as constituted since 1 January 2007.
3 OECD figure includes 2004 data for Australia, Hungary, Japan, Luxembourg and the Netherlands.  EU27 figure includes 2004 data for Cyprus, Estonia, Hungary, Latvia, Lithuania, Luxembourg, Malta, the Netherlands and Slovenia. EU15 figure includes 2004 data for Luxembourg and the Netherlands.
- Not available.
GDP = Gross Domestic Product.
*Sources:*  OECD Health Database (OECD).
World Development Indicators (World Bank).
World Health Report: Core Health Indicators (WHO).
For sources of UK health expenditure data refer to Table 2.1.
Economic Trends (ONS).

Table 2.15   Index (2000=100) of public health expenditure[1] as a percentage of GDP at market prices in OECD and EU countries, 1960 - 2005

**Index of public health expenditure as a percentage of GDP (2000=100)**

| | Year | | | | | | | | | | |
|---|---|---|---|---|---|---|---|---|---|---|---|
| | 1960 | 1970 | 1980 | 1990 | 1995 | 2000 | 2001 | 2002 | 2003 | 2004 | 2005[3] |
| OECD[2] | 30 | 54 | 76 | 86 | 101 | 100 | 105 | 109 | 112 | 113 | 114 |
| EU27[2] | 42 | 62 | 86 | 89 | 102 | 100 | 102 | 105 | 110 | 110 | 112 |
| EU15[2] | 41 | 61 | 85 | 89 | 102 | 100 | 102 | 105 | 110 | 110 | 112 |
| | | | | | | | | | | | |
| Australia | 33 | 48 | 71 | 85 | 89 | 100 | 101 | 103 | 104 | 107 | - |
| Austria | 39 | 43 | 68 | 68 | 93 | 100 | 100 | 101 | 102 | 103 | 103 |
| Belgium | 32 | 52 | 79 | 98 | 98 | 100 | 102 | 103 | 110 | 114 | 113 |
| Bulgaria | - | - | - | - | - | 100 | 110 | 122 | 133 | 126 | 131 |
| Canada | 37 | 77 | 86 | 106 | 104 | 100 | 105 | 107 | 110 | 110 | 111 |
| Cyprus | - | - | - | - | - | 100 | 103 | 114 | 130 | 123 | - |
| Czech Republic | - | - | - | 77 | 108 | 100 | 102 | 108 | 113 | 110 | 107 |
| Denmark | 46 | 73 | 115 | 101 | 98 | 100 | 104 | 107 | 112 | 114 | 113 |
| Estonia | - | - | - | - | - | 100 | 94 | 90 | 96 | 98 | - |
| Finland | 42 | 83 | 100 | 126 | 114 | 100 | 103 | 109 | 113 | 115 | 119 |
| France | 31 | 54 | 75 | 85 | 103 | 100 | 101 | 105 | 115 | 116 | 118 |
| Germany | 38 | 53 | 81 | 77 | 100 | 100 | 101 | 103 | 104 | 99 | 100 |
| Greece | 34 | 49 | 69 | 75 | 95 | 100 | 113 | 111 | 113 | 104 | 105 |
| Hungary | - | - | - | - | 124 | 100 | 101 | 108 | 120 | 116 | - |
| Iceland | 25 | 40 | 73 | 89 | 90 | 100 | 99 | 109 | 111 | 108 | 103 |
| Ireland | 61 | 90 | 147 | 95 | 105 | 100 | 112 | 118 | 122 | 127 | 127 |
| Italy | 51 | 75 | 94 | 105 | 88 | 100 | 105 | 106 | 107 | 113 | 117 |
| Japan | 29 | 51 | 75 | 74 | 91 | 100 | 104 | 104 | 105 | 105 | - |
| Korea, Republic of | - | - | - | 71 | 66 | 100 | 128 | 122 | 126 | 129 | 141 |
| Latvia | - | - | - | - | - | 100 | 96 | 99 | 99 | 100 | - |
| Lithuania | - | - | - | - | - | 100 | 101 | 107 | 111 | 108 | - |
| Luxembourg | - | 53 | 92 | 95 | 99 | 100 | 107 | 117 | 135 | 143 | - |
| Malta | - | - | - | - | - | 100 | 102 | 119 | 122 | 118 | - |
| Mexico | - | - | - | 75 | 92 | 100 | 103 | 104 | 108 | 116 | 113 |
| Netherlands | 25 | 95 | 104 | 107 | 118 | 100 | 104 | 110 | 115 | 114 | - |
| New Zealand | 57 | 68 | 85 | 94 | 92 | 100 | 99 | 106 | 104 | 111 | 117 |
| Norway | 32 | 58 | 85 | 91 | 96 | 100 | 106 | 118 | 121 | 116 | 109 |
| Poland | - | - | - | 114 | 103 | 100 | 109 | 117 | 113 | 110 | 112 |
| Portugal | - | 23 | 53 | 60 | 76 | 100 | 98 | 101 | 111 | 109 | 115 |
| Romania | - | - | - | - | - | 100 | 101 | 107 | 113 | 103 | 113 |
| Slovak Republic | - | - | - | - | - | 100 | 100 | 102 | 106 | 109 | 108 |
| Slovenia | - | - | - | - | - | 100 | 104 | 102 | 100 | 101 | - |
| Spain | 17 | 44 | 82 | 100 | 104 | 100 | 100 | 100 | 107 | 111 | 114 |
| Sweden | 45 | 83 | 117 | 105 | 98 | 100 | 104 | 110 | 112 | 108 | 108 |
| Switzerland | 42 | 57 | 81 | 75 | 90 | 100 | 107 | 111 | 116 | 116 | 119 |
| Turkey | - | 52 | 51 | 87 | 57 | 100 | 122 | 125 | 130 | 134 | 130 |
| UK | 56 | 64 | 82 | 85 | 97 | 100 | 105 | 111 | 119 | 123 | 129 |
| USA | 21 | 44 | 62 | 81 | 104 | 100 | 108 | 114 | 117 | 118 | 120 |

*Notes:*   Trends over time should be interpreted with caution as there are several breaks in series (see OECD Health Database for further information).
1 Including patient payments (e.g. prescription charges).
2 Weighted average. EU15 as constituted before 1 May 2004 and EU27 as constituted since 1 January 2007.
3 OECD figure includes 2004 data for Australia, Hungary, Japan, Luxembourg and the Netherlands. EU27 figure includes 2004 data for Cyprus, Estonia, Hungary, Latvia, Lithuania, Luxembourg, Malta, the Netherlands and Slovenia. EU15 figure includes 2004 data for Luxembourg and the Netherlands.
- Not available.
GDP = Gross Domestic Product.
*Sources:*   OECD Health Database (OECD).
World Development Indicators (World Bank).
World Health Report: Core Health Indicators (WHO).
For sources of UK health expenditure data refer to Table 2.1.
Economic Trends (ONS).

# Cost of the NHS

Figure 2.14 **Public health expenditure as a percentage of GDP[1] in selected OECD and EU countries, 1960 and 2005**

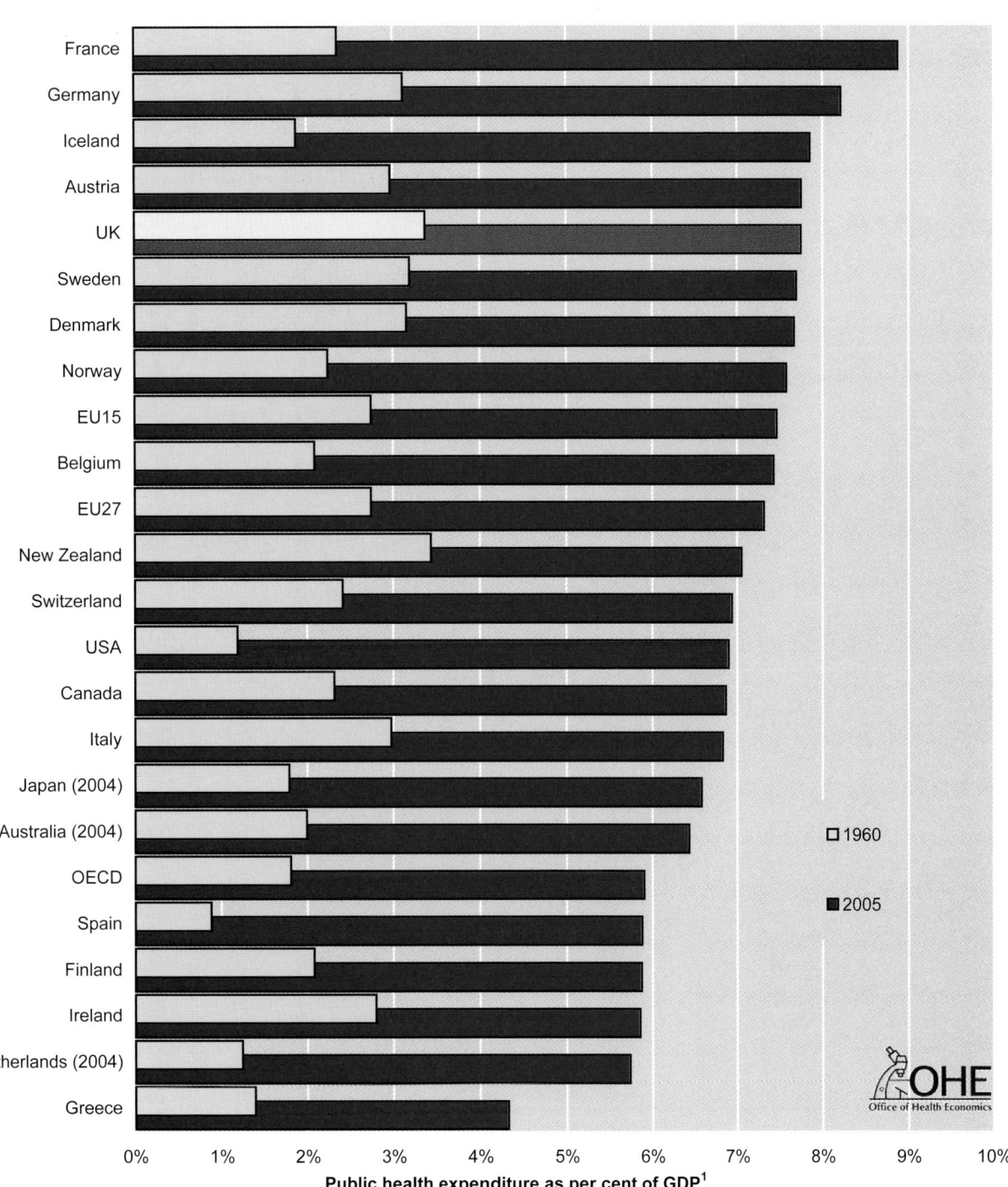

**Public health expenditure as per cent of GDP[1]**

*Notes:*   1 GDP = Gross Domestic Product at market prices.
　　　　Figures for OECD, EU27 and EU15 are weighted averages.
　　　　EU15 as constituted before 1 May 2004 and EU27 as constituted since 1 January 2007.
　　　　Those countries with no health care expenditure information for 1960 have not been included.
　　　　Year is 2005 unless otherwise stated.
　　　　Including patient payments (e.g. prescription charges).
*Sources:* OECD Health Database (OECD).
　　　　World Development Indicators (World Bank).
　　　　World Health Reports: Core Health Indicators (WHO).
　　　　For sources of UK health expenditure data refer to Table 2.1.
　　　　Economic Trends (ONS).

Table 2.16   Public[1] health expenditure per capita (£ cash) in OECD and EU countries, 1960 - 2005

**Public health expenditure per capita (£ cash)**

| | Year | | | | | | | | | | |
|---|---|---|---|---|---|---|---|---|---|---|---|
| | 1960 | 1970 | 1980 | 1990 | 1995 | 2000 | 2001 | 2002 | 2003 | 2004 | 2005[3] |
| OECD[2] | 10 | 42 | 211 | 506 | 854 | 899 | 977 | 1,007 | 1,067 | 1,058 | 1,125 |
| EU27[2] | - | - | - | - | - | 760 | 826 | 888 | 1,028 | 1,057 | 1,128 |
| EU15[2] | 11 | 41 | 254 | 657 | 1,023 | 941 | 1,017 | 1,089 | 1,260 | 1,293 | 1,375 |
| Australia | 13 | 42 | 212 | 530 | 717 | 827 | 822 | 889 | 1,044 | 1,151 | - |
| Austria | 10 | 28 | 237 | 610 | 1,326 | 1,187 | 1,249 | 1,303 | 1,472 | 1,510 | 1,585 |
| Belgium | 9 | 39 | 285 | 733 | 1,150 | 976 | 1,044 | 1,097 | 1,312 | 1,401 | 1,452 |
| Bulgaria | - | - | - | - | - | 38 | 48 | 58 | 76 | 79 | 91 |
| Canada | 19 | 81 | 250 | 776 | 824 | 964 | 1,041 | 1,039 | 1,147 | 1,161 | 1,324 |
| Cyprus | - | - | - | - | - | 185 | 207 | 237 | 310 | 302 | - |
| Czech Republic | - | - | - | 78 | 216 | 215 | 252 | 315 | 366 | 375 | 423 |
| Denmark | 15 | 70 | 459 | 1,021 | 1,478 | 1,348 | 1,473 | 1,566 | 1,850 | 1,918 | 2,011 |
| Estonia | - | - | - | - | - | 112 | 122 | 133 | 170 | 190 | - |
| Finland | 9 | 41 | 236 | 981 | 918 | 765 | 853 | 932 | 1,073 | 1,116 | 1,207 |
| France | 12 | 49 | 312 | 787 | 1,333 | 1,112 | 1,190 | 1,280 | 1,575 | 1,617 | 1,720 |
| Germany | 15 | 58 | 392 | 880 | 1,617 | 1,247 | 1,319 | 1,376 | 1,532 | 1,469 | 1,533 |
| Greece | 3 | 13 | 77 | 183 | 351 | 364 | 443 | 473 | 570 | 557 | 609 |
| Hungary | - | - | - | - | 172 | 152 | 179 | 232 | 300 | 315 | - |
| Iceland | 10 | 33 | 347 | 946 | 1,146 | 1,546 | 1,438 | 1,678 | 1,943 | 2,005 | 2,343 |
| Ireland | 7 | 25 | 179 | 332 | 570 | 767 | 965 | 1,126 | 1,346 | 1,437 | 1,567 |
| Italy | 9 | 38 | 196 | 684 | 647 | 737 | 828 | 879 | 995 | 1,071 | 1,148 |
| Japan | 3 | 26 | 181 | 634 | 1,512 | 1,517 | 1,451 | 1,328 | 1,336 | 1,294 | - |
| Korea, Republic of | - | - | - | 55 | 108 | 160 | 202 | 209 | 219 | 223 | 283 |
| Latvia | - | - | - | - | - | 71 | 77 | 86 | 95 | 106 | - |
| Lithuania | - | - | - | - | - | 97 | 110 | 131 | 163 | 173 | - |
| Luxembourg | - | 49 | 341 | 918 | 1,634 | 1,596 | 1,771 | 2,073 | 2,750 | 3,004 | - |
| Malta | - | - | - | - | - | 394 | 412 | 489 | 542 | 521 | - |
| Mexico | - | - | - | 35 | 47 | 101 | 116 | 115 | 107 | 107 | 116 |
| Netherlands | 5 | 54 | 283 | 591 | 1,014 | 798 | 902 | 1,002 | 1,163 | 1,161 | - |
| New Zealand | 21 | 40 | 161 | 414 | 586 | 543 | 560 | 651 | 776 | 886 | 1,037 |
| Norway | 12 | 55 | 396 | 982 | 1,435 | 1,718 | 1,934 | 2,302 | 2,529 | 2,479 | 2,716 |
| Poland | - | - | - | 42 | 91 | 114 | 146 | 156 | 152 | 154 | 188 |
| Portugal | - | 6 | 47 | 164 | 355 | 464 | 491 | 532 | 648 | 647 | 715 |
| Romania | - | - | - | - | - | 39 | 45 | 53 | 64 | 67 | 97 |
| Slovak Republic | - | - | - | - | - | 123 | 134 | 152 | 194 | 228 | 256 |
| Slovenia | - | - | - | - | - | 423 | 473 | 503 | 569 | 591 | - |
| Spain | 1 | 11 | 110 | 388 | 515 | 490 | 534 | 573 | 707 | 758 | 842 |
| Sweden | 23 | 107 | 563 | 1,184 | 1,257 | 1,278 | 1,281 | 1,412 | 1,648 | 1,630 | 1,673 |
| Switzerland | 15 | 50 | 348 | 852 | 1,483 | 1,311 | 1,498 | 1,627 | 1,801 | 1,800 | 1,868 |
| Turkey | - | 5 | 14 | 55 | 38 | 81 | 75 | 92 | 113 | 129 | 150 |
| UK | 17 | 36 | 200 | 497 | 721 | 969 | 1,064 | 1,177 | 1,324 | 1,444 | 1,576 |
| USA | 12 | 53 | 189 | 605 | 1,050 | 1,317 | 1,522 | 1,578 | 1,547 | 1,473 | 1,585 |

*Notes:*   Trends over time should be interpreted with caution as there are several breaks in series (see OECD Health Database for further information).
Figures are dependent on exchange rates between national currencies and £ sterling over time.
1 Excluding patient payments (e.g. prescription charges).
2 Weighted average. EU15 as constituted before 1 May 2004 and EU27 as constituted since 1 January 2007.
3 OECD figure includes 2004 data for Australia, Hungary, Japan, Luxembourg and the Netherlands. EU27 figure includes 2004 data for Cyprus, Estonia, Hungary, Latvia, Lithuania, Luxembourg, Malta, the Netherlands and Slovenia. EU15 figure includes 2004 data for Luxembourg and the Netherlands.
- Not available.

*Sources:*  OECD Health Database (OECD).
World Development Indicators (World Bank).
World Health Report: Core Health Indicators (WHO).
World Health Organisation National Health Accounts Series (WHO).
For sources of UK data refer to Table 2.1.

Table 2.17  Index of (£) public[1] health expenditure per capita (2000=100) in OECD and EU countries, 1960 - 2005

**Index of public health expenditure per capita (2000=100)**

| | Year | | | | | | | | | | |
|---|---|---|---|---|---|---|---|---|---|---|---|
| | 1960 | 1970 | 1980 | 1990 | 1995 | 2000 | 2001 | 2002 | 2003 | 2004 | 2005[3] |
| OECD[2] | 1 | 5 | 23 | 56 | 95 | 100 | 109 | 112 | 119 | 118 | 125 |
| EU27[2] | 1 | 5 | 33 | 77 | 118 | 100 | 109 | 117 | 135 | 139 | 148 |
| EU15[2] | 1 | 4 | 27 | 70 | 109 | 100 | 108 | 116 | 134 | 138 | 146 |
| | | | | | | | | | | | |
| Australia | 2 | 5 | 26 | 64 | 87 | 100 | 99 | 108 | 126 | 139 | - |
| Austria | 1 | 2 | 20 | 51 | 112 | 100 | 105 | 110 | 124 | 127 | 134 |
| Belgium | 1 | 4 | 29 | 75 | 118 | 100 | 107 | 112 | 134 | 143 | 149 |
| Bulgaria | - | - | - | - | - | 100 | 126 | 154 | 200 | 206 | 238 |
| Canada | 2 | 8 | 26 | 80 | 85 | 100 | 108 | 108 | 119 | 120 | 137 |
| Cyprus | - | - | - | - | - | 100 | 112 | 128 | 167 | 163 | - |
| Czech Republic | - | - | - | 36 | 100 | 100 | 117 | 146 | 170 | 174 | 196 |
| Denmark | 1 | 5 | 34 | 76 | 110 | 100 | 109 | 116 | 137 | 142 | 149 |
| Estonia | - | - | - | - | - | 100 | 108 | 118 | 151 | 169 | - |
| Finland | 1 | 5 | 31 | 128 | 120 | 100 | 112 | 122 | 140 | 146 | 158 |
| France | 1 | 4 | 28 | 71 | 120 | 100 | 107 | 115 | 142 | 145 | 155 |
| Germany | 1 | 5 | 31 | 71 | 130 | 100 | 106 | 110 | 123 | 118 | 123 |
| Greece | 1 | 4 | 21 | 50 | 96 | 100 | 122 | 130 | 157 | 153 | 167 |
| Hungary | - | - | - | - | 113 | 100 | 118 | 152 | 197 | 207 | - |
| Iceland | 1 | 2 | 22 | 61 | 74 | 100 | 93 | 109 | 126 | 130 | 152 |
| Ireland | 1 | 3 | 23 | 43 | 74 | 100 | 126 | 147 | 175 | 187 | 204 |
| Italy | 1 | 5 | 27 | 93 | 88 | 100 | 112 | 119 | 135 | 145 | 156 |
| Japan | 0 | 2 | 12 | 42 | 100 | 100 | 96 | 88 | 88 | 85 | - |
| Korea, Republic of | - | - | - | 34 | 67 | 100 | 126 | 130 | 137 | 139 | 176 |
| Latvia | - | - | - | - | - | 100 | 108 | 121 | 135 | 149 | - |
| Lithuania | - | - | - | - | - | 100 | 113 | 135 | 168 | 178 | - |
| Luxembourg | - | 3 | 21 | 58 | 102 | 100 | 111 | 130 | 172 | 188 | - |
| Malta | - | - | - | - | - | 100 | 104 | 124 | 137 | 132 | - |
| Mexico | - | - | - | 35 | 47 | 100 | 115 | 114 | 106 | 107 | 115 |
| Netherlands | 1 | 7 | 35 | 74 | 127 | 100 | 113 | 126 | 146 | 146 | - |
| New Zealand | 4 | 7 | 30 | 76 | 108 | 100 | 103 | 120 | 143 | 163 | 191 |
| Norway | 1 | 3 | 23 | 57 | 84 | 100 | 113 | 134 | 147 | 144 | 158 |
| Poland | - | - | - | 37 | 80 | 100 | 128 | 136 | 133 | 135 | 165 |
| Portugal | - | 1 | 10 | 35 | 76 | 100 | 106 | 115 | 140 | 139 | 154 |
| Romania | - | - | - | - | - | 100 | 116 | 134 | 164 | 170 | 246 |
| Slovak Republic | - | - | - | - | - | 100 | 109 | 124 | 159 | 186 | 209 |
| Slovenia | - | - | - | - | - | 100 | 112 | 119 | 135 | 140 | - |
| Spain | 0 | 2 | 22 | 79 | 105 | 100 | 109 | 117 | 144 | 155 | 172 |
| Sweden | 2 | 8 | 44 | 93 | 98 | 100 | 100 | 111 | 129 | 128 | 131 |
| Switzerland | 1 | 4 | 27 | 65 | 113 | 100 | 114 | 124 | 137 | 137 | 142 |
| Turkey | - | 6 | 17 | 68 | 47 | 100 | 93 | 114 | 140 | 160 | 186 |
| UK | 2 | 4 | 21 | 51 | 74 | 100 | 110 | 121 | 137 | 149 | 163 |
| USA | 1 | 4 | 14 | 46 | 80 | 100 | 116 | 120 | 117 | 112 | 120 |

Notes:   Figures are dependent on exchange rates between national currencies and £ sterling over time.
Trends over time should be interpreted with caution as there are several breaks in series (see OECD Health Database for further information).
0 = non-zero but less than 0.5.
1 Excluding patient payments (e.g. prescription charges).
2 Weighted average. EU15 as constituted before 1 May 2004 and EU27 as constituted since 1 January 2007.
3 OECD figure includes 2004 data for Australia, Hungary, Japan, Luxembourg and the Netherlands.  EU27 figure includes 2004 data for Cyprus, Estonia, Hungary, Latvia, Lithuania, Luxembourg, Malta, the Netherlands and Slovenia.  EU15 figure includes 2004 data for Luxembourg and the Netherlands.
- Not available.

Sources:   OECD Health Database (OECD).
World Development Indicators (World Bank).
World Health Report: Core Health Indicators (WHO).
World Health Organisation National Health Accounts Series (WHO).
For sources of UK data refer to Table 2.1.

Figure 2.15  **Relationship between per capita public health spending and per capita GDP [1], OECD and EU countries, circa 2005**

**Public health spending per capita (£ cash)**

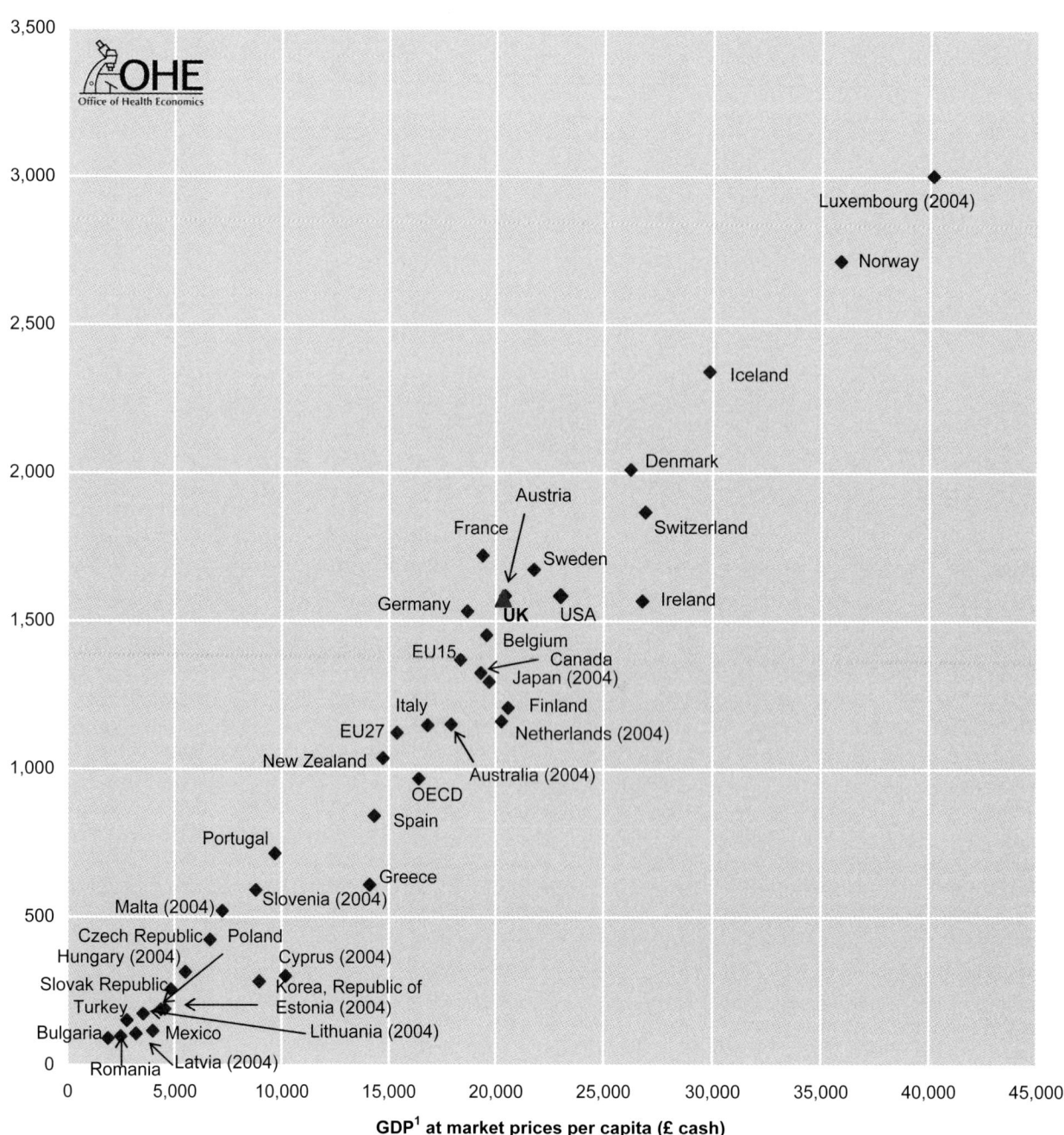

**GDP[1] at market prices per capita (£ cash)**

*Notes:*   1 GDP = Gross Domestic Product at market prices.
Figures are dependent on exchange rates between national currencies and £ sterling over time.
OECD, EU27 and EU15 are weighted averages.

*Sources:*  OECD Health Database (OECD).
World Development Indicators (World Bank).
World Health Report: Core Health Indicators (WHO).
World Health Organisation National Health Accounts Series (WHO).
For sources of UK health expenditure refer to Table 2.1.
Economic Trends (ONS).

Table 2.18 **Hospital and Community Health Services gross expenditure by age, England, 1980/81 - 2003/04**

**HCHS gross expenditure per capita**

| Year | Age group All births | 0-4 | 5-15 | 16-64 | 65-74 | >=75 | All ages |
|---|---|---|---|---|---|---|---|
| 1980/81 | 790 | 145 | 60 | 80 | 285 | 705 | **145** |
| 1983/84 | 1,025 | 160 | 75 | 95 | 370 | 875 | **185** |
| 1984/85 | 1,075 | 175 | 80 | 100 | 395 | 925 | **195** |
| 1985/86 | 1,110 | 187 | 90 | 105 | 405 | 975 | **205** |
| 1986/87 | 1,185 | 195 | 95 | 110 | 415 | 1,030 | **215** |
| 1987/88 | 1,255 | 225 | 100 | 115 | 437 | 1,095 | **231** |
| 1988/89 | 1,385 | 186 | 110 | 146 | 520 | 1,119 | **262** |
| 1989/90 | 1,360 | 205 | 105 | 161 | 545 | 1,199 | **280** |
| 1990/91 | 1,436 | 296 | 132 | 194 | 502 | 1,160 | **307** |
| 1991/92 | 1,606 | 342 | 162 | 228 | 616 | 1,377 | **364** |
| 1992/93 | 1,776 | 388 | 191 | 262 | 729 | 1,593 | **420** |
| 1993/94 | 1,792 | 421 | 198 | 277 | 761 | 1,675 | **440** |
| 1994/95 | 1,869 | 439 | 215 | 293 | 821 | 1,690 | **461** |
| 1995/96 | 1,969 | 541 | 226 | 308 | 846 | 1,749 | **488** |
| 1996/97 | 1,962 | 469 | 199 | 304 | 807 | 1,664 | **468** |
| 1997/98 | 2,013 | 466 | 202 | 336 | 786 | 1,628 | **486** |
| 1998/99 | 2,147 | 609 | 173 | 359 | 837 | 1,723 | **519** |
| 1999/00 | 2,674 | 802 | 187 | 383 | 947 | 1,955 | **580** |
| 2000/01 | 2,484 | 718 | 203 | 399 | 1,053 | 2,195 | **611** |
| 2001/02 | 2,570 | 679 | 284 | 441 | 1,047 | 2,180 | **646** |
| 2002/03 | 2,506 | 750 | 233 | 419 | 1,395 | 2,829 | **707** |
| 2003/04 | 2,654 | 835 | 233 | 496 | 1,414 | 2,790 | **766** |

*Notes:* All figures relate to financial years ending 31 March.
From 1989/90, figures have been estimated by the DH based on a method slightly different from that of previous years.
Since 2003/04 age breakdowns are no longer available.

*Sources:* The Government's Expenditure Plans (DH).
Public Expenditure on Health and Personal Social Services (House of Commons Health Committee).
Government Actuary's Department (GAD).

Table 2.19 **Percentage distribution of HCHS gross expenditure by age, England, 1980/81 - 2003/04**

| Year | Age group All births | 0-4 | 5-15 | 16-64 | 65-74 | >=75 | All ages |
|---|---|---|---|---|---|---|---|
| 1980/81 | 7 | 6 | 6 | 35 | 18 | 28 | **100** |
| 1983/84 | 7 | 6 | 6 | 34 | 18 | 29 | **100** |
| 1984/85 | 7 | 6 | 5 | 34 | 18 | 30 | **100** |
| 1985/86 | 7 | 6 | 6 | 34 | 17 | 30 | **100** |
| 1986/87 | 7 | 6 | 6 | 33 | 17 | 31 | **100** |
| 1987/88 | 7 | 6 | 5 | 33 | 17 | 31 | **100** |
| 1988/89 | 7 | 5 | 5 | 37 | 18 | 29 | **100** |
| 1989/90 | 7 | 5 | 5 | 38 | 17 | 29 | **100** |
| 1990/91 | 7 | 5 | 4 | 40 | 17 | 28 | **100** |
| 1991/92 | 6 | 5 | 5 | 39 | 17 | 29 | **100** |
| 1992/93 | 6 | 5 | 5 | 38 | 17 | 30 | **100** |
| 1993/94 | 5 | 5 | 5 | 37 | 18 | 31 | **100** |
| 1994/95 | 5 | 6 | 6 | 41 | 16 | 25 | **100** |
| 1995/96 | 5 | 7 | 6 | 41 | 15 | 25 | **100** |
| 1996/97 | 5 | 6 | 5 | 42 | 15 | 26 | **100** |
| 1997/98 | 5 | 6 | 5 | 45 | 14 | 25 | **100** |
| 1998/99 | 5 | 7 | 4 | 45 | 14 | 25 | **100** |
| 1999/00 | 6 | 9 | 4 | 43 | 14 | 25 | **100** |
| 2000/01 | 5 | 7 | 4 | 43 | 14 | 27 | **100** |
| 2001/02 | 5 | 6 | 6 | 45 | 13 | 25 | **100** |
| 2002/03 | 4 | 6 | 4 | 39 | 16 | 30 | **100** |
| 2003/04 | 4 | 6 | 4 | 43 | 15 | 28 | **100** |

*Notes:* All figures relate to financial years ending 31 March.
From 1989/90, figures have been estimated by the DH based on a method slightly different from that of previous years.

*Sources:* The Government's Expenditure Plans (DH).
Public Expenditure on Health and Personal Social Services (House of Commons Health Committee).

Figure 2.16  **Estimated Hospital and Community Health Services expenditure per capita by age group, England, 2003/04**

**HCHS expenditure per capita (£ cash)**

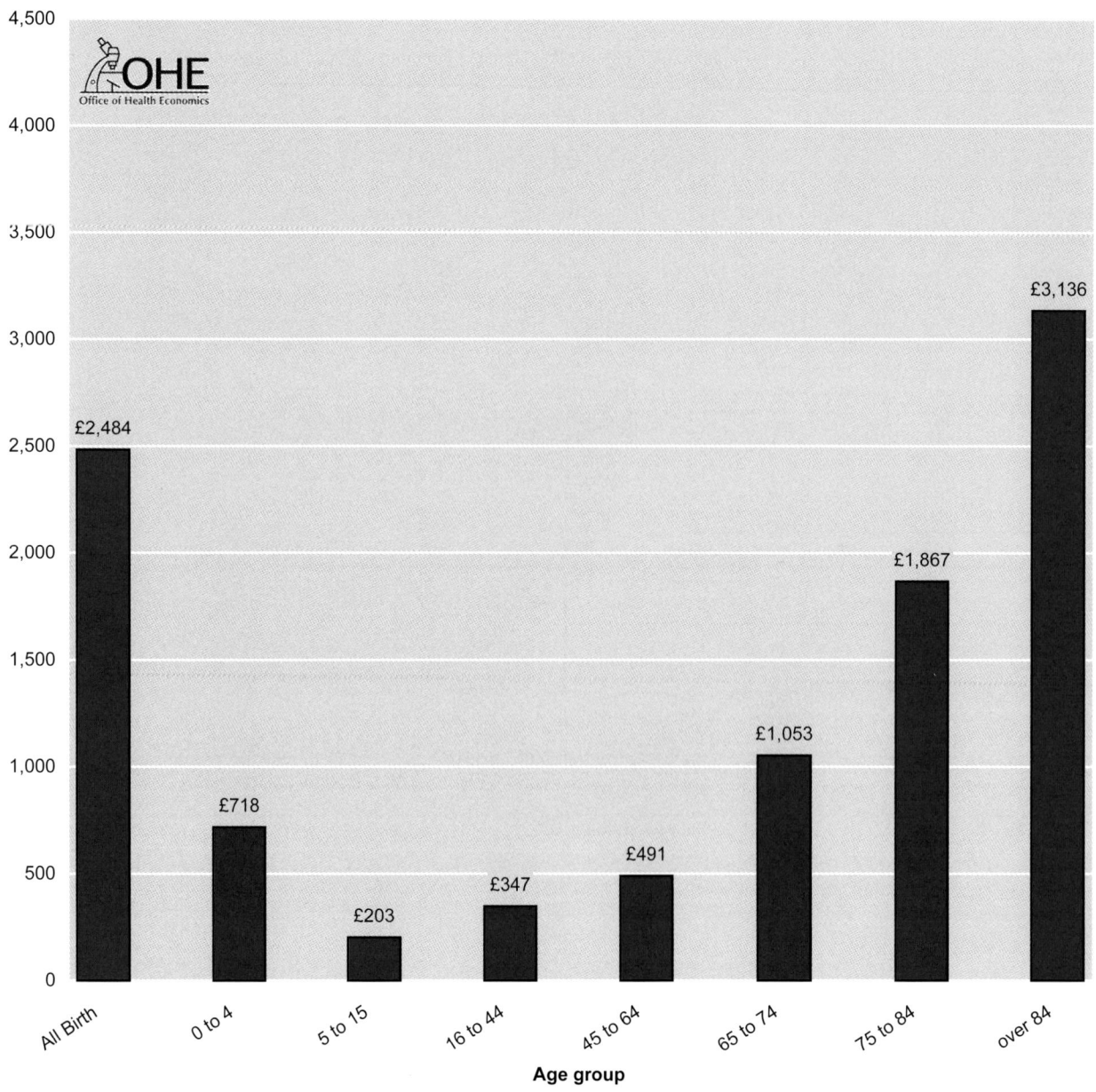

*Note:*  Since 2003/04 data for HCHS expenditure by age group are no longer available.
*Sources:*  The Government's Expenditure Plans (DH).
     Public Expenditure on Health and Personal Social Services (House of Commons Health Committee).
     Government Actuary's Department (GAD).

Table 2.20  **Revenue expenditure of strategic health authorities, NHS Trusts and primary care trusts, England, 1984/85 - 2004/05**

**£ million (cash)**

| | Financial year ending | | | | | | | | |
|---|---|---|---|---|---|---|---|---|---|
| | **1985** | **1990** | **1995** | **2000** | **2001** | **2002** | **2003** | **2004** | **2005** |
| **Revenue expenditure[1]** | **9,135** | **13,573** | **22,573** | **30,622** | **34,009** | **37,229** | **44,236** | **48,427** | **49,574** |
| Salaries and wages [2] | 6,778 | 10,255 | 14,303 | 18,708 | 20,532 | 23,212 | 25,912 | 28,560 | 29,973 |
| Clinical supplies and services [3] | 835 | 1,191 | 2,219 | 3,433 | 3,885 | 4,305 | 4,814 | 5,325 | 4,235 |
| General supplies and services [4] | 293 | 372 | 482 | 755 | 803 | 874 | 944 | 980 | 786 |
| Establishment expenses [5] | 306 | 421 | 670 | 956 | 1,079 | 1,195 | 1,297 | 1,406 | 1,319 |
| Transport and movable plant [6] | 54 | 91 | 121 | - | - | - | - | - | - |
| Premises and fixed plant [7] | 809 | 982 | 1,576 | 1,549 | 1,780 | 1,864 | 1,932 | 1,978 | 1,860 |
| Miscellaneous costs [8] | 185 | 425 | 1,391 | 2,151 | 3,107 | 2,559 | 6,017 | 5,017 | 1,418 |
| SHA Workforce Development Confederation | - | - | - | - | - | - | - | - | 1,058 |
| Capital charges [9] | - | - | 1,107 | 1,639 | 1,125 | 1,218 | 1,541 | 1,617 | 1,526 |
| Non-NHS purchases [10] | - | - | 586 | 1,301 | 1,549 | 1,793 | 1,550 | 3,316 | 3,666 |
| External contracts [11][12] | 54 | 108 | 118 | 128 | 149 | 209 | 228 | 228 | 207 |
| Purchases from Foundation Trusts [13] | - | - | - | - | - | - | - | - | 3,526 |

**Percentage breakdown of revenue expenditure[1]**

| | **1985** | **1990** | **1995** | **2000** | **2001** | **2002** | **2003** | **2004** | **2005** |
|---|---|---|---|---|---|---|---|---|---|
| Salaries and wages [2] | 74% | 76% | 63% | 61% | 60% | 62% | 59% | 59% | 60% |
| Clinical supplies and services [3] | 9% | 9% | 10% | 11% | 11% | 12% | 11% | 11% | 9% |
| General supplies and services [4] | 3% | 3% | 2% | 2% | 2% | 2% | 2% | 2% | 2% |
| Establishment expenses [5] | 3% | 3% | 3% | 3% | 3% | 3% | 3% | 3% | 3% |
| Transport and movable plant [6] | 1% | 1% | 1% | - | - | - | - | - | - |
| Premises and fixed plant [7] | 9% | 7% | 7% | 5% | 5% | 5% | 4% | 4% | 4% |
| Miscellaneous costs [8] | 2% | 3% | 6% | 7% | 9% | 7% | 14% | 10% | 3% |
| SHA Workforce Development Confederation | - | - | - | - | - | - | - | - | 2% |
| Capital charges [9] | - | - | 5% | 5% | 3% | 3% | 3% | 3% | 3% |
| Non-NHS purchases [10] | - | - | 3% | 4% | 5% | 5% | 4% | 7% | 7% |
| External contracts [11][12] | 1% | 1% | 1% | 0% | 0% | 1% | 1% | 0% | 0% |
| Purchases from Foundation Trusts [13] | - | - | - | - | - | - | - | - | 7% |

*Notes:*   All figures relate to financial years ending 31 March. Figures exclude NHS Foundation Trusts expenditure.
1  Figures relate to gross value of goods and services, including capital charges.
2  Including general managers, medical, dental, nurses, professional and technical staff, ambulance, administrative and clerical staff etc.
3  Including medicines, dressings, medical, surgical and laboratory equipment, patient appliances etc.
4  Including purchases of provisions, staff uniforms, patient clothing, laundry, linen etc.
5  Including printing and stationery, postage, telephone, advertising, travel and subsistence etc.
6  Including fuel and oil, maintenance, hire of transport etc.
7  Including energy, furniture, office and computer equipment, rent and rates, engineering maintenance etc.
8  Including student bursaries, redundancy payments, auditors' remuneration and other expenditure. Prior to 2005 Miscellaneous costs included Workforce Development Confederations Expenditure.
9  Capital charges for HAs include depreciation and interest charges. For NHS trusts they are made up of depreciation charges only.
10 Figures relate to the purchase of health care from non-NHS bodies.
11 Figures include consultancy services.
12 Figures for 1985 and 1990 relate to agency services.
13 Purchase of health care and services from NHS Foundation Trusts.
- Not applicable, percentages less than 0.5% are displayed as 0%.

*Sources:*   Health and Personal Social Services Statistics for England (DH).
Private communication with the Department of Health (DH).

# Cost of the NHS

Figure 2.17  **Revenue expenditure of strategic health authorities, NHS trusts and primary care trusts, England, 1984/85 - 2004/05**

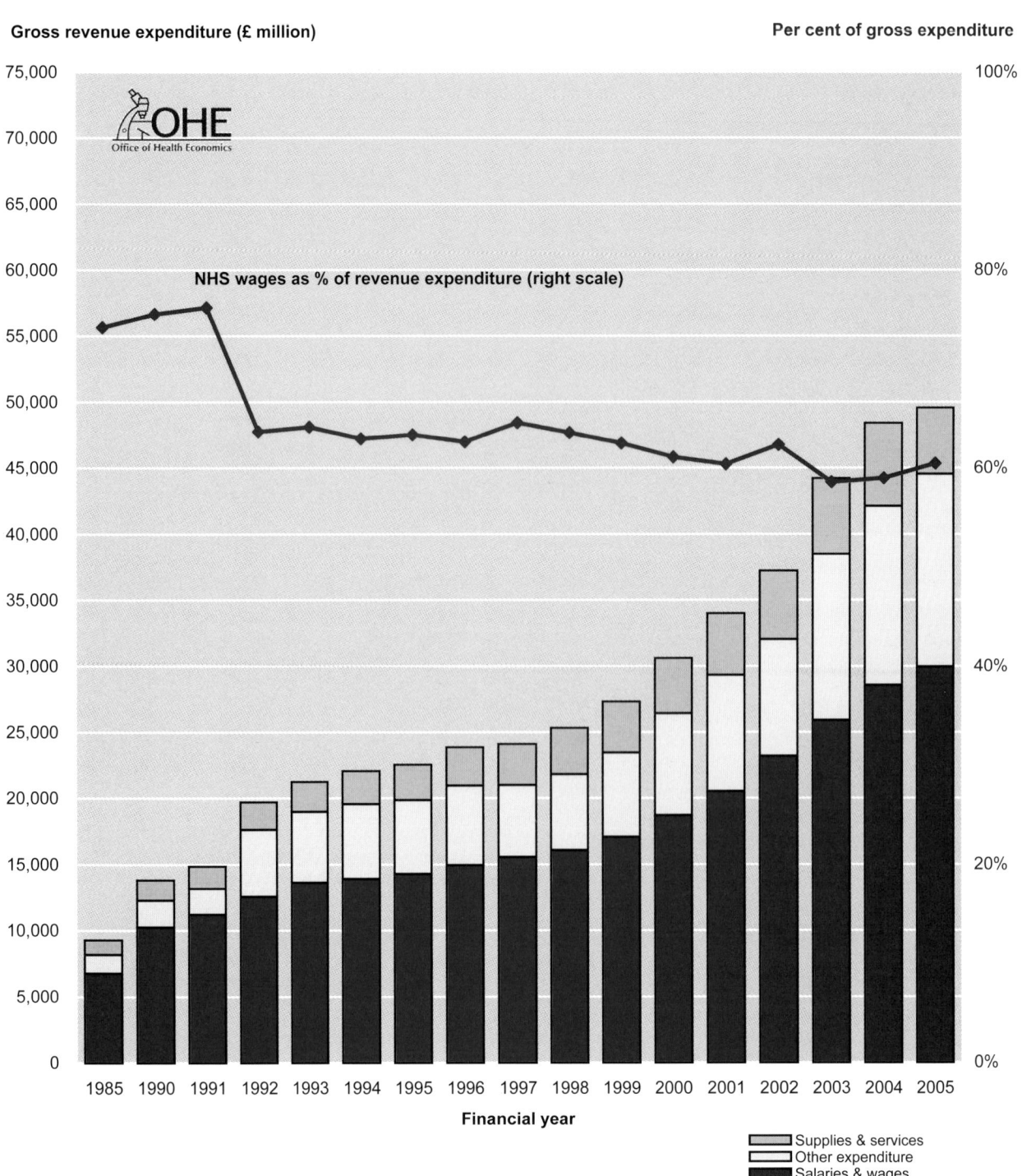

**Gross revenue expenditure (£ million)**

**Per cent of gross expenditure**

NHS wages as % of revenue expenditure (right scale)

Supplies & services
Other expenditure
Salaries & wages

**Financial year**

*Notes:*  All figures relate to financial years ending 31 March. Figures exclude NHS Foundation Trusts, the first of which were created in 2004/05.
The introduction of NHS capital charges in 1991/92 and their inclusion in measured revenue expenditure is the cause of the step change drop in the per cent of total revenue expenditure accounted for by salaries and wages and the increase in "other expenditure".
The step change in other expenditure between 2004 and 2005 is due to the inclusion of provider subcontracted healthcare, the purchase of healthcare from foundation trusts and workforce development confederation.

*Sources:*  Health and Personal Social Services Statistics for England (DH).
Private communication with the Department of Health (DH).

# Cost of the NHS

Table 2.21  **UK public employees in selected sectors, 1961 - 2007**

**Thousands**

| Year | Central government | | | Local authorities | | Nationalised industries[2] | Total public sector[3] | NHS as a % total public sector |
|---|---|---|---|---|---|---|---|---|
| | HM Forces | NHS | Other | Education | HSS[1] | | | |
| 1961 | 474 | 575 | 741 | 785 | 170 | 2,152 | 5,859 | 10% |
| 1965 | 423 | 650 | 743 | 962 | 209 | 1,894 | 5,995 | 11% |
| 1970 | 372 | 741 | 818 | 1,241 | 265 | 1,879 | 6,515 | 11% |
| 1975 | 332 | 1,042 | 917 | 1,508 | 309 | 1,816 | 7,249 | 14% |
| 1980 | 323 | 1,174 | 897 | 1,501 | 346 | 1,816 | 7,387 | 16% |
| 1985 | 326 | 1,223 | 811 | 1,429 | 376 | 1,131 | 6,569 | 19% |
| 1990 | 303 | 1,221 | 776 | 1,431 | 417 | 675 | 6,052 | 20% |
| 1991 | 311 | 1,220 | 805 | 1,314 | 446 | 497 | 5,979 | 20% |
| 1992 | 304 | 1,225 | 823 | 1,293 | 443 | 457 | 5,909 | 21% |
| 1993 | 285 | 1,204 | 812 | 1,131 | 428 | 437 | 5,598 | 22% |
| 1994 | 262 | 1,189 | 790 | 1,105 | 438 | 382 | 5,435 | 22% |
| 1995 | 241 | 1,193 | 751 | 1,126 | 440 | 345 | 5,372 | 22% |
| 1996 | 230 | 1,197 | 721 | 1,127 | 436 | 287 | 5,273 | 23% |
| 1997 | 220 | 1,190 | 697 | 1,131 | 436 | 242 | 5,179 | 23% |
| 1998 | 219 | 1,202 | 690 | 1,141 | 424 | 248 | 5,168 | 23% |
| 1999 | 218 | 1,212 | 685 | 1,163 | 417 | 247 | 5,208 | 23% |
| 2000 | 217 | 1,239 | 698 | 1,219 | 414 | 245 | 5,289 | 23% |
| 2001 | 214 | 1,285 | 733 | 1,247 | 400 | 242 | 5,383 | 24% |
| 2002 | 214 | 1,348 | 762 | 1,256 | 392 | 242 | 5,490 | 25% |
| 2003 | 223 | 1,417 | 794 | 1,312 | 374 | - | 5,645 | 25% |
| 2004 | 218 | 1,475 | 813 | 1,349 | 388 | - | 5,762 | 26% |
| 2005 | 210 | 1,528 | 825 | 1,371 | 393 | - | 5,859 | 26% |
| 2006 | 204 | 1,522 | 811 | 1,397 | 385 | - | 5,825 | 26% |
| 2007 | 197 | 1,501 | 793 | 1,407 | 386 | - | 5,781 | 26% |
| **Index (1961=100)** | | | | | | | | |
| 1961 | 100 | 100 | 100 | 100 | 100 | 100 | 100 | 100 |
| 1965 | 89 | 113 | 100 | 123 | 123 | 88 | 102 | 110 |
| 1970 | 78 | 129 | 110 | 158 | 156 | 87 | 111 | 116 |
| 1975 | 70 | 181 | 124 | 192 | 182 | 84 | 124 | 146 |
| 1980 | 68 | 204 | 121 | 191 | 204 | 84 | 126 | 162 |
| 1985 | 69 | 213 | 109 | 182 | 221 | 53 | 112 | 190 |
| 1990 | 64 | 212 | 105 | 182 | 245 | 31 | 103 | 206 |
| 1991 | 66 | 212 | 109 | 167 | 262 | 23 | 102 | 208 |
| 1992 | 64 | 213 | 111 | 165 | 261 | 21 | 101 | 211 |
| 1993 | 60 | 209 | 110 | 144 | 252 | 20 | 96 | 219 |
| 1994 | 55 | 207 | 107 | 141 | 258 | 18 | 93 | 223 |
| 1995 | 51 | 207 | 101 | 143 | 259 | 16 | 92 | 226 |
| 1996 | 49 | 208 | 97 | 144 | 256 | 13 | 90 | 231 |
| 1997 | 46 | 207 | 94 | 144 | 256 | 11 | 88 | 234 |
| 1998 | 46 | 209 | 93 | 145 | 249 | 12 | 88 | 237 |
| 1999 | 46 | 211 | 92 | 148 | 245 | 11 | 89 | 237 |
| 2000 | 46 | 215 | 94 | 155 | 244 | 11 | 90 | 239 |
| 2001 | 45 | 223 | 99 | 159 | 235 | 11 | 92 | 243 |
| 2002 | 45 | 234 | 103 | 160 | 231 | 11 | 94 | 250 |
| 2003 | 47 | 246 | 107 | 167 | 220 | - | 96 | 256 |
| 2004 | 46 | 257 | 110 | 172 | 228 | - | 98 | 261 |
| 2005 | 44 | 266 | 111 | 175 | 231 | - | 100 | 266 |
| 2006 | 43 | 265 | 109 | 178 | 226 | - | 99 | 266 |
| 2007 | 42 | 261 | 107 | 179 | 227 | - | 99 | 265 |

*Notes:* All figures are based on headcount and relate to June.
Data from 1991 from Public Sector Employment (ONS).
Figures from 1999 onwards are seasonally adjusted.
1 HSS = Health and Social Services.
2 Including Post Office.
3 Central government, local authorities and nationalised industries.
- Not available.

*Sources:* Economic Trends (Annual Supplement) (ONS).
Public Sector Employment (ONS).

Figure 2.18  **Indices of UK public employees in selected sectors, 1975 - 2007**

**Index (1975=100)**

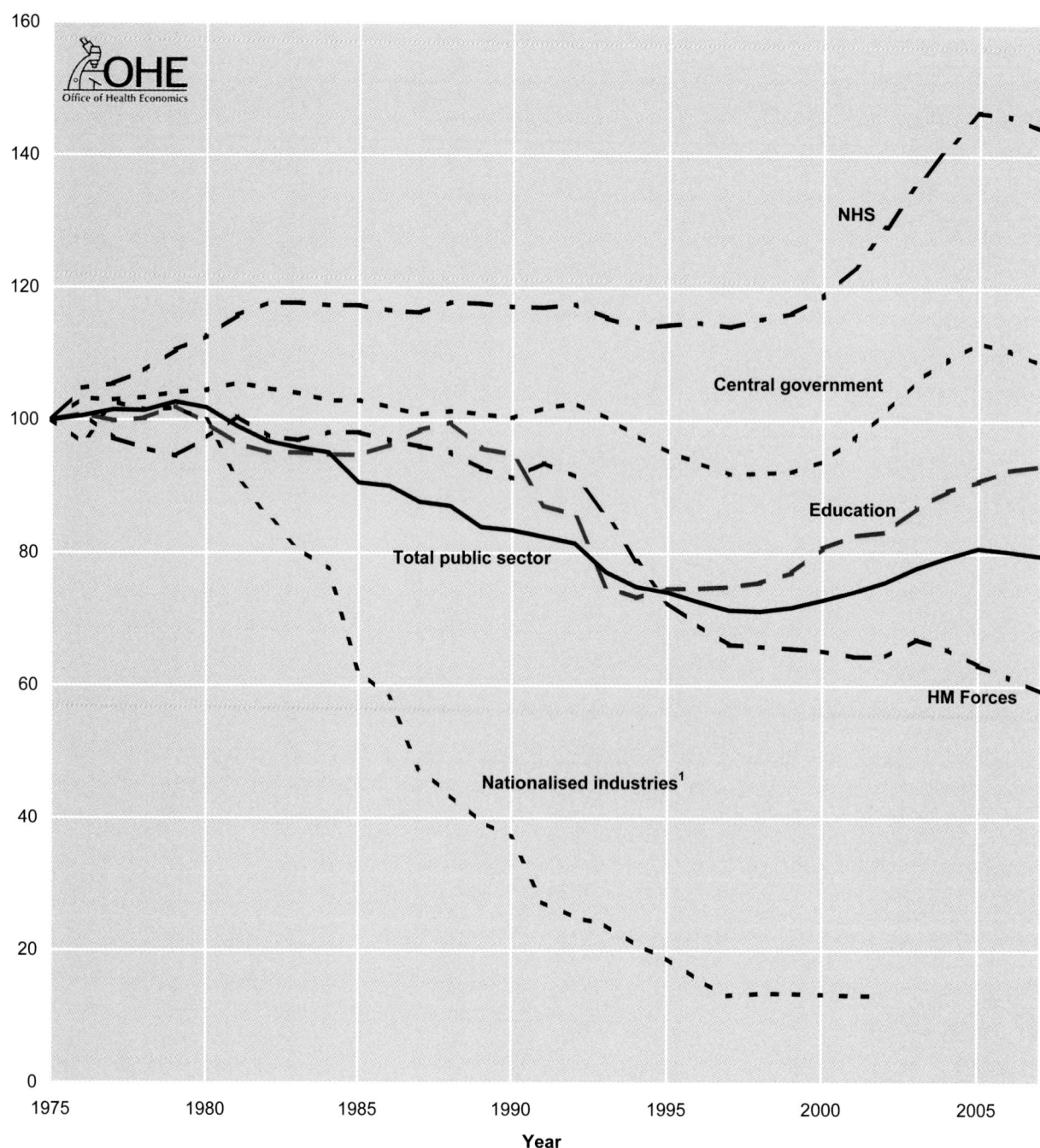

**Year**

Notes:    All figures are based on headcount relate to June (see Table 2.21).
            From 1999 onwards figures are seasonally adjusted.
            1 Including the Post Office.  Data from 2003 onwards is no longer available.
Sources:  Economic Trends (Annual Supplement) (ONS).
            Public Sector Employmont (ONS).

# Cost of the NHS

Table 2.22 **NHS net expenditure[1] (revenue and capital) per capita and per household, UK, 1975/76 - 2005/06**

| Financial year | England | Wales | Scotland | N Ireland | UK | England | Wales | Scotland | N Ireland | UK |
|---|---|---|---|---|---|---|---|---|---|---|
| | | | | | *NHS expenditure per person (£ cash)* | | | | | |
| | | | *(£ cash)* | | | *At constant prices[2] (Index 1975/76=100)* | | | | |
| 1975/76 | 91 | 97 | 108 | 102 | 93 | 100 | 100 | 100 | 100 | 100 |
| 1979/80 | 156 | 164 | 189 | 193 | 160 | 102 | 101 | 105 | 113 | 103 |
| 1980/81 | 200 | 210 | 240 | 246 | 205 | 111 | 109 | 112 | 122 | 111 |
| 1983/84 | 256 | 279 | 298 | 317 | 263 | 116 | 119 | 114 | 128 | 116 |
| 1984/85 | 277 | 299 | 342 | 332 | 286 | 119 | 121 | 124 | 127 | 120 |
| 1985/86 | 293 | 319 | 383 | 342 | 303 | 119 | 122 | 132 | 124 | 121 |
| 1986/87 | 314 | 344 | 393 | 368 | 324 | 124 | 127 | 131 | 130 | 125 |
| 1987/88 | 343 | 376 | 423 | 433 | 354 | 128 | 132 | 133 | 144 | 129 |
| 1988/89 | 382 | 416 | 473 | 473 | 395 | 134 | 136 | 139 | 148 | 135 |
| 1989/90 | 412 | 448 | 538 | 509 | 428 | 134 | 137 | 148 | 148 | 136 |
| 1990/91 | 467 | 497 | 587 | 573 | 482 | 141 | 141 | 149 | 155 | 142 |
| 1991/92 | 529 | 598 | 659 | 598 | 546 | 151 | 160 | 158 | 152 | 152 |
| 1992/93 | 582 | 668 | 766 | 671 | 605 | 161 | 173 | 178 | 165 | 163 |
| 1993/94 | 601 | 690 | 808 | 737 | 628 | 162 | 174 | 183 | 177 | 165 |
| 1994/95 | 633 | 727 | 848 | 753 | 660 | 168 | 181 | 189 | 178 | 171 |
| 1995/96 | 660 | 766 | 861 | 801 | 687 | 170 | 185 | 186 | 184 | 173 |
| 1996/97 | 680 | 799 | 858 | 799 | 705 | 169 | 187 | 180 | 177 | 171 |
| 1997/98 | 712 | 779 | 857 | 681 | 727 | 172 | 177 | 174 | 147 | 172 |
| 1998/99 | 749 | 836 | 904 | 734 | 766 | 177 | 185 | 180 | 154 | 176 |
| 1999/00 | 819 | 913 | 975 | 797 | 836 | 189 | 198 | 190 | 164 | 189 |
| 2000/01 | 891 | 991 | 1,063 | 901 | 911 | 203 | 212 | 204 | 183 | 203 |
| 2001/02 | 990 | 1,079 | 1,232 | 1,042 | 1,017 | 220 | 225 | 231 | 207 | 221 |
| 2002/03 | 1,121 | 1,180 | 1,319 | 1,203 | 1,143 | 242 | 239 | 240 | 232 | 241 |
| 2003/04 | 1,286 | 1,223 | 1,417 | 1,296 | 1,294 | 270 | 241 | 250 | 242 | 265 |
| 2004/05 | 1,376 | 1,344 | 1,612 | 1,442 | 1,396 | 281 | 257 | 277 | 263 | 278 |
| 2005/06 | 1,500 | 1,422 | 1,745 | 1,569 | 1,519 | 300 | 267 | 294 | 280 | 296 |
| | | | | | *NHS expenditure per household (£ cash)* | | | | | |
| | | | *(£ cash)* | | | *At constant prices[2] (Index 1975/76=100)* | | | | |
| 1975/76 | 258 | 281 | 320 | 316 | 266 | 100 | 100 | 100 | 100 | 100 |
| 1979/80 | 429 | 461 | 538 | 571 | 444 | 100 | 98 | 100 | 108 | 100 |
| 1980/81 | 546 | 585 | 677 | 749 | 565 | 107 | 105 | 107 | 120 | 107 |
| 1983/84 | 681 | 756 | 803 | 962 | 702 | 109 | 111 | 103 | 125 | 109 |
| 1984/85 | 731 | 803 | 908 | 1,003 | 757 | 111 | 112 | 111 | 124 | 111 |
| 1985/86 | 766 | 846 | 1,007 | 1,028 | 798 | 110 | 112 | 117 | 121 | 111 |
| 1986/87 | 815 | 905 | 1,021 | 1,102 | 845 | 114 | 116 | 115 | 125 | 114 |
| 1987/88 | 883 | 981 | 1,086 | 1,294 | 916 | 117 | 119 | 115 | 139 | 117 |
| 1988/89 | 975 | 1,076 | 1,202 | 1,407 | 1,011 | 120 | 122 | 119 | 142 | 121 |
| 1989/90 | 1,041 | 1,147 | 1,352 | 1,497 | 1,085 | 120 | 121 | 125 | 141 | 121 |
| 1990/91 | 1,173 | 1,264 | 1,466 | 1,669 | 1,216 | 125 | 124 | 126 | 145 | 126 |
| 1991/92 | 1,321 | 1,508 | 1,637 | 1,732 | 1,368 | 133 | 139 | 132 | 142 | 133 |
| 1992/93 | 1,448 | 1,678 | 1,890 | 1,918 | 1,511 | 141 | 150 | 148 | 153 | 143 |
| 1993/94 | 1,490 | 1,723 | 1,977 | 2,085 | 1,560 | 142 | 150 | 151 | 162 | 144 |
| 1994/95 | 1,565 | 1,806 | 2,061 | 2,081 | 1,635 | 146 | 155 | 155 | 159 | 148 |
| 1995/96 | 1,627 | 1,896 | 2,075 | 2,214 | 1,695 | 148 | 158 | 152 | 164 | 149 |
| 1996/97 | 1,671 | 1,970 | 2,051 | 2,206 | 1,733 | 147 | 159 | 145 | 158 | 148 |
| 1997/98 | 1,747 | 1,913 | 2,032 | 1,959 | 1,786 | 149 | 150 | 140 | 136 | 148 |
| 1998/99 | 1,834 | 2,046 | 2,128 | 2,055 | 1,877 | 153 | 156 | 143 | 140 | 151 |
| 1999/00 | 2,001 | 2,226 | 2,278 | 2,184 | 2,041 | 163 | 167 | 150 | 145 | 161 |
| 2000/01 | 2,164 | 2,400 | 2,466 | 2,431 | 2,210 | 174 | 177 | 160 | 160 | 172 |
| 2001/02 | 2,383 | 2,593 | 2,835 | 2,795 | 2,444 | 187 | 187 | 179 | 179 | 186 |
| 2002/03 | 2,683 | 2,814 | 3,011 | 3,196 | 2,732 | 204 | 197 | 185 | 199 | 202 |
| 2003/04 | 3,065 | 2,899 | 3,214 | 3,414 | 3,079 | 227 | 197 | 191 | 206 | 221 |
| 2004/05 | 3,271 | 3,169 | 3,633 | 3,773 | 3,311 | 236 | 209 | 211 | 222 | 231 |
| 2005/06 | 3,552 | 3,330 | 3,911 | 4,093 | 3,587 | 251 | 216 | 222 | 236 | 245 |

*Notes:* All figures include Hospital and Community Health Services, Family Health and Other Services.

1 Figures pre 1999/00 are on a cash resource basis, from 1999/00 - 2002/03 on a stage 1 resource budgeting basis and from 2003/04 on a stage 2 Resource Budgeting basis. Figures for Wales, Scotland and Northern Ireland exclude expenditure on departmental administration

2 As adjusted by the Gross Domestic Product (GDP) deflator at market prices.

Growth in NHS expenditure for England between 2002/03 and 2003/04 is distorted by a switch from the Exchequers Annually managed Expenditure to cover the increased cost of pensions.

*Sources:* The Government's Expenditure Plans (DH).

Health Statistics Wales (NAW).

Scottish Health Service Costs (ISD).

Main Estimate (DHSSPS).

Household Estimates and Projections (DCLG).

Household Projections (GROS).

Household Data (NISRA).

# Cost of the NHS

Table 2.23   **UK NHS gross expenditure (£) per capita, by service, 1950 - 2004/05**

| Year | Hospital Services | Community Health Services[1] | Family Health Services | | | | Other Services[3] | Total NHS Cost |
| | | | Pharma-ceutical[2] | General Medical | General Dental | General Ophthalmic | | |
| --- | --- | --- | --- | --- | --- | --- | --- | --- |
| 1950 | 5 | 1 | 1 | 1 | 1 | 0 | 0 | 9 |
| 1960 | 9 | 2 | 2 | 2 | 1 | 0 | 1 | 17 |
| 1970 | 23 | 3 | 4 | 3 | 2 | 0 | 1 | 36 |
| 1975[4] | 57 | 6 | 8 | 6 | 4 | 1 | 10 | 91 |
| 1980 | 120 | 12 | 19 | 13 | 8 | 2 | 27 | 200 |
| 1990/91 | 245 | 42 | 57 | 41 | 22 | 2 | 100 | 509 |
| 1991/92 | 305 | 53 | 63 | 47 | 26 | 3 | 78 | 575 |
| 1992/93 | 331 | 60 | 71 | 51 | 27 | 4 | 85 | 629 |
| 1993/94 | 365 | 67 | 78 | 53 | 25 | 4 | 59 | 650 |
| 1994/95[5] | 366 | 67 | 83 | 54 | 26 | 4 | 96 | 698 |
| 1995/96 | 387 | 73 | 89 | 57 | 27 | 5 | 91 | 729 |
| 1996/97[6] | 374 | 72 | 97 | 60 | 27 | 5 | 120 | 755 |
| 1997/98 | 392 | 74 | 104 | 63 | 28 | 5 | 127 | 792 |
| 1998/99 | 414 | 83 | 109 | 65 | 30 | 5 | 127 | 833 |
| 1999/00 | 446 | 91 | 120 | 70 | 31 | 6 | 147 | 910 |
| 2000/01 | 486 | 98 | 127 | 76 | 32 | 6 | 163 | 989 |
| 2001/02 | 523 | 95 | 139 | 79 | 34 | 6 | 213 | 1,089 |
| 2002/03 | 571 | 117 | 152 | 83 | 36 | 6 | 242 | 1,207 |
| 2003/04 | 620 | 129 | 165 | 93 | 37 | 7 | 313 | 1,363 |
| 2004/05 | 684 | 143 | 172 | 135 | 39 | 7 | 290 | 1,470 |
| **Per capita spending at constant prices**[7] **(Index 1975=100)** | | | | | | | | |
| 1975[4] | 100 | 100 | 100 | 100 | 100 | 100 | 100 | 100 |
| 1980 | 106 | 109 | 121 | 106 | 101 | 78 | 130 | 109 |
| 1990/91 | 105 | 184 | 177 | 167 | 139 | 45 | 238 | 135 |
| 1991/92 | 123 | 218 | 186 | 181 | 159 | 54 | 174 | 144 |
| 1992/93 | 129 | 240 | 201 | 190 | 160 | 63 | 184 | 152 |
| 1993/94 | 139 | 259 | 216 | 192 | 146 | 69 | 124 | 154 |
| 1994/95[5] | 138 | 257 | 228 | 195 | 150 | 75 | 200 | 163 |
| 1995/96 | 141 | 271 | 237 | 196 | 147 | 76 | 184 | 165 |
| 1996/97[6] | 132 | 257 | 249 | 200 | 145 | 78 | 235 | 165 |
| 1997/98 | 134 | 258 | 259 | 205 | 144 | 78 | 241 | 168 |
| 1998/99 | 138 | 283 | 266 | 207 | 150 | 75 | 236 | 173 |
| 1999/00 | 146 | 301 | 286 | 219 | 151 | 85 | 266 | 185 |
| 2000/01 | 157 | 322 | 299 | 233 | 157 | 87 | 292 | 198 |
| 2001/02 | 165 | 304 | 319 | 238 | 162 | 87 | 372 | 213 |
| 2002/03 | 175 | 362 | 339 | 242 | 164 | 85 | 409 | 229 |
| 2003/04 | 184 | 389 | 358 | 264 | 165 | 87 | 514 | 251 |
| 2004/05 | 198 | 421 | 362 | 373 | 171 | 89 | 465 | 264 |

*Notes:*      All figures include income received and charges paid by patients. Prior to 1990 figures relate to calendar years.

1 Prior to 1974, figures relate to former Local Authority Services.  From 1991/92, HCHS figures include capital charges, depreciation and certain other expenditure not previously included.

2 Figures include costs of prescription medicines dispensed by chemists and appliance contractors, dispensing fees and other allowances.

3 Figures include headquarters administration (at district and regional levels), central administration, ambulance services, mass radiography services and centrally financed items such as laboratory, vaccine, research and development costs not falling within the finance of any one of the services listed.

4 Reorganisation of the NHS in 1974.  Administration of certain NHS community health services transferred from local authorities to new Area Health Authorities.  School health services formerly administered by the Department of Education and Science were transferred to the NHS.

5 There is a break in the statistical series at 1994, as a result of changes in NHS accounting policy (see also footnotes to Table 2.24).

6 The apparent reduction in HCHS expenditure since 1995-96 was due to changes to accounting practice and the structure of the NHS.

7 As adjusted by the Gross Domestic Product (GDP) deflator at market prices.

*Sources:*    The Government's Expenditure Plans (DH).

Annual Abstract of Statistics (ONS).

Health Statistics Wales (NAW).

# Cost of the NHS

Table 2.24 **NHS gross expenditure - proportion spent on each service, UK, 1949 - 2005/06**

| Year | Hospital Services | Community Health Services[1] | Family Health Services | | | | Other Services[2] |
| | | | Pharma-ceutical | General Medical | General Dental | General Ophthalmic | |
| | % | % | % | % | % | % | % |
| 1949 | 51.3 | 7.3 | 7.6 | 10.1 | 10.3 | 5.3 | 8.2 |
| 1950 | 54.9 | 7.8 | 8.4 | 10.1 | 9.9 | 5.2 | 3.8 |
| 1960 | 57.2 | 9.1 | 10.1 | 10.0 | 6.3 | 2.0 | 5.3 |
| 1970[3] | 65.4 | 7.1 | 10.2 | 8.7 | 5.0 | 1.4 | 2.4 |
| 1975 | 62.0 | 6.1 | 8.5 | 6.5 | 4.1 | 1.4 | 11.2 |
| 1980 | 60.0 | 6.1 | 9.4 | 6.3 | 3.8 | 1.0 | 13.3 |
| 1981 | 60.2 | 6.1 | 9.3 | 6.5 | 3.9 | 1.0 | 13.0 |
| 1982 | 61.6 | 6.4 | 10.1 | 6.9 | 4.1 | 1.1 | 9.8 |
| 1983 | 57.6 | 6.0 | 9.9 | 6.7 | 3.9 | 1.6 | 14.3 |
| 1984 | 57.6 | 6.2 | 10.0 | 7.1 | 4.1 | 1.1 | 13.9 |
| 1985 | 57.1 | 6.4 | 10.1 | 7.2 | 4.2 | 0.9 | 14.1 |
| 1986 | 56.4 | 6.7 | 10.2 | 7.2 | 4.1 | 0.8 | 14.6 |
| 1987 | 55.1 | 7.5 | 10.5 | 7.5 | 4.2 | 0.8 | 14.3 |
| 1988 | 54.9 | 8.2 | 10.7 | 7.4 | 4.4 | 0.8 | 13.6 |
| 1989 | 54.1 | 8.4 | 10.4 | 7.6 | 4.2 | 0.6 | 14.5 |
| 1990/91 | 53.0 | 8.4 | 10.3 | 8.1 | 4.1 | 0.5 | 15.7 |
| 1991/92[5] | 53.0 | 9.2 | 11.0 | 8.2 | 4.5 | 0.5 | 13.6 |
| 1992/93 | 52.6 | 9.6 | 11.2 | 8.1 | 4.3 | 0.6 | 13.5 |
| 1993/94 | 56.0 | 10.3 | 12.0 | 8.1 | 3.9 | 0.6 | 9.1 |
| 1994/95[6] | 52.5 | 9.6 | 11.9 | 7.8 | 3.8 | 0.6 | 13.8 |
| 1995/96 | 53.1 | 10.0 | 12.3 | 7.8 | 3.7 | 0.6 | 12.5 |
| 1996/97[7] | 49.5 | 9.5 | 12.8 | 7.9 | 3.6 | 0.7 | 16.0 |
| 1997/98 | 49.5 | 9.4 | 13.1 | 7.9 | 3.5 | 0.6 | 16.0 |
| 1998/99 | 49.6 | 10.0 | 13.1 | 7.8 | 3.6 | 0.6 | 15.3 |
| 1999/00 | 49.0 | 10.0 | 13.2 | 7.7 | 3.4 | 0.6 | 16.1 |
| 2000/01 | 49.2 | 9.9 | 12.9 | 7.7 | 3.2 | 0.6 | 16.5 |
| 2001/02 | 48.0 | 8.7 | 12.7 | 7.3 | 3.1 | 0.6 | 19.6 |
| 2002/03 | 47.4 | 9.7 | 12.6 | 6.9 | 2.9 | 0.5 | 20.0 |
| 2003/04 | 45.5 | 9.5 | 12.1 | 6.8 | 2.7 | 0.5 | 23.0 |
| 2004/05 | 46.5 | 9.8 | 11.7 | 9.2 | 2.7 | 0.5 | 19.7 |
| 2005/06 | 46.1 | 9.8 | 10.7 | 9.3 | 2.7 | 0.5 | 21.0 |

*Notes:* All figures include income received and charges paid by patients.

1 Prior to 1974, figures relate to former Local Authority Services (see also note 5).

2 Figures include headquarters administration (at district and regional levels), central administration, ambulance services, mass radiography services and centrally financed items such as laboratory, vaccine, research and development costs not falling within the finance of any one of the services listed (see also note 4).

3 Change in definition of NHS. Certain local authority services were transferred from the NHS to Social Services in 1969.

4 Reorganisation of the NHS. Administration of certain NHS community health services transferred in 1974 from local authorities to new Area Health Authorities. School health services formerly administrated by the Department of Education and Science were also transferred to the NHS.

5 From 1991/92, HCHS figures include capital charges, depreciation and certain other expenditure not previously included.

6 There is a break in the statistical series at 1994, as a result of changes in NHS accounting policy.

7 The apparent reduction in HCHS expenditure since 1995-96 was due to changes to accounting practice and the changing structure of the NHS.

*Sources:* The Government's Expenditure Plans (DH).
Annual Abstract of Statistics (ONS).
Health Statistics Wales (NAW).

Table 2.25    **UK NHS sources of finance, 1949 - 2006**

| Year | Taxation | | NHS contribution | | LHA[1] | | Patients' payments[2] | | Total NHS income | NHS income as a % of UK government receipts[3] |
|---|---|---|---|---|---|---|---|---|---|---|
| | £m | %NHS | £m | %NHS | £m | %NHS | £m | %NHS | £m | |
| 1949 | 437 | 100.0 | - | - | - | - | - | - | 437 | 8.2 |
| 1950 | 477 | 100.0 | - | - | - | - | - | - | 477 | 8.7 |
| 1951 | 414 | 83.3 | 42 | 8.5 | 41 | 8.2 | 15 | 3.1 | 497 | 8.5 |
| 1955 | 489 | 84.0 | 42 | 7.2 | 51 | 8.8 | 28 | 4.8 | 582 | 8.2 |
| 1960 | 671 | 77.5 | 118 | 13.6 | 77 | 8.9 | 43 | 5.0 | 866 | 9.8 |
| 1961 | 706 | 75.5 | 142 | 15.2 | 87 | 9.3 | 48 | 5.2 | 935 | 9.6 |
| 1962 | 718 | 73.6 | 163 | 16.7 | 95 | 9.7 | 51 | 5.3 | 976 | 9.2 |
| 1963 | 772 | 74.2 | 165 | 15.9 | 104 | 10.0 | 52 | 5.0 | 1,041 | 9.5 |
| 1964 | 854 | 75.1 | 169 | 14.9 | 113 | 9.9 | 53 | 4.6 | 1,137 | 9.5 |
| 1965 | 981 | 77.0 | 166 | 13.0 | 127 | 10.0 | 34 | 2.7 | 1,274 | 9.5 |
| 1966 | 1,102 | 78.6 | 166 | 11.8 | 134 | 9.6 | 30 | 2.1 | 1,402 | 9.6 |
| 1967 | 1,207 | 79.2 | 164 | 10.8 | 153 | 10.0 | 31 | 2.0 | 1,524 | 9.4 |
| 1968 | 1,310 | 79.1 | 178 | 10.7 | 168 | 10.1 | 42 | 2.6 | 1,656 | 9.0 |
| 1969 | 1,416 | 81.7 | 186 | 10.7 | 131 | 7.6 | 55 | 3.2 | 1,733 | 8.4 |
| 1970 | 1,635 | 82.6 | 209 | 10.6 | 135 | 6.8 | 60 | 3.0 | 1,979 | 8.7 |
| 1971 | 1,862 | 82.8 | 232 | 10.3 | 154 | 6.9 | 74 | 3.3 | 2,248 | 9.3 |
| 1972 | 2,179 | 84.0 | 236 | 9.1 | 178 | 6.9 | 87 | 3.4 | 2,593 | 10.1 |
| 1973 | 2,499 | 84.5 | 239 | 8.1 | 204 | 6.9 | 98 | 3.3 | 2,956 | 10.3 |
| 1974 | 3,491 | 91.0 | 235 | 6.1 | - | - | 109 | 2.8 | 3,835 | 10.7 |
| 1975 | 4,565 | 89.0 | 451 | 8.8 | - | - | 111 | 2.2 | 5,126 | 11.2 |
| 1976 | 5,331 | 88.0 | 597 | 9.9 | - | - | 127 | 2.1 | 6,054 | 11.2 |
| 1977 | 5,919 | 87.9 | 671 | 10.0 | - | - | 144 | 2.1 | 6,734 | 11.0 |
| 1978 | 6,684 | 88.0 | 761 | 10.0 | - | - | 155 | 2.0 | 7,600 | 11.2 |
| 1979 | 7,782 | 87.9 | 882 | 10.0 | - | - | 191 | 2.2 | 8,855 | 11.2 |
| 1980 | 9,951 | 88.4 | 1,042 | 9.3 | - | - | 264 | 2.3 | 11,257 | 11.5 |
| 1981 | 11,261 | 87.1 | 1,344 | 10.4 | - | - | 331 | 2.6 | 12,936 | 11.4 |
| 1982 | 12,122 | 85.9 | 1,594 | 11.3 | - | - | 390 | 2.8 | 14,106 | 11.1 |
| 1983 | 12,945 | 85.5 | 1,754 | 11.6 | - | - | 435 | 2.9 | 15,134 | 11.1 |
| 1984 | 13,746 | 85.5 | 1,861 | 11.6 | - | - | 473 | 2.9 | 16,080 | 11.1 |
| 1985 | 14,635 | 85.3 | 2,032 | 11.8 | - | - | 487 | 2.8 | 17,154 | 11.0 |
| 1986 | 15,805 | 85.0 | 2,244 | 12.1 | - | - | 546 | 2.9 | 18,595 | 11.4 |
| 1987 | 17,034 | 83.5 | 2,741 | 13.4 | - | - | 631 | 3.1 | 20,406 | 11.8 |
| 1988 | 19,425 | 82.1 | 3,435 | 14.5 | - | - | 787 | 3.3 | 23,646 | 12.3 |
| 1989 | 20,601 | 80.2 | 4,139 | 16.1 | - | - | 950 | 3.7 | 25,690 | 12.3 |
| 1990 | 22,992 | 80.9 | 4,288 | 15.1 | - | - | 1,146 | 4.0 | 28,426 | 12.9 |
| 1991 | 26,300 | 82.0 | 4,513 | 14.1 | - | - | 1,265 | 3.9 | 32,078 | 14.1 |
| 1992 | 29,548 | 83.4 | 4,612 | 13.0 | - | - | 1,276 | 3.6 | 35,436 | 15.4 |
| 1993 | 31,347 | 84.2 | 4,717 | 12.7 | - | - | 1,167 | 3.1 | 37,231 | 16.0 |
| 1994 | 33,875 | 85.3 | 4,869 | 12.3 | - | - | 971 | 2.4 | 39,715 | 15.9 |
| 1995 | 35,833 | 85.6 | 5,101 | 12.2 | - | - | 919 | 2.2 | 41,853 | 15.4 |
| 1996 | 37,284 | 85.7 | 5,360 | 12.3 | - | - | 879 | 2.0 | 43,522 | 15.3 |
| 1997 | 39,064 | 85.6 | 5,691 | 12.5 | - | - | 906 | 2.0 | 45,660 | 15.0 |
| 1998 | 41,037 | 85.3 | 6,162 | 12.8 | - | - | 939 | 1.9 | 48,138 | 14.5 |
| 1999 | 44,569 | 85.3 | 6,690 | 12.8 | - | - | 1,006 | 1.9 | 52,264 | 14.9 |
| 2000 | 49,103 | 86.0 | 6,905 | 12.1 | - | - | 1,058 | 1.9 | 57,067 | 15.2 |
| 2001 | 54,116 | 86.0 | 7,610 | 12.1 | - | - | 1,166 | 1.9 | 62,892 | 16.1 |
| 2002 | 60,136 | 86.1 | 8,452 | 12.1 | - | - | 1,263 | 1.8 | 69,851 | 17.7 |
| 2003 | 61,422 | 77.9 | 16,087 | 20.4 | - | - | 1,349 | 1.7 | 78,859 | 19.0 |
| 2004 | 66,562 | 77.0 | 18,580 | 21.5 | - | - | 1,278 | 1.5 | 86,420 | 19.5 |
| 2005 | 74,525 | 78.5 | 19,181 | 20.2 | - | - | 1,251 | 1.3 | 94,958 | 20.0 |
| 2006 | 82,247 | 80.3 | 18,838 | 18.4 | - | - | 1,297 | 1.3 | 102,382 | 20.1 |

*Notes:*    All figures relate to calendar years.
%NHS refers to the percentage of NHS funding from each source.
1 LHA = Former Local Health Authorities. From 1974 onwards, services provided by LHAs were transferred to the NHS.
2 Patient charges for 2004 onwards are not comparable to earlier years, see Table 2.26 for further information.
3 UK government receipts include taxes and social security contributions.

*Sources:*    Economic Trends (ONS).
Economic and Labour Market Review (ONS).
Annual Abstract of Statistics (ONS).
The Government's Expenditure Plans (DH).

Table 2.26   **NHS patient charges, UK, 1950/51 - 2006/07**

| Financial year | Hospital[1] £m | Prescriptions[2] £m | Dental[3] £m | Ophthalmic £m | Total charges Cash (£m) | Total charges Index[4] (1951/52=100) |
|---|---|---|---|---|---|---|
| 1950/51 | 4 | - | 1 | 2 | 7 | 40 |
| 1955/56 | 5 | 8 | 9 | 6 | 28 | 128 |
| 1960/61 | 7 | 21 | 11 | 7 | 46 | 174 |
| 1961/62 | 8 | 23 | 11 | 7 | 49 | 182 |
| 1962/63 | 8 | 24 | 12 | 8 | 52 | 187 |
| 1963/64 | 7 | 25 | 12 | 8 | 52 | 180 |
| 1964/65 | 8 | 25 | 12 | 8 | 53 | 181 |
| 1965/66 | 7 - | | 13 | 8 | 28 | 91 |
| 1966/67 | 8 - | | 13 | 9 | 30 | 94 |
| 1967/68 | 8 - | | 14 | 9 | 31 | 94 |
| 1968/69 | 9 | 12 | 16 | 9 | 46 | 133 |
| 1969/70 | 11 | 19 | 17 | 11 | 58 | 159 |
| 1970/71 | 11 | 19 | 19 | 12 | 61 | 155 |
| 1971/72 | 13 | 25 | 26 | 14 | 78 | 181 |
| 1972/73 | 16 | 28 | 30 | 16 | 90 | 193 |
| 1973/74 | 19 | 29 | 34 | 18 | 100 | 200 |
| 1974/75 | 20 | 32 | 39 | 21 | 112 | 188 |
| 1975/76 | 25 | 27 | 37 | 21 | 110 | 147 |
| 1976/77 | 32 | 27 | 47 | 26 | 132 | 155 |
| 1977/78 | 33 | 27 | 61 | 27 | 148 | 153 |
| 1978/79 | 34 | 28 | 65 | 30 | 157 | 146 |
| 1979/80 | 42 | 49 | 78 | 33 | 202 | 161 |
| 1980/81 | 57 | 88 | 106 | 34 | 285 | 192 |
| 1981/82 | 69 | 107 | 132 | 38 | 346 | 213 |
| 1982/83 | 72 | 125 | 163 | 45 | 405 | 233 |
| 1983/84 | 81 | 134 | 179 | 51 | 445 | 245 |
| 1984/85 | 84 | 149 | 197 | 52 | 482 | 252 |
| 1985/86 | 92 | 158 | 225 | 14 | 489 | 242 |
| 1986/87 | 99 | 204 | 261 | 1 | 565 | 271 |
| 1987/88 | 106 | 256 | 290 | 1 | 653 | 297 |
| 1988/89 | 347 | 202 | 282 | - | 831 | 353 |
| 1989/90 | 407 | 242 | 340 | - | 989 | 392 |
| 1990/91 | 510 | 247 | 441 | - | 1198 | 440 |
| 1991/92 | 540 | 270 | 477 | - | 1287 | 446 |
| 1992/93 | 505 | 297 | 470 | - | 1272 | 427 |
| 1993/94 | 368 | 324 | 440 | - | 1132 | 370 |
| 1994/95 | 111 | 342 | 464 | - | 917 | 295 |
| 1995/96 | 42 | 383 | 494 | - | 919 | 287 |
| 1996/97 | 42 | 376 | 447 | - | 865 | 261 |
| 1997/98 | 48 | 396 | 475 | - | 919 | 270 |
| 1998/99 | 84 | 391 | 470 | - | 945 | 271 |
| 1999/00 | 138 | 405 | 483 | - | 1026 | 288 |
| 2000/01 | 138 | 425 | 506 | - | 1069 | 296 |
| 2001/02 | 155 | 478 | 565 | - | 1198 | 324 |
| 2002/03 | 172 | 528 | 584 | - | 1284 | 337 |
| 2003/04 | 194 | 596 | 581 | - | 1371 | 349 |
| 2004/05[2,3] | 205 | 513 | 558 | - | 1277 | 317 |
| 2005/06 | 211 | 522 | 511 | - | 1243 | 302 |
| 2006/07 | 213 | 530 | 572 | - | 1315 | 311 |

*Notes:*   Figures relate to year ending  31 March.
Prescription charges were not introduced until 1952, then temporarily abolished in 1966 - 1968.
The Ophthalmic Services were part-privatised in 1985.
1 From 1994 pay bed and similar income collected locally by NHS trusts no longer included under hospital charges.
2 Figures prior to 2004/05 are taken from the Annual Abstract of Statistics and relate to payments by patients for pharmaceutical services, this data was last published for2003/2004. As such, comparable data is not available since 2003/04 and data shown relates to prescription charge revenue, including income received by pharmacists and dispensing doctors and income from the sale of pre-payment certificates.
3 Data for 2004/05 onwards are not strictly comparable with earlier data, as reliable data for PDS in England and Wales are not available before 2004/05 and therefore data prior to 2004/05 is based on GDS patient charges alone. In 2005/06 there was a  shortfall in patient charge income, in part attributable to PDS pilots income being based on the old GDS system of patient charges in England and Wales.
4 At constant prices, as adjusted by the Gross Domestic Product (GDP) deflator at market prices.

*Sources:*   Annual Abstract of Statistics (ONS).
Economic Data (HM Treasury).

Table 2.27    **Distribution of UK public[1] expenditure by selected sectors, 1950 - 2006/07**

| Year | Public expenditure[2] £ million | Health % | Defence[3] % | Education % | Housing[4] % | Social security benefits[5] % | Other[6] % |
|---|---|---|---|---|---|---|---|
| 1950 | 4,039 | 11.8 | 21.3 | 9.2 | 8.4 | 16.7 | 32.6 |
| 1955 | 6,153 | 9.5 | 25.9 | 8.9 | 8.4 | 16.1 | 31.3 |
| 1960 | 8,291 | 10.4 | 19.8 | 11.0 | 6.0 | 17.9 | 34.7 |
| 1961 | 9,050 | 10.3 | 19.1 | 11.2 | 6.1 | 18.0 | 35.3 |
| 1962 | 9,742 | 10.0 | 18.9 | 12.0 | 5.4 | 17.9 | 35.7 |
| 1963 | 10,365 | 10.0 | 18.3 | 12.4 | 5.7 | 19.2 | 34.4 |
| 1964 | 11,389 | 10.0 | 17.5 | 12.4 | 7.1 | 18.4 | 34.5 |
| 1965 | 12,666 | 10.1 | 16.6 | 12.5 | 7.6 | 19.0 | 34.2 |
| 1966 | 13,736 | 10.2 | 16.1 | 12.9 | 7.1 | 18.8 | 35.0 |
| 1967 | 15,783 | 9.7 | 15.3 | 12.5 | 7.0 | 18.4 | 37.2 |
| 1968 | 17,185 | 9.6 | 14.2 | 12.7 | 6.6 | 19.4 | 37.5 |
| 1969 | 17,754 | 9.8 | 12.9 | 12.7 | 6.8 | 20.1 | 37.8 |
| 1970 | 18,570 | 10.7 | 13.2 | 13.6 | 7.1 | 21.1 | 34.2 |
| 1971 | 21,045 | 10.7 | 13.1 | 13.8 | 6.2 | 20.5 | 35.8 |
| 1972 | 23,702 | 10.9 | 12.9 | 14.4 | 6.4 | 21.6 | 33.8 |
| 1973 | 27,311 | 10.8 | 12.7 | 14.6 | 8.5 | 20.3 | 33.1 |
| 1974 | 35,012 | 11.0 | 11.7 | 13.3 | 12.0 | 19.5 | 32.5 |
| 1975 | 46,550 | 11.1 | 11.1 | 14.2 | 9.5 | 19.1 | 34.8 |
| 1976 | 52,162 | 11.8 | 11.9 | 14.0 | 9.8 | 21.5 | 30.9 |
| 1977 | 54,694 | 12.5 | 12.5 | 15.3 | 10.0 | 27.7 | 22.0 |
| 1978 | 64,107 | 12.2 | 11.8 | 14.3 | 9.4 | 27.9 | 24.4 |
| 1979 | 75,624 | 12.0 | 11.9 | 13.6 | 9.6 | 27.8 | 25.2 |
| 1980 | 91,654 | 12.7 | 12.5 | 13.9 | 9.2 | 27.8 | 23.9 |
| 1981 | 102,434 | 13.1 | 12.3 | 14.0 | 7.0 | 30.4 | 23.3 |
| 1982 | 112,786 | 12.5 | 12.8 | 13.6 | 5.8 | 32.3 | 23.0 |
| 1983 | 122,232 | 13.0 | 13.0 | 13.4 | 6.1 | 32.1 | 22.4 |
| 1984 | 129,361 | 13.0 | 13.2 | 13.1 | 6.2 | 32.6 | 21.9 |
| 1985/86 | 139,400 | 13.0 | 12.9 | 12.1 | 3.0 | 30.9 | 28.1 |
| 1986/87 | 147,300 | 13.2 | 12.4 | 12.6 | 2.8 | 31.4 | 27.7 |
| 1987/88 | 176,000 | 11.6 | 10.8 | 11.6 | 2.6 | 31.2 | 32.2 |
| 1988/89 | 182,200 | 12.3 | 10.6 | 12.1 | 2.0 | 31.1 | 31.9 |
| 1989/90 | 200,100 | 12.1 | 10.4 | 12.3 | 2.6 | 30.4 | 32.0 |
| 1990/91 | 217,300 | 12.5 | 10.0 | 12.4 | 2.8 | 31.2 | 31.1 |
| 1991/92 | 236,400 | 13.2 | 9.7 | 12.6 | 2.9 | 28.7 | 33.0 |
| 1992/93 | 259,200 | 13.3 | 8.9 | 12.4 | 2.7 | 30.8 | 31.9 |
| 1993/94 | 270,400 | 13.6 | 8.3 | 12.4 | 2.3 | 36.2 | 27.3 |
| 1994/95 | 282,900 | 14.0 | 7.9 | 12.4 | 2.2 | 35.9 | 27.6 |
| 1995/96 | 294,500 | 14.1 | 7.4 | 12.2 | 2.0 | 36.4 | 27.9 |
| 1996/97 | 301,000 | 14.2 | 7.1 | 12.1 | 1.9 | 37.2 | 27.5 |
| 1997/98 | 307,000 | 14.6 | 6.8 | 12.2 | 1.6 | 37.0 | 27.9 |
| 1998/99 | 316,800 | 14.9 | 7.5 | 12.2 | 1.7 | 36.1 | 27.6 |
| 1999/00 | 329,800 | 15.0 | 7.3 | 12.4 | 1.4 | 37.0 | 26.8 |
| 2000/01 | 350,000 | 15.5 | 7.1 | 12.7 | 1.6 | 36.4 | 26.7 |
| 2001/02 | 373,200 | 16.1 | 6.6 | 13.3 | 1.7 | 36.5 | 25.8 |
| 2002/03 | 399,800 | 16.6 | 6.5 | 13.3 | 1.4 | 36.2 | 25.9 |
| 2003/04 | 436,500 | 17.2 | 6.3 | 13.6 | 1.6 | 35.5 | 25.9 |
| 2004/05 | 471,500 | 17.5 | 6.3 | 13.5 | 1.7 | 34.7 | 26.2 |
| 2005/06 | 502,400 | 17.8 | 6.2 | 13.5 | 2.2 | 33.9 | 26.4 |
| 2006/07e | 524,800 | 18.1 | 6.2 | 13.6 | 2.2 | 33.8 | 26.2 |

*Notes:*    From 1987-88, expenditure on services has been amended to conform to United Nations Classification of Functions of Government (CONFOG) definitions.

1 Figures relate to central government and local authority expenditure, excluding user charges (e.g. prescription charges).
2 Before debt interest.
3 Military and civil defence.
4 Including community amenities, including water, sewage and others.
5 From 1997, "Social Security" comes under "Social Protection" classification in the new European System of Accounts (ESA 95).
6 Including Public order and safety, transport etc.
e = Estimate from Public Expenditure Statistical Analyses.

*Sources:*    UK National Accounts (ONS).
Public Expenditure Statistical Analyses (HM Treasury).

Figure 2.19 **Indices of UK public expenditure at constant prices[1], 1986/87 - 2006/07**

**Index (1986/87 = 100)**

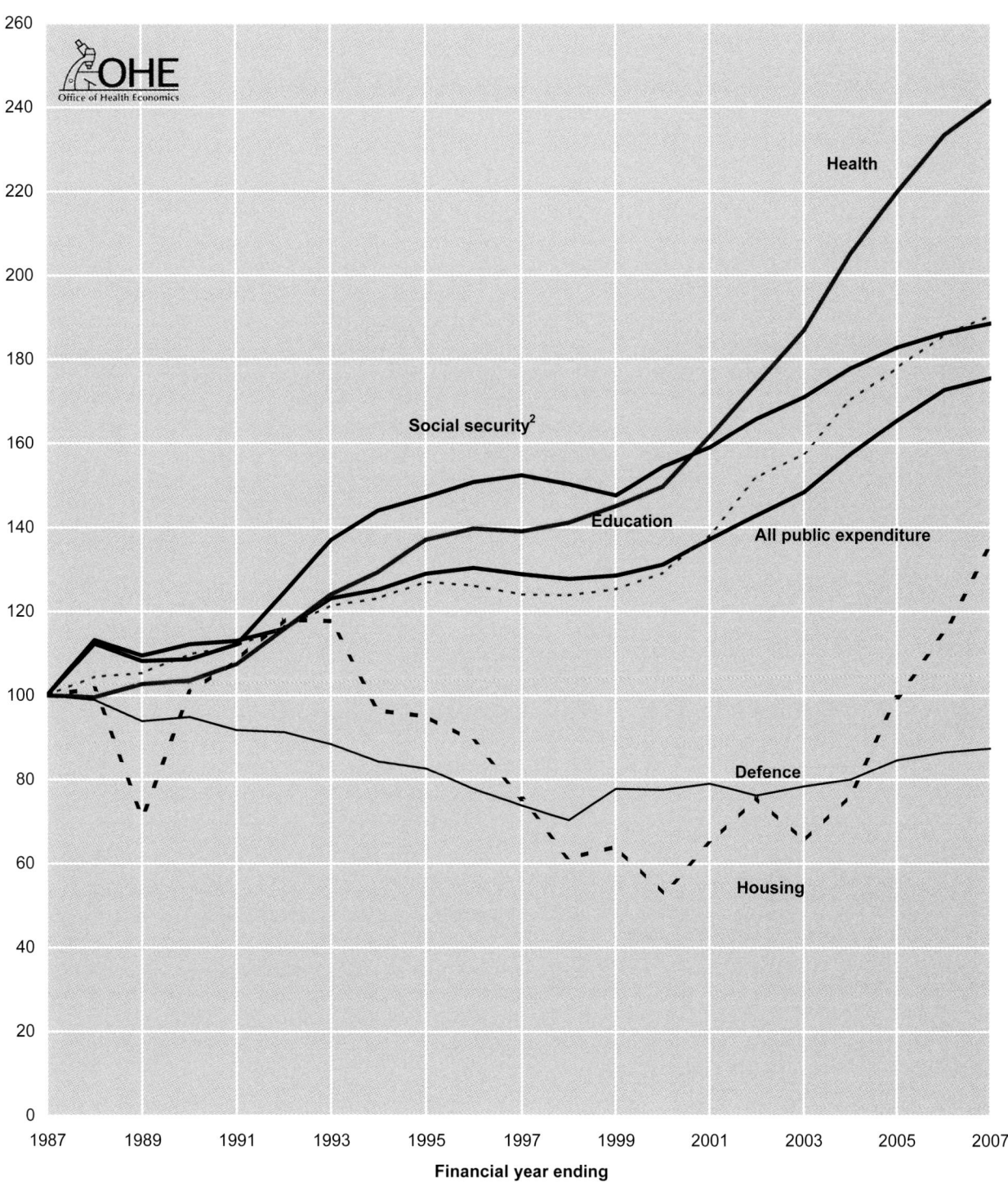

**Financial year ending**

Notes: 1 As adjusted by the Gross Domestic Product (GDP) deflator at market prices.
2 From 1997, "Social security" comes under "Social protection" in the European System of Accounts (ESA 95).
Figures relate to financial year ending 31st March i.e. 2000=1999/2000
Sources: UK National Accounts (ONS).
Public Expenditure Statistical Analyses (HM Treasury).
Economic Data (HM Treasury).

Table 2.28   **The Government's Expenditure Plans for the NHS, England, 1999/2000 - 2007/08**

**England**

| | Year | | | | | | |
|---|---|---|---|---|---|---|---|
| | 1999/00 | 2000/01 | 2003/04 | 2004/05 | 2005/06 | 2006/07 estimated outturn | 2007/08 plan |
| **NHS cash spending - £ million** | | | | | | | |
| HCFHS[1] | 37,607 | 41,229 | 60,723 | 65,575 | 72,405 | 79,140 | 88,166 |
| FHS (non-discretionary)[2] | 1,796 | 1,875 | 2,141 | 2,129 | 2,131 | 1,002 | 987 |
| Central and Administration[3] | 797 | 827 | 1,321 | 1,373 | 1,293 | 1,530 | 1,550 |
| **Total NHS** | **40,200** | **43,931** | **64,184** | **69,078** | **75,829** | **81,672** | **90,702** |
| **Real[4] NHS spending (Index 1999/00=100)** | | | | | | | |
| HCFHS[1] | 100 | 108 | 147 | 154 | 167 | 177 | 192 |
| FHS (non-discretionary)[2] | 100 | 103 | 108 | 105 | 103 | 47 | 45 |
| Central and Administration[3] | 100 | 102 | 150 | 152 | 140 | 162 | 159 |
| **Total NHS** | **100** | **108** | **145** | **152** | **163** | **171** | **185** |
| **Distribution of NHS spending** | | | | | | | |
| HCFHS[1] | 94% | 94% | 95% | 95% | 95% | 97% | 97% |
| FHS (non-discretionary)[2] | 4% | 4% | 3% | 3% | 3% | 1% | 1% |
| Central and Administration[3] | 2% | 2% | 2% | 2% | 2% | 2% | 2% |
| **Total NHS** | **100%** | **100%** | **100%** | **100%** | **100%** | **100%** | **100%** |
| **NHS spending per capita (£) at 2005/06 prices** | | | | | | | |
| HCFHS[1] | 886 | 954 | 1,276 | 1,334 | 1,433 | 1,514 | 1,631 |
| FHS (non-discretionary)[2] | 42 | 43 | 45 | 43 | 42 | 19 | 18 |
| Central and Administration[3] | 19 | 19 | 28 | 28 | 26 | 29 | 29 |
| **Total NHS** | **947** | **1,016** | **1,349** | **1,405** | **1,500** | **1,563** | **1,679** |
| *GDP deflator (1999/2000 = 100)* | *100* | *101* | *110* | *113* | *116* | *119* | *122* |

*Notes:*   All figures relate to financial years ending 31 March and exclude charges and receipts.
Constituent items may not add up to totals due to rounding.
1 HCFHS = Hospital and Community Health Services, Ambulance Services etc; figures include capital expenditure, Family Health Services (discretionary) expenditure and Trusts' expenditure.
2 FHS = Non-discretionary Family Health Services (see also Section 4). These figures have been revised to take into account the introduction of the Primary Medical Services allocation in 2004-05 when all GMS funding is discretionary.  Funding for General Dental Services is partially transferred from FHS non-discretionary to HCFHS in 2005/06.  Funding for Primary Dental Services and General Dental Services is included in HCFHS provision in 2006/07 onwards.
3 Figures relate to miscellaneous health services and departmental administration.
4 As adjusted by the Gross Domestic Product (GDP) deflator at market prices.

*Sources:*   The Government's Expenditure Plans (DH).
Government Actuary's Department (GAD).
Economic Data (HM Treasury).

Table 2.29 **Gross NHS expenditure[6] by Programme Budget categories, England, 2002/03 - 2005/06**

| | £ million (2005/06 prices[7]) | | | | As % of groups shown[8] | | | |
|---|---|---|---|---|---|---|---|---|
| | 2002/03 | 2003/04 | 2004/05 | 2005/06 | 2002/03 | 2003/04 | 2004/05 | 2005/06 |
| **Total below[8]** | **50,773** | **52,400** | **56,203** | **59,971** | **100%** | **100%** | **100%** | **100%** |
| Mental Health Problems[1] | 6,618 | 7,749 | 8,071 | 8,539 | 13.0% | 14.8% | 14.4% | 14.2% |
| Circulation Problems (CHD) | 6,236 | 5,996 | 6,318 | 6,362 | 12.3% | 11.4% | 11.2% | 10.6% |
| Cancers & Tumours | 3,596 | 3,552 | 3,852 | 4,303 | 7.1% | 6.8% | 6.9% | 7.2% |
| Gastro Intestinal System Problems | 3,808 | 3,320 | 3,600 | 3,976 | 7.5% | 6.3% | 6.4% | 6.6% |
| Trauma & Injuries (including burns) | 3,554 | 3,344 | 3,666 | 3,853 | 7.0% | 6.4% | 6.5% | 6.4% |
| Musculo Skeletal System Problems[2] | 3,467 | 3,291 | 3,652 | 3,769 | 6.8% | 6.3% | 6.5% | 6.3% |
| Genito Urinary System Disorders[3] | 2,885 | 2,947 | 3,163 | 3,508 | 5.7% | 5.6% | 5.6% | 5.8% |
| Respiratory System Problems | 3,076 | 2,887 | 3,137 | 3,459 | 6.1% | 5.5% | 5.6% | 5.8% |
| Maternity & Reproductive Health | 3,214 | 2,697 | 2,672 | 2,930 | 6.3% | 5.1% | 4.8% | 4.9% |
| Dental Problems | 2,452 | 2,486 | 2,476 | 2,760 | 4.8% | 4.7% | 4.4% | 4.6% |
| Learning Disability Problems | 1,794 | 2,385 | 2,405 | 2,596 | 3.5% | 4.6% | 4.3% | 4.3% |
| Neurological System Problems | 1,582 | 1,647 | 1,817 | 2,120 | 3.1% | 3.1% | 3.2% | 3.5% |
| Endocrine, Nutritional and Metabolic | 1,475 | 1,590 | 1,633 | 1,895 | 2.9% | 3.0% | 2.9% | 3.2% |
| Social Care Needs | 198 | 1,557 | 1,646 | 1,745 | 0.4% | 3.0% | 2.9% | 2.9% |
| Eye/Vision Problems | 1,384 | 1,262 | 1,330 | 1,356 | 2.7% | 2.4% | 2.4% | 2.3% |
| Healthy Individuals | 881 | 1,163 | 1,182 | 1,341 | 1.7% | 2.2% | 2.1% | 2.2% |
| Skin Problems | 1,160 | 1,123 | 1,239 | 1,335 | 2.3% | 2.1% | 2.2% | 2.2% |
| Infectious Diseases | 891 | 1,025 | 1,649 | 1,258 | 1.8% | 2.0% | 2.9% | 2.1% |
| Blood Disorders | 763 | 868 | 964 | 1,051 | 1.5% | 1.7% | 1.7% | 1.8% |
| Neonate Conditions | 811 | 687 | 793 | 786 | 1.6% | 1.3% | 1.4% | 1.3% |
| Poisoning | 615 | 507 | 611 | 708 | 1.2% | 1.0% | 1.1% | 1.2% |
| Hearing Problems | 311 | 316 | 326 | 322 | 0.6% | 0.6% | 0.6% | 0.5% |
| **Other Areas of Spend/Conditions:** | | | | | | | | |
| GMS/PMS[4] | 3,542 | 5,252 | 6,511 | 7,308 | | | | |
| Strategic Health Authorities (inc WDC[5]) | 3,937 | 4,218 | 4,130 | 3,818 | | | | |
| Miscellaneous | 6,486 | 9,058 | 6,588 | 9,081 | | | | |

*Notes:* Figures are based on financial years.
1 Including Alzheimer's syndrome.
2 Excluding Trauma.
3 Except infertility.
4 General Medical Services/Personal Medical Services.
5 Workforce Development Confederation.
6 Gross spending of resource allocation between the 23 programme budget categories. Figures for 2002/03 are based on NHS spend apportioned across the programme budget categories using reference costs and prescribing information. Figures for 2003/04 onwards are based on an aggregation of PCT returns of allocated spending at local level across the programme budget categories.
Figures include the totality of PCT expenditure including inpatient, outpatient and FHS prescribing costs,
GMS/PMS expenditure on consulting is included but not broken down into the different programme budget categories.
7 As adjusted by the Gross Domestic Product (GDP) deflator at market prices.
8 Excluding other areas of spend/conditions.

*Source:* Department of Health Resource Accounts (DH).

# Cost of the NHS

Table 2.30  **Gross NHS expenditure by Programme Budget categories, Wales, 2003/04 - 2005/06**

| | £ million (2005/06 prices[4]) | | | As % of groups shown[5] | | |
|---|---|---|---|---|---|---|
| | 2003/04 | 2004/05 | 2005/06 | 2003/04 | 2004/05 | 2005/06 |
| **Total below[5]** | **3,784** | **4,052** | **4,244** | **100%** | **100%** | **100%** |
| Mental Health Problems[1] | 450 | 480 | 510 | 13.8% | 13.7% | 13.8% |
| Circulation Problems (CHD) | 401 | 426 | 429 | 12.3% | 12.2% | 11.6% |
| Trauma & Injuries (including burns) | 233 | 258 | 294 | 7.1% | 7.4% | 8.0% |
| Gastro Intestinal System Problems | 252 | 267 | 276 | 7.7% | 7.6% | 7.5% |
| Respiratory System Problems | 253 | 254 | 273 | 7.8% | 7.3% | 7.4% |
| Cancers & Tumours | 237 | 250 | 266 | 7.3% | 7.2% | 7.2% |
| Musculo Skeletal System Problems[2] | 172 | 212 | 225 | 5.3% | 6.1% | 6.1% |
| Genito Urinary System Disorders[3] | 167 | 177 | 193 | 5.1% | 5.0% | 5.2% |
| Maternity & Reproductive Health | 160 | 154 | 161 | 4.9% | 4.4% | 4.4% |
| Dental Problems | 143 | 145 | 156 | 4.4% | 4.1% | 4.2% |
| Endocrine, Nutritional and Metabolic | 118 | 126 | 142 | 3.6% | 3.6% | 3.8% |
| Neurological System Problems | 112 | 118 | 132 | 3.4% | 3.4% | 3.6% |
| Healthy Individuals | 94 | 124 | 124 | 2.9% | 3.5% | 3.4% |
| Skin Problems | 85 | 89 | 89 | 2.6% | 2.5% | 2.4% |
| Learning Disability Problems | 79 | 81 | 87 | 2.4% | 2.3% | 2.4% |
| Eye/Vision Problems | 82 | 84 | 87 | 2.5% | 2.4% | 2.4% |
| Infectious Diseases | 54 | 58 | 58 | 1.6% | 1.7% | 1.6% |
| Poisoning | 36 | 41 | 48 | 1.1% | 1.2% | 1.3% |
| Social Care Needs | 47 | 53 | 45 | 1.4% | 1.5% | 1.2% |
| Blood Disorders | 38 | 42 | 38 | 1.2% | 1.2% | 1.0% |
| Neonate Conditions | 28 | 34 | 36 | 0.9% | 1.0% | 1.0% |
| Hearing Problems | 21 | 26 | 25 | 0.6% | 0.7% | 0.7% |
| **Other Areas of Spend/Conditions:** | | | | | | |
| Other | 544 | 580 | 575 | | | |

Notes:  Figures are based on financial years.
1 Including Alzheimer's syndrome.
2 Excluding Trauma.
3 Except infertility.
4 As adjusted by the Gross Domestic Product (GDP) deflator at market prices.
5 Excluding other areas of spend/conditions.
Figures include expenditure by Health Commission Wales and Dental Practice Board.

Source:  Programme budget returns from NHS Wales (NAW).

# Private Health Care

Although every UK citizen is entitled to receive NHS health care services that are for the most part free at the point of delivery, 11% of the population are also covered by private medical insurance (PMI). Among the major users of private health care are subscribers to provident schemes and other commercial organisations, which make limited payments for private health care in return for annual subscriptions. According to Laing's Healthcare Market Review 2006/07 (Laing and Buisson), there were 8 provident and 13 commercial PMI insurers operating in the UK market in July 2006. Two associations: BUPA (British United Provident Association), and AXA PPP (Private Patients Plan), continued to dominate the market in 2005, with a combined share of over 65 per cent, followed by Norwich Union and Standard Life Healthcare with a combined share of over 15 per cent.

Over the past 20 years there has been an expansion of both the NHS (**Table 2.1**) and the private health care sector, which includes consumer expenditure on private medical insurance, treatment and other out-of-pocket health care expenditure. The latter includes over-the-counter (OTC) medicines and therapeutic equipment such as prescription spectacles, contact lenses and hearing aids. **Figure 2.5** shows that spending on private health care continued to rise in real terms in 2007. Spending on non-prescription OTC medicines and therapeutic equipment, however, stopped rising in real terms in 2003 (**Table 2.32**).

In 2005, the general public spent £8.8 billion on private health care[1] (**Table 2.31**). **Figure 2.21** indicates that the previously steep increase in private health expenditure as a percentage of total consumer spending has levelled off since 2002.

Although private health care expenditure in the UK has increased steadily since 1973, it still only represented 1.2 per cent of GDP in 2005. This is well below the average observed across OECD and EU countries. In contrast, private health care represented 8.4 per cent of GDP in the USA and over 2% of GDP in France and Germany (**Table 2.33**). UK expenditure per capita on private health care was £254 in 2005, towards the lower end of the range across OECD and EU countries (**Table 2.33**).

The number of individuals subscribing to private medical insurance (PMI) totalled 3.6 million in 2005 (**Table 2.30**), with about two individuals insured per subscriber on average so that a total of 6.5 million people were covered by PMI. The number of individuals covered by PMI in the UK decreased marginally during 2005 to 4.8% below the peak level observed in 2000. (**Figure 2.19**). However, examining the numbers insured through PMI alone may fail to give the full picture as since 1990 the numbers of people covered through self insured Third Party Administrators business has increased substantially, with 557,000 subscribers to company paid

self-insurance medical schemes in 2005 (Laing and Buisson).

*Note:*

1.  This is defined as part of consumer spending not involving NHS statutory charges (prescription charges, dental charges, etc). It includes expenditure on subscriptions to private medical insurance carriers, out of pocket payments for private hospital care and consultations with family doctors not covered by health insurance and payments for private beds in NHS hospitals.

# Private Health Care

Table 2.31    Number of private medical insurance subscribers, people covered and payments, UK, 1955 - 2005

**United Kingdom**

| Year | Subscribers[1] 000s | People insured[1] 000s | Subscriptions paid £m | Benefits paid £m | People insured: per subscriber | as % of UK population | Subscriptions paid as % of total private health care spending | Total private health care spending £m |
|---|---|---|---|---|---|---|---|---|
| 1955 | 274 | 585 | 2 | 2 | 2.1 | 1.2 | - | - |
| 1960 | 467 | 995 | 5 | 4 | 2.1 | 1.9 | - | - |
| 1965 | 680 | 1,445 | 9 | 8 | 2.1 | 2.7 | - | - |
| 1966 | 735 | 1,565 | 11 | 9 | 2.1 | 2.9 | - | - |
| 1967 | 784 | 1,670 | 13 | 11 | 2.1 | 3.1 | - | - |
| 1968 | 831 | 1,770 | 15 | 12 | 2.1 | 3.2 | - | - |
| 1969 | 886 | 1,887 | 17 | 15 | 2.1 | 3.4 | - | - |
| 1970 | 930 | 1,982 | 20 | 17 | 2.1 | 3.6 | - | - |
| 1971 | 986 | 2,102 | 24 | 20 | 2.1 | 3.8 | - | - |
| 1972 | 1,021 | 2,176 | 29 | 25 | 2.1 | 3.9 | - | - |
| 1973 | 1,064 | 2,265 | 36 | 29 | 2.1 | 4.1 | 35 | 102 |
| 1974 | 1,096 | 2,334 | 45 | 36 | 2.1 | 4.2 | 38 | 120 |
| 1975 | 1,087 | 2,315 | 55 | 46 | 2.1 | 4.1 | 41 | 134 |
| 1976 | 1,057 | 2,251 | 71 | 53 | 2.1 | 4.0 | 43 | 166 |
| 1977 | 1,057 | 2,254 | 91 | 65 | 2.1 | 4.0 | 44 | 205 |
| 1978 | 1,118 | 2,388 | 105 | 68 | 2.1 | 4.3 | 46 | 231 |
| 1979 | 1,292 | 2,765 | 122 | 84 | 2.1 | 5.0 | 46 | 263 |
| 1980 | 1,647 | 3,577 | 154 | 128 | 2.2 | 6.4 | 43 | 355 |
| 1981 | 1,863 | 4,063 | 205 | 195 | 2.2 | 7.3 | 44 | 463 |
| 1982 | 1,917 | 4,182 | 286 | 245 | 2.2 | 7.5 | 48 | 593 |
| 1983 | 1,954 | 4,254 | 355 | 291 | 2.2 | 7.6 | 53 | 672 |
| 1984 | 2,010 | 4,367 | 413 | 341 | 2.2 | 7.8 | 66 | 623 |

**Laing and Buisson survey estimates for all insurers**

| Year | Subscribers[1] 000s | People insured[1] 000s | Subscriptions paid £m | Benefits paid £m | People insured: per subscriber | as % of UK population | Subscriptions paid as % of total private health care spending | Total private health care spending £m |
|---|---|---|---|---|---|---|---|---|
| 1985 | 2,380 | 5,057 | 520 | 456 | 2.1 | 8.9 | 70 | 738 |
| 1986 | 2,428 | 4,951 | 609 | 513 | 2.0 | 8.7 | 72 | 846 |
| 1987 | 2,590 | 5,283 | 711 | 581 | 2.0 | 9.3 | 67 | 1,066 |
| 1988 | 2,809 | 5,918 | 819 | 689 | 2.1 | 10.4 | 66 | 1,246 |
| 1989 | 3,083 | 6,254 | 951 | 815 | 2.0 | 11.0 | 70 | 1,353 |
| 1990 | 3,300 | 6,692 | 1,110 | 984 | 2.0 | 11.7 | 68 | 1,623 |
| 1991 | 3,300 | 6,651 | 1,284 | 1,128 | 2.0 | 11.6 | 65 | 1,969 |
| 1992 | 3,366 | 6,670 | 1,464 | 1,202 | 2.0 | 11.6 | 73 | 2,015 |
| 1993 | 3,392 | 6,351 | 1,551 | 1,226 | 1.9 | 11.0 | 73 | 2,138 |
| 1994 | 3,390 | 6,613 | 1,617 | 1,295 | 2.0 | 11.4 | 68 | 2,391 |
| 1995 | 3,430 | 6,673 | 1,718 | 1,388 | 1.9 | 11.5 | 68 | 2,533 |
| 1996 | 3,484 | 6,772 | 1,873 | 1,502 | 1.9 | 11.6 | 62 | 3,043 |
| 1997 | 3,486 | 6,679 | 2,000 | 1,586 | 1.9 | 11.5 | 56 | 3,548 |
| 1998 | 3,585 | 6,824 | 2,072 | 1,704 | 1.9 | 11.7 | 51 | 4,057 |
| 1999 | 3,560 | 6,536 | 2,223 | 1,834 | 1.8 | 11.1 | 51 | 4,353 |
| 2000 | 3,677 | 6,867 | 2,450 | 1,937 | 1.9 | 11.7 | 48 | 5,087 |
| 2001 | 3,718 | 6,663 | 2,653 | 2,063 | 1.8 | 11.3 | 46 | 5,785 |
| 2002 | 3,701 | 6,711 | 2,854 | 2,189 | 1.8 | 11.3 | 43 | 6,655 |
| 2003 | 3,661 | 6,615 | 2,970 | 2,269 | 1.8 | 11.1 | 40 | 7,348 |
| 2004 | 3,623 | 6,553 | 3,041 | 2,356 | 1.8 | 10.9 | 38 | 8,055 |
| 2005 | 3,607 | 6,536 | 3,156 | 2,432 | 1.8 | 10.9 | 36 | 8,777 |

*Notes:*    The apparent decreases in some quantities in 1986 and 1993 are due to the revision of BUPA's multiplier which converts the number of subscribers to the number of people covered.
Self insured TPA business is not included.
1 Figures relate to 31 December.

*Sources:*    Lee Donaldson Associates (for data from 1955-84).
Laing's Healthcare Market Review (Laing and Buisson, for data from 1985 onwards).

Figure 2.20  **Number of private medical insurance subscribers and people insured, UK, 1955 - 2005**

**Millions of people insured or subscribers**

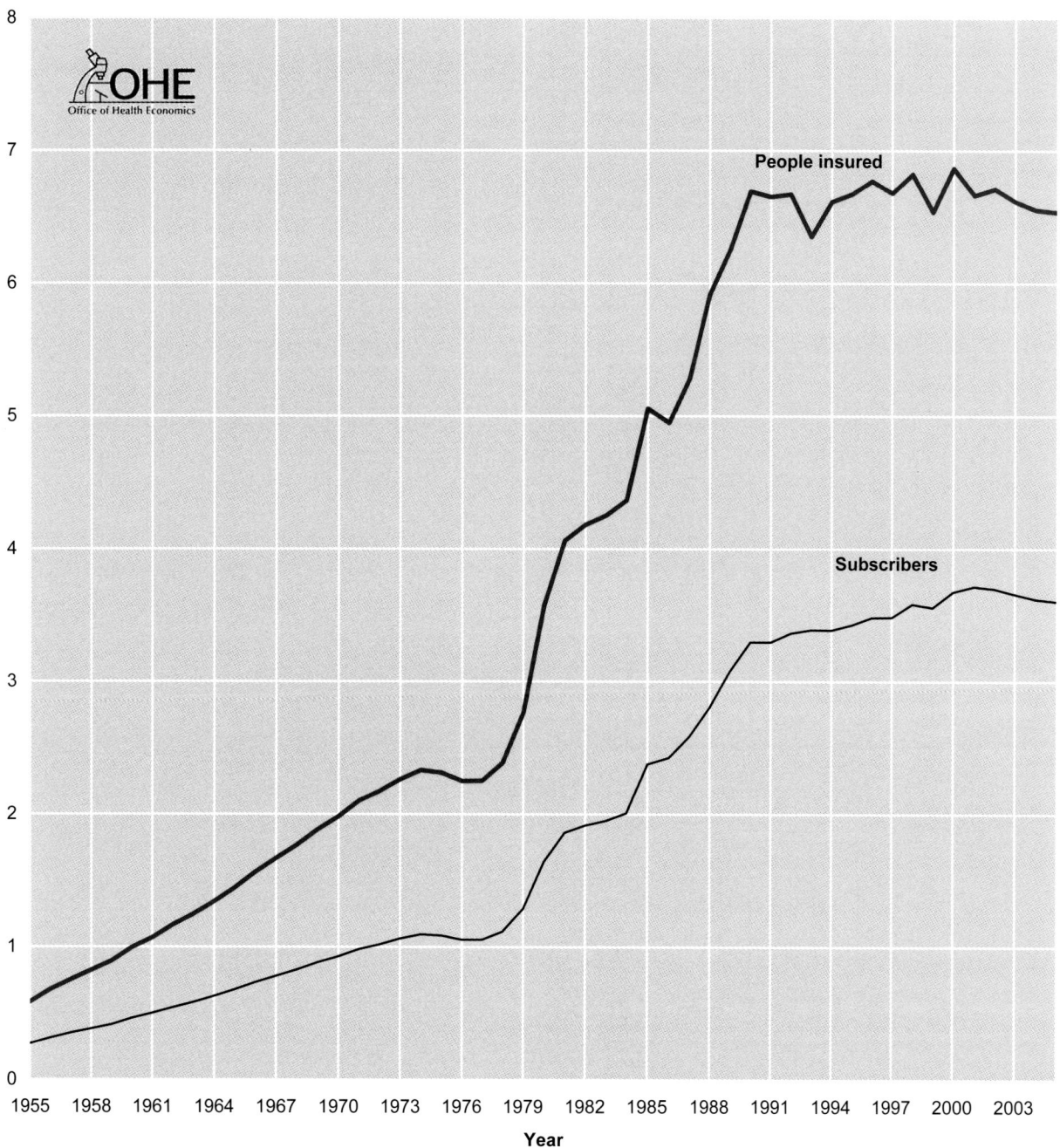

Year

*Note:*     There is a break in the time series between 1984 and 1985; see Table 2.30.
*Sources:*  Lee Donaldson Associates (for data from 1955 to 1984).
            Laing's Healthcare Market Review (Laing and Buisson, for data from 1985 onwards).

Table 2.32   **Private health care and gross NHS expenditure per household, UK, 1973 - 2006**

| Year | Expenditure per household | | | Index[1] of real expenditure per household | | | Total private health expenditure as % of total consumer spending[5] |
|---|---|---|---|---|---|---|---|
| | Private health[2] £(cash) | Private medical products[3] | NHS[4] £(cash) | Private health[2] 1973=100 | Private medical products[3] 1973=100 | NHS[4] 1973=100 | |
| 1973 | 5 | 10 | 148 | 100 | 100 | 100 | 0.7 |
| 1974 | 6 | 12 | 197 | 104 | 99 | 114 | 0.7 |
| 1975 | 7 | 14 | 261 | 91 | 91 | 120 | 0.6 |
| 1976 | 8 | 16 | 305 | 97 | 90 | 122 | 0.6 |
| 1977 | 10 | 17 | 337 | 105 | 88 | 119 | 0.6 |
| 1978 | 11 | 20 | 378 | 104 | 89 | 118 | 0.6 |
| 1979 | 13 | 25 | 437 | 103 | 96 | 120 | 0.6 |
| 1980 | 17 | 30 | 551 | 117 | 99 | 128 | 0.7 |
| 1981 | 22 | 33 | 624 | 135 | 98 | 130 | 0.7 |
| 1982 | 28 | 38 | 676 | 161 | 105 | 133 | 0.8 |
| 1983 | 32 | 43 | 719 | 172 | 113 | 133 | 0.8 |
| 1984 | 29 | 51 | 757 | 151 | 128 | 135 | 0.9 |
| 1985 | 34 | 55 | 799 | 168 | 133 | 135 | 0.9 |
| 1986 | 39 | 63 | 858 | 185 | 146 | 140 | 0.9 |
| 1987 | 49 | 65 | 931 | 219 | 145 | 145 | 0.9 |
| 1988 | 56 | 72 | 1,066 | 238 | 149 | 156 | 0.9 |
| 1989 | 60 | 80 | 1,144 | 237 | 153 | 155 | 1.0 |
| 1990 | 72 | 85 | 1,254 | 261 | 151 | 158 | 1.0 |
| 1991 | 86 | 100 | 1,401 | 297 | 170 | 167 | 1.1 |
| 1992 | 87 | 118 | 1,537 | 291 | 193 | 177 | 1.2 |
| 1993 | 92 | 127 | 1,605 | 299 | 202 | 179 | 1.3 |
| 1994 | 102 | 162 | 1,701 | 327 | 254 | 187 | 1.5 |
| 1995 | 108 | 167 | 1,782 | 335 | 254 | 191 | 1.5 |
| 1996 | 129 | 178 | 1,841 | 386 | 261 | 191 | 1.5 |
| 1997 | 150 | 185 | 1,926 | 437 | 265 | 194 | 1.6 |
| 1998 | 170 | 197 | 2,018 | 485 | 275 | 199 | 1.6 |
| 1999 | 181 | 208 | 2,176 | 508 | 286 | 211 | 1.7 |
| 2000 | 210 | 217 | 2,356 | 582 | 295 | 225 | 1.7 |
| 2001 | 236 | 233 | 2,561 | 635 | 308 | 238 | 1.8 |
| 2002 | 268 | 253 | 2,818 | 699 | 323 | 253 | 2.0 |
| 2003 | 294 | 262 | 3,153 | 742 | 324 | 275 | 2.0 |
| 2004 | 319 | 268 | 3,428 | 786 | 323 | 291 | 2.1 |
| 2005 | 344 | 256 | 3,726 | 829 | 302 | 309 | 2.0 |
| 2006 | 369 | 273 | 3,976 | 867 | 315 | 322 | 2.1 |

*Notes:*   1 At constant prices, as adjusted by the GDP deflator at market prices.
2 Consumer expenditure on Private Medical Insurance (PMI) and private medical treatment.
3 Figures relate to consumer expenditure on medical goods including medicines not purchased on NHS prescription, and expenditure on therapeutic equipments such as spectacles, contact lenses and hearing aids.
4 Including charges paid by patients.
5 Consumer spending includes purchases of all goods and services.
GDP = Gross Domestic Product.

*Sources:*   Consumer Trends (ONS).
Annual Abstract of Statistics (ONS).
The Government's Expenditure Plans (DH).
Lee Donaldson Associates (for data from 1973-84).
Laing's Healthcare Market Review (Laing and Buisson).
Regional Trends (ONS).
Northern Ireland Statistics and Research Agency (NISRA).
Economic Trends (ONS).
UK dentistry market research report (MBD).

# Private Health Care

Figure 2.21 **UK consumer expenditure on private health care at 2006 prices [1], 1973 - 2006**

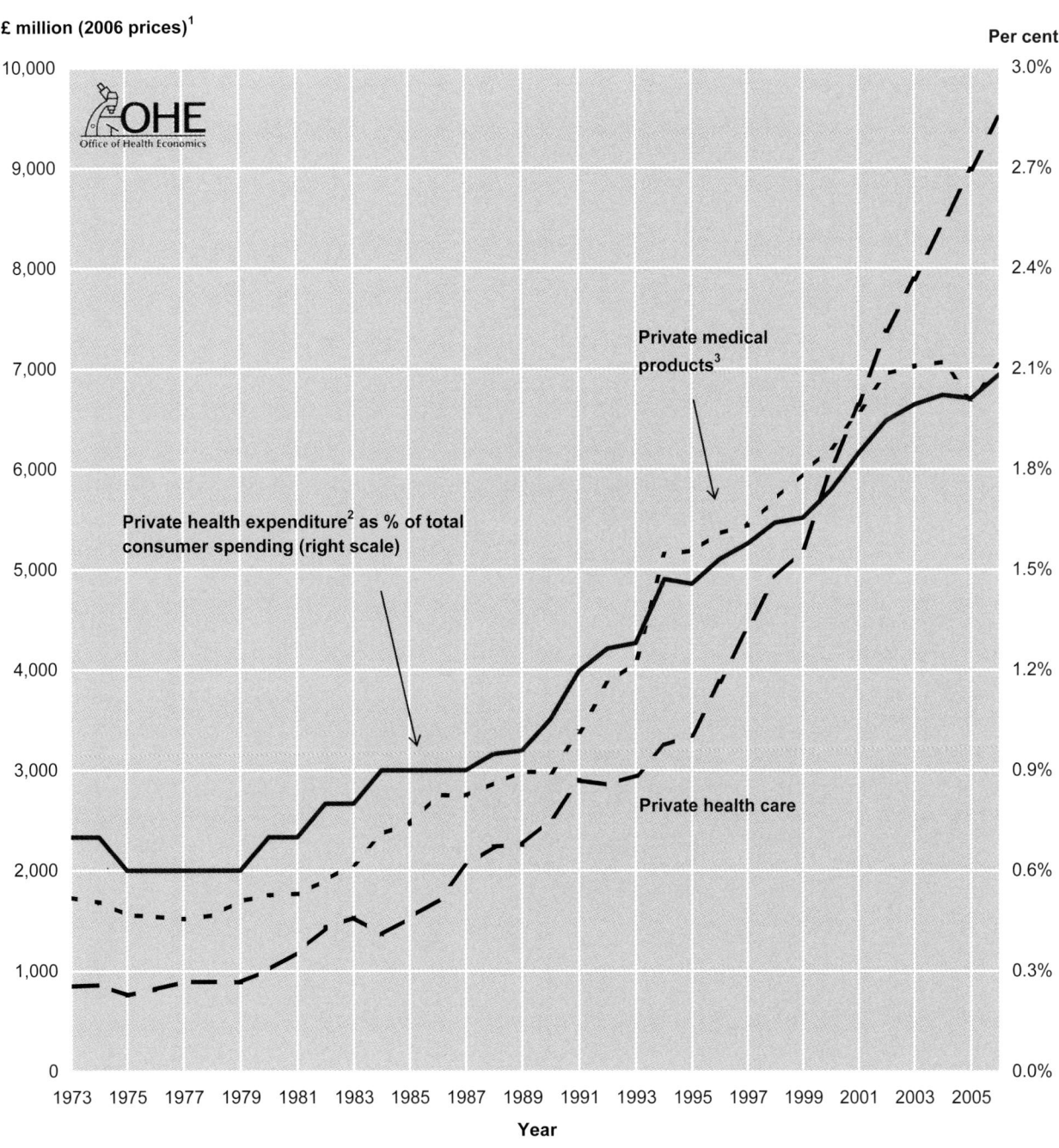

**£ million (2006 prices)[1]**

**Per cent**

Private medical products[3]

Private health expenditure[2] as % of total consumer spending (right scale)

Private health care

**Year**

*Notes:*  1 As adjusted by the Gross Domestic Product (GDP) deflator.
2 Including pharmaceuticals (see Table 2.1).
3 Figures relate to consumer expenditure on medical goods including medicines not purchased on NHS prescription, and expenditure on therapeutic equipment such as spectacles, contact lenses and hearing aids.

*Sources:*  Consumer Trends (ONS).
Annual Abstract of Statistics (ONS).
Economic Trends (ONS).
The Government's Expenditure Plans (DH).
Department of Health Departmental Report (DH).
Health Statistics Wales (NAW).
NHS Board Operating Costs and Capital Expenditure, ISD Scotland (ISD).
Public Expenditure Statistical Analyses (HM Treasury).
Lee Donaldson Associates (for data from 1955 - 1984).
Laing's Healthcare Market Review (Laing and Buisson).
Regional Trends (ONS).
Northern Ireland Statistics and Research Agency (NISRA).
Population Projections Database (GAD).
UK dentistry market research report (MBD).

Table 2.33   **Private[1] health care expenditure as a percentage of GDP in OECD and EU countries, 1960 - 2005**

Per cent

|  | Year | | | | | | | | | | |
|---|---|---|---|---|---|---|---|---|---|---|---|
|  | 1960 | 1970 | 1980 | 1990 | 1995 | 2000 | 2001 | 2002 | 2003 | 2004 | 2005[3] |
| **OECD[2]** | **2.7** | **2.8** | **2.8** | **3.5** | **3.4** | **4.0** | **4.3** | **4.4** | **4.4** | **4.4** | **4.4** |
| **EU27[2]** | **1.0** | **1.1** | **1.2** | **1.5** | **1.7** | **1.8** | **1.8** | **1.9** | **2.0** | **2.0** | **2.2** |
| **EU15[2]** | **1.1** | **1.1** | **1.4** | **1.6** | **1.9** | **2.0** | **2.0** | **2.1** | **2.2** | **2.2** | **2.2** |
| Australia | 2.0 | 1.3 | 2.5 | 2.5 | 2.7 | 2.8 | 2.9 | 3.0 | 3.0 | 3.1 | - |
| Austria | 1.3 | 1.9 | 2.3 | 1.8 | 2.8 | 2.4 | 2.4 | 2.5 | 2.5 | 2.5 | 2.5 |
| Belgium | 1.3 | 0.5 | 1.1 | 0.8 | 1.8 | 2.1 | 2.0 | 2.2 | 2.9 | 2.8 | 2.8 |
| Bulgaria | - | - | - | - | - | 2.5 | 3.2 | 3.0 | 3.0 | 3.4 | 3.5 |
| Canada | 3.1 | 2.1 | 1.7 | 2.3 | 2.6 | 2.6 | 2.8 | 2.9 | 2.9 | 2.9 | 2.9 |
| Cyprus | - | - | - | - | - | 3.4 | 3.4 | 3.4 | 3.3 | 3.2 | - |
| Czech Republic | - | - | - | 0.1 | 0.6 | 0.6 | 0.7 | 0.7 | 0.8 | 0.8 | 0.8 |
| Denmark | 0.4 | 0.8 | 1.1 | 1.4 | 1.4 | 1.5 | 1.5 | 1.5 | 1.4 | 1.4 | 1.4 |
| Estonia | - | - | - | - | - | 1.2 | 1.1 | 1.1 | 1.2 | 1.3 | - |
| Finland | 1.8 | 1.4 | 1.3 | 1.5 | 1.8 | 1.6 | 1.6 | 1.7 | 1.7 | 1.7 | 1.7 |
| France | 1.4 | 1.3 | 1.4 | 2.0 | 2.1 | 2.1 | 2.1 | 2.1 | 2.2 | 2.3 | 2.2 |
| Germany | 1.6 | 1.6 | 1.8 | 2.0 | 1.9 | 2.1 | 2.2 | 2.2 | 2.3 | 2.4 | 2.5 |
| Greece | - | 2.7 | 2.3 | 2.7 | 3.6 | 5.2 | 5.2 | 5.2 | 5.4 | 5.3 | 5.8 |
| Hungary | - | - | - | - | 1.2 | 2.0 | 2.2 | 2.3 | 2.4 | 2.4 | - |
| Iceland | 1.1 | 1.7 | 0.8 | 1.0 | 1.3 | 1.7 | 1.7 | 1.7 | 1.8 | 1.8 | 1.7 |
| Ireland | 0.9 | 0.9 | 1.5 | 1.7 | 1.9 | 1.7 | 1.8 | 1.7 | 1.7 | 1.6 | 1.7 |
| Italy | 0.6 | 0.7 | 1.3 | 1.6 | 2.1 | 2.2 | 2.1 | 2.1 | 2.1 | 2.1 | 2.1 |
| Japan | 1.2 | 1.4 | 1.9 | 1.3 | 1.2 | 1.4 | 1.5 | 1.5 | 1.5 | 1.5 | - |
| Korea, Republic of | - | - | - | 2.8 | 2.7 | 2.5 | 2.5 | 2.6 | 2.6 | 2.6 | 2.8 |
| Latvia | - | - | - | - | - | 2.7 | 3.0 | 3.0 | 3.1 | 3.1 | - |
| Lithuania | - | - | - | - | - | 2.0 | 1.7 | 1.6 | 1.6 | 1.6 | - |
| Luxembourg | - | 0.3 | 0.4 | 0.4 | 0.4 | 0.6 | 0.8 | 0.7 | 0.7 | 0.8 | - |
| Malta | - | - | - | - | - | 1.9 | 1.8 | 1.8 | 1.9 | 2.0 | - |
| Mexico | - | - | - | 2.9 | 3.3 | 3.0 | 3.3 | 3.5 | 3.5 | 3.5 | 3.5 |
| Netherlands | 2.5 | 0.9 | 2.3 | 2.6 | 2.4 | 2.9 | 3.1 | 3.3 | 3.4 | 3.5 | - |
| New Zealand | 0.8 | 1.0 | 0.7 | 1.2 | 1.6 | 1.7 | 1.8 | 1.8 | 1.7 | 1.9 | 2.0 |
| Norway | 0.6 | 0.4 | 1.0 | 1.3 | 1.2 | 1.5 | 1.4 | 1.6 | 1.6 | 1.6 | 1.5 |
| Poland | - | - | - | 0.4 | 1.5 | 1.7 | 1.6 | 1.8 | 1.9 | 2.0 | 1.9 |
| Portugal | - | 1.0 | 1.9 | 2.0 | 2.9 | 2.4 | 2.5 | 2.5 | 2.6 | 2.8 | 2.8 |
| Romania | - | - | - | - | - | 1.7 | 1.8 | 1.9 | 1.0 | 1.4 | 1.3 |
| Slovak Republic | - | - | - | - | - | 0.6 | 0.6 | 0.6 | 0.7 | 1.9 | 1.8 |
| Slovenia | - | - | - | - | - | 1.9 | 2.1 | 2.1 | 2.1 | 2.0 | - |
| Spain | 0.6 | 1.2 | 1.1 | 1.4 | 2.1 | 2.0 | 2.1 | 2.1 | 2.3 | 2.3 | 2.4 |
| Sweden | 1.2 | 1.0 | 0.7 | 0.8 | 1.1 | 1.3 | 1.3 | 1.4 | 1.4 | 1.4 | 1.4 |
| Switzerland | 2.5 | 2.2 | 2.7 | 3.9 | 4.5 | 4.6 | 4.7 | 4.7 | 4.8 | 4.8 | 4.7 |
| Turkey | - | 0.3 | 1.2 | 0.3 | 1.0 | 2.5 | 2.4 | 2.2 | 2.2 | 2.1 | 2.2 |
| UK | 0.5 | 0.6 | 0.4 | 0.6 | 0.9 | 1.1 | 1.2 | 1.2 | 1.3 | 1.3 | 1.2 |
| USA | 3.9 | 4.5 | 5.2 | 7.2 | 7.2 | 7.4 | 7.7 | 8.1 | 8.4 | 8.4 | 8.4 |

*Notes:*   Trends over time should be interpreted with caution as there are several breaks in series (see OECD Health Database for further information).
1 Private health care is calculated by subtracting public expenditure on health from total health care spending.
2 Weighted average. EU15 as constituted before 1 May 2004 and EU27 as constituted since 1 January 2007. Figures exclude Cyprus.
3 OECD figure includes 2004 data for Australia, Hungary, Japan, Luxembourg and the Netherlands. EU27 figure includes 2004 data for Cyprus, Estonia, Hungary, Latvia, Lithuania, Luxembourg, Malta, the Netherlands and Slovenia. EU15 figure includes 2004 data for Luxembourg and the Netherlands.
2005 figures for Belgium, Cyprus, Denmark, Estonia, Japan, Latvia, Lithuania, Malta, Slovak Republic and Slovenia are WHO provisional estimates.
GDP = Gross Domestic Product.
- Not available.

*Sources:*   OECD Health Database (OECD).
World Development Indicators (World Bank).
World Health Report: Core Health Indicators (WHO).
World Health Organisation National Health Accounts Series (WHO).
For sources of UK data refer to Table 2.1.
Economic Trends (ONS).

# Private Health Care

Table 2.34    Private[1] health care expenditure per capita (£ cash) in OECD and EU countries, 1960 - 2005

**Private health care expenditure per capita (£ cash)**

| | Year | | | | | | | | | | |
|---|---|---|---|---|---|---|---|---|---|---|---|
| | 1960 | 1970 | 1980 | 1990 | 1995 | 2000 | 2001 | 2002 | 2003 | 2004 | 2005[3] |
| OECD[2] | 16 | 34 | 119 | 338 | 486 | 606 | 664 | 688 | 705 | 682 | 723 |
| EU27[2] | 4 | 12 | 61 | 156 | 248 | 227 | 245 | 264 | 306 | 293 | 336 |
| EU15[2] | 4 | 12 | 61 | 178 | 284 | 279 | 300 | 321 | 374 | 388 | 406 |
| | | | | | | | | | | | |
| Australia | 13 | 19 | 125 | 260 | 359 | 382 | 396 | 428 | 503 | 555 | - |
| Austria | 4 | 16 | 107 | 220 | 529 | 377 | 400 | 424 | 481 | 489 | 508 |
| Belgium | 6 | 6 | 59 | 90 | 314 | 308 | 319 | 362 | 520 | 516 | 556 |
| Bulgaria | - | - | - | - | - | 26 | 38 | 40 | 46 | 58 | 67 |
| Canada | 25 | 35 | 81 | 265 | 331 | 406 | 446 | 455 | 487 | 492 | 561 |
| Cyprus | - | - | - | - | - | 260 | 282 | 290 | 322 | 330 | - |
| Czech Republic | - | - | - | 2 | 22 | 23 | 29 | 33 | 42 | 46 | 54 |
| Denmark | 2 | 11 | 64 | 213 | 313 | 287 | 309 | 322 | 346 | 356 | 380 |
| Estonia | - | - | - | - | - | 33 | 33 | 40 | 50 | 60 | - |
| Finland | 7 | 15 | 63 | 231 | 297 | 253 | 271 | 289 | 335 | 330 | 345 |
| France | 7 | 16 | 78 | 241 | 363 | 307 | 329 | 348 | 410 | 419 | 434 |
| Germany | 8 | 22 | 106 | 275 | 365 | 319 | 344 | 361 | 415 | 441 | 461 |
| Greece | - | 18 | 61 | 158 | 323 | 459 | 492 | 533 | 659 | 692 | 813 |
| Hungary | - | - | - | - | 33 | 63 | 81 | 98 | 121 | 132 | - |
| Iceland | 6 | 18 | 47 | 145 | 221 | 341 | 317 | 351 | 413 | 428 | 496 |
| Ireland | 2 | 6 | 41 | 131 | 223 | 285 | 346 | 363 | 409 | 401 | 442 |
| Italy | 2 | 6 | 47 | 176 | 267 | 280 | 281 | 301 | 338 | 342 | 351 |
| Japan | 2 | 11 | 73 | 183 | 309 | 349 | 326 | 302 | 304 | 289 | - |
| Korea, Republic of | - | - | - | 95 | 194 | 182 | 179 | 196 | 203 | 201 | 252 |
| Latvia | - | - | - | - | - | 58 | 73 | 79 | 91 | 99 | - |
| Lithuania | - | - | - | - | - | 42 | 42 | 44 | 52 | 57 | - |
| Luxembourg | - | 6 | 27 | 69 | 133 | 191 | 245 | 222 | 285 | 311 | - |
| Malta | - | - | - | - | - | 121 | 118 | 125 | 135 | 145 | - |
| Mexico | - | - | - | 52 | 65 | 115 | 142 | 147 | 135 | 124 | 139 |
| Netherlands | 9 | 10 | 125 | 290 | 413 | 467 | 534 | 602 | 683 | 708 | - |
| New Zealand | 5 | 10 | 22 | 88 | 173 | 153 | 173 | 184 | 214 | 257 | 291 |
| Norway | 3 | 5 | 69 | 204 | 269 | 365 | 381 | 456 | 492 | 488 | 534 |
| Poland | - | - | - | 4 | 34 | 49 | 57 | 63 | 65 | 70 | 83 |
| Portugal | - | 4 | 26 | 87 | 212 | 176 | 195 | 205 | 235 | 256 | 269 |
| Romania | - | - | - | - | - | 19 | 24 | 28 | 17 | 27 | 32 |
| Slovak Republic | - | - | - | - | - | 15 | 16 | 19 | 26 | 81 | 88 |
| Slovenia | - | - | - | - | - | 121 | 142 | 154 | 180 | 174 | - |
| Spain | 1 | 6 | 28 | 105 | 199 | 194 | 216 | 231 | 299 | 312 | 338 |
| Sweden | 9 | 17 | 45 | 134 | 194 | 227 | 228 | 247 | 282 | 297 | 304 |
| Switzerland | 15 | 33 | 203 | 775 | 1,275 | 1,046 | 1,125 | 1,183 | 1,279 | 1,276 | 1,261 |
| Turkey | - | 1 | 8 | 5 | 16 | 48 | 35 | 39 | 45 | 49 | 60 |
| UK | 3 | 6 | 17 | 62 | 111 | 176 | 195 | 218 | 233 | 247 | 254 |
| USA | 40 | 93 | 270 | 928 | 1,266 | 1,699 | 1,893 | 1,953 | 1,931 | 1,823 | 1,933 |

Notes:    Trends over time should be interpreted with caution as there are several breaks in series (see OECD Health Database for further information).
1 Private health care is calculated by subtracting public expenditure on health from total health care spending.
2 Weighted average. EU15 as constituted before 1 May 2004 and EU27 as constituted since 1 January 2007. Figures exclude Cyprus.
3 OECD figure includes 2004 data for Australia, Hungary, Japan, Luxembourg and the Netherlands. EU27 figure includes 2004 data for Cyprus, Estonia, Hungary, Latvia, Lithuania, Luxembourg, Malta, the Netherlands and Slovenia. EU15 figure includes 2004 data for Luxembourg and the Netherlands.
2005 figures for Belgium, Cyprus, Denmark, Estonia, Japan, Latvia, Lithuania, Malta, Slovak Republic and Slovenia are WHO provisional estimates.
GDP = Gross Domestic Product.
- Not available.

Sources:   OECD Health Database (OECD).
World Development Indicators (World Bank).
World Health Report: Core Health Indicators (WHO).

Figure 2.22 **Private health care expenditure per capita in OECD and EU countries, 2005**

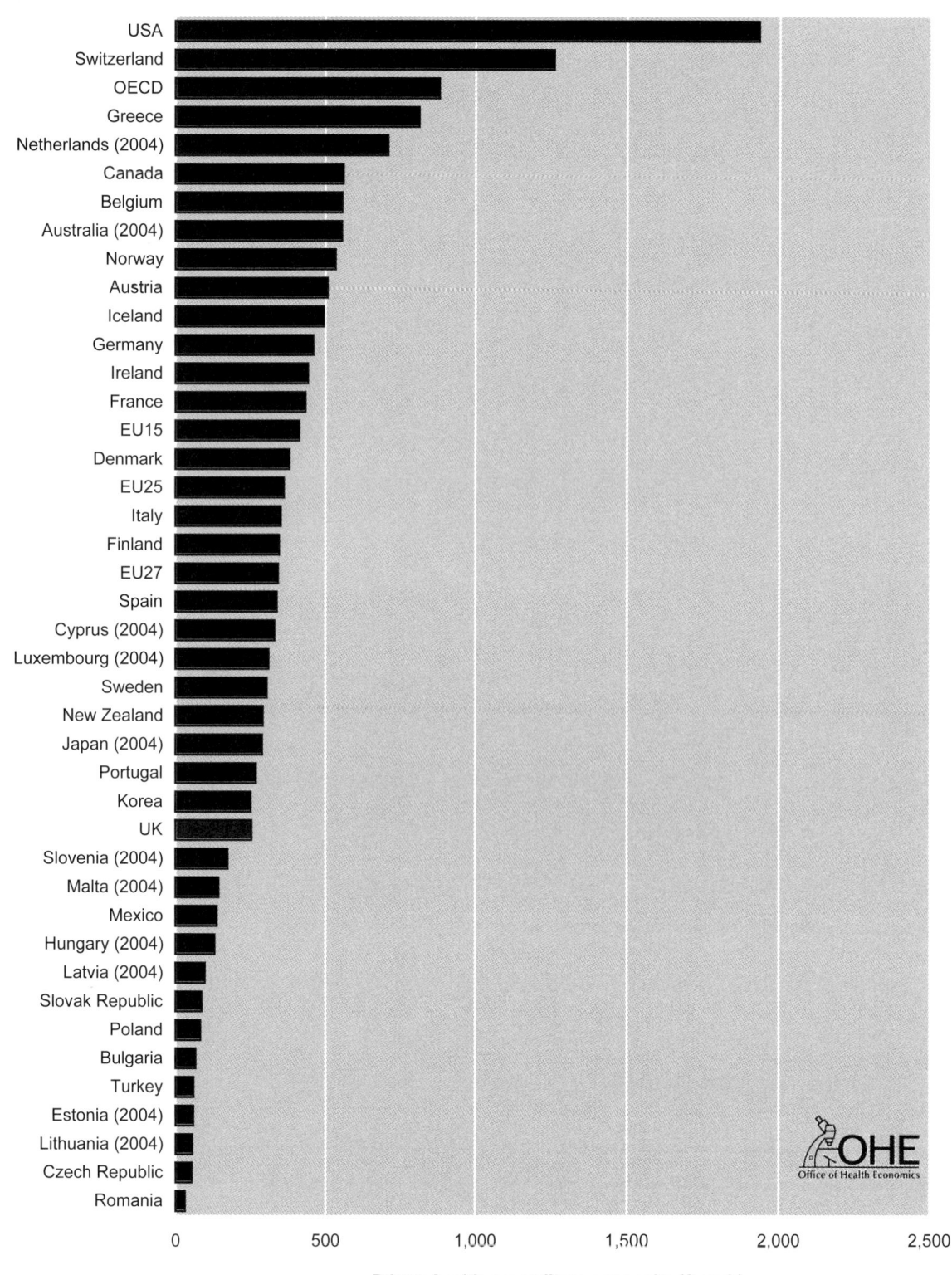

**Private health expenditure per capita (£ cash)**

*Notes:*  Figures are dependent on exchange rates between national currencies and £ sterling.

2005 figures for Belgium, Cyprus, Denmark, Estonia, Japan, Latvia, Lithuania, Malta, Slovak Republic and Slovenia are WHO  provisional estimates,

*Sources:*  OECD Health Database (OECD).

World Development Indicators (World Bank).

World Health Report: Core Health Indicators (WHO).

World Health Organisation National Health Accounts Series (WHO).

For sources of UK data refer to Table 2.1.

# Hospital Services

## Main Points

- The number of available acute NHS hospital beds has been little changed for more than a decade and is still low by international standards at 2.2 acute beds per 1,000 population in Great Britain.

- The total number of finished consultant episodes/discharges and deaths in the UK NHS in 2005/06 was 17.1 million, which was 15.2% higher than in 2000/01. But over the same five year period, hospital and community health staffing increased 23.3%

- Waiting lists for NHS admission have fallen dramatically by 32% (334,000) over the past five years. Average waiting times have also fallen, with only a tiny percentage of patients now recorded as waiting greater than 6 months.

This section of the Compendium deals mainly with NHS hospital activities, excluding community health and other non-hospital services unless otherwise stated.

### Cost of hospital services

In the UK in 2005/06 the gross cost of NHS hospital services was £44.9 billion, 54% higher in real terms than just ten years earlier (**Table 3.1**). Since the NHS was first established, NHS hospital expenditure has grown in most years, even after allowing for general inflation (**Figure 3.1**). Despite these increases, growth in expenditure on Family Health Services (FHS) has exceeded that of the hospital sector for the past three decades (**Box 1**).

| Box 1 Real[1] decadal growth in UK NHS expenditure | | | |
|---|---|---|---|
| **Decade** | **Hospital** | **FHS** | **All NHS** |
| 1965 – 1975 | 71 | 33 | 67 |
| 1975 – 1985 | 14 | 42 | 23 |
| 1985 – 1995 | 40 | 53 | 55 |
| 1995 – 2005 | 53 | 68 | 76 |

*Notes:* 1 As adjusted by the GDP deflator.
FHS = Family Health Services.
All figures include patient charges and capital expenditure.
*Sources:* The Government Expenditure Plans.
Public Expenditure Statistical Analyses (HM Treasury).
NHS Board Operating Costs and Capital Expenditure, ISD Scotland (ISD).
Department of Health Departmental Report (DH).
NHS Summarised Accounts (House of Commons).
Scottish Health Statistics (ISD).
Health Statistics Wales (NAW).
Annual Abstract of Statistics (ONS).
Population Projections Database (GAD).
Economic Trends (ONS).

This slower relative growth of the hospital sector reflects a deliberate political switch towards primary and community based health care. As a result, the share of NHS resources given to the hospital services has fallen from 69% in 1972/73 to 46% in 2005/06 (**Figure 3.1**). The UK still devotes proportionally more of its health care resources to hospital services than do many other developed countries (**Figure 3.3**).

UK per capita expenditure on NHS hospital services rose to £744 in 2005/06, however, this was not consistent across the UK (**Table 3.2**). In 2005/06, per capita spending on NHS hospital services was much higher in Scotland, standing at £882 than in any other part of the UK.

There has been a large difference between "volume" and "real" hospital expenditure growth in the UK (**Figure 3.4**). This is mainly due to the relatively greater impact of wage inflation on the labour intensive hospital sector as compared to other areas of the economy.

### Hospital workforce

In 2005 there were over 1.2 million staff employed in NHS hospitals and community health services, the highest ever number (**Table 3.3**). However, at times there have been apparent reductions in some sectors of the hospital workforce. The exclusion of Project 2000 nurses in 1990 (a then new university-based system of nurse education), produced an apparent reduction in numbers and, since 1982, contracting out of domestic and ancillary services has significantly reduced the number directly employed by NHS hospitals in that category. The interpretation of workforce data based on headcount numbers rather than full-time equivalents should be made with caution as this does not take account of possible shifts in working patterns from full-time to part-time status.

| Box 2 Numbers of NHS hospital general and senior managers (England) | |
|---|---|
| **Year** | **Hospital managers** |
| 1996 | 20,588 |
| 1997 | 21,433 |
| 1998 | 21,853 |
| 1999 | 23,378 |
| 2000 | 24,253 |
| 2001 | 26,285 |
| 2002 | 30,914 |
| 2003 | 33,809 |
| 2004 | 36,007 |
| 2005 | 37,549 |
| 2006 | 35,040 |

*Note:* Figures refer to full-time equivalents at 30th September. The apparent drop between 2005 and 2006 may in part be due to additional validation resulting in the identification of duplicate records.
*Sources:* Health and Personal Social Services Statistics for England (DH).
NHS hospital and community heath services non-medical staff in England (IC).

The most rapid increases in staffing levels have been in the non-medical, non-nursing, professional and technical areas; followed by administrative and clerical staff (**Figure 3.5**). The latter group includes general and senior managers, whose measured numbers have grown by 70% over the last ten years, despite a fall in 2005/06 (**Box 2**).

The number of medical and dental staff working in NHS hospitals, measured by full-time equivalents (FTE), has increased in every year but one (1987) since 1951 (**Box 3** and **Table 3.3**). In 2005, the number of hospital medical and dental staff employed in NHS hospitals rose above 100,000, which equates to 167 per 100,000 population in the UK, almost six times the ratio in 1951 (**Table 3.4**). Despite the rises, the number of doctors per 100,000 population in the UK remains well below that for most OECD countries, although comparisons should be made with caution due to differences in definitions (see also **Section 4**).

Box 3   **Decadal change (%) in numbers of hospital medical and dental staff[1], UK**

| Decade | Total medical and dental staff | Staff per 100,000 population | FCEs[2] per staff |
|---|---|---|---|
| 1965 - 1975 | 50 | 45 | -27 |
| 1975 - 1985 | 32 | 31 | -2 |
| 1985 - 1995 | 36 | 33 | 22 |
| 1995 - 2005 | 56 | 50 | -19 |

Notes:    1 Figures relate to full-time equivalent staff numbers.
2 Prior to 1987/88 figures relate to discharges and deaths.
Sources: Population Projections database (GAD).
Annual Abstract of Statistics (ONS).
The Government Expenditure Plans (DH).
Health Statistics Wales (NAW).
Scottish Health Statistics (ISD).
Hospital Episode Statistics (DH).

In England 36% of all NHS hospital medical and dental staff were Consultants in 2006. This proportion has increased slightly in recent years. The NHS in England had 86 thousand FTE hospital and community medical staff in 2006, 59% more than a decade earlier (**Table 3.8**). There are, however, large differences between specialties in the rates of increase (**Tables 3.11** and **3.12**). Some of these apparent differences are the results of changes in classification only. For instance, Consultants in the specialty of General Medicine were reclassified in 1994 using their second specialty instead of the first. This resulted in the recorded number of FTE Consultants in General Medicine falling from 1,179 in 1994 to 238 in 1995. Other specialties within the General Medicine area, such as Cardiology and Gastroenterology, saw sharply increased numbers recorded as a result of this reclassification. The number of hospital and community medical and dental staff differs between the constituent countries (**Table 3.10**). In England there were 158 staff per 1,000 population compared to 182 in Scotland.

In 2005, the number of WTE NHS hospital Consultants per 10,000 population was 578 in Great Britain, however, there were considerably more hospital consultants per population than this in Scotland and fewer in Wales (**Table 3.12**).

In 2005 there were 506,000 hospital nurses and midwives in the UK. The number remains below the peak level reported in 1989 (**Table 3.6** and **Figure 3.6**) but has increased by 87,000 since 1997.

In parallel with the increased number of nursing and midwifery staff and the reduced number of hospital beds in the UK, there has been a steady reduction in the number of NHS beds per nurse since 1951 (**Table 3.7**). In contrast, nurses and midwives have experienced an increase in caseload over the past decade in terms of inpatient finished consultant episodes (FCEs) **(Box 4).**

Box 4   **Decadal change (%) in nursing and midwifery staff[1], UK**

| Decade | Total numbers | Per 100,000 population | FCE's[2] per staff[1] |
|---|---|---|---|
| 1965 - 1975 | 52 | 47 | -28 |
| 1975 - 1985 | 14 | 14 | 13 |
| 1985 - 1995 | -16 | -18 | 99 |
| 1995 - 2005 | 20 | 16 | 5 |

Notes:    1 Figures relate to whole-time equivalent staff.
2 Prior to 1987/88, figures relate to discharges and deaths. At least part of the change in trend direction is due to the difference between discharges and deaths and FCEs.
Sources: Population Projections Database (GAD).
Annual Abstract of Statistics (ONS).
The Government Expenditure Plans (DH).
Health Statistics Wales (NAW).
Scottish Health Statistics (ISD).
Hospital Episode Statistics (DH).

## Hospital activities

### Hospital beds

Whilst NHS hospital medical staff numbers continue to increase and the population is rising, NHS hospital bed numbers are continuing to fall, although at a much slower rate than previously (**Table 3.13**), this pattern is true throughout the constituent countries of the UK. The number of NHS hospital beds per thousand population in the UK has dropped from a peak of 11.0 in the 1950s to 3.7 in 2005/06. **Box 5** shows the particularly steep decadal change in NHS available beds between 1985 and 1995.

The UK has fewer hospital inpatient acute beds per capita than most other economically developed countries (**Figure 3.7**). However, such differences are difficult to interpret. For some OECD countries, private hospitals and/or nursing homes are included in the figures, but they are not in the UK figures.

Most of the historic reduction in NHS hospital beds has occurred in mental health wards, where bed numbers have fallen 78% since 1959 in Great Britain (**Table 3.14**). This dramatic change is largely due to a marked shift in attitudes towards mental health and a change to providing care in the community, facilitated by development of new medicines in the area.

# Hospital Services

**Box 5  Decadal change (%) in number of NHS available beds, UK**

| Decade | Total | Per head of population |
|--------|-------|------------------------|
| 1965 – 1975 | -10 | -13 |
| 1975 – 1985 | -15 | -16 |
| 1985 – 1995 | -35 | -37 |
| 1995 – 2005 | -17 | -20 |

*Notes:* Including psychiatric hospitals.
Data for 1995 relates to 1995/96 and data for 2005 relates to 2005/06.
*Sources:* Health and Personal Social Services for England (DH).
Health Statistics Wales (NAW).
Scottish Health Statistics (ISD).
Annual Abstract of Statistics (ONS).
Hospital Activity Statistics (DH).
Population Projections Database (GAD).

In 2005/06 there were 129,000 beds in the acute (surgical and non-surgical) specialty group in Great Britain, 59% of all NHS hospital beds. This corresponds to 22 acute beds per 10,000 population (**Table 3.14**).

The occupancy of NHS acute beds in England at 84% in 2006/07 is slightly below the peak level reached a few years before but is still somewhat higher than in the 1990s. (**Table 3.16**). High bed occupancy accompanied by shorter lengths of stay in hospital, indicates that NHS beds are being used intensively. For the UK as a whole, the average (acute and non-acute) bed occupancy rate has ranged between 79% and 88% for the last 50 years and is currently 84% (**Table 3.16**).

Until 1985, the Hospital Inpatient Enquiry (HIPE) gave a detailed account of NHS hospital activity in England. These data were collected under the Hospital Activity Analysis system (HAA) and based on a 10% sample of inpatient and day case records. Together with the Mental Health Enquiry, HIPE was officially replaced on 1st April 1987 by the Hospital Episode Statistics (HES), which are based on the Körner data collection system. This brought major changes to the way hospital information is collected and compiled in England including the use of finished consultant episodes (FCEs see **Glossary**), instead of deaths and discharges, and the introduction of the 4th revision of the OPCS classification of surgical operations. Data for Wales are based on discharges and deaths, although, they too changed to the HES system in April 1991. Comparisons over time and between countries should be made with caution due to organisational changes, reviews of best practice within the medical community, data quality problems that are often year specific and differences in definition. see **Note 1** on page 139 for further information on current definitions for FCEs/discharges and deaths in the four countries of the UK. Throughout the Compendium, FCE is used as a shorthand to refer to both measures.

The number of inpatient and day cases treated in NHS hospitals as measured by finished consultant episodes (England since 1987/88) and discharges and deaths (Wales, Scotland and Northern Ireland, and in England prior to 1987/88; also see **Glossary**) rose to 17.1 million in the UK in 2005/06, compared with 3.8 million in 1951 (**Table 3.17**). The ratio of FCEs/discharges and deaths annually per hospital bed rose to 76 in 2005/06, 10 times as many as 50 years earlier. The ratio of FCEs per available hospital bed has accelerated particularly steeply since the mid 1980s (**Box 6**). The change in unit of measurement from "deaths and discharges" to FCEs in England (while other parts of the UK still measure hospital activity in terms of deaths and discharges) has boosted measured throughput since 1987/88 relative to the years before then.

**Box 6  Growth in FCEs[1] (%), UK**

| Decade | FCEs[1] | FCEs[1] per available bed |
|--------|---------|---------------------------|
| 1965 - 1975 | 10 | 22 |
| 1975 - 1985 | 30 | 53 |
| 1985 - 1995 | 66 | 157 |
| 1995 - 2005 | 26 | 52 |

*Notes:* 1 Figures relate to inpatient FCEs in England and Wales from 1987/88 onwards but otherwise to discharges and deaths.
Available bed data for 1995 relates to 1995/96 and data for 2005 relates to 2005/06.
*Sources:* Annual Abstract of Statistics (ONS).
The Government Expenditure Plans (DH).
Health Statistics Wales (NAW).
Scottish Health Statistics (ISD).
Hospital Episode Statistics (DH).

In Great Britain 81% of hospital inpatient admissions are for acute medicine or surgery (**Table 3.18**). Hospital acute admissions and discharges per 1,000 population in the UK are in the middle of the range for economically developed countries **(Figure 3.8),** despite the relatively small number of UK acute hospital beds.

During 2005/06 there were 14,424 million FCEs, including both ordinary admissions and day cases, in England alone, 31% higher than just a decade earlier (**Table 3.20**). In 1995/96 pregnancy and childbirth were the single largest cause of hospital episodes, but now diseases of the digestive system and neoplasms are the most common causes of hospital admissions, each accounting for over one in ten of all FCEs in 2005/06. FCEs per capita vary considerably between diagnostic groups, ranging from two per 1,000 population for conditions relating to congenital anomalies to 127 per 1,000 female population aged 15-44 for pregnancy and childbirth (**Table 3.21a**).

Considering only ordinary admissions and excluding day cases, pregnancy and childbirth etc. contributed 12.0% of all hospital inpatient admissions in England in 2005/06, followed by circulatory conditions at 10.1% (**Table 3.22**). **Table 3.25** gives a detailed breakdown of total FCEs, excluding day cases, for the most frequently occurring diagnoses. These causes led between them to 73% of all finished consultant episodes in 2005/06 and account for 60% of total hospital beds (**Table 3.26**).

Twenty nine per cent of total NHS FCEs in England were on a day cases basis in 2005/06 (**Table 3.33**). About 91% of all day cases involved a surgical operation compared to 34% of ordinary admission episodes (HES IC). The number of surgical operations performed in NHS hospitals in England was 7.2 million, an increase of 20% compared to just a decade earlier (**Table 3.27**). Considering all surgical procedures combined, 40% are now performed on a day case basis (**Table 3.33**). The number of surgical procedures carried out, based on the OPCS classification (OPCS4), varies markedly between sites and the rate per 10,000 population increases with patient age (**Table 3.28**). In 2005/06 the most common site for operations in the 75s and over, was the eye, with 554 per 10,000 population of that age, compared to just 19 eye operations per 10,000 population in the 0-14 age group. A more detailed breakdown is given in **Table 3.29**, which shows that the most frequent procedures considering all ages combined were endoscopic operations on the upper gastrointestinal tract and colon, followed by normal deliveries.

There were over 113,585 Caesarean sections without complications done in England in 2005/06, each costing an average of £2,309 (**Table 3.35**). This compares with the cost of £1,013 for a normal delivery without complications. Together with 21,083 complicated cases, Caesarean sections cost the NHS £323 million in 2005/06.

| Box 7 Change (%) in average length of stay in NHS hospitals, UK | | |
|---|---|---|
| Decade | % change in average length of stay[1] | % change in number of available hospital beds |
| 1955 - 1965 | -29 | -2 |
| 1965 - 1975 | -23 | -10 |
| 1975 - 1985 | -30 | -15 |
| 1985 - 1995 | -54 | -35 |
| 1995 - 2005 | -41 | -17 |

*Notes:* 1 Including patients for all specialties other than mental illness and learning disabilities.
Data for 1995 relate to 1995/96 and data for 2005 relates to 2005/06.
*Sources:* Hospital Episode Statistics (DH).
Health Statistics Wales (NAW).
Scottish Health Statistics (ISD).
Hospital Statistics (DHSSPS, Northern Ireland).

**Length of stay**

The average length of stay for all specialties bar mental illness and learning disabilities was 4.4 days in 2005/06 in the UK, continuing the trend for shorter stays. In contrast, the average stay was 45 days in 1951 (**Table 3.19**).

**Box 7** shows the decline in the average length of stay through each of the last five decades. It must, however, be

emphasised that changes in definitions in England since 1997/98, especially in the calculation of duration of episodes, compilation of hospital information, and changes in case-mix do not allow strict comparability across time. Sizeable reductions in average length of stay have been achieved in all acute specialties but may now be bottoming out (**Figure 3.9**). **Table 3.23** shows the average length of stay in England by main cause. Mental disorders accounted for only 2.1% of hospital admissions in 2005/06, but with a mean length of stay per episode of 46 days they accounted for 13.7% of all bed days (**Tables 3.22, 3.23** and **3.24**).

**Treatment costs**

The Department of Health in England publishes annually a set of unit costs for a range of surgical procedures and medical treatments compiled from NHS Trusts in England. Since 2003 these Reference Costs also include cost information on NHS patients treated in non-NHS hospitals. To allow for differences in case-mix and ensure that costs are consistent and comparable, the unit costs are based on Healthcare Resource Groups[2] (HRGs). **Table 3.34** lists the 40 HRGs for elective inpatient admissions that cost NHS Trusts the most in 2005/06. Primary knee replacement topped the list with a mean cost per episode of £5,843 and an estimated total cost in England, in the NHS, of £306 million. This is followed by primary hip replacement which cost about £173 million a year for elective inpatient care in NHS hospitals.

There were over quarter of a million cataract replacements carried out as day cases in 2005/06, at an average cost of £764 each in England (**Table 3.36**). This compares with £1,188 when done as an elective inpatient.

In 2005/06 there were over 4,000 primary knee replacements and over 3,000 primary hip replacements carried out at private hospitals for NHS patients in England. The average costs for these operations were 19% and 12% more expensive respectively than at NHS hospitals (**Table 3.34** and **3.37**). On average it cost around £6,641 for a coronary bypass at private hospitals for NHS patients compared with £8,172 at NHS hospitals in 2005/06. In 2005/06 over 30,000 surgical terminations of pregnancy carried out for NHS patients at private hospitals as day cases, each costing £347 compared with 36,400 costing £564 each at NHS hospitals (**Tables 3.38** and **Table 3.36**).

**Waiting times**

There were 701,000 thousand people waiting for non-emergency admission to NHS hospitals in England on 31 March 2007 (**Table 3.30**). The specialty with most people waiting is orthopaedic surgery, accounting for 25% of the total list on 31st March 2007. Total numbers of patients on inpatient and day case waiting lists for all specialties peaked in 1998 at 1.3 million (**Figure 3.10**). The percentage of patients waiting who had been doing so for more than 12 months fell sharply from 9% in 1992 to under

# Hospital Services

1% by 31 March 1996 but then rose to 5% two years later. A rush to meet the 12 month waiting time target in England by the end of the 2002/03 financial year, saw a sharp fall again to nearly zero. This level of zero 12-month waits has been maintained since 2003 and greater than six-month waits fell almost to zero in England in 2006.

**Table 3.31** shows that according to the latest available figures, patients in 2005/06 in England had waited 180 days on average for primary knee replacement and 165 days on average for primary hip replacement. Nearly 119,000 patients were admitted to hospital for arthroscopies, and on average they had waited 131 days.

The waiting time for the first outpatient appointment is measured as the interval between the date the GP written request is received by the hospital and the date when the patient is seen at the outpatient clinic. Significant variations in waiting times for first outpatient appointments are found between specialties (**Table 3.32**). For restorative dentistry, 5% waited longer than 13 weeks but less than 1% did so in geriatric medicine, for example.

### Outpatients

The total number of NHS hospital outpatient attendances in the UK grew to over 81 million in 2005/06 (**Table 3.39**). This represents an increase of 13.8 million (20%) over the past 10 years. Most of this increase can be attributed to growth in the number of new outpatient cases, i.e. first attendances (**Table 3.40**), which rose by 9.8 million (35%) over the decade to 2005/06. According to the General Household Survey, the proportion of the population in Great Britain who attended a hospital as an outpatient in 2005 has remained relatively constant over the past two decades, standing at 14% **(Table 3.41)**, with an estimated 67,689 outpatient attendances in the UK in 2005.

## *Notes*

1. In England, hospital discharges and deaths are identified as "finished consultant episodes" or FCEs. A consultant episode is a period of care spent under one consultant within one NHS trust. Patients may experience more than one FCE in an admission. The transfer of a patient from one hospital to another with the same consultant and within the same NHS Trust does not end the episode in England. Data for Wales are based on discharges and deaths. In Northern Ireland transfers between consultants do not count as a discharge. In Scotland "discharges" can be the result of several types of change during the course of a patient's care, including transfers from one consultant to another within the same hospital (provided there is a change of specialty or a significant change in facilities), a change in location or the end of treatment. Transfers from one hospital to another with the same consultant do count as a discharge in Scotland. In all four countries deaths count as discharges. Scottish figures also include

NHS activity in joint-user and contractual hospitals, although these hospitals account for only a small proportion of total NHS activity. Other differences between hospital activity data also exist between the four countries, for example, well new-born babies are included for Northern Ireland but excluded from England, Wales and Scotland.

2. Modelled on the US Diagnostic Related Groups (DRGs), treatments are assigned to a particular Healthcare Resource Group (HRG) on the basis of procedure (as defined by OPCS4 codes) and diagnosis (as defined by ICD10 codes), while taking into account the patient's age, length of stay and outcome (death/discharge). Such groupings should contain treatments that are clinically similar and that use the same level of resources. (For details see http://www.ic.nhs.uk/casemix).

# Cost of Hospital Services

Table 3.1    **Gross cost of hospital services and Family Health Services (FHS), UK, 1949/50 - 2005/06**

| Year | Gross cost: (£ million cash) | | | Gross cost per capita: (£ cash) | | | As % of NHS cost: | |
|---|---|---|---|---|---|---|---|---|
| | Hospital | FHS | All NHS | Hospital | FHS | All NHS | Hospital | FHS |
| 1949/50 | 234 | 159 | 447 | 5 | 3 | 9 | 52 | 36 |
| 1950/51 | 266 | 158 | 482 | 5 | 3 | 10 | 55 | 33 |
| 1955/56 | 356 | 157 | 596 | 7 | 3 | 12 | 60 | 26 |
| 1960/61 | 527 | 248 | 883 | 10 | 5 | 17 | 60 | 28 |
| 1965/66 | 809 | 351 | 1,306 | 15 | 6 | 24 | 62 | 27 |
| 1970/71 | 1,387 | 544 | 2,046 | 25 | 10 | 37 | 68 | 27 |
| 1975/76 | 3,373 | 1,141 | 5,358 | 60 | 20 | 95 | 63 | 21 |
| 1980/81 | 7,181 | 2,584 | 11,677 | 127 | 46 | 207 | 61 | 22 |
| 1985/86 | 10,254 | 4,278 | 17,514 | 181 | 76 | 310 | 59 | 24 |
| 1990/91 | 15,651 | 6,968 | 29,178 | 273 | 122 | 509 | 54 | 24 |
| 1995/96 | 22,490 | 10,290 | 42,326 | 387 | 177 | 729 | 53 | 24 |
| 1996/97 | 21,750 | 10,989 | 43,921 | 374 | 189 | 755 | 50 | 25 |
| 1997/98 | 22,871 | 11,634 | 46,240 | 392 | 199 | 792 | 49 | 25 |
| 1998/99 | 24,213 | 12,229 | 48,770 | 414 | 209 | 833 | 50 | 25 |
| 1999/00 | 26,193 | 13,288 | 53,429 | 446 | 226 | 910 | 49 | 25 |
| 2000/01 | 28,669 | 14,199 | 58,279 | 486 | 241 | 989 | 49 | 24 |
| 2001/02 | 30,935 | 15,268 | 64,430 | 523 | 258 | 1,089 | 48 | 24 |
| 2002/03 | 33,934 | 16,440 | 71,657 | 571 | 277 | 1,207 | 47 | 23 |
| 2003/04 | 36,945 | 17,980 | 81,259 | 620 | 302 | 1,363 | 45 | 22 |
| 2004/05 | 40,996 | 21,146 | 88,141 | 684 | 353 | 1,470 | 47 | 24 |
| 2005/06 | 44,870 | 22,488 | 97,230 | 744 | 373 | 1,612 | 46 | 23 |

## Expenditure at constant prices[1] (Index 1975/76=100)

| Year | Hospital | FHS | All NHS | Hospital | FHS | All NHS | Hospital | FHS |
|---|---|---|---|---|---|---|---|---|
| 1949/50 | 26 | 51 | 31 | 29 | 57 | 34 | 83 | 167 |
| 1950/51 | 29 | 50 | 33 | 32 | 56 | 36 | 88 | 154 |
| 1955/56 | 30 | 40 | 32 | 34 | 44 | 35 | 95 | 124 |
| 1960/61 | 37 | 52 | 39 | 40 | 55 | 42 | 95 | 132 |
| 1965/66 | 50 | 64 | 51 | 52 | 66 | 52 | 98 | 126 |
| 1970/71 | 69 | 80 | 64 | 70 | 81 | 65 | 108 | 125 |
| 1975/76 | 100 | 100 | 100 | 100 | 100 | 100 | 100 | 100 |
| 1980/81 | 102 | 109 | 105 | 102 | 109 | 105 | 98 | 104 |
| 1985/86 | 98 | 121 | 105 | 97 | 120 | 105 | 93 | 115 |
| 1990/91 | 113 | 149 | 133 | 111 | 146 | 130 | 85 | 112 |
| 1995/96 | 134 | 181 | 159 | 130 | 175 | 154 | 84 | 114 |
| 1996/97 | 126 | 188 | 160 | 122 | 182 | 155 | 79 | 117 |
| 1997/98 | 128 | 192 | 163 | 123 | 185 | 157 | 79 | 118 |
| 1998/99 | 132 | 197 | 168 | 127 | 190 | 161 | 79 | 118 |
| 1999/00 | 140 | 210 | 180 | 134 | 201 | 172 | 78 | 117 |
| 2000/01 | 151 | 221 | 193 | 144 | 210 | 184 | 78 | 114 |
| 2001/02 | 160 | 233 | 210 | 152 | 222 | 199 | 76 | 111 |
| 2002/03 | 170 | 244 | 227 | 161 | 231 | 215 | 75 | 108 |
| 2003/04 | 179 | 258 | 248 | 169 | 243 | 234 | 72 | 104 |
| 2004/05 | 193 | 295 | 262 | 181 | 276 | 245 | 74 | 113 |
| 2005/06 | 206 | 306 | 281 | 192 | 285 | 262 | 73 | 109 |

*Notes:*    All figures relate to calendar years and include capital expenditure and charges paid by patients. From 1991/92, hospital expenditure includes capital charges.
         1 As adjusted by the Gross Domestic Product (GDP) deflator, at market prices.

*Sources:*    The Government's Expenditure Plans (DH).
         Public Expenditure Statistical Analyses (HM Treasury).
         NHS Board Operating Costs and Capital Expenditure, ISD Scotland (ISD).
         Department of Health Departmental Report (DH).
         NHS Summarised Accounts (House of Commons).
         Scottish Health Statistics (ISD)
         Health Statistics Wales (NAW).
         Annual Abstract of Statistics (ONS).
         Population Projections Database (GAD).
         Economic Trends (ONS).

# Cost of Hospital Services

Table 3.2 **NHS hospital gross expenditure (revenue and capital) per capita and household, UK, 1975/76 - 2005/06**

| Year | England | Wales | Scotland | Northern Ireland | UK | England | Wales | Scotland | Northern Ireland | UK |
|---|---|---|---|---|---|---|---|---|---|---|
| | Hospital expenditure per capita | | | | | | | | | |
| | (£ cash) | | | | | At constant prices[1] (Index 1975/76=100) | | | | |
| 1975/76 | 60 | 62 | 75 | 71 | 60 | 100 | 100 | 100 | 100 | 100 |
| 1980/81 | 131 | 132 | 170 | 165 | 127 | 110 | 108 | 115 | 117 | 107 |
| 1985/86 | 183 | 197 | 254 | 236 | 181 | 113 | 118 | 126 | 123 | 112 |
| 1990/91 | 267 | 288 | 373 | 330 | 273 | 123 | 128 | 137 | 128 | 125 |
| 1991/92 | 290 | 347 | 426 | 278 | 305 | 125 | 145 | 147 | 102 | 132 |
| 1992/93 | 318 | 355 | 457 | 295 | 331 | 133 | 144 | 153 | 104 | 139 |
| 1993/94 | 358 | 289 | 479 | 319 | 365 | 146 | 114 | 156 | 110 | 149 |
| 1994/95 | 358 | 298 | 497 | 339 | 366 | 144 | 116 | 160 | 115 | 147 |
| 1995/96 | 375 | 383 | 512 | 366 | 387 | 146 | 144 | 160 | 121 | 151 |
| 1996/97 | 360 | 363 | 514 | 375 | 374 | 136 | 132 | 155 | 120 | 141 |
| 1997/98 | 378 | 386 | 527 | 403 | 392 | 139 | 137 | 154 | 125 | 144 |
| 1998/99 | 401 | 420 | 532 | 414 | 414 | 143 | 145 | 152 | 125 | 148 |
| 1999/00 | 436 | 448 | 537 | 450 | 446 | 153 | 152 | 150 | 133 | 156 |
| 2000/01 | 477 | 505 | 568 | 488 | 486 | 165 | 169 | 157 | 142 | 168 |
| 2001/02 | 512 | 545 | 615 | 530 | 523 | 173 | 178 | 166 | 151 | 176 |
| 2002/03 | 562 | 603 | 643 | 583 | 571 | 184 | 191 | 168 | 161 | 187 |
| 2003/04[2] | 605 | 638 | 745 | *636* | 620 | 192 | 196 | 190 | *171* | 197 |
| 2004/05[2] | 668 | 706 | 825 | *690* | 684 | 207 | 211 | 204 | *181* | 212 |
| 2005/06 | 729 | 754 | 882 | 742 | 744 | 221 | 221 | 214 | 190 | 225 |
| | Hospital expenditure per household | | | | | | | | | |
| | (£ cash) | | | | | At constant prices[1] (Index 1975/76=100) | | | | |
| 1975/76 | 170 | 180 | 223 | 224 | 172 | 100 | 100 | 100 | 100 | 100 |
| 1980/81 | 359 | 369 | 480 | 495 | 352 | 107 | 104 | 109 | 112 | 104 |
| 1985/86 | 480 | 525 | 669 | 711 | 478 | 105 | 108 | 111 | 118 | 103 |
| 1990/91 | 673 | 780 | 970 | 846 | 690 | 109 | 119 | 120 | 104 | 111 |
| 1991/92 | 726 | 877 | 1,061 | 811 | 765 | 111 | 126 | 123 | 94 | 116 |
| 1992/93 | 791 | 892 | 1,129 | 846 | 827 | 117 | 124 | 127 | 95 | 121 |
| 1993/94 | 890 | 724 | 1,176 | 911 | 908 | 128 | 98 | 129 | 99 | 129 |
| 1994/95 | 885 | 742 | 1,212 | 936 | 908 | 125 | 99 | 131 | 101 | 128 |
| 1995/96 | 926 | 948 | 1,237 | 1,019 | 957 | 127 | 123 | 130 | 106 | 131 |
| 1996/97 | 885 | 895 | 1,230 | 1,022 | 920 | 118 | 113 | 125 | 103 | 121 |
| 1997/98 | 929 | 949 | 1,251 | 1,167 | 965 | 120 | 116 | 123 | 114 | 124 |
| 1998/99 | 984 | 1,029 | 1,253 | 1,164 | 1,015 | 124 | 123 | 121 | 111 | 127 |
| 1999/00 | 1,068 | 1,094 | 1,256 | 1,240 | 1,091 | 132 | 128 | 118 | 116 | 134 |
| 2000/01 | 1,162 | 1,227 | 1,320 | 1,319 | 1,184 | 142 | 141 | 123 | 122 | 143 |
| 2001/02 | 1,235 | 1,314 | 1,417 | 1,427 | 1,260 | 147 | 148 | 129 | 129 | 149 |
| 2002/03 | 1,348 | 1,441 | 1,472 | 1,555 | 1,369 | 155 | 157 | 130 | 136 | 157 |
| 2003/04[2] | 1,445 | 1,515 | 1,694 | *1,681* | 1,477 | 162 | 161 | 145 | *143* | 164 |
| 2004/05[2] | 1,592 | 1,669 | 1,865 | *1,812* | 1,626 | 174 | 172 | 155 | *150* | 176 |
| 2005/06 | 1,731 | 1,769 | 1,980 | 1,940 | 1,761 | 185 | 179 | 161 | 157 | 187 |

*Notes:* All figures include patient payments, capital expenditure, and capital charges from 1991/92.
1 As adjusted by the Gross Domestic Product (GDP) deflator, at market prices.
2 Figures in italics for Northern Ireland for 2003/04 and 2004/05 are OHE estimates and are interpolated based on available data.

*Sources:* The Government's Expenditure Plans (DH).
Annual Abstract of Statistics (ONS).
Health Statistics Wales (NAW).
Scottish Health Statistics (ISD).
Economic Data (HM Treasury).
Population Projections Database (GAD).
Household Estimates and projections (DCLG).
Household projections (GROS).
Household data (NISRA).

# Cost of Hospital Services

Figure 3.1 **Gross cost of hospital services £ cash and as a percentage of NHS cost, UK, 1949/50 - 2005/06**

**Hospital services (gross cost £ million at 2005/06 prices[1])**

**Percentage of gross NHS cost**

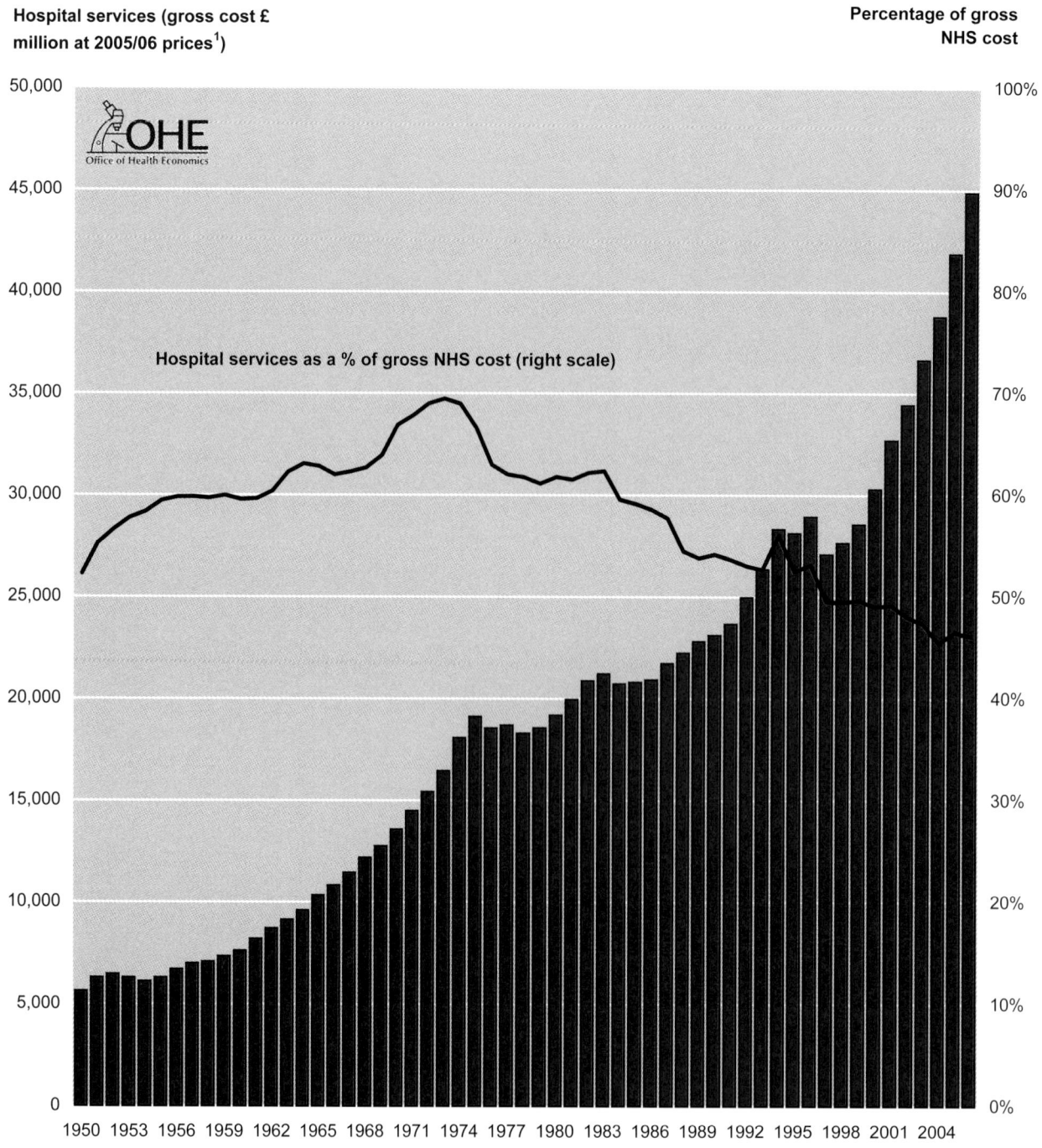

Hospital services as a % of gross NHS cost (right scale)

**Financial year ending**

Notes: All figures include capital expenditure and charges paid by patients.
Year ending 31 March (i.e. 2004 = 2003/04).
1 As adjusted by the Gross Domestic Product (GDP) deflator, at market prices.

Sources: NHS Summarised Accounts (House of Commons).
Health Statistics Wales (NAW).
Scottish Health Statistics (ISD).
Annual Abstract of Statistics (ONS).
The Government's Expenditure Plans (DH).
Economic Trends (ONS).

# Cost of Hospital Services

Figure 3.2 **Relationship between NHS expenditure on Family Health Services (FHS)[1] and on hospital services, UK, 1975/76 - 2005/06**

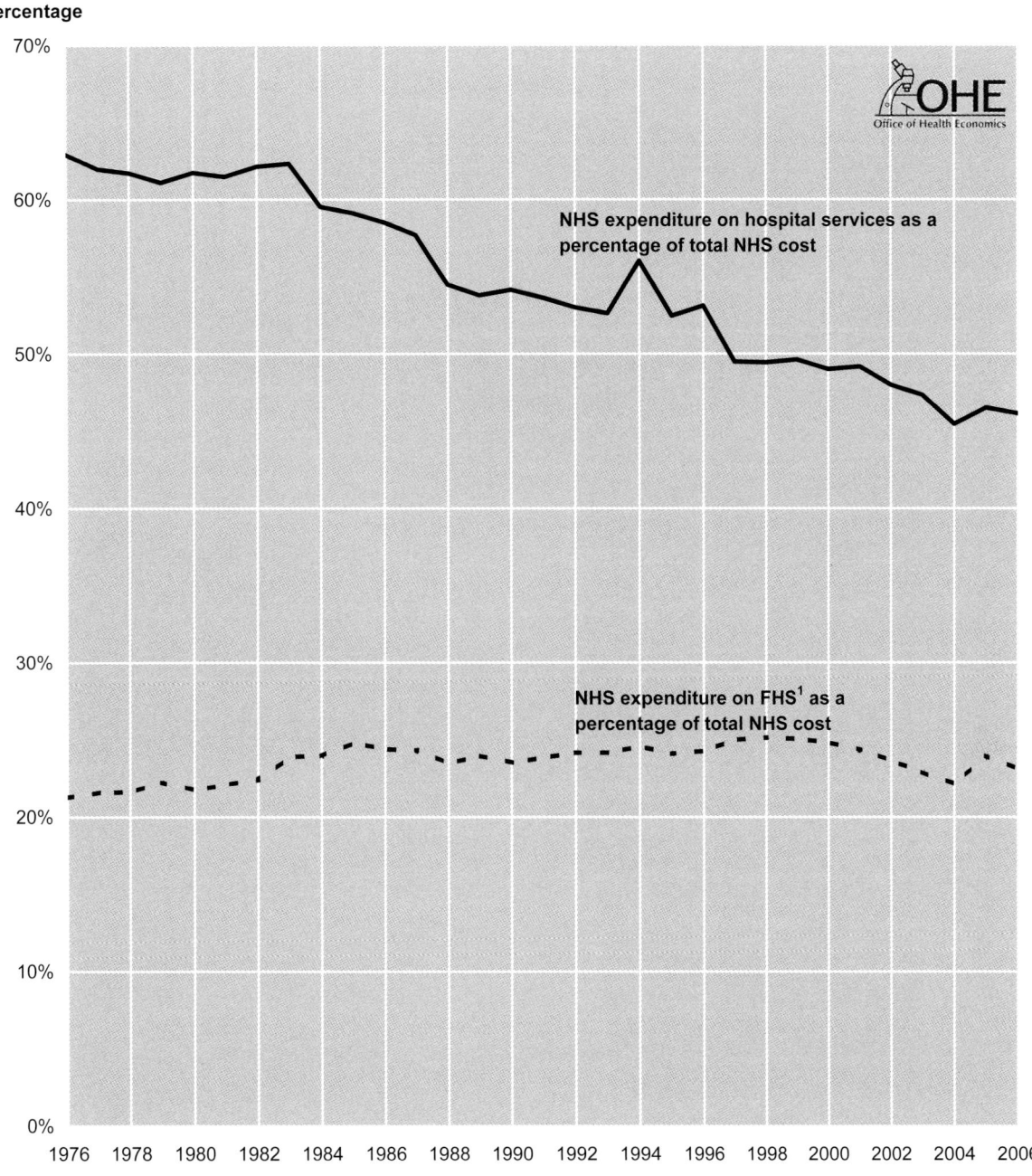

**Percentage**

NHS expenditure on hospital services as a percentage of total NHS cost

NHS expenditure on FHS[1] as a percentage of total NHS cost

**Financial year ending**

*Notes:* Year ending 31st March (i.e. 2004=2003/04).
All figures relate to gross expenditure, including capital charges and patient payments. Hospital expenditure includes psychiatric services but not community health and other related services, e.g. ambulance and blood transfusion units.
1 Figures relate to gross costs of the General Medical, Pharmaceutical, Dental and Ophthalmic Services, including payments by patients.
*Sources:* NHS Summarised Accounts (House of Commons).
Annual Abstract of Statistics (ONS).
Health and Personal Social Services Statistics for England (DH).
Health Statistics Wales (NAW).
Scottish Health Statistics (ISD).

Figure 3.3 **Hospital expenditure as a percentage of total health spending and hospital expenditure per capita (£) in selected OECD countries, circa 2005**

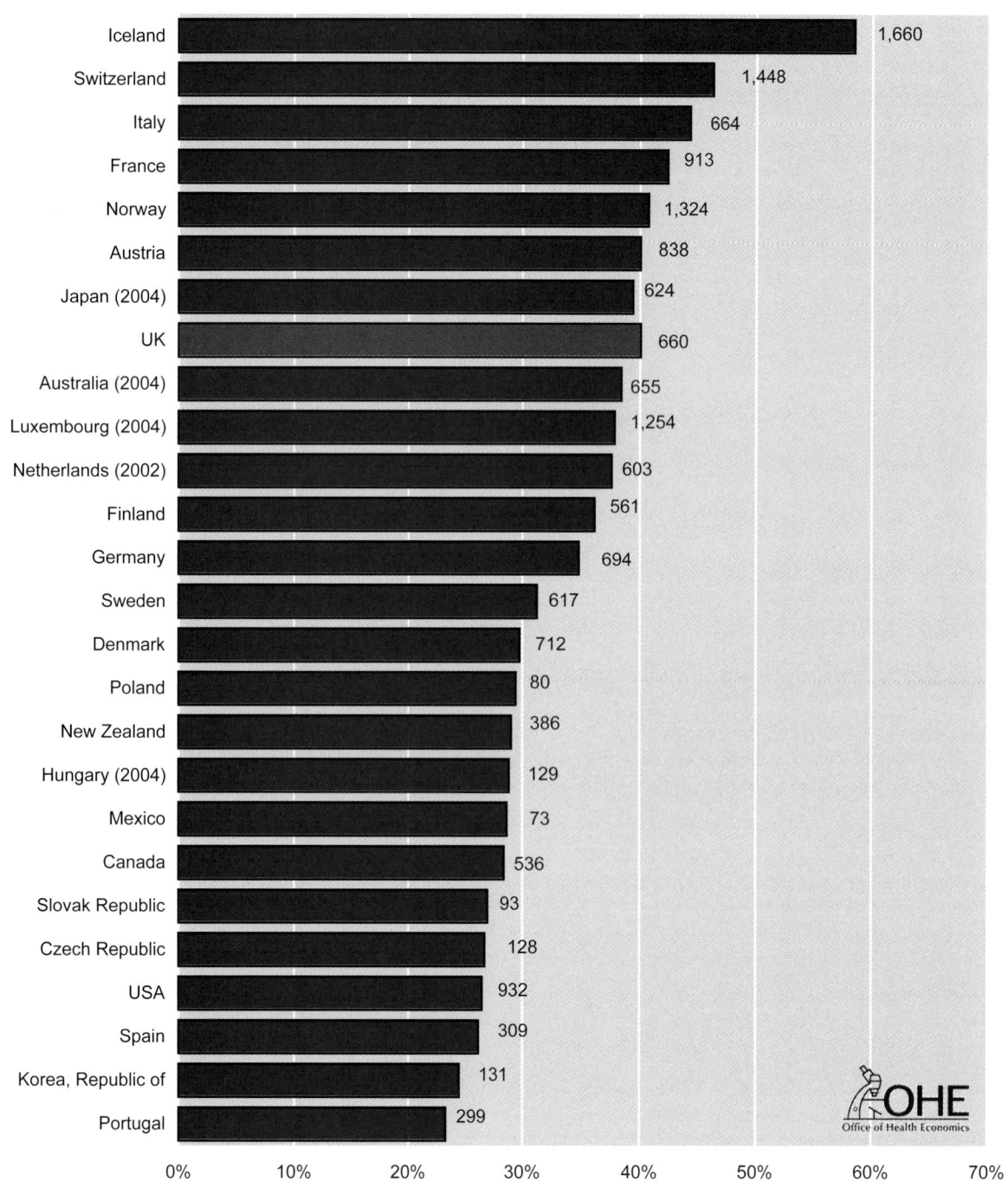

**Hospital expenditure as a percentage of total health spending**

*Notes:* Year is 2005 unless stated otherwise.
Figures at end of bars relate to hospital expenditure per capita in £ (money of the day).
Cross-country comparison should be carried out with caution as figures may be based on different definitions.
*Sources:* OECD Health Database.
UK figure see Table 3.1 and Table 2.2.

# Cost of Hospital Services

Figure 3.4  **Comparison of 'volume' and 'real' growth in NHS hospital gross expenditure, UK, 1975/76 - 2005/06**

**Index 1975/76=100**

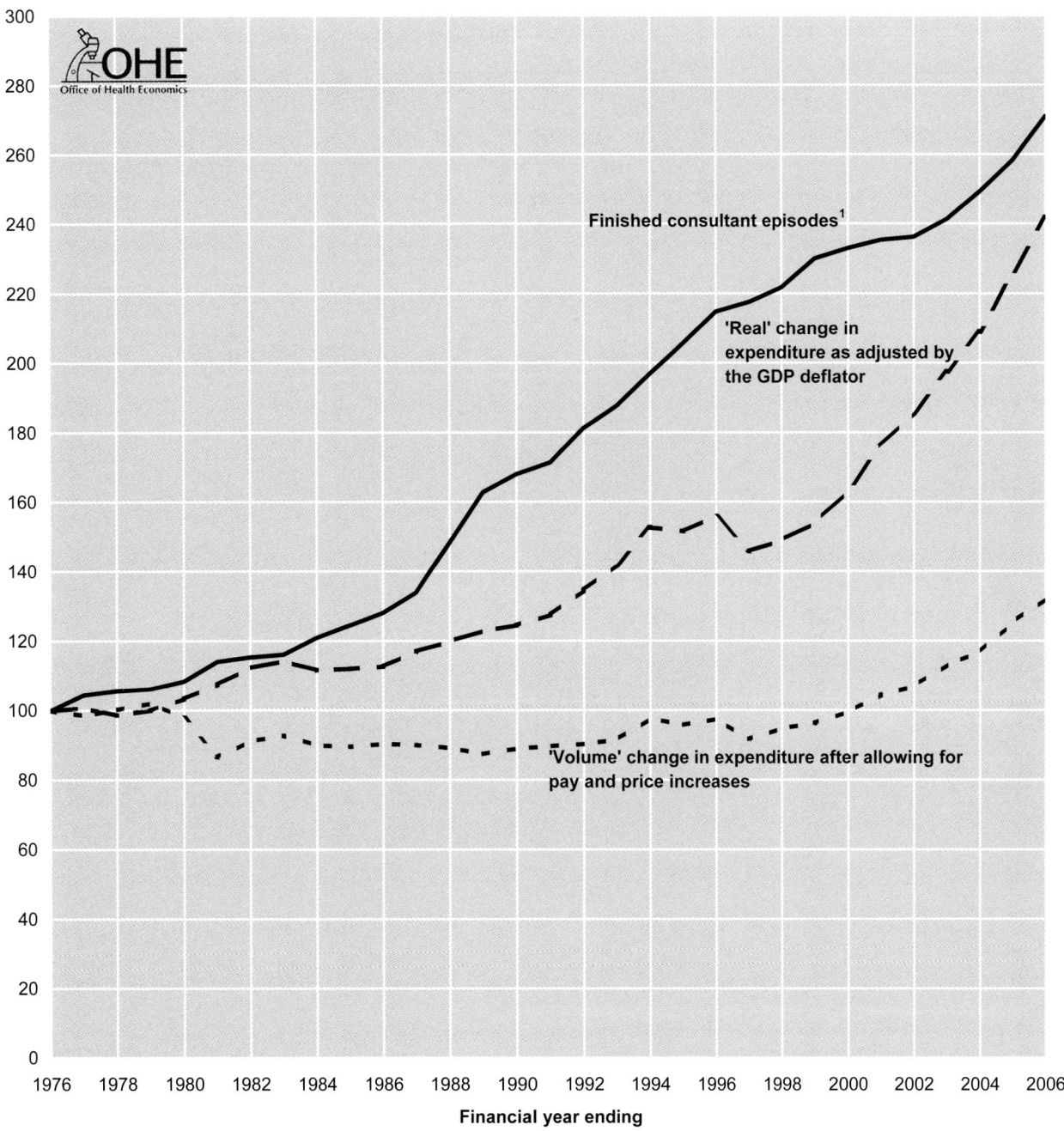

**Financial year ending**

*Notes:*    All figures relate to financial years ending 31st March (e.g. 2006=2005/06) and include income from charges to patients.
　　　　  GDP = Gross Domestic Product.
　　　　  1 Prior to 1987/88, all figures relate to discharges and deaths. From 1987/88 onwards data for England relates to FCEs.
*Sources:*  NHS Summarised Accounts (House of Commons).
　　　　  Annual Abstract of Statistics (ONS).
　　　　  Hospital Episode Statistics (DH).
　　　　  Economic Trends (ONS).
　　　　  Public Expenditure Team, Finance Directorate (DH).
　　　　  Scottish Health Statistics (ISD).
　　　　  Health Statistics Wales (NAW).
　　　　  Hospital Statistics for Northern Ireland (DHSSPS).

Table 3.3 **Number of staff employed in NHS hospitals and community services by category, UK, 1951 - 2005**

30th September

| Year | Medical and dental[1] | Nursing and midwifery[2] | Professional and technical[3] | Admin. and clerical[4] | Domestic ancillary[1] | Total[5] |
|---|---|---|---|---|---|---|
| 1951 | 15,102 | 188,580 | 14,110 | 29,021 | 163,666 | 410,479 |
| 1955 | 16,870 | 206,567 | 19,404 | 33,421 | 157,917 | 434,179 |
| 1960 | 20,651 | 242,164 | 24,002 | 38,450 | 202,968 | 528,235 |
| 1961 | 21,184 | 249,571 | 27,460 | 40,877 | 210,308 | 549,400 |
| 1962 | 21,956 | 264,657 | 28,555 | 42,675 | 215,528 | 573,371 |
| 1963 | 22,584 | 267,725 | 29,850 | 44,075 | 215,245 | 579,479 |
| 1964 | 23,069 | 275,537 | 31,060 | 45,667 | 217,410 | 592,743 |
| 1965 | 23,860 | 290,338 | 32,720 | 47,872 | 218,191 | 612,981 |
| 1966 | 24,545 | 303,338 | 34,353 | 50,110 | 224,005 | 636,351 |
| 1967 | 25,704 | 315,896 | 36,112 | 51,902 | 229,596 | 659,210 |
| 1968 | 26,719 | 320,142 | 36,929 | 51,434 | 227,039 | 662,263 |
| 1969 | 27,625 | 330,684 | 38,763 | 54,097 | 227,461 | 678,630 |
| 1970 | 28,511 | 343,664 | 41,696 | 56,877 | 229,313 | 700,061 |
| 1971 | 29,944 | 361,980 | 43,089 | 60,050 | 235,642 | 730,705 |
| 1972 | 31,536 | 382,652 | 45,343 | 64,551 | 236,940 | 761,022 |
| 1973 | 32,650 | 392,387 | 47,785 | 69,184 | 231,050 | 773,056 |
| 1974 | 34,210 | 408,146 | 47,015 | 99,111 | 230,944 | 819,426 |
| 1975 | 35,899 | 440,981 | 57,011 | 110,429 | 235,209 | 879,529 |
| 1976 | 36,838 | 448,336 | 65,204 | 117,674 | 242,212 | 910,264 |
| 1977 | 37,895 | 447,973 | 65,357 | 118,688 | 241,823 | 911,736 |
| 1978 | 39,069 | 445,647 | 69,024 | 120,390 | 258,569 | 932,699 |
| 1979 | 40,519 | 453,500 | 72,390 | 123,616 | 256,893 | 946,918 |
| 1980 | 41,760 | 467,500 | 74,558 | 126,124 | 258,368 | 968,310 |
| 1981 | 42,562 | 493,700 | 78,269 | 130,221 | 259,765 | 1,004,517 |
| 1982 | 45,184 | 500,500 | 80,543 | 130,767 | 258,031 | 1,015,025 |
| 1983 | 45,876 | 500,500 | 82,505 | 132,266 | 252,371 | 1,013,518 |
| 1984 | 46,353 | 501,100 | 89,437 | 132,812 | 235,698 | 1,005,400 |
| 1985 | 47,308 | 504,000 | 91,471 | 137,982 | 221,334 | 1,002,095 |
| 1986 | 47,602 | 507,300 | 93,705 | 138,929 | 204,169 | 991,705 |
| 1987 | 47,596 | 508,300 | 97,047 | 142,662 | 192,259 | 987,864 |
| 1988 | 49,229 | 509,000 | 98,270 | 143,941 | 180,327 | 980,767 |
| 1989 | 50,795 | 510,900 | 99,956 | 150,400 | 168,717 | 980,768 |
| 1990 | 55,838 | 507,100 | 103,097 | 164,370 | 156,995 | 987,400 |
| 1991 | 57,187 | 500,300 | 106,580 | 172,964 | 142,600 | 979,631 |
| 1992 | 58,153 | 482,700 | 110,444 | 187,027 | 132,916 | 971,240 |
| 1993 | 59,908 | 459,800 | 112,584 | 188,746 | 128,313 | 949,351 |
| 1994 | 61,059 | 446,400 | 114,865 | 194,764 | 117,706 | 934,794 |
| 1995 | 64,466 | 421,983 | 118,415 | 193,210 | 123,289 | 921,362 |
| 1996 | 67,093 | 421,521 | 121,933 | 191,615 | 127,451 | 929,613 |
| 1997 | 70,347 | 419,142 | 124,008 | 191,652 | 123,571 | 928,721 |
| 1998 | 72,238 | 420,924 | 127,604 | 193,396 | 123,758 | 937,919 |
| 1999 | 74,079 | 428,011 | 132,029 | 199,397 | 122,871 | 956,387 |
| 2000 | 75,682 | 436,557 | 136,355 | 206,483 | 123,541 | 978,618 |
| 2001 | 78,036 | 449,970 | 142,931 | 218,422 | 128,732 | 1,018,090 |
| 2002 | 83,356 | 467,556 | 151,678 | 234,479 | 132,860 | 1,069,930 |
| 2003 | 87,723 | 487,469 | 160,640 | 252,169 | 136,070 | 1,124,071 |
| 2004 | 94,790 | 498,261 | 169,986 | 267,573 | 139,109 | 1,169,718 |
| 2005 | 100,355 | 506,249 | 177,117 | 280,692 | 141,758 | 1,206,172 |

*Notes:* All figures are based on aggregates of England, Wales, Scotland and Northern Ireland, and may be based on different definitions and timing of coverage. The totals include staff working in the personal social services in Northern Ireland.

1 All figures relate to full-time equivalents, medical and dental staff include Hospital and Community Health Services staff from 1990 onwards.

2 Full-time and part-time, including Community Health Services staff in England. The exclusion of nurses on Project 2000 training courses produced an apparent reduction in numbers since 1990.

3 Excluding works, maintenance, ancillary, ambulance and transport staff and part-time staff in Scotland.

4 Including general and senior managers.

5 These are totals of the columns shown. As some categories of employment are not shown, these totals are underestimates of the total NHS hospital workforce.

*Sources:* NHS Hospital, Public Health Medicine and Community Health Service Medical and Dental Workforce Census (IC).

NHS Hospital and Community Health Services non-medical staff in England (IC).

Health Statistics Wales (NAW).

Scottish Health Statistics (ISD).

Annual Abstract of Statistics (ONS).

# Hospital Workforce

Figure 3.5 **Index of NHS hospital and community workforce per 100,000 population, UK, 1951 - 2005**

**Index (1951=100)**

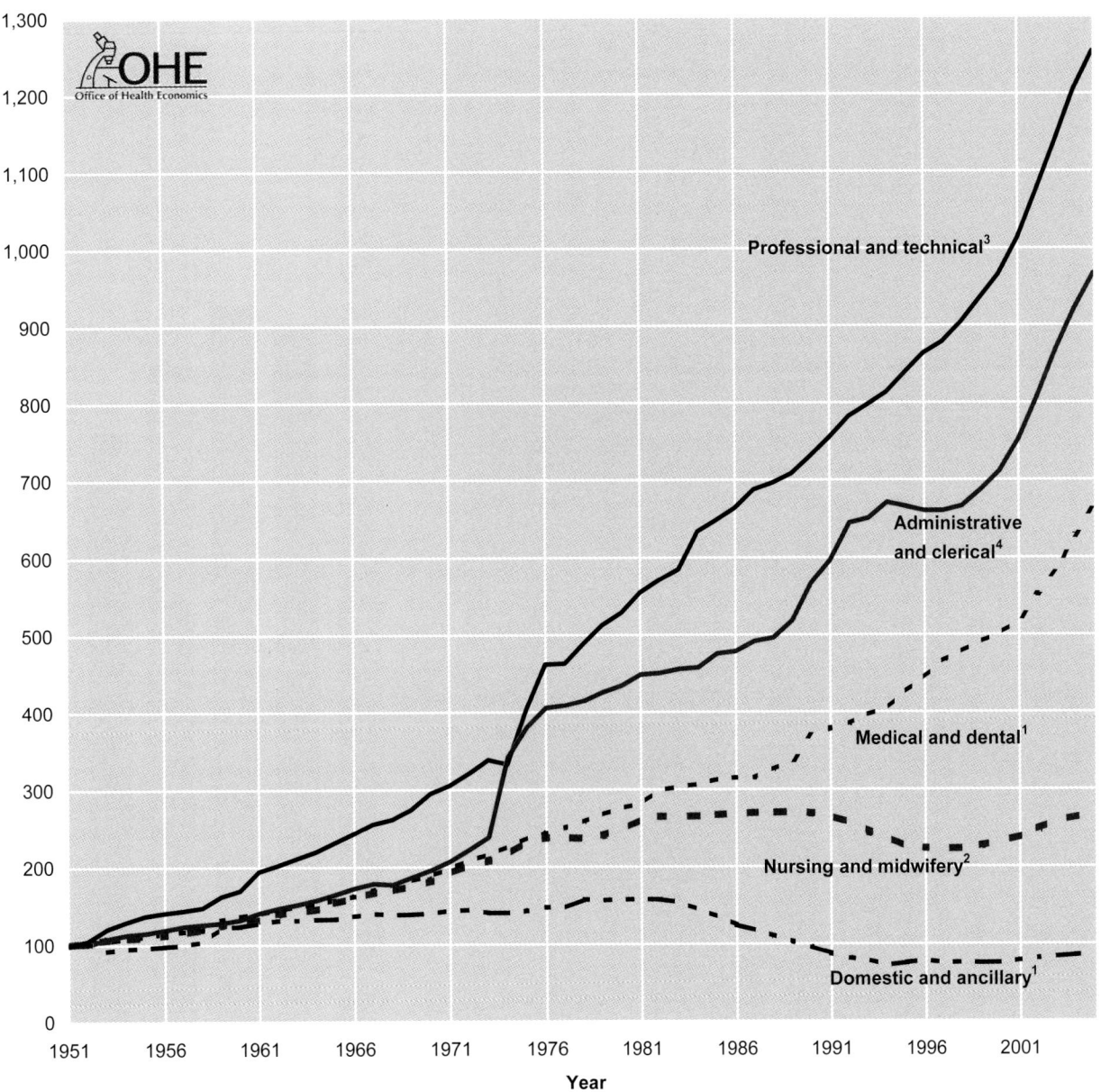

*Notes:* All figures are based on aggregates of England, Wales, Scotland and Northern Ireland, and may be based on different definitions and timing of coverage. The totals include staff working in personal social services in Northern Ireland.
1 All figures relate to full-time equivalents, medical and dental staff include Hospital and Community Health Services staff from 1990 onwards.
2 Full-time ad part-time, including Community Health Services staff in England. The exclusion of nurses on Project 2000 training courses produced an apparent reduction in numbers since 1990.
3 Excluding works, maintenance, ancillary, ambulance and transport staff and part-time staff in Scotland.
4 Including general and senior managers.
*Sources:* NHS Hospital, Public Health Medicine and Community Health Services Medical and Dental Workforce Census (IC).
NHS Hospital and Community Health Services non-medical staff in England (IC).
Health Statistics Wales (NAW).
Scottish Health Statistics (ISD).
Annual Abstract of Statistics (ONS).

Table 3.4 **Medical and dental staff employed in NHS hospitals, UK, 1951 - 2005**
30th September

| Year | Number of medical and dental staff[1] | | | | Staff per 100,000 population | | | |
|---|---|---|---|---|---|---|---|---|
| | England and Wales[2] | Scotland | Northern Ireland[3] | United Kingdom | England and Wales[2] | Scotland | Northern Ireland[3] | United Kingdom |
| 1951 | 13,639 | 757 | 381 | 14,777 | 31 | 15 | 28 | 29 |
| 1955 | 15,028 | 977 | 456 | 16,461 | 34 | 19 | 33 | 32 |
| 1960 | 17,045 | 2,248 | 560 | 19,853 | 37 | 43 | 39 | 38 |
| 1961 | 17,391 | 2,370 | 584 | 20,345 | 38 | 46 | 41 | 39 |
| 1962 | 18,063 | 2,452 | 580 | 21,095 | 39 | 47 | 40 | 40 |
| 1963 | 18,515 | 2,553 | 616 | 21,684 | 39 | 49 | 43 | 41 |
| 1964 | 18,928 | 2,581 | 639 | 22,148 | 40 | 50 | 44 | 41 |
| 1965 | 19,483 | 2,785 | 666 | 22,934 | 41 | 53 | 45 | 42 |
| 1966 | 20,142 | 2,787 | 676 | 23,605 | 42 | 54 | 46 | 43 |
| 1967 | 21,057 | 2,912 | 682 | 24,651 | 44 | 56 | 46 | 45 |
| 1968 | 21,927 | 3,050 | 702 | 25,679 | 45 | 59 | 47 | 47 |
| 1969 | 22,724 | 3,136 | 744 | 26,604 | 47 | 60 | 49 | 48 |
| 1970 | 23,299 | 3,224 | 826 | 27,349 | 48 | 62 | 54 | 49 |
| 1971 | 24,559 | 3,481 | 812 | 28,852 | 50 | 66 | 53 | 52 |
| 1972 | 25,808 | 3,673 | 882 | 30,363 | 52 | 70 | 57 | 54 |
| 1973 | 26,934 | 3,797 | 939 | 31,670 | 54 | 73 | 61 | 56 |
| 1974 | 27,924 | 4,581 | 1,280 | 33,785 | 56 | 87 | 84 | 60 |
| 1975 | 29,337 | 4,680 | 1,464 | 35,481 | 59 | 89 | 96 | 63 |
| 1976 | 30,169 | 4,762 | 1,483 | 36,414 | 61 | 91 | 97 | 65 |
| 1977 | 30,991 | 4,886 | 1,585 | 37,462 | 63 | 93 | 104 | 67 |
| 1978 | 31,978 | 4,953 | 1,711 | 38,642 | 65 | 95 | 112 | 69 |
| 1979 | 33,168 | 5,105 | 1,810 | 40,083 | 67 | 98 | 118 | 71 |
| 1980 | 34,298 | 5,163 | 1,864 | 41,325 | 69 | 99 | 122 | 73 |
| 1981 | 35,111 | 5,159 | 1,874 | 42,144 | 71 | 100 | 122 | 75 |
| 1982 | 37,631 | 5,222 | 1,935 | 44,788 | 76 | 101 | 125 | 80 |
| 1983 | 38,337 | 5,155 | 1,988 | 45,480 | 77 | 100 | 128 | 81 |
| 1984 | 38,616 | 5,285 | 2,044 | 45,945 | 78 | 103 | 131 | 81 |
| 1985 | 39,278 | 5,588 | 2,027 | 46,893 | 79 | 109 | 129 | 83 |
| 1986 | 39,654 | 5,486 | 2,040 | 47,180 | 79 | 107 | 130 | 83 |
| 1987 | 39,602 | 5,497 | 2,065 | 47,164 | 79 | 108 | 131 | 83 |
| 1988 | 40,958 | 5,749 | 2,091 | 48,798 | 82 | 113 | 132 | 86 |
| 1989 | 42,386 | 5,787 | 2,218 | 50,391 | 84 | 114 | 139 | 88 |
| 1990 | 44,041 | 5,940 | 2,238 | 52,219 | 87 | 117 | 140 | 91 |
| 1991 | 45,335 | 5,969 | 2,262 | 53,566 | 89 | 117 | 141 | 93 |
| 1992 | 46,387 | 6,133 | 2,226 | 54,746 | 91 | 121 | 137 | 95 |
| 1993 | 51,091 | 6,275 | 2,541 | 59,908 | 100 | 123 | 155 | 104 |
| 1994 | 51,806 | 6,478 | 2,774 | 61,059 | 101 | 127 | 169 | 106 |
| 1995 | 55,078 | 6,642 | 2,745 | 64,466 | 107 | 130 | 166 | 111 |
| 1996 | 56,873 | 7,457 | 2,763 | 67,093 | 111 | 146 | 166 | 115 |
| 1997 | 59,796 | 7,771 | 2,781 | 70,347 | 116 | 153 | 166 | 121 |
| 1998 | 61,605 | 7,831 | 2,801 | 72,238 | 119 | 154 | 167 | 124 |
| 1999 | 63,254 | 7,986 | 2,839 | 74,079 | 122 | 157 | 169 | 126 |
| 2000 | 65,078 | 8,032 | 2,572 | 75,682 | 125 | 159 | 153 | 129 |
| 2001 | 67,064 | 8,333 | 2,639 | 78,036 | 128 | 165 | 156 | 132 |
| 2002 | 71,639 | 8,931 | 2,787 | 83,356 | 136 | 177 | 164 | 141 |
| 2003 | 75,601 | 9,143 | 2,979 | 87,723 | 143 | 181 | 175 | 147 |
| 2004 | 82,241 | 9,424 | 3,125 | 94,790 | 155 | 186 | 183 | 158 |
| 2005 | 87,427 | 9,643 | 3,285 | 100,355 | 164 | 189 | 191 | 167 |

*Notes:* Figures from 1990 onwards for England and Wales and from 1996 for Scotland includes community staff.

1 All figures relate to full-time equivalents.

2 In England, figures include principals in general practice who are working in hospitals, or medical and dental officers to whom paragraph 94 and 106-107 of the Terms and Conditions of Service apply.

3 From 1974 onwards, figures relate to 31 December and include health and social services staff.

*Sources:* Health and Personal Social Services Statistics for England (DH).

Health Statistics Wales (NAW).

Scottish Health Statistics (ISD).

Annual Abstract of Statistics (ONS)

NHS Hospital, Public Health Medicine and Community Health Service Medical and Dental Workforce Census (IC).

Population Projections Database (GAD).

Table 3.5   **NHS available hospital beds and FCEs[1] per medical and dental staff[2], UK, 1951 - 2005/06**

| | Available beds per medical and dental staff[2] | | | | Finished consultant episodes (FCEs) per staff[2] | | | |
|---|---|---|---|---|---|---|---|---|
| Year | England and Wales | Scotland | Northern Ireland[3] | United Kingdom | England and Wales | Scotland | Northern Ireland[3] | United Kingdom |
| 1951 | 34.2 | 62.8 | 30.5 | 36.0 | 239 | 456 | 211 | 252 |
| 1955 | 32.1 | 50.3 | 27.2 | 33.3 | 243 | 394 | 217 | 253 |
| 1960 | 28.1 | 22.2 | 23.5 | 27.1 | 243 | 198 | 201 | 235 |
| 1961 | 27.5 | 21.1 | 22.5 | 26.4 | 245 | 192 | 206 | 236 |
| 1962 | 26.2 | 20.0 | 21.4 | 25.2 | 243 | 190 | 218 | 235 |
| 1963 | 25.5 | 19.2 | 20.1 | 24.4 | 247 | 187 | 215 | 237 |
| 1964 | 24.9 | 19.3 | 20.6 | 24.0 | 250 | 188 | 219 | 240 |
| 1965 | 24.1 | 18.2 | 19.9 | 23.1 | 247 | 181 | 222 | 237 |
| 1966 | 23.2 | 17.9 | 19.1 | 22.3 | 243 | 181 | 221 | 234 |
| 1967 | 22.2 | 17.1 | 18.7 | 21.3 | 238 | 176 | 224 | 228 |
| 1968 | 21.2 | 16.3 | 18.1 | 20.4 | 235 | 176 | 222 | 226 |
| 1969 | 20.3 | 16.1 | 17.2 | 19.6 | 232 | 177 | 216 | 224 |
| 1970 | 19.6 | 15.2 | 15.8 | 18.8 | 229 | 169 | 202 | 219 |
| 1971 | 18.3 | 14.6 | 15.8 | 17.7 | 224 | 169 | 203 | 215 |
| 1972 | 17.2 | 13.8 | 15.7 | 16.6 | 215 | 159 | 202 | 206 |
| 1973 | 16.2 | 13.8 | 14.8 | 15.8 | 202 | 157 | 186 | 196 |
| 1974 | 15.3 | 13.5 | 10.6 | 14.8 | 197 | 157 | 131 | 188 |
| 1975 | 14.3 | 13.0 | 9.0 | 13.8 | 181 | 149 | 117 | 173 |
| 1976 | 13.7 | 12.6 | 8.9 | 13.3 | 185 | 156 | 121 | 178 |
| 1977 | 13.0 | 12.1 | 8.4 | 12.7 | 184 | 151 | 114 | 176 |
| 1978 | 12.4 | 11.9 | 8.0 | 12.1 | 178 | 151 | 111 | 171 |
| 1979 | 11.7 | 11.4 | 7.6 | 11.4 | 173 | 145 | 107 | 166 |
| 1980 | 11.2 | 11.2 | 7.4 | 11.0 | 176 | 171 | 107 | 172 |
| 1981 | 10.8 | 11.2 | 7.4 | 10.7 | 175 | 173 | 113 | 171 |
| 1982 | 10.0 | 11.1 | 7.3 | 10.0 | 162 | 171 | 111 | 160 |
| 1983 | 9.7 | 11.1 | 7.1 | 9.7 | 167 | 173 | 113 | 165 |
| 1984 | 9.2 | 10.8 | 6.9 | 9.3 | 171 | 174 | 112 | 168 |
| 1985 | 8.9 | 10.2 | 7.0 | 8.9 | 173 | 176 | 119 | 170 |
| 1986 | 8.5 | 10.1 | 6.5 | 8.6 | 173 | 183 | 118 | 171 |
| 1987 | 8.0 | 9.9 | 6.2 | 8.1 | 203 | 188 | 118 | 197 |
| 1988/89[4] | 7.4 | 9.3 | 5.8 | 7.6 | 217 | 184 | 123 | 208 |
| 1989/90 | 6.8 | 9.0 | 5.4 | 7.0 | 217 | 187 | 121 | 209 |
| 1990/91 | 5.8 | 8.5 | 5.2 | 6.1 | 198 | 188 | 126 | 194 |
| 1991/92 | 5.4 | 8.2 | 4.8 | 5.7 | 204 | 193 | 130 | 200 |
| 1992/93 | 5.1 | 7.6 | 4.6 | 5.3 | 208 | 193 | 135 | 203 |
| 1993/94 | 4.6 | 7.0 | 4.3 | 4.9 | 211 | 197 | 145 | 207 |
| 1994/95 | 4.4 | 6.5 | 3.7 | 4.6 | 218 | 199 | 140 | 212 |
| 1995/96 | 4.0 | 6.1 | 3.7 | 4.2 | 215 | 199 | 146 | 210 |
| 1996/97 | 3.8 | 5.2 | 3.4 | 3.9 | 210 | 181 | 144 | 204 |
| 1997/98 | 3.5 | 4.9 | 3.2 | 3.6 | 204 | 179 | 147 | 199 |
| 1998/99 | 3.3 | 4.6 | 3.1 | 3.5 | 205 | 181 | 160 | 201 |
| 1999/00 | 3.2 | 4.3 | 3.0 | 3.3 | 203 | 175 | 159 | 198 |
| 2000/01 | 3.1 | 4.1 | 3.3 | 3.2 | 199 | 175 | 177 | 196 |
| 2001/02 | 3.0 | 3.8 | 3.2 | 3.1 | 195 | 165 | 174 | 191 |
| 2002/03 | 2.8 | 3.4 | 3.0 | 2.8 | 187 | 148 | 167 | 183 |
| 2003/04 | 2.6 | 3.3 | 2.8 | 2.7 | 184 | 149 | 162 | 179 |
| 2004/05 | 2.4 | 3.1 | 2.7 | 2.5 | 175 | 146 | 157 | 172 |
| 2005/06 | 2.2 | 2.9 | 2.5 | 2.3 | 173 | 149 | 152 | 170 |

*Notes:*   1 Finished consultant episodes.
2 All figures relate to full-time equivalents, Medical and dental staff include Hospital and Community Health Services staff from 1990 onwards.
3 From 1974 onwards, figures relate to 31 December and include health and social services staff.
4 From 1988, figures for available beds relate to financial year ending 31 March and hence the ratios are not strictly comparable with earlier years Figures prior to 1988 relate to 30 September.
Prior to 1987/88 and for Wales, Scotland and N Ireland, figures for FCEs relate to discharges and deaths.  FCE data for England for 2004/05 and 2005/06 have not been adjusted to take into account shortfalls in the number of records received or for missing/invalid clinical data.

*Sources:*   See Table 3.4.
Hospital Activity Statistics: England (DH).
Hospital Episode Statistics (DH).
Hospital Statistics for Northern Ireland (DHSSPS).
Health and Personal Social Services Statistics for England (DH).
NHS Hospital, Public Health Medicine and Community Health Services Medical and Dental Workforce Census (IC).

Table 3.6   **NHS hospital and community nursing and midwifery staff[1], UK, 1951 - 2005**

30th September

| Year | Nursing and midwifery staff[1] ('000s) | | | | Staff[1] per 100,000 population | | | |
|------|------------------------------|------------------------|-------------------------------|-------------------|----------------------------|------------------------|-------------------------------|-------------------|
|      | England and Wales[2] | Scotland[3] | Northern Ireland[4] | United Kingdom | England and Wales[2] | Scotland[3] | Northern Ireland[4] | United Kingdom |
| 1951 | 162.0 | 22.0 | 4.6 | 188.6 | 370 | 431 | 335 | 375 |
| 1955 | 176.2 | 25.1 | 5.3 | 206.6 | 396 | 491 | 380 | 406 |
| 1960 | 206.3 | 29.4 | 6.4 | 242.1 | 451 | 568 | 451 | 462 |
| 1961 | 212.7 | 30.2 | 6.6 | 249.5 | 460 | 583 | 462 | 472 |
| 1962 | 226.0 | 31.6 | 7.1 | 264.7 | 485 | 608 | 494 | 497 |
| 1963 | 228.4 | 32.1 | 7.2 | 267.7 | 487 | 617 | 498 | 500 |
| 1964 | 234.5 | 33.4 | 7.6 | 275.5 | 496 | 641 | 521 | 510 |
| 1965 | 246.9 | 35.1 | 8.3 | 290.3 | 518 | 674 | 565 | 534 |
| 1966 | 258.7 | 36.0 | 8.7 | 303.4 | 539 | 692 | 589 | 555 |
| 1967 | 268.1 | 38.7 | 9.1 | 315.9 | 555 | 745 | 611 | 575 |
| 1968 | 271.6 | 39.4 | 9.1 | 320.1 | 560 | 758 | 605 | 580 |
| 1969 | 279.2 | 40.8 | 10.6 | 330.6 | 573 | 783 | 700 | 596 |
| 1970 | 290.4 | 43.1 | 10.2 | 343.7 | 594 | 827 | 668 | 618 |
| 1971 | 304.9 | 46.2 | 10.9 | 362.0 | 620 | 882 | 707 | 647 |
| 1972 | 322.3 | 48.7 | 11.7 | 382.7 | 653 | 931 | 760 | 682 |
| 1973 | 328.5 | 50.4 | 13.5 | 392.4 | 664 | 963 | 882 | 698 |
| 1974 | 339.9 | 52.4 | 15.9 | 408.2 | 687 | 1,000 | 1,041 | 726 |
| 1975 | 371.6 | 52.5 | 16.8 | 440.9 | 751 | 1,003 | 1,103 | 784 |
| 1976 | 378.4 | 53.4 | 16.6 | 448.4 | 765 | 1,020 | 1,089 | 798 |
| 1977 | 377.6 | 53.2 | 17.1 | 447.9 | 764 | 1,018 | 1,123 | 797 |
| 1978 | 373.4 | 54.4 | 17.9 | 445.7 | 755 | 1,044 | 1,175 | 793 |
| 1979 | 381.5 | 53.3 | 18.8 | 453.6 | 771 | 1,024 | 1,230 | 807 |
| 1980 | 394.4 | 53.3 | 19.8 | 467.5 | 795 | 1,026 | 1,292 | 830 |
| 1981 | 417.1 | 55.7 | 20.8 | 493.6 | 840 | 1,075 | 1,353 | 876 |
| 1982 | 423.0 | 56.4 | 21.2 | 500.6 | 853 | 1,092 | 1,373 | 889 |
| 1983 | 423.1 | 56.3 | 21.1 | 500.5 | 853 | 1,094 | 1,361 | 889 |
| 1984 | 423.9 | 56.3 | 20.8 | 501.0 | 853 | 1,096 | 1,336 | 888 |
| 1985 | 428.2 | 55.2 | 20.6 | 504.0 | 859 | 1,076 | 1,316 | 891 |
| 1986 | 429.9 | 56.9 | 20.6 | 507.4 | 860 | 1,113 | 1,309 | 895 |
| 1987 | 431.8 | 55.9 | 20.6 | 508.3 | 861 | 1,096 | 1,302 | 895 |
| 1988 | 431.8 | 56.3 | 20.8 | 508.9 | 859 | 1,109 | 1,312 | 894 |
| 1989 | 433.2 | 56.8 | 20.9 | 510.9 | 859 | 1,119 | 1,314 | 895 |
| 1990 | 430.0 | 56.2 | 20.9 | 507.1 | 850 | 1,106 | 1,310 | 886 |
| 1991 | 423.7 | 56.0 | 20.6 | 500.3 | 835 | 1,102 | 1,282 | 871 |
| 1992 | 408.5 | 54.4 | 19.8 | 482.7 | 803 | 1,070 | 1,220 | 838 |
| 1993 | 387.9 | 52.5 | 19.4 | 459.8 | 761 | 1,031 | 1,186 | 797 |
| 1994 | 374.0 | 46.6 | 19.7 | 440.3 | 732 | 912 | 1,199 | 761 |
| 1995 | 354.5 | 52.4 | 15.1 | 422.0 | 691 | 1,027 | 916 | 727 |
| 1996 | 354.6 | 51.9 | 15.0 | 421.5 | 690 | 1,019 | 901 | 725 |
| 1997 | 353.3 | 51.5 | 14.3 | 419.1 | 685 | 1,013 | 858 | 719 |
| 1998 | 355.4 | 51.1 | 14.5 | 420.9 | 687 | 1,007 | 862 | 720 |
| 1999 | 362.0 | 51.4 | 14.6 | 428.0 | 697 | 1,013 | 872 | 729 |
| 2000 | 370.3 | 51.3 | 14.9 | 436.6 | 710 | 1,013 | 886 | 741 |
| 2001 | 382.7 | 52.2 | 15.0 | 450.0 | 731 | 1,031 | 890 | 761 |
| 2002 | 398.5 | 53.2 | 15.8 | 467.6 | 758 | 1,052 | 933 | 788 |
| 2003 | 416.8 | 54.1 | 16.5 | 487.5 | 789 | 1,070 | 971 | 818 |
| 2004 | 426.6 | 54.6 | 17.1 | 498.3 | 804 | 1,074 | 998 | 833 |
| 2005 | 433.3 | 55.5 | 17.4 | 506.2 | 811 | 1,089 | 1,011 | 840 |

*Notes:*   1 Staff numbers are in whole-time equivalents and include unqualified staff.
2 From 1968 onwards, figures include community health services and hospital staff, and from 1971 onwards they include headquarters, blood transfusion units and agency staff.
3 Figures relate to hospital and community nurses and midwives including unqualified nursing staff from 1994 onwards.
4 Figures include whole-time and part-time staff.  From 1974 onwards, figures include personal social services staff.  Figures from 2000 onwards exclude all home helps and all agency/bank staff. Prior to 1995 figures relate to headcount.

*Sources:*   Health and Personal Social Services Statistics for England (DH).
Health Statistics Wales (NAW).
Scottish Health Statistics (ISD).
Annual Abstract of Statistics (ONS).
Population Projections Database (GAD).

# Hospital Workforce

Figure 3.6 **Trends in NHS medical and nursing staff numbers, FCEs and available beds, UK, 1951 - 2005**

**Index (1951=100)**

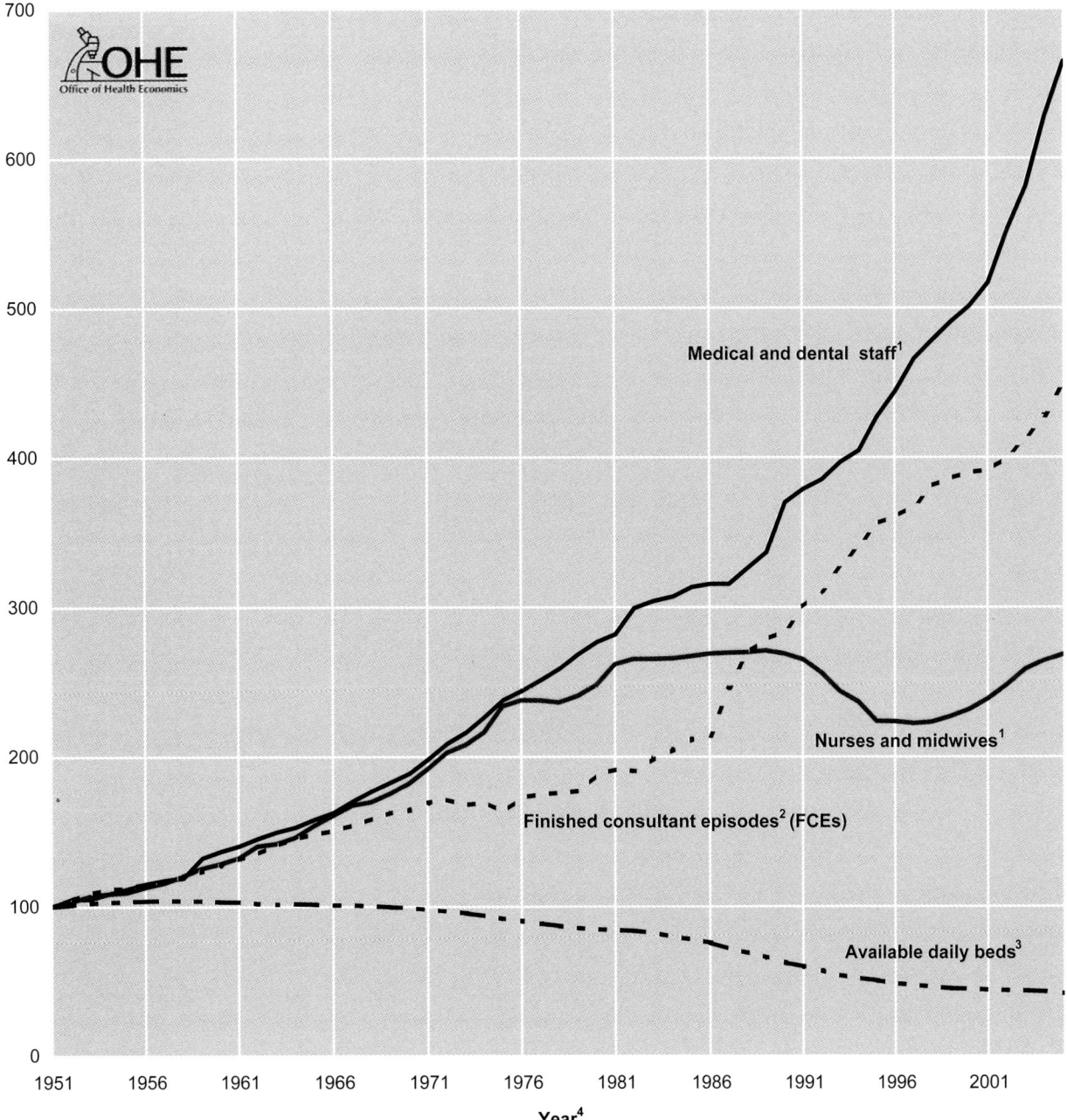

**Year[4]**

Notes:    1 Staff numbers at 30 September.  Northern Ireland figures relate to full-time and part-time equivalents and include unqualified staff and
from  1974 onwards, include personal social services staff.  From 1968 onwards, figures in England and Wales include community health
services and hospital staff, and from 1971 onwards they include headquarters,  blood transfusion units and agency staff.  Figures for
Scotland relate to hospital nurses and midwives including unqualified nurses and, from 1994 onwards, excluding teaching staff and student
nurses.
2 Prior to 1987/88, England figures relate to discharges and deaths but from 1987/88 they relate to finished consultant episodes (FCEs).
3 Available beds include those in all NHS hospitals for all specialties.
4 From 1987/88 onwards are for financial year.  Prior to 1987 figures relate to calendar year.

Sources:    Health and Personal Social Services Statistics for England (DH).
Health Statistics Wales (NAW).
Scottish Health Statistics (ISD).
Annual Abstract of Statistics (ONS).
NHS Hospital, Public Health Medicine and Community Health Services Medical and Dental Workforce Census (IC).

Table 3.7 **NHS available hospital beds and FCEs per nursing and midwifery staff[1], 1951 - 2005/06**

30th September

| | Available beds per staff[1] | | | | Finished consultant episodes (FCEs) per staff[1] | | | |
|---|---|---|---|---|---|---|---|---|
| Year | England and Wales[2] | Scotland[3] | Northern Ireland[4] | United Kingdom | England and Wales[2] | Scotland[3] | Northern Ireland[4] | United Kingdom |
| 1951 | 2.88 | 2.77 | 3.26 | 2.88 | 20.1 | 20.1 | 22.6 | 20.2 |
| 1955 | 2.74 | 2.51 | 3.02 | 2.72 | 20.7 | 19.7 | 24.2 | 20.7 |
| 1960 | 2.32 | 2.18 | 2.66 | 2.31 | 20.0 | 19.4 | 22.7 | 20.0 |
| 1961 | 2.25 | 2.12 | 2.58 | 2.24 | 20.1 | 19.3 | 23.5 | 20.1 |
| 1962 | 2.10 | 1.99 | 2.25 | 2.09 | 19.4 | 18.9 | 23.0 | 19.5 |
| 1963 | 2.07 | 1.96 | 2.22 | 2.06 | 20.0 | 19.1 | 23.8 | 20.0 |
| 1964 | 2.01 | 1.92 | 2.24 | 2.01 | 20.1 | 18.7 | 23.8 | 20.1 |
| 1965 | 1.90 | 1.82 | 2.05 | 1.90 | 19.5 | 18.1 | 22.8 | 19.4 |
| 1966 | 1.81 | 1.75 | 1.95 | 1.81 | 18.9 | 17.7 | 22.6 | 18.9 |
| 1967 | 1.74 | 1.65 | 1.87 | 1.73 | 18.7 | 17.0 | 22.3 | 18.6 |
| 1968 | 1.71 | 1.60 | 1.87 | 1.70 | 19.0 | 17.2 | 22.9 | 18.9 |
| 1969 | 1.65 | 1.54 | 1.60 | 1.64 | 18.9 | 17.0 | 20.1 | 18.7 |
| 1970 | 1.57 | 1.46 | 1.67 | 1.56 | 18.4 | 16.2 | 21.4 | 18.2 |
| 1971 | 1.48 | 1.36 | 1.56 | 1.46 | 18.0 | 15.8 | 20.1 | 17.8 |
| 1972 | 1.37 | 1.29 | 1.54 | 1.37 | 17.2 | 14.9 | 19.8 | 17.0 |
| 1973 | 1.33 | 1.23 | 1.33 | 1.32 | 16.6 | 14.0 | 16.8 | 16.3 |
| 1974 | 1.26 | 1.18 | 1.13 | 1.24 | 16.2 | 13.7 | 14.1 | 15.8 |
| 1975 | 1.13 | 1.16 | 1.01 | 1.13 | 14.3 | 13.3 | 13.1 | 14.1 |
| 1976 | 1.09 | 1.12 | 1.02 | 1.09 | 14.8 | 13.9 | 13.9 | 14.6 |
| 1977 | 1.07 | 1.11 | 0.99 | 1.07 | 15.1 | 13.9 | 13.5 | 14.9 |
| 1978 | 1.06 | 1.08 | 0.95 | 1.06 | 15.3 | 13.8 | 13.2 | 15.0 |
| 1979 | 1.02 | 1.09 | 0.90 | 1.02 | 15.1 | 13.8 | 12.8 | 14.8 |
| 1980 | 0.97 | 1.09 | 0.86 | 0.98 | 15.3 | 16.6 | 12.4 | 15.3 |
| 1981 | 0.91 | 1.04 | 0.82 | 0.92 | 14.7 | 16.0 | 12.5 | 14.8 |
| 1982 | 0.89 | 1.03 | 0.80 | 0.90 | 14.4 | 15.9 | 12.2 | 14.5 |
| 1983 | 0.88 | 1.01 | 0.81 | 0.89 | 15.2 | 15.8 | 12.8 | 15.1 |
| 1984 | 0.84 | 1.01 | 0.82 | 0.86 | 15.5 | 16.4 | 13.2 | 15.5 |
| 1985 | 0.81 | 1.03 | 0.83 | 0.84 | 15.8 | 17.8 | 14.1 | 16.0 |
| 1986 | 0.79 | 0.97 | 0.78 | 0.81 | 15.9 | 17.6 | 14.1 | 16.0 |
| 1987 | 0.74 | 0.97 | 0.75 | 0.76 | 18.6 | 18.5 | 14.3 | 18.4 |
| 1988/89[5] | 0.70 | 0.95 | 0.71 | 0.73 | 20.6 | 18.8 | 14.9 | 20.2 |
| 1989/90 | 0.67 | 0.92 | 0.67 | 0.70 | 21.2 | 19.0 | 15.1 | 20.7 |
| 1990/91 | 0.64 | 0.90 | 0.65 | 0.67 | 21.8 | 19.9 | 15.5 | 21.3 |
| 1991/92 | 0.62 | 0.87 | 0.61 | 0.65 | 23.4 | 20.5 | 16.5 | 22.8 |
| 1992/93 | 0.61 | 0.86 | 0.59 | 0.64 | 25.2 | 21.8 | 17.3 | 24.5 |
| 1993/94 | 0.61 | 0.84 | 0.56 | 0.63 | 27.9 | 23.6 | 19.0 | 27.0 |
| 1994/95 | 0.61 | 0.91 | 0.53 | 0.64 | 30.2 | 27.6 | 19.7 | 29.5 |
| 1995/96 | 0.63 | 0.77 | 0.67 | 0.65 | 33.3 | 25.3 | 26.5 | 32.1 |
| 1996/97 | 0.61 | 0.74 | 0.63 | 0.62 | 33.7 | 26.0 | 26.6 | 32.5 |
| 1997/98 | 0.59 | 0.74 | 0.63 | 0.61 | 34.5 | 27.1 | 28.6 | 33.3 |
| 1998/99 | 0.58 | 0.71 | 0.61 | 0.59 | 35.5 | 27.7 | 31.0 | 34.4 |
| 1999/00 | 0.55 | 0.68 | 0.59 | 0.57 | 35.5 | 27.2 | 30.9 | 34.3 |
| 2000/01 | 0.54 | 0.65 | 0.57 | 0.56 | 35.0 | 27.3 | 30.6 | 34.0 |
| 2001/02 | 0.52 | 0.61 | 0.56 | 0.53 | 34.1 | 26.3 | 30.5 | 33.1 |
| 2002/03 | 0.50 | 0.58 | 0.52 | 0.51 | 33.7 | 24.9 | 29.4 | 32.5 |
| 2003/04 | 0.48 | 0.55 | 0.51 | 0.49 | 33.3 | 25.1 | 29.2 | 32.2 |
| 2004/05 | 0.46 | 0.53 | 0.49 | 0.47 | 33.8 | 25.3 | 28.7 | 32.7 |
| 2005/06 | 0.44 | 0.51 | 0.47 | 0.45 | 34.9 | 25.9 | 28.7 | 33.7 |

*Notes:*   1 Staff numbers are in full-time equivalents and include unqualified staff.
2 From 1968 onwards, figures for Wales include community health care and hospital staff, and from 1971 headquarters staff of hospital boards
3 Figures relate to hospital nurses and midwives including unqualified nursing staff and, from 1994 onwards, excluding teaching staff and student nurses.
4 From 1974 onwards, figures include personal social services staff. Figures from 2000 onwards exclude all home helps and all agency/bank staff. Prior to 1995 figures relate to headcount.
5 From 1988, figures for available beds relate to financial years ending 31 March and hence the ratios are not strictly comparable with earlier years. Prior to 1987/88, and for Wales, Scotland and Northern Ireland, figures for FCEs relate to discharges and deaths.

*Sources:*   Health and Personal Social Services Statistics for England (DH).
Health Statistics Wales (NAW).
Scottish Health Statistics (ISD).
Annual Abstract of Statistics (ONS).

Table 3.8    Number of hospital and community medical and dental staff (full-time equivalents), by grade, England, 1996 - 2006

30th September

| | Year | | | | | | | | |
|---|---|---|---|---|---|---|---|---|---|
| | 1996 | 1999 | 2000 | 2001 | 2002 | 2003 | 2004 | 2005 | 2006 |
| **Total** | **54,233** | **60,338** | **62,094** | **64,055** | **68,260** | **72,260** | **78,462** | **82,568** | **85,975** |
| of which medical staff | 49,709 | 56,071 | 57,941 | 59,920 | 64,170 | 68,106 | 74,281 | 79,638 | 84,203 |
| Consultant[1] | 18,603 | 21,410 | 22,186 | 23,064 | 24,756 | 26,341 | 28,141 | 29,613 | 30,619 |
| Associate specialist | 2,009 | 3,343 | 3,855 | 4,105 | 4,799 | 4,828 | 4,948 | 4,966 | 5,325 |
| Staff grade | 1,074 | 1,336 | 1,381 | 1,408 | 1,578 | 1,780 | 2,029 | 2,260 | 2,495 |
| Registrar group[2] | 10,717 | 12,085 | 12,199 | 12,629 | 13,031 | 13,989 | 16,112 | 17,313 | 18,180 |
| Senior house officer | 14,084 | 14,866 | 15,322 | 15,642 | 16,912 | 18,419 | 20,283 | 21,337 | 22,352 |
| House officer | 3,264 | 3,548 | 3,683 | 3,733 | 3,989 | 3,994 | 4,259 | 4,645 | 4,890 |
| Other grades[3] | 4,483 | 3,750 | 3,468 | 3,474 | 3,194 | 2,909 | 2,689 | 2,435 | 2,114 |

## Index number of hospital medical and dental staff, England (1996 = 100)

30th September

| | Year | | | | | | | | |
|---|---|---|---|---|---|---|---|---|---|
| | 1996 | 1999 | 2000 | 2001 | 2002 | 2003 | 2004 | 2005 | 2006 |
| **Total** | **100** | **111** | **114** | **118** | **126** | **133** | **145** | **152** | **159** |
| of which medical staff | 100 | 113 | 117 | 121 | 129 | 137 | 149 | 160 | 169 |
| Consultant[1] | 100 | 115 | 119 | 124 | 133 | 142 | 151 | 159 | 165 |
| Associate specialist | 100 | 124 | 129 | 131 | 147 | 166 | 189 | 210 | 232 |
| Staff grade | 100 | 166 | 192 | 204 | 239 | 240 | 246 | 247 | 265 |
| Registrar group[2] | 100 | 113 | 114 | 118 | 122 | 131 | 150 | 162 | 170 |
| Senior house officer[3] | 100 | 106 | 109 | 111 | 120 | 131 | 144 | 151 | 159 |
| House officer[4] | 100 | 109 | 113 | 114 | 122 | 122 | 130 | 142 | 150 |
| Other grades[5] | 100 | 84 | 77 | 77 | 71 | 65 | 60 | 54 | 47 |

## Percentage distribution of hospital medical and dental staff, England

30th September

| | Year | | | | | | | | |
|---|---|---|---|---|---|---|---|---|---|
| | 1996 | 1999 | 2000 | 2001 | 2002 | 2003 | 2004 | 2005 | 2006 |
| **Total** | **100** | **100** | **100** | **100** | **100** | **100** | **100** | **100** | **100** |
| of which medical staff | 92 | 93 | 93 | 94 | 94 | 94 | 95 | 96 | 98 |
| Consultant[1] | 34 | 35 | 36 | 36 | 36 | 36 | 36 | 36 | 36 |
| Associate specialist | 4 | 6 | 6 | 6 | 7 | 7 | 6 | 6 | 6 |
| Staff grade | 2 | 2 | 2 | 2 | 2 | 2 | 3 | 3 | 3 |
| Registrar group[2] | 20 | 20 | 20 | 20 | 19 | 19 | 21 | 21 | 21 |
| Senior house officer[3] | 26 | 25 | 25 | 24 | 25 | 25 | 26 | 26 | 26 |
| House officer[4] | 6 | 6 | 6 | 6 | 6 | 6 | 5 | 6 | 6 |
| Other grades[5] | 8 | 6 | 6 | 5 | 5 | 4 | 3 | 3 | 2 |

Notes:     Figures relate to NHS doctors and dentists working outside general practice.
    1 Including Directors of Public Health.
    2 This group comprises of doctors in the specialist registrar, senior registrar and registrar grades.
    3 In 2006 this group includes Foundation House Officer 2 (FHO2).
    4 In 2006 this group includes Foundation House Officer 1 (FHO1).
    5 This includes hospital practitioner, clinical assistant and other staff.
Source:    NHS Hospital, Public Health Medicine and Community Health Service Medical and Dental Workforce Census (IC).

Table 3.9  **Number of full-time equivalent hospital and community medical staff by selected specialty, England, 1990 - 2006**
30th September

| | Year | | | | | | | | | | | |
|---|---|---|---|---|---|---|---|---|---|---|---|---|
| | 1990 | 1996 | 1997 | 1998 | 1999 | 2000 | 2001 | 2002 | 2003 | 2004 | 2005 | 2006 |
| **All specialties** | 40,253 | 49,709 | 52,651 | 54,416 | 56,071 | 57,941 | 59,920 | 64,170 | 68,106 | 74,281 | 79,638 | 84,203 |
| *per 10,000 population* | *844* | *1,025* | *1,082* | *1,115* | *1,144* | *1,177* | *1,212* | *1,292* | *1,366* | *1,482* | *1,578* | *1,659* |
| Accident and emergency | 1,886 | 2,452 | 2,558 | 2,718 | 2,762 | 2,859 | 2,928 | 3,183 | 3,370 | 3,842 | 4,181 | 4,523 |
| Anaesthetics | 4,497 | 5,779 | 6,137 | 6,357 | 6,587 | 6,814 | 7,043 | 7,880 | 8,405 | 9,194 | 9,609 | 10,004 |
| Cardiology[1] | 437 | 864 | 936 | 1,056 | 1,065 | 1,154 | 1,233 | 1,395 | 1,549 | 1,749 | 1,834 | 1,890 |
| Cardiothoracic surgery | 353 | 465 | 474 | 507 | 535 | 560 | 587 | 603 | 631 | 726 | 729 | 704 |
| Chemical pathology | 263 | 210 | 223 | 208 | 220 | 199 | 202 | 198 | 206 | 212 | 224 | 236 |
| Child and adolescent psychiatry | 478 | 608 | 644 | 651 | 670 | 709 | 695 | 693 | 750 | 838 | 922 | 945 |
| Clinical genetics | 47 | 94 | 87 | 88 | 106 | 102 | 116 | 129 | 144 | 142 | 146 | 172 |
| Clinical neuro-physiology | 62 | 57 | 62 | 76 | 77 | 77 | 84 | 98 | 106 | 106 | 94 | 95 |
| Clinical pharmacology | 60 | 132 | 73 | 78 | 82 | 93 | 98 | 91 | 133 | 122 | 102 | 162 |
| Dermatology | 432 | 525 | 554 | 565 | 606 | 628 | 650 | 687 | 733 | 773 | 774 | 774 |
| Diabetes and endocrinology[1] | 86 | 421 | 507 | 585 | 608 | 725 | 793 | 832 | 891 | 1,006 | 1,021 | 1,045 |
| Forensic psychiatry | 66 | 197 | 252 | 310 | 289 | 320 | 383 | 357 | 401 | 431 | 467 | 499 |
| Gastroenterology[1] | 139 | 520 | 633 | 758 | 800 | 934 | 999 | 1,177 | 1,210 | 1,395 | 1,334 | 1,412 |
| General medicine[1] | 4,643 | 4,139 | 4,308 | 3,977 | 4,132 | 3,770 | 3,865 | 3,998 | 4,203 | 4,424 | 5,204 | 5,411 |
| General surgery | 3,523 | 4,059 | 4,187 | 4,241 | 4,351 | 4,506 | 4,712 | 5,079 | 5,354 | 5,777 | 6,205 | 6,338 |
| Genito-urinary medicine | 336 | 447 | 458 | 486 | 520 | 544 | 568 | 620 | 626 | 662 | 721 | 731 |
| Geriatric medicine | 1,897 | 2,041 | 2,127 | 2,178 | 2,121 | 2,206 | 2,203 | 2,382 | 2,549 | 2,685 | 2,688 | 2,762 |
| Haematology | 633 | 763 | 768 | 789 | 834 | 805 | 861 | 1,020 | 1,052 | 1,128 | 1,144 | 1,206 |
| Histopathology[2] | 878 | 872 | 895 | 979 | 1,015 | 1,068 | 1,180 | 1,276 | 1,382 | 1,490 | 1,533 | 1,559 |
| Immuno-pathology | 45 | 42 | 43 | 53 | 55 | 65 | 63 | 93 | 93 | 112 | 91 | 99 |
| Infectious diseases | 77 | 127 | 162 | 140 | 144 | 164 | 187 | 191 | 184 | 200 | 237 | 260 |
| Learning disabilities | 369 | 325 | 318 | 338 | 359 | 359 | 347 | 397 | 407 | 421 | 405 | 444 |
| Medical microbiology and virology[3] | 402 | 471 | 463 | 475 | 488 | 510 | 527 | 580 | 559 | 618 | 585 | 592 |
| Medical oncology | 70 | 213 | 215 | 265 | 317 | 341 | 367 | 428 | 522 | 487 | 520 | 537 |
| Mental illness | 3,354 | 3,440 | 3,620 | 3,760 | 3,953 | 4,156 | 4,058 | 4,345 | 4,550 | 5,057 | 5,351 | 5,573 |
| Nephrology | 219 | 443 | 494 | 521 | 523 | 565 | 607 | 667 | 757 | 829 | 819 | 888 |
| Neurology | 376 | 529 | 555 | 544 | 551 | 580 | 624 | 631 | 702 | 774 | 824 | 892 |
| Neurosurgery | 246 | 352 | 344 | 360 | 352 | 389 | 405 | 455 | 471 | 518 | 543 | 541 |
| Nuclear medicine | 38 | 43 | 43 | 45 | 43 | 36 | 44 | 50 | 57 | 62 | 56 | 67 |
| Obstetrics and gynaecology | 2,815 | 3,541 | 3,608 | 3,685 | 3,684 | 3,677 | 3,696 | 3,898 | 4,069 | 4,286 | 4,580 | 4,658 |
| Occupational health | 63 | 93 | 93 | 102 | 106 | 111 | 123 | 137 | 137 | 144 | 148 | 149 |
| Old age psychiatry | 103 | 512 | 570 | 627 | 679 | 720 | 759 | 812 | 910 | 1,116 | 1,134 | 1,155 |
| Ophthalmology | 1,156 | 1,498 | 1,599 | 1,643 | 1,704 | 1,749 | 1,757 | 1,852 | 1,953 | 2,019 | 2,108 | 2,106 |
| Other | 189 | 225 | 210 | 265 | 260 | 263 | 381 | 449 | 400 | 594 | 450 | 878 |
| Otolaryngology | 943 | 1,113 | 1,182 | 1,162 | 1,165 | 1,182 | 1,180 | 1,256 | 1,313 | 1,446 | 1,519 | 1,533 |
| Paediatric cardiology | - | 38 | 37 | 53 | 49 | 49 | 65 | 106 | 102 | 101 | 82 | 119 |
| Paediatric surgery | 128 | 213 | 219 | 259 | 226 | 269 | 261 | 287 | 247 | 314 | 328 | 297 |
| Paediatrics | 2,316 | 3,617 | 3,953 | 4,119 | 4,279 | 4,496 | 4,492 | 5,048 | 5,414 | 5,893 | 6,239 | 6,484 |
| Palliative medicine | 26 | 97 | 138 | 146 | 155 | 195 | 211 | 279 | 296 | 288 | 300 | 313 |
| Plastic surgery | 259 | 418 | 448 | 456 | 465 | 487 | 540 | 578 | 626 | 709 | 750 | 749 |
| Psychotherapy | 122 | 128 | 135 | 131 | 124 | 122 | 123 | 128 | 130 | 143 | 142 | 135 |
| Public health medicine | - | 783 | 815 | 818 | 161 | 138 | 112 | 1,198 | 1,227 | 1,204 | 1,324 | 1,268 |
| Radiology | 1,552 | 1,793 | 1,895 | 1,935 | 2,028 | 2,134 | 2,255 | 2,371 | 2,505 | 2,654 | 2,842 | 2,966 |
| Radiotherapy (clinical oncology) | 451 | 529 | 568 | 597 | 623 | 634 | 696 | 721 | 734 | 868 | 912 | 979 |
| Rehabilitation | 18 | 108 | 123 | 146 | 152 | 158 | 168 | 203 | 209 | 192 | 182 | 211 |
| Rheumatology | 471 | 536 | 586 | 618 | 624 | 659 | 687 | 714 | 748 | 767 | 810 | 829 |
| Thoracic medicine[1] | 284 | 540 | 632 | 725 | 725 | 852 | 920 | 1,001 | 1,103 | 1,230 | 1,258 | 1,368 |
| Traumatic and orthopaedic surgery | 2,199 | 2,958 | 3,178 | 3,271 | 3,389 | 3,463 | 3,602 | 3,864 | 4,185 | 4,536 | 4,750 | 5,039 |
| Urology | 500 | 759 | 836 | 914 | 969 | 999 | 1,040 | 1,114 | 1,166 | 1,293 | 1,327 | 1,364 |

*Notes:*  All figures include principals in general practice who are working in hospitals, or medical and dental officers to whom paragraph 94 and 106-107 of the Terms and Conditions of Service apply.  As a result of reclassification of specialties, figures may not be strictly comparable over time.
  1 From 1994, consultants in specialty of general medicine were reclassified using their second specialty if available.
  2 Figures for staff for neuropathology are included under histopathology.
  3 Figures for staff for virology are included under medical microbiology and virology.
  - Specialties not classified at that time.

*Sources:*  Health and Personal Social Services Statistics for England (DH).
  NHS Hospital, Public Health Medicine and Community Health Service Medical and Dental Workforce Census (DH).
  Population Projections Database (GAD).
  Population Estimates (ONS).

Table 3.10   **Full-time equivalent hospital and community medical staff by selected specialty and country, number and per 10,000 population, Great Britain, 2005**

30th September

| | Number of full-time equivalents | | | | Per 10,000 population | | | |
|---|---|---|---|---|---|---|---|---|
| | England | Wales | Scotland | Great Britain | England | Wales | Scotland | Great Britain |
| **All specialties** | **79,638** | **4,546** | **9,262** | **93,445** | **1,578.1** | **1,539.0** | **1,817.9** | **1,597.0** |
| Accident and emergency | 4,181 | 221 | 398 | 4,800 | 82.8 | 74.9 | 78.1 | 82.0 |
| Anaesthetics | 9,609 | 596 | 1,071 | 11,276 | 190.4 | 201.8 | 210.2 | 192.7 |
| Cardiology | 1,834 | 70 | 175 | 2,079 | 36.3 | 23.6 | 34.3 | 35.5 |
| Cardio-thoracic surgery | 729 | 32 | 84 | 844 | 14.4 | 10.7 | 16.4 | 14.4 |
| Chemical pathology | 224 | 18 | 37 | 279 | 4.4 | 6.1 | 7.3 | 4.8 |
| Child and adolescent psychiatry | 922 | 53 | 88 | 1,063 | 18.3 | 17.9 | 17.2 | 18.2 |
| Clinical genetics | 146 | 17 | 19 | 183 | 2.9 | 5.8 | 3.8 | 3.1 |
| Dermatology | 774 | 43 | 112 | 929 | 15.3 | 14.5 | 21.9 | 15.9 |
| Diabetes and endocrinology | 1,021 | 34 | 104 | 1,160 | 20.2 | 11.6 | 20.5 | 19.8 |
| Forensic psychiatry | 467 | 17 | 49 | 533 | 9.3 | 5.7 | 9.7 | 9.1 |
| Gastroenterology | 1,334 | 43 | 134 | 1,512 | 26.4 | 14.7 | 26.4 | 25.8 |
| General medicine | 5,204 | 459 | 799 | 6,462 | 103.1 | 155.5 | 156.7 | 110.4 |
| General surgery | 6,205 | 385 | 809 | 7,399 | 123.0 | 130.4 | 158.7 | 126.4 |
| Genito-urinary medicine | 721 | 27 | 26 | 773 | 14.3 | 9.0 | 5.0 | 13.2 |
| Geriatric medicine | 2,688 | 199 | 403 | 3,290 | 53.3 | 67.5 | 79.1 | 56.2 |
| Haematology | 1,144 | 74 | 154 | 1,372 | 22.7 | 25.2 | 30.2 | 23.5 |
| Histopathology | 1,533 | 63 | 196 | 1,792 | 30.4 | 21.3 | 38.5 | 30.6 |
| Learning disabilities | 405 | 31 | 63 | 499 | 8.0 | 10.4 | 12.4 | 8.5 |
| Medical microbiology and virology | 585 | 40 | 82 | 707 | 11.6 | 13.7 | 16.0 | 12.1 |
| Medical oncology | 520 | 10 | 48 | 578 | 10.3 | 3.5 | 9.3 | 9.9 |
| Mental illness | 5,351 | 242 | 670 | 6,262 | 106.0 | 81.9 | 131.4 | 107.0 |
| Nephrology | 819 | 42 | 117 | 978 | 16.2 | 14.1 | 23.0 | 16.7 |
| Neurology | 824 | 31 | 83 | 938 | 16.3 | 10.6 | 16.2 | 16.0 |
| Neurosurgery | 543 | 20 | 58 | 621 | 10.8 | 6.8 | 11.3 | 10.6 |
| Obstetrics and gynaecology | 4,580 | 286 | 500 | 5,366 | 90.8 | 96.8 | 98.2 | 91.7 |
| Occupational health | 148 | 10 | 35 | 194 | 2.9 | 3.5 | 6.9 | 3.3 |
| Old age psychiatry | 1,134 | 70 | 118 | 1,322 | 22.5 | 23.6 | 23.2 | 22.6 |
| Ophthalmology | 2,108 | 124 | 197 | 2,429 | 41.8 | 42.0 | 38.7 | 41.5 |
| Otolaryngology | 1,519 | 105 | 166 | 1,789 | 30.1 | 35.4 | 32.5 | 30.6 |
| Paediatric surgery | 328 | 9 | 58 | 395 | 6.5 | 3.1 | 11.3 | 6.7 |
| Paediatrics | 6,239 | 392 | 493 | 7,124 | 123.6 | 132.8 | 96.7 | 121.7 |
| Palliative medicine | 300 | 35 | 48 | 383 | 5.9 | 11.9 | 9.4 | 6.5 |
| Plastic surgery | 750 | 35 | 78 | 864 | 14.9 | 12.0 | 15.4 | 14.8 |
| Radiology | 2,842 | 148 | 320 | 3,310 | 56.3 | 50.0 | 62.8 | 56.6 |
| Radiotherapy (clinical oncology) | 912 | 61 | 113 | 1,086 | 18.1 | 20.5 | 22.2 | 18.6 |
| Rehabilitation | 182 | 9 | 47 | 239 | 3.6 | 3.2 | 9.3 | 4.1 |
| Rheumatology | 810 | 39 | 74 | 922 | 16.1 | 13.0 | 14.5 | 15.8 |
| Thoracic medicine | 1,258 | 71 | 138 | 1,467 | 24.9 | 24.1 | 27.1 | 25.1 |
| Traumatic and orthopaedic surgery | 4,750 | 260 | 441 | 5,451 | 94.1 | 88.1 | 86.5 | 93.2 |
| Urology | 1,327 | 76 | 112 | 1,515 | 26.3 | 25.6 | 22.0 | 25.9 |

*Notes:*   All figures relate to full-time equivalents, and include principals in general practice who are working in hospitals, or medical and dental officers to whom paragraph 94 and 106-107 of the Terms and Conditions of Service apply.
Anaesthetics for England include intensive care.
Due to differences in definitions, figures may not be comparable across countries.

*Sources:*   Health and Personal Social Services Statistics for England (DH).
NHS Hospital, Public Health Medicine and Community Health Service Medical and Dental Workforce Census (DH).
Health Statistics Wales (NAW).
Scottish Health Statistics (ISD).
Population Projections Database (GAD).

Table 3.11　**Number of full-time equivalent hospital and community medical consultants by selected specialty, England, 1990 - 2006**
30th September

| | Year | | | | | | | | | | | |
|---|---|---|---|---|---|---|---|---|---|---|---|---|
| | 1990 | 1996 | 1997 | 1998 | 1999 | 2000 | 2001 | 2002 | 2003 | 2004 | 2005 | 2006 |
| **All specialties** | 14,188 | 17,625 | 18,618 | 19,379 | 20,336 | 21,077 | 21,954 | 24,585 | 26,105 | 27,914 | 28,995 | 30,049 |
| *per 10,000 population* | *297* | *363* | *383* | *397* | *415* | *428* | *444* | *495* | *524* | *557* | *575* | *592* |
| Accident and emergency | 196 | 343 | 378 | 408 | 428 | 441 | 468 | 511 | 544 | 596 | 665 | 697 |
| Anaesthetics | 1,986 | 2,498 | 2,641 | 2,821 | 3,024 | 3,148 | 3,321 | 3,712 | 3,958 | 4,191 | 4,353 | 4,559 |
| Audiological medicine | 11 | 20 | 26 | 27 | 29 | 28 | 27 | 36 | 35 | 40 | 38 | 35 |
| Cardiology[1] | 133 | 349 | 364 | 415 | 425 | 483 | 512 | 561 | 609 | 663 | 677 | 705 |
| Cardiothoracic surgery | 116 | 145 | 147 | 159 | 172 | 183 | 185 | 197 | 207 | 219 | 231 | 232 |
| Chemical pathology | 158 | 145 | 158 | 149 | 152 | 147 | 151 | 150 | 149 | 149 | 148 | 149 |
| Child and adolescent psychiatry | 327 | 360 | 390 | 400 | 422 | 419 | 417 | 401 | 444 | 490 | 539 | 547 |
| Clinical genetics | 29 | 50 | 46 | 49 | 52 | 57 | 69 | 79 | 91 | 88 | 91 | 107 |
| Clinical neuro-physiology | 50 | 46 | 47 | 52 | 51 | 54 | 58 | 74 | 80 | 80 | 68 | 76 |
| Clinical pharmacology | 25 | 53 | 35 | 36 | 35 | 43 | 43 | 38 | 44 | 40 | 37 | 37 |
| Dermatology | 223 | 264 | 276 | 289 | 308 | 315 | 319 | 339 | 359 | 378 | 386 | 400 |
| Diabetes and endocrinology[1] | 17 | 237 | 262 | 295 | 292 | 365 | 376 | 416 | 446 | 483 | 456 | 453 |
| Forensic psychiatry | 43 | 91 | 114 | 136 | 141 | 151 | 187 | 177 | 212 | 209 | 225 | 227 |
| Gastroenterology[1] | 34 | 268 | 291 | 360 | 358 | 437 | 458 | 551 | 581 | 614 | 617 | 595 |
| General medicine[1] | 1,156 | 400 | 393 | 219 | 326 | 31 | 75 | 39 | 19 | 93 | 285 | 486 |
| General surgery | 879 | 1,083 | 1,122 | 1,138 | 1,199 | 1,258 | 1,275 | 1,386 | 1,457 | 1,548 | 1,637 | 1,671 |
| Genito-urinary medicine | 158 | 212 | 223 | 229 | 229 | 238 | 252 | 256 | 271 | 294 | 318 | 317 |
| Geriatric medicine | 484 | 624 | 653 | 686 | 693 | 733 | 738 | 814 | 849 | 867 | 880 | 873 |
| Haematology | 334 | 392 | 408 | 415 | 430 | 430 | 450 | 532 | 548 | 584 | 599 | 619 |
| Histopathology[2] | 568 | 664 | 688 | 744 | 755 | 778 | 827 | 882 | 939 | 995 | 1,012 | 1,018 |
| Immuno-pathology | 25 | 30 | 29 | 29 | 31 | 38 | 39 | 65 | 64 | 73 | 54 | 56 |
| Infectious diseases | 27 | 44 | 52 | 52 | 46 | 57 | 57 | 63 | 67 | 72 | 93 | 90 |
| Learning disabilities | 155 | 146 | 146 | 159 | 168 | 172 | 163 | 169 | 186 | 194 | 197 | 204 |
| Medical microbiology and virology[3] | 243 | 333 | 320 | 332 | 340 | 358 | 363 | 394 | 393 | 417 | 383 | 402 |
| Medical oncology | 23 | 67 | 68 | 79 | 87 | 103 | 120 | 152 | 167 | 164 | 185 | 202 |
| Mental illness | 1,093 | 1,175 | 1,243 | 1,325 | 1,418 | 1,493 | 1,461 | 1,523 | 1,604 | 1,776 | 1,907 | 1,924 |
| Nephrology | 59 | 165 | 183 | 194 | 190 | 207 | 231 | 253 | 278 | 303 | 311 | 324 |
| Neurology | 167 | 229 | 246 | 262 | 261 | 279 | 298 | 309 | 355 | 403 | 436 | 455 |
| Neurosurgery | 87 | 114 | 118 | 124 | 132 | 129 | 141 | 153 | 157 | 171 | 179 | 179 |
| Nuclear medicine | 22 | 25 | 27 | 28 | 27 | 25 | 32 | 39 | 43 | 44 | 38 | 39 |
| Obstetrics and gynaecology | 736 | 910 | 965 | 967 | 983 | 1,049 | 1,105 | 1,211 | 1,253 | 1,306 | 1,370 | 1,426 |
| Occupational health | 27 | 51 | 47 | 48 | 50 | 53 | 60 | 61 | 63 | 68 | 78 | 81 |
| Old age psychiatry | 79 | 222 | 231 | 253 | 290 | 305 | 324 | 321 | 382 | 470 | 468 | 482 |
| Ophthalmology | 408 | 516 | 539 | 556 | 582 | 606 | 613 | 661 | 702 | 734 | 766 | 771 |
| Otolaryngology | 353 | 383 | 402 | 389 | 407 | 422 | 419 | 440 | 462 | 497 | 514 | 529 |
| Paediatric cardiology | - | 13 | 16 | 17 | 17 | 22 | 27 | 58 | 61 | 57 | 41 | 58 |
| Paediatric surgery | 36 | 63 | 70 | 82 | 93 | 99 | 93 | 96 | 92 | 100 | 102 | 98 |
| Paediatrics | 685 | 1,032 | 1,094 | 1,156 | 1,206 | 1,258 | 1,278 | 1,480 | 1,581 | 1,681 | 1,828 | 1,927 |
| Palliative medicine | 13 | 44 | 61 | 64 | 73 | 88 | 94 | 125 | 138 | 151 | 151 | 155 |
| Plastic surgery | 93 | 136 | 147 | 156 | 159 | 174 | 179 | 187 | 204 | 228 | 241 | 236 |
| Psychotherapy | 68 | 82 | 82 | 86 | 85 | 82 | 81 | 83 | 91 | 92 | 97 | 89 |
| Public health medicine | - | 418 | 442 | 453 | 65 | 56 | 49 | 363 | 357 | 431 | 732 | 687 |
| Radiology | 1,055 | 1,310 | 1,364 | 1,387 | 1,414 | 1,460 | 1,492 | 1,582 | 1,669 | 1,746 | 1,892 | 1,945 |
| Radiotherapy (clinical oncology) | 182 | 237 | 265 | 277 | 283 | 279 | 299 | 295 | 325 | 364 | 407 | 450 |
| Rehabilitation | 9 | 54 | 62 | 62 | 67 | 71 | 75 | 100 | 107 | 107 | 101 | 98 |
| Rheumatology | 222 | 289 | 304 | 319 | 331 | 340 | 361 | 380 | 403 | 421 | 452 | 459 |
| Thoracic medicine[1] | 84 | 273 | 286 | 322 | 316 | 402 | 429 | 493 | 523 | 556 | 556 | 546 |
| Traumatic and orthopaedic surgery | 697 | 947 | 1,010 | 1,023 | 1,099 | 1,148 | 1,189 | 1,266 | 1,367 | 1,459 | 1,544 | 1,651 |
| Urology | 206 | 300 | 327 | 340 | 372 | 365 | 398 | 435 | 457 | 485 | 488 | 495 |

*Notes:*　All figures include principals in general practice who are working in hospitals, or medical and dental officers to whom paragraph 94 and 106-107 of the Terms and Conditions of Service apply.　As a result of reclassification of specialties, figures may not be strictly comparable over time.
　　　　1 From 1994, consultants in specialty of general medicine were reclassified using their second specialty if available.
　　　　2 Figures for staff for neuropathology are included under histopathology.
　　　　3 Figures for staff for virology are included under medical microbiology and virology.
　　　　- Specialties not classified at that time.

*Sources:*　Health and Personal Social Services Statistics for England (DH).
　　　　NHS Hospital, Public Health Medicine and Community Health Service Medical and Dental Workforce Census (DH).
　　　　Population Projections Database (GAD).
　　　　Population Estimates (ONS).

Table 3.12   **Full-time equivalent hospital and community consultants by selected specialty and country, number and per 10,000 population, Great Britain, 2005**
30th September

| | Number of full-time equivalents | | | | Per 10,000 population | | | |
|---|---|---|---|---|---|---|---|---|
| | England | Wales | Scotland | Great Britain | England | Wales | Scotland | Great Britain |
| **All specialties** | **28,995** | **1,584** | **3,265** | **33,844** | **574.5** | **536.4** | **640.8** | **578.4** |
| Accident and emergency | 665 | 32 | 71 | 768 | 13.2 | 10.9 | 13.9 | 13.1 |
| Anaesthetics | 4,353 | 264 | 529 | 5,145 | 86.3 | 89.3 | 103.7 | 87.9 |
| Audiological medicine | 38 | 1 | 1 | 40 | 0.8 | 0.3 | 0.2 | 0.7 |
| Cardiology | 677 | 26 | 72 | 775 | 13.4 | 8.7 | 14.2 | 13.2 |
| Cardio-thoracic surgery | 231 | 12 | 27 | 270 | 4.6 | 4.1 | 5.2 | 4.6 |
| Chemical pathology | 148 | 11 | 25 | 184 | 2.9 | 3.7 | 4.9 | 3.1 |
| Child and adolescent psychiatry | 539 | 26 | 55 | 620 | 10.7 | 8.9 | 10.7 | 10.6 |
| Clinical genetics | 91 | 9 | 11 | 111 | 1.8 | 3.1 | 2.2 | 1.9 |
| Clinical neurological physiology | 68 | 3 | 5 | 76 | 1.3 | 0.8 | 1.0 | 1.3 |
| Clinical pharmacology and therapeutics | 37 | 2 | 11 | 50 | 0.7 | 0.5 | 2.2 | 0.8 |
| Dermatology | 386 | 18 | 47 | 451 | 7.6 | 6.0 | 9.2 | 7.7 |
| Diabetes and endocrinology | 456 | 8 | 65 | 528 | 9.0 | 2.6 | 12.7 | 9.0 |
| Forensic psychiatry | 225 | 6 | 33 | 265 | 4.5 | 2.1 | 6.5 | 4.5 |
| Gastroenterology | 617 | 12 | 74 | 703 | 12.2 | 4.1 | 14.5 | 12.0 |
| General medicine | 285 | 97 | 23 | 405 | 5.6 | 32.7 | 4.6 | 6.9 |
| General surgery | 1,637 | 105 | 215 | 1,958 | 32.4 | 35.7 | 42.3 | 33.5 |
| Genito-urinary medicine | 318 | 11 | 14 | 343 | 6.3 | 3.7 | 2.8 | 5.9 |
| Geriatric medicine | 880 | 51 | 117 | 1,049 | 17.4 | 17.4 | 23.0 | 17.9 |
| Haematology | 599 | 39 | 80 | 718 | 11.9 | 13.2 | 15.7 | 12.3 |
| Histopathology | 1,012 | 46 | 123 | 1,182 | 20.1 | 15.7 | 24.2 | 20.2 |
| Immuno-pathology | 54 | 2 | - | 56 | 1.1 | 0.7 | - | 1.0 |
| Infectious diseases | 93 | 0 | 20 | 113 | 1.8 | 0.0 | 4.0 | 1.9 |
| Learning disabilities | 197 | 13 | 27 | 237 | 3.9 | 4.3 | 5.4 | 4.1 |
| Medical microbiology and virology | 383 | 32 | 50 | 465 | 7.6 | 10.8 | 9.9 | 8.0 |
| Medical oncology | 185 | 5 | 15 | 205 | 3.7 | 1.7 | 2.9 | 3.5 |
| Mental illness | 1,907 | 81 | 242 | 2,229 | 37.8 | 27.3 | 47.4 | 38.1 |
| Nephrology | 311 | 6 | 46 | 363 | 6.2 | 2.0 | 9.0 | 6.2 |
| Neurology | 436 | 13 | 43 | 492 | 8.6 | 4.4 | 8.4 | 8.4 |
| Neurosurgery | 179 | 8 | 21 | 208 | 3.5 | 2.7 | 4.1 | 3.6 |
| Nuclear medicine | 38 | 0 | 6 | 44 | 0.8 | 0.0 | 1.1 | 0.7 |
| Obstetrics and gynaecology | 1,370 | 82 | 153 | 1,605 | 27.1 | 27.9 | 30.0 | 27.4 |
| Occupational health | 78 | 6 | 20 | 104 | 1.5 | 2.1 | 3.8 | 1.8 |
| Old age psychiatry | 468 | 29 | 62 | 559 | 9.3 | 9.9 | 12.1 | 9.5 |
| Ophthalmology | 766 | 49 | 81 | 896 | 15.2 | 16.6 | 15.8 | 15.3 |
| Other | 107 | 3 | - | 110 | 2.1 | 0.9 | - | 1.9 |
| Otolaryngology | 514 | 35 | 67 | 617 | 10.2 | 12.0 | 13.2 | 10.5 |
| Paediatrics | 1,828 | 106 | 127 | 2,061 | 36.2 | 35.8 | 25.0 | 35.2 |
| Palliative medicine | 151 | 11 | 17 | 179 | 3.0 | 3.6 | 3.4 | 3.1 |
| Plastic surgery | 241 | 9 | 26 | 277 | 4.8 | 3.2 | 5.1 | 4.7 |
| Psychotherapy | 97 | 1 | 15 | 113 | 1.9 | 0.3 | 3.0 | 1.9 |
| Public Health Medicine | 732 | - | 99 | 831 | 14.5 | - | 19.5 | 14.2 |
| Radiology | 1,892 | 108 | 211 | 2,211 | 37.5 | 36.5 | 41.4 | 37.8 |
| Radiotherapy (clinical oncology) | 407 | 27 | 46 | 480 | 8.1 | 9.1 | 9.1 | 8.2 |
| Rehabilitation | 101 | 5 | 21 | 127 | 2.0 | 1.7 | 4.1 | 2.2 |
| Rheumatology | 452 | 19 | 38 | 509 | 9.0 | 6.4 | 7.5 | 8.7 |
| Thoracic medicine | 556 | 23 | 64 | 643 | 11.0 | 7.8 | 12.6 | 11.0 |
| Traumatic and orthopaedic surgery | 1,544 | 86 | 154 | 1,784 | 30.6 | 29.1 | 30.2 | 30.5 |
| Urology | 488 | 25 | 50 | 563 | 9.7 | 8.5 | 9.7 | 9.6 |

*Notes:*   All figures relate to full-time equivalents, and include principals in general practice who are working in hospitals, or medical and dental officers to whom paragraph 94 and 106-107 of the Terms and Conditions of Service apply.
Anaesthetics for England include intensive care.
Due to differences in definitions, figures may not be comparable across countries.

*Sources:*   Health and Personal Social Services Statistics for England (DH).
NHS Hospital, Public Health Medicine and Community Health Service Medical and Dental Workforce Census (IC).
Health Statistics Wales (NAW).
Scottish Health Statistics (ISD).
Population Projections Database (GAD).

Table 3.13 **Average daily number of available NHS hospital beds, UK, 1951 - 2005/06**

| Year | Available beds '000s | | | | Per 1,000 population | | | |
|------|---------------------|---------|---------------------|-------------------|---------------------|---------|---------------------|-------------------|
| | England and Wales[1] | Scotland[2] | Northern Ireland[3] | United Kingdom | England and Wales[1] | Scotland[2] | Northern Ireland[3] | United Kingdom |
| 1951 | 467 | 61 | 15 | 543 | 10.7 | 12.0 | 10.9 | 10.8 |
| 1955 | 482 | 63 | 16 | 561 | 10.8 | 12.3 | 11.5 | 11.0 |
| 1960 | 479 | 64 | 17 | 560 | 10.5 | 12.4 | 12.0 | 10.7 |
| 1961 | 478 | 64 | 17 | 559 | 10.3 | 12.3 | 11.9 | 10.6 |
| 1962 | 474 | 63 | 16 | 553 | 10.2 | 12.1 | 11.1 | 10.4 |
| 1963 | 472 | 63 | 16 | 551 | 10.1 | 12.1 | 11.1 | 10.3 |
| 1964 | 472 | 64 | 17 | 553 | 10.0 | 12.3 | 11.7 | 10.2 |
| 1965 | 470 | 64 | 17 | 551 | 9.9 | 12.3 | 11.6 | 10.1 |
| 1966 | 468 | 63 | 17 | 548 | 9.8 | 12.1 | 11.5 | 10.0 |
| 1967 | 467 | 64 | 17 | 548 | 9.7 | 12.3 | 11.4 | 10.0 |
| 1968 | 465 | 63 | 17 | 545 | 9.6 | 12.1 | 11.3 | 9.9 |
| 1969 | 461 | 63 | 17 | 541 | 9.5 | 12.1 | 11.2 | 9.8 |
| 1970 | 456 | 63 | 17 | 536 | 9.3 | 12.1 | 11.1 | 9.6 |
| 1971 | 450 | 63 | 17 | 530 | 9.2 | 12.0 | 11.0 | 9.5 |
| 1972 | 443 | 63 | 18 | 524 | 9.0 | 12.0 | 11.7 | 9.3 |
| 1973 | 437 | 62 | 18 | 517 | 8.8 | 11.8 | 11.8 | 9.2 |
| 1974 | 427 | 62 | 18 | 507 | 8.6 | 11.8 | 11.8 | 9.0 |
| 1975 | 419 | 61 | 17 | 497 | 8.5 | 11.7 | 11.2 | 8.8 |
| 1976 | 412 | 60 | 17 | 489 | 8.3 | 11.5 | 11.2 | 8.7 |
| 1977 | 404 | 59 | 17 | 480 | 8.2 | 11.3 | 11.2 | 8.5 |
| 1978 | 395 | 59 | 17 | 471 | 8.0 | 11.3 | 11.2 | 8.4 |
| 1979 | 388 | 58 | 17 | 463 | 7.8 | 11.1 | 11.1 | 8.2 |
| 1980 | 383 | 58 | 17 | 458 | 7.7 | 11.2 | 11.1 | 8.1 |
| 1981 | 380 | 58 | 17 | 455 | 7.7 | 11.2 | 11.1 | 8.1 |
| 1982 | 378 | 58 | 17 | 453 | 7.6 | 11.2 | 11.0 | 8.0 |
| 1983 | 372 | 57 | 17 | 446 | 7.5 | 11.1 | 11.0 | 7.9 |
| 1984 | 357 | 57 | 17 | 431 | 7.2 | 11.1 | 10.9 | 7.6 |
| 1985 | 348 | 57 | 17 | 422 | 7.0 | 11.1 | 10.9 | 7.5 |
| 1986 | 338 | 55 | 16 | 409 | 6.8 | 10.8 | 10.2 | 7.2 |
| 1987/88 | 318 | 55 | 15 | 388 | 6.3 | 10.7 | 9.7 | 6.8 |
| 1988/89 | 304 | 53 | 15 | 372 | 6.0 | 10.5 | 9.3 | 6.5 |
| 1989/90 | 290 | 52 | 14 | 356 | 5.7 | 10.3 | 8.9 | 6.2 |
| 1990/91 | 274 | 51 | 13 | 338 | 5.4 | 10.0 | 8.4 | 5.9 |
| 1991/92 | 262 | 49 | 13 | 323 | 5.2 | 9.6 | 7.8 | 5.6 |
| 1992/93 | 250 | 47 | 12 | 308 | 4.9 | 9.2 | 7.2 | 5.4 |
| 1993/94 | 236 | 44 | 11 | 292 | 4.6 | 8.7 | 6.7 | 5.0 |
| 1994/95 | 229 | 42 | 10 | 282 | 4.5 | 8.3 | 6.3 | 4.9 |
| 1995/96 | 222 | 41 | 10 | 273 | 4.3 | 8.0 | 6.1 | 4.7 |
| 1996/97 | 215 | 38 | 9 | 262 | 4.2 | 7.5 | 5.7 | 4.5 |
| 1997/98 | 209 | 38 | 9 | 256 | 4.1 | 7.5 | 5.4 | 4.4 |
| 1998/99 | 205 | 36 | 9 | 250 | 4.0 | 7.2 | 5.3 | 4.3 |
| 1999/00 | 201 | 35 | 9 | 244 | 3.9 | 6.8 | 5.1 | 4.2 |
| 2000/01 | 201 | 33 | 9 | 242 | 3.8 | 6.5 | 5.1 | 4.1 |
| 2001/02 | 199 | 32 | 8 | 240 | 3.8 | 6.3 | 5.0 | 4.1 |
| 2002/03 | 198 | 31 | 8 | 237 | 3.8 | 6.1 | 4.9 | 4.0 |
| 2003/04 | 198 | 30 | 8 | 236 | 3.7 | 5.9 | 4.9 | 4.0 |
| 2004/05 | 196 | 29 | 8 | 233 | 3.7 | 5.7 | 4.9 | 3.9 |
| 2005/06 | 189 | 28 | 8 | 226 | 3.5 | 5.5 | 4.8 | 3.7 |

*Notes:* From 1987/88 onwards, all figures relate to financial years ending 31 March. Before that, all figures are for calendar years.

1 Figures for England relate to average number of open and staffed beds on wards open overnight in NHS hospitals. Figures for Wales relate to average daily number of staffed beds.

2 Figures relate to average available staffed beds including temporary and borrowed beds. Figures exclude NHS beds in joint-user and contractual hospitals. From 1968 to 1986, figures relate to 30 September.

3 Figures relate to average available beds in wards open overnight during year. From 1974 to 1986, figures relate to 31 December.

*Sources:* Health and Personal Social Services Statistics for England (DH).
Health Statistics Wales (NAW).
Scottish Health Statistics (ISD).
Annual Abstract of Statistics (ONS).
Hospital Activity Statistics: England (DH).
Population Projections Database (GAD).

Table 3.14   **Average daily available acute beds in NHS hospitals, Great Britain, 1959 - 2005/06**

Thousands

| Year | Acute total | Mental illness | Learning disabilities | Geriatrics | All beds[1] | Per 10,000 population | |
|---|---|---|---|---|---|---|---|
| | | | | | | Total acute | All beds |
| 1959 | 183 | 178 | 64 | 62 | 546 | 36.2 | 108.0 |
| 1960 | 182 | 175 | 66 | 63 | 543 | 35.7 | 106.6 |
| 1965 | 177 | 164 | 69 | 65 | 534 | 33.5 | 101.0 |
| 1966 | 176 | 162 | 68 | 65 | 531 | 33.1 | 99.9 |
| 1967 | 175 | 160 | 69 | 66 | 531 | 32.7 | 99.3 |
| 1968 | 174 | 157 | 69 | 67 | 528 | 32.4 | 98.3 |
| 1969 | 172 | 154 | 69 | 68 | 524 | 31.9 | 97.1 |
| 1970 | 171 | 151 | 69 | 69 | 519 | 31.6 | 95.9 |
| 1971 | 180 | 146 | 68 | 70 | 513 | 33.1 | 94.3 |
| 1972 | 176 | 141 | 67 | 70 | 506 | 32.3 | 92.7 |
| 1973 | 170 | 135 | 66 | 70 | 499 | 31.1 | 91.2 |
| 1974 | 169 | 130 | 65 | 69 | 489 | 30.9 | 89.4 |
| 1975 | 165 | 124 | 64 | 70 | 480 | 30.2 | 87.7 |
| 1976 | 168 | 121 | 63 | 70 | 472 | 30.7 | 86.3 |
| 1977 | 164 | 117 | 62 | 71 | 463 | 30.0 | 84.7 |
| 1978 | 163 | 112 | 60 | 72 | 454 | 29.8 | 83.1 |
| 1979 | 157 | 111 | 59 | 71 | 446 | 28.7 | 81.5 |
| 1980 | 158 | 110 | 58 | 71 | 441 | 28.8 | 80.5 |
| 1981 | 153 | 107 | 57 | 71 | 438 | 27.9 | 79.9 |
| 1982 | 151 | 106 | 56 | 72 | 436 | 27.6 | 79.6 |
| 1983 | 167 | 104 | 55 | 72 | 429 | 30.5 | 78.3 |
| 1984 | 162 | 100 | 53 | 72 | 414 | 29.5 | 75.5 |
| 1985 | 160 | 97 | 50 | 72 | 405 | 29.1 | 73.7 |
| 1986 | 157 | 93 | 47 | 71 | 394 | 28.5 | 71.5 |
| 1987/88 | 153 | 87 | 41 | 71 | 373 | 27.7 | 67.5 |
| 1988/89 | 147 | 82 | 37 | 67 | 357 | 26.5 | 64.5 |
| 1989/90 | 146 | 78 | 33 | 65 | 342 | 26.3 | 61.6 |
| 1990/91 | 142 | 73 | 29 | 61 | 325 | 25.5 | 58.4 |
| 1991/92 | 139 | 50 | 21 | 57 | 310 | 24.9 | 55.5 |
| 1992/93 | 137 | 47 | 18 | 55 | 297 | 24.5 | 53.0 |
| 1993/94 | 130 | 53 | 22 | 51 | 281 | 23.2 | 50.1 |
| 1994/95 | 129 | 50 | 18 | 50 | 271 | 22.9 | 48.2 |
| 1995/96 | 129 | 53 | 17 | 48 | 264 | 22.8 | 46.8 |
| 1996/97 | 129 | 50 | 14 | 44 | 254 | 22.8 | 45.0 |
| 1997/98 | 129 | 48 | 12 | 42 | 247 | 22.7 | 43.6 |
| 1998/99 | 129 | 47 | 11 | 39 | 241 | 22.7 | 42.4 |
| 1999/00 | 128 | 45 | 9 | 38 | 236 | 22.5 | 41.3 |
| 2000/01 | 129 | 44 | 9 | 37 | 234 | 22.5 | 40.8 |
| 2001/02 | 129 | 43 | 7 | 37 | 231 | 22.5 | 40.2 |
| 2002/03 | 130 | 42 | 6 | 37 | 229 | 22.5 | 39.7 |
| 2003/04 | 131 | 42 | 6 | 36 | 228 | 22.5 | 39.4 |
| 2004/05 | 130 | 40 | 5 | 35 | 224 | 22.4 | 38.5 |
| 2005/06 | 129 | 38 | 5 | 33 | 218 | 22.0 | 37.2 |

*Notes:*   In this table figures have been added together which are not based on precisely the same basis in definition or timing. The differences do not affect the broad picture of the health services for Great Britain.
From 1987/88 onwards, all figures relate to financial years ending 31 March.  Prior to 1987/88, all figures are for calendar years.
1 Figures include obstetrics and other departments not shown in the table.

*Sources:*   Health and Personal Social Services Statistics for England (DH).
Health Statistics Wales (NAW).
Scottish Health Statistics (ISD).
Hospital Activity Statistics: England (DH).
Population Projections Database (GAD).

Table 3.15   **Average daily available NHS beds: number, per 100,000 population and occupancy, England, 1996/97 - 2006/07**

| | Year | | | | | | | | |
|---|---|---|---|---|---|---|---|---|---|
| | 1996/97 | 1999/00 | 2000/01 | 2001/02 | 2002/03 | 2003/04 | 2004/05 | 2005/06 | 2006/07 |
| **Number of available beds** | | | | | | | | | |
| A  Intensive care | 4,185 | 4,347 | 4,507 | 4,939 | 5,021 | 5,013 | 5,223 | 5,463 | 5,615 |
| B  Terminally ill/palliative care | 493 | 457 | 509 | 440 | 478 | 386 | 436 | 427 | 395 |
| C  Younger physically disabled | 1,296 | 1,176 | 1,163 | 1,043 | 1,013 | 914 | 859 | 792 | 566 |
| D  Other general and acute: Elderly | 31,647 | 27,862 | 27,839 | 28,047 | 27,973 | 27,431 | 26,619 | 24,920 | 22,897 |
| E  Other general and acute: Other | 102,895 | 101,237 | 101,776 | 102,115 | 102,193 | 103,534 | 102,986 | 101,432 | 97,503 |
| F  Maternity (inc GP, consultant and mixed) | 11,000 | 10,203 | 9,767 | 9,812 | 9,356 | 9,309 | 9,081 | 8,883 | 8,643 |
| G  Mental illness (excluding residential care) | 37,640 | 34,172 | 34,214 | 32,783 | 32,752 | 32,410 | 31,286 | 29,803 | 27,915 |
| H  Patients with learning disabilities | 9,693 | 6,834 | 6,316 | 5,695 | 5,037 | 5,211 | 4,416 | 3,926 | 3,487 |
| Acute (A+B+C+E) | 108,869 | 107,217 | 107,955 | 108,537 | 108,705 | 109,847 | 109,504 | 108,114 | 104,079 |
| General and Acute (A+B+C+D+E) | 140,516 | 135,079 | 135,794 | 136,584 | 136,678 | 137,278 | 136,123 | 133,034 | 126,976 |
| **Available beds per 100,000 population** | | | | | | | | | |
| A  Intensive care | 8.6 | 8.9 | 9.1 | 10.0 | 10.1 | 10.0 | 10.4 | 10.8 | 11.0 |
| B  Terminally ill/palliative care | 1.0 | 0.9 | 1.0 | 0.9 | 1.0 | 0.8 | 0.9 | 0.8 | 0.8 |
| C  Younger physically disabled | 2.7 | 2.4 | 2.4 | 2.1 | 2.0 | 1.8 | 1.7 | 1.6 | 1.1 |
| D  Other general and acute: Elderly[1] | 409.0 | 358.8 | 357.1 | 357.3 | 354.0 | 344.9 | 332.4 | 309.2 | 282.6 |
| E  Other general and acute: Other | 211.3 | 206.3 | 206.5 | 206.3 | 205.6 | 207.4 | 205.2 | 200.7 | 191.8 |
| F  Maternity (inc GP, consultant and mixed)[2] | 108.3 | 99.9 | 95.2 | 95.2 | 90.5 | 89.7 | 87.0 | 84.5 | 82.0 |
| G  Mental illness (excluding residential care) | 77.3 | 69.6 | 69.4 | 66.2 | 65.9 | 64.9 | 62.3 | 59.0 | 54.9 |
| H  Patients with learning disabilities | 19.9 | 13.9 | 12.8 | 11.5 | 10.1 | 10.4 | 8.8 | 7.8 | 6.9 |
| Acute (A+B+C+E) | 223.53 | 218.4 | 219.0 | 219.3 | 218.7 | 220.0 | 218.1 | 213.9 | 204.7 |
| General and Acute (A+B+C+D+E) | 288.51 | 275.2 | 275.5 | 275.9 | 275.0 | 275.0 | 271.2 | 263.2 | 249.7 |
| **Percentage occupancy** | | | | | | | | | |
| A  Intensive care | 72% | 74% | 75% | 75% | 75% | 77% | 78% | 76% | 78% |
| B  Terminally ill/palliative care | 77% | 75% | 77% | 80% | 80% | 78% | 78% | 75% | 78% |
| C  Younger physically disabled | 77% | 76% | 74% | 77% | 77% | 81% | 81% | 82% | 79% |
| D  Other general and acute: Elderly | 87% | 89% | 91% | 92% | 91% | 92% | 91% | 91% | 91% |
| E  Other general and acute: Other | 79% | 82% | 84% | 85% | 86% | 86% | 85% | 85% | 84% |
| F  Maternity (inc GP, consultant and mixed) | 63% | 61% | 60% | 60% | 61% | 63% | 63% | 65% | 64% |
| G  Mental illness (excluding residential care) | 87% | 87% | 87% | 89% | 87% | 88% | 88% | 86% | 87% |
| H  Patients with learning disabilities | 88% | 85% | 87% | 87% | 86% | 84% | 85% | 84% | 85% |
| Acute (A+B+C+E) | 79% | 82% | 83% | 84% | 85% | 86% | 85% | 84% | 84% |
| General and Acute (A+B+C+D+E) | 81% | 83% | 85% | 86% | 87% | 86% | 86% | 86% | 85% |

*Notes:*   1 Per 100,000 population aged 65 or over.
2 Per female population aged 15 - 44.

*Sources:*  Hospital Activity Statistics: England (DH).
Population Projections Database (GAD).
Population estimates (ONS).

Table 3.16    **Average daily occupied beds[1] in NHS hospitals, by country, UK, 1951 - 2005/06**

| Year | Average daily occupied beds[1] '000s | | | | | Bed occupancy rate as % of available beds[1] | | | | |
|---|---|---|---|---|---|---|---|---|---|---|
| | England[2] | Wales | Scotland | Northern Ireland | United Kingdom | England[2] | Wales | Scotland | Northern Ireland | United Kingdom |
| 1951 | 407.0 | - | 52.0 | 13.0 | 472.0 | 87 | - | 86 | 89 | 87 |
| 1955 | 426.0 | - | 55.0 | 15.0 | 496.0 | 88 | - | 88 | 92 | 88 |
| 1956 | 424.0 | - | 54.0 | 15.0 | 493.0 | 88 | - | 86 | 91 | 88 |
| 1957 | 420.0 | - | 55.0 | 15.0 | 489.0 | 87 | - | 85 | 90 | 87 |
| 1958 | 418.0 | - | 54.0 | 15.0 | 487.0 | 87 | - | 85 | 90 | 86 |
| 1959 | 413.0 | - | 53.0 | 14.0 | 480.0 | 86 | - | 83 | 84 | 85 |
| 1960 | 410.0 | - | 53.0 | 15.0 | 478.0 | 86 | - | 83 | 88 | 85 |
| 1961 | 404.0 | - | 53.0 | 15.0 | 471.0 | 85 | - | 83 | 89 | 84 |
| 1962 | 403.0 | - | 54.0 | 14.0 | 471.0 | 85 | - | 84 | 88 | 85 |
| 1963 | 404.0 | - | 53.0 | 15.0 | 472.0 | 86 | - | 84 | 89 | 86 |
| 1964 | 400.0 | - | 53.0 | 15.0 | 468.0 | 85 | - | 84 | 86 | 85 |
| 1965 | 397.0 | - | 54.0 | 15.0 | 466.0 | 84 | - | 85 | 88 | 85 |
| 1966 | 393.0 | - | 54.0 | 15.0 | 462.0 | 84 | - | 85 | 88 | 84 |
| 1967 | 390.0 | - | 54.0 | 15.0 | 459.0 | 84 | - | 84 | 88 | 84 |
| 1968 | 385.0 | - | 54.0 | 15.0 | 454.0 | 83 | - | 85 | 86 | 83 |
| 1969 | 380.0 | - | 55.0 | 15.0 | 450.0 | 82 | - | 88 | 87 | 83 |
| 1970 | 372.0 | - | 54.0 | 15.0 | 441.0 | 82 | - | 85 | 87 | 82 |
| 1971 | 368.0 | - | 53.0 | 14.0 | 436.0 | 82 | - | 85 | 83 | 82 |
| 1972 | 362.0 | - | 53.0 | 15.0 | 429.0 | 82 | - | 84 | 81 | 82 |
| 1973 | 348.0 | - | 52.0 | 14.0 | 414.0 | 80 | - | 83 | 80 | 80 |
| 1974 | 341.0 | - | 52.0 | 14.0 | 407.0 | 80 | - | 84 | 80 | 80 |
| 1975 | 332.0 | - | 51.0 | 14.0 | 396.0 | 79 | - | 83 | 80 | 80 |
| 1976 | 330.0 | - | 50.0 | 14.0 | 394.0 | 80 | - | 84 | 81 | 81 |
| 1977 | 325.0 | - | 50.0 | 14.0 | 389.0 | 80 | - | 84 | 80 | 81 |
| 1978 | 318.0 | - | 50.0 | 14.0 | 381.0 | 81 | - | 84 | 80 | 81 |
| 1979 | 311.0 | - | 49.0 | 14.0 | 373.0 | 80 | - | 84 | 80 | 81 |
| 1980 | 307.0 | - | 48.0 | 14.0 | 369.0 | 80 | - | 84 | 80 | 81 |
| 1981 | 304.0 | - | 48.0 | 13.0 | 365.0 | 80 | - | 83 | 78 | 80 |
| 1982 | 298.0 | - | 48.0 | 13.0 | 359.0 | 79 | - | 83 | 78 | 79 |
| 1983 | 294.0 | - | 47.0 | 13.0 | 354.0 | 79 | - | 82 | 78 | 79 |
| 1984 | 287.0 | - | 47.0 | 13.0 | 347.0 | 80 | - | 82 | 78 | 81 |
| 1985 | 281.0 | - | 46.0 | 13.0 | 340.0 | 81 | - | 82 | 79 | 81 |
| 1986 | 272.0 | - | 45.0 | 12.0 | 329.0 | 80 | - | 82 | 78 | 81 |
| 1987/88 | 260.0 | - | 44.0 | 12.0 | 316.0 | 82 | - | 81 | 79 | 82 |
| 1988/89 | 263.0 | - | 44.0 | 12.0 | 319.0 | 86 | - | 81 | 80 | 86 |
| 1989/90 | 231.8 | 15.2 | 43.0 | 11.0 | 301.0 | 85 | 77 | 81 | 79 | 85 |
| 1990/91 | 232.2 | 14.8 | 41.0 | 10.0 | 280.0 | 83 | 76 | 82 | 78 | 83 |
| 1991/92 | 232.7 | 14.3 | 40.0 | 10.0 | 264.0 | 82 | 77 | 81 | 77 | 82 |
| 1992/93 | 233.2 | 13.8 | 38.0 | 9.0 | 250.0 | 81 | 76 | 81 | 78 | 81 |
| 1993/94 | 178.0 | 13.5 | 37.0 | 8.0 | 236.5 | 81 | 77 | 84 | 73 | 81 |
| 1994/95 | 172.5 | 12.9 | 34.0 | 8.0 | 227.4 | 81 | 77 | 80 | 77 | 81 |
| 1995/96 | 167.2 | 12.4 | 33.9 | 7.8 | 221.2 | 81 | 78 | 83 | 78 | 81 |
| 1996/97 | 162.0 | 12.2 | 32.0 | 7.5 | 213.7 | 81 | 78 | 83 | 79 | 81 |
| 1997/98 | 157.0 | 12.0 | 30.6 | 7.3 | 206.9 | 81 | 79 | 81 | 81 | 81 |
| 1998/99 | 156.7 | 11.8 | 29.3 | 7.2 | 205.0 | 82 | 79 | 81 | 82 | 82 |
| 1999/00 | 154.1 | 11.8 | 28.0 | 7.0 | 201.0 | 83 | 82 | 81 | 82 | 82 |
| 2000/01 | 156.3 | 11.7 | 26.8 | 7.0 | 201.8 | 84 | 80 | 81 | 82 | 83 |
| 2001/02 | 157.3 | 11.7 | 26.0 | 7.0 | 202.0 | 85 | 81 | 81 | 83 | 84 |
| 2002/03 | 156.9 | 11.8 | 25.1 | 7.0 | 200.8 | 85 | 83 | 82 | 84 | 85 |
| 2003/04 | 157.9 | 11.8 | 24.0 | 7.0 | 200.7 | 86 | 83 | 80 | 84 | 85 |
| 2004/05 | 154.8 | 11.6 | 23.3 | 7.0 | 196.7 | 85 | 83 | 80 | 84 | 84 |
| 2005/06 | 148.6 | 11.4 | 22.8 | 6.9 | 189.8 | 85 | 83 | 81 | 84 | 84 |

*Notes:*    From 1987/88 onwards, all figures relate to financial years ending 31 March.  Before that, all figures are for calendar years.
1 Figures include all NHS hospital trusts in England, Wales and Scotland, figures include NHS beds in joint-user and contractual hospitals.
2 Prior to 1989/90 data for England and Wales combined.

*Sources:*    Annual Abstract of Statistics (ONS).
Health Statistics Wales (NAW).
Scottish Health Statistics (ISD).
Hospital Activity Statistics: England (DH).

**Figure 3.7  Hospital inpatient acute beds per 1,000 population in selected OECD countries, circa 2005**

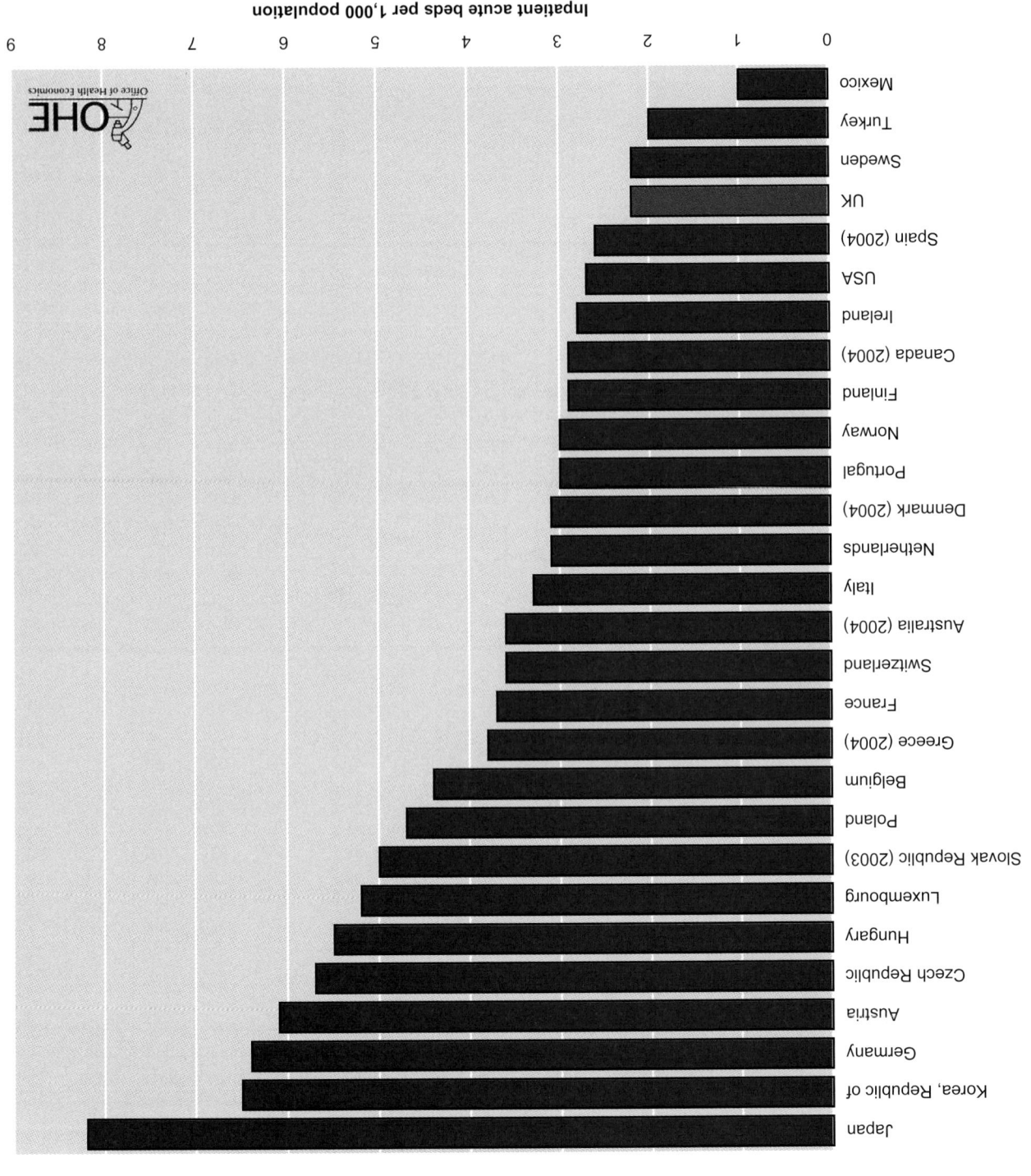

**Inpatient acute beds per 1,000 population**

*Notes:*    Year is 2005 unless stated otherwise.
Cross-country comparison should be carried out with caution as figures may be based on different definitions.
*Sources:*    OECD Health Database (OECD).
Health and Personal Social Services Statistics for England (DH).
Health Statistics Wales (NAW).
Scottish Health Statistics (ISD).
Hospital Activity Statistics: England (DH).
Hospital Statistics for Northern Ireland (DHSSPS).

Table 3.17   **Number of NHS hospital finished consultant episodes (FCEs) [1]/discharges and deaths, UK, 1951 - 2005/06**

| Year | FCEs/discharges and deaths '000s | | | | | FCEs/discharges and deaths per available bed [1] | | | | |
|------|----------------------|-------|----------|---------------------|-------------------|----------------------|-------|----------|---------------------|-------------------|
|      | England[2] | Wales | Scotland | Northern Ireland | United Kingdom | England[2] | Wales | Scotland | Northern Ireland | United Kingdom |
| 1951 | 3,259 | - | 443 | 104 | 3,806 | 7.0 | - | 7.3 | 7.2 | 7.2 |
| 1955 | 3,652 | - | 494 | 128 | 4,274 | 7.6 | - | 7.8 | 8.1 | 7.6 |
| 1960 | 4,136 | - | 571 | 145 | 4,852 | 8.6 | - | 9.0 | 8.7 | 8.7 |
| 1965 | 4,818 | - | 637 | 189 | 5,644 | 10.3 | - | 10.0 | 11.0 | 10.2 |
| 1966 | 4,898 | - | 637 | 197 | 5,732 | 10.5 | - | 10.1 | 11.5 | 10.5 |
| 1967 | 5,012 | - | 657 | 203 | 5,872 | 10.7 | - | 10.3 | 11.8 | 10.7 |
| 1968 | 5,150 | - | 679 | 208 | 6,037 | 11.1 | - | 10.7 | 11.9 | 11.1 |
| 1969 | 5,282 | - | 693 | 213 | 6,188 | 11.5 | - | 11.0 | 12.2 | 11.4 |
| 1970 | 5,329 | - | 699 | 218 | 6,246 | 11.7 | - | 11.1 | 12.6 | 11.6 |
| 1971 | 5,494 | - | 728 | 219 | 6,441 | 12.2 | - | 11.6 | 12.6 | 12.1 |
| 1972 | 5,550 | - | 727 | 232 | 6,509 | 12.5 | - | 11.6 | 13.0 | 12.4 |
| 1973 | 5,452 | - | 706 | 227 | 6,385 | 12.5 | - | 11.4 | 12.7 | 12.4 |
| 1974 | 5,501 | - | 718 | 224 | 6,443 | 12.9 | - | 11.7 | 12.8 | 12.7 |
| 1975 | 5,296 | - | 697 | 220 | 6,213 | 12.6 | - | 11.5 | 12.7 | 12.5 |
| 1976 | 5,593 | - | 743 | 231 | 6,567 | 13.6 | - | 12.5 | 13.5 | 13.4 |
| 1977 | 5,688 | - | 737 | 231 | 6,656 | 14.1 | - | 12.5 | 13.4 | 13.9 |
| 1978 | 5,700 | - | 749 | 237 | 6,686 | 14.4 | - | 12.7 | 13.9 | 14.2 |
| 1979 | 5,750 | - | 738 | 241 | 6,729 | 14.8 | - | 12.7 | 14.1 | 14.5 |
| 1980 | 6,036 | - | 774 | 246 | 7,056 | 15.8 | - | 13.4 | 14.4 | 15.4 |
| 1981 | 6,135 | - | 793 | 249 | 7,177 | 16.1 | - | 13.7 | 14.6 | 15.8 |
| 1982 | 6,090 | - | 794 | 249 | 7,133 | 16.1 | - | 13.8 | 14.6 | 15.8 |
| 1983 | 6,412 | - | 791 | 258 | 7,461 | 17.2 | - | 13.8 | 15.2 | 16.7 |
| 1984 | 6,591 | - | 810 | 261 | 7,662 | 18.5 | - | 14.1 | 15.6 | 17.8 |
| 1985 | 6,780 | - | 822 | 274 | 7,876 | 19.5 | - | 14.5 | 16.5 | 18.7 |
| 1986 | 6,848 | - | 837 | 269 | 7,954 | 20.3 | - | 14.9 | 16.8 | 19.4 |
| 1987/88 | 7,500 | 526 | 1,032 | 295 | 9,353 | 25.3 | 25.0 | 18.9 | 19.2 | 24.1 |
| 1988/89 | 8,351 | 543 | 1,058 | 309 | 10,261 | 29.5 | 26.2 | 19.8 | 21.0 | 27.6 |
| 1989/90 | 8,637 | 556 | 1,082 | 316 | 10,591 | 32.0 | 28.0 | 20.8 | 22.4 | 29.7 |
| 1990/91 | 8,782 | 584 | 1,116 | 324 | 10,806 | 34.4 | 30.1 | 22.1 | 24.0 | 31.9 |
| 1991/92 | 9,302 | 633 | 1,150 | 339 | 11,424 | 38.4 | 34.0 | 23.6 | 26.9 | 35.5 |
| 1992/93 | 9,635 | 668 | 1,184 | 343 | 11,831 | 41.5 | 37.0 | 25.4 | 29.3 | 38.4 |
| 1993/94 | 10,094 | 710 | 1,237 | 369 | 12,410 | 46.1 | 40.6 | 28.0 | 33.9 | 42.6 |
| 1994/95 | 10,539 | 753 | 1,287 | 389 | 12,968 | 49.7 | 44.8 | 30.3 | 37.6 | 46.1 |
| 1995/96 | 11,037 | 778 | 1,324 | 400 | 13,539 | 53.6 | 48.7 | 32.6 | 39.8 | 49.7 |
| 1996/97 | 11,275 | 690 | 1,349 | 398 | 13,712 | 56.7 | 44.3 | 35.1 | 42.0 | 52.2 |
| 1997/98 | 11,530 | 643 | 1,393 | 410 | 13,975 | 59.4 | 42.3 | 36.7 | 45.5 | 54.5 |
| 1998/99 | 11,984 | 649 | 1,415 | 449 | 14,497 | 63.1 | 43.6 | 38.9 | 50.9 | 58.0 |
| 1999/00 | 12,197 | 639 | 1,399 | 452 | 14,687 | 65.5 | 44.3 | 40.3 | 52.3 | 60.2 |
| 2000/01 | 12,265 | 711 | 1,403 | 456 | 14,835 | 65.9 | 48.8 | 42.3 | 53.2 | 61.2 |
| 2001/02 | 12,357 | 701 | 1,374 | 458 | 14,891 | 66.8 | 48.6 | 43.0 | 54.4 | 62.1 |
| 2002/03 | 12,756 | 671 | 1,325 | 465 | 15,217 | 69.4 | 47.0 | 43.0 | 56.1 | 64.2 |
| 2003/04 | 13,174 | 702 | 1,359 | 482 | 15,718 | 71.6 | 49.4 | 45.5 | 57.7 | 66.5 |
| 2004/05 | 13,707 | 709 | 1,379 | 490 | 16,284 | 75.4 | 50.6 | 47.4 | 58.9 | 69.8 |
| 2005/06 | 14,424 | 722 | 1,438 | 500 | 17,084 | 82.1 | 52.3 | 50.8 | 60.7 | 75.6 |

*Notes:*   From 1987/88 onwards, all figures relate to financial years ending 31 March.  Before that, all figures are for calendar years.
Figures include inpatients and day cases.
Data for Wales are based on discharges and deaths.
Data from 1996 onwards for Northern Ireland is based on admissions data.
Data for Scotland and Northern Ireland are based on a system where transfers between consultants don't count as discharges, except in Scotland where figures include patients transferred from one consultant to another within the same hospital, provided there is a change of specialty or significant facilities.
Scotland, figures include NHS beds in joint-user and contractual hospitals.
1 In England, figures from 1987/88 relate to finished consultant episodes (FCEs) in all NHS hospital trusts.  FCE data for England for 2004/05 and 2005/06 have not been adjusted to take into account shortfalls in the number of records received or for missing/invalid clinical data.
2 From 1951 - 1986 figures are for England and Wales.

*Sources:* Annual Abstract of Statistics (ONS).
The Government's Expenditure Plans (DH).
Health Statistics Wales (NAW).
Scottish Health Statistics (ISD).
Hospital Episode Statistics (IC).

Table 3.18    **Inpatient finished consultant episodes (FCEs), discharges and deaths [1] in NHS hospitals, by selected specialties, Great Britain, 1959 - 2005/06**

Thousands

| Year | Acute services | | | Mental illness | Learning disabilities | Geriatrics | All FCEs[3] | FCEs per 10,000 population | |
|---|---|---|---|---|---|---|---|---|---|
| | Medical | Surgical | Total[2] | | | | | Total acute | All FCEs |
| 1959 | 987 | 2,175 | 3,162 | 160 | 7 | 145 | 4,558 | 63 | 90 |
| 1960 | 1,021 | 2,249 | 3,270 | 165 | 9 | 151 | 4,707 | 64 | 92 |
| 1965 | 1,160 | 2,591 | 3,751 | 192 | 12 | 173 | 5,455 | 71 | 103 |
| 1966 | 1,184 | 2,609 | 3,793 | 196 | 13 | 181 | 5,535 | 71 | 104 |
| 1967 | 1,202 | 2,684 | 3,886 | 200 | 12 | 180 | 5,669 | 73 | 106 |
| 1968 | 1,243 | 2,753 | 3,996 | 207 | 14 | 194 | 5,829 | 74 | 109 |
| 1969 | 1,290 | 2,816 | 4,106 | 213 | 14 | 195 | 5,975 | 76 | 111 |
| 1970 | 1,314 | 2,917 | 4,231 | 212 | 15 | 201 | 6,028 | 78 | 111 |
| 1971 | 1,332 | 3,030 | 4,362 | 213 | 17 | 203 | 6,222 | 80 | 114 |
| 1972 | 1,394 | 3,062 | 4,456 | 218 | 18 | 218 | 6,277 | 82 | 115 |
| 1973 | 1,392 | 2,987 | 4,379 | 217 | 18 | 220 | 6,158 | 80 | 113 |
| 1974 | 1,425 | 3,042 | 4,467 | 213 | 18 | 223 | 6,219 | 82 | 114 |
| 1975 | 1,439 | 2,841 | 4,280 | 215 | 19 | 234 | 5,993 | 78 | 110 |
| 1976 | 1,476 | 3,050 | 4,526 | 219 | 19 | 259 | 6,336 | 83 | 116 |
| 1977 | 1,504 | 3,138 | 4,642 | 214 | 22 | 266 | 6,425 | 85 | 118 |
| 1978 | 1,531 | 3,109 | 4,640 | 210 | 23 | 281 | 6,449 | 85 | 118 |
| 1979 | 1,546 | 3,132 | 4,678 | 207 | 25 | 284 | 6,488 | 86 | 119 |
| 1980 | 1,620 | 3,304 | 4,923 | 220 | 29 | 311 | 6,810 | 90 | 124 |
| 1981 | 1,676 | 3,359 | 5,035 | 224 | 32 | 331 | 6,928 | 92 | 126 |
| 1982 | 1,718 | 3,232 | 4,951 | 221 | 34 | 350 | 6,884 | 90 | 126 |
| 1983 | 1,791 | 3,478 | 5,269 | 227 | 40 | 384 | 7,203 | 96 | 131 |
| 1984 | 1,846 | 3,551 | 5,396 | 233 | 46 | 414 | 7,401 | 98 | 135 |
| 1985 | 1,935 | 3,583 | 5,518 | 246 | 49 | 445 | 7,602 | 100 | 138 |
| 1986 | 1,952 | 3,609 | 5,561 | 247 | 54 | 474 | 7,685 | 101 | 139 |
| 1987/88 | 2,283 | 3,705 | 5,988 | 248 | 47 | 474 | 7,940 | 108 | 143 |
| 1988/89 | 2,906 | 3,735 | 6,641 | 256 | 50 | 489 | 8,677 | 120 | 156 |
| 1989/90 | 2,983 | 3,762 | 6,745 | 260 | 60 | 531 | 8,843 | 121 | 159 |
| 1990/91 | 3,047 | 3,736 | 6,783 | 265 | 60 | 553 | 8,913 | 121 | 159 |
| 1991/92 | 3,145 | 3,823 | 6,968 | 269 | 60 | 600 | 9,170 | 124 | 163 |
| 1992/93 | 3,216 | 3,809 | 7,025 | 282 | 61 | 624 | 9,273 | 125 | 164 |
| 1993/94 | 3,348 | 3,773 | 7,121 | 285 | 59 | 652 | 9,361 | 120 | 166 |
| 1994/95 | 3,588 | 3,797 | 7,385 | 284 | 64 | 698 | 9,449 | 116 | 167 |
| 1995/96 | 3,162 | 3,685 | 6,848 | 295 | 61 | 648 | 9,752 | 121 | 173 |
| 1996/97 | 3,303 | 3,575 | 6,877 | 290 | 61 | 640 | 9,854 | 122 | 174 |
| 1997/98 | 3,542 | 3,555 | 7,097 | 286 | 62 | 617 | 9,963 | 125 | 176 |
| 1998/99[4] | 4,023 | 3,875 | 7,898 | 264 | 43 | 629 | 10,067 | 139 | 177 |
| 1999/00 | 4,106 | 3,846 | 7,952 | 258 | 39 | 616 | 10,072 | 139 | 177 |
| 2000/01 | 4,222 | 3,790 | 8,013 | 252 | 40 | 601 | 10,119 | 140 | 177 |
| 2001/02 | 4,372 | 3,778 | 8,150 | 246 | 38 | 607 | 10,228 | 142 | 178 |
| 2002/03 | 4,505 | 3,834 | 8,339 | 243 | 40 | 631 | 10,476 | 145 | 182 |
| 2003/04 | 4,772 | 3,930 | 8,702 | 227 | 32 | 639 | 10,891 | 150 | 188 |
| 2004/05 | 4,964 | 4,094 | 9,059 | 223 | 28 | 674 | 11,337 | 156 | 195 |
| 2005/06 | 5,242 | 4,328 | 9,570 | 203 | 24 | 676 | 11,826 | 163 | 202 |

*Notes:*    In this table figures have been added together which are not all based on precisely the same definition or timing. The differences do not affect the broad picture of the health services in Great Britain.

Figures for England for 1987/88 onwards are FCEs.  Earlier English and all Scottish and Welsh figures are for discharges and deaths.

Figures for England from 1994/95, are based on all FCEs.  Figures for previous years are based on a 25 per cent sample of FCEs.

Finished Consultant Episode data for England for 2004/05 and 2005/06 have not been adjusted to take into account shortfalls in the number of records received or for missing/invalid clinical data.

1 All figures exclude day cases. Prior to 1987/88, figures relate to calendar years, but from then on to financial years ending 31 March.

2 Including pre-convalescent department and gynaecology.

3 Figures include obstetrics and other departments not shown in the table.

4 The reduction in mental illness and learning disabilities FCEs was due to change in definition.

*Sources:*  Hospital Episode Statistics (IC).

Health Statistics Wales (NAW).

Scottish Health Statistics (ISD).

Population Projections Database (GAD).

Figure 3.8  **Relationship between acute bed provision and hospital discharge rate in selected OECD countries, circa 2005**

**Discharge rate per 1,000 population**

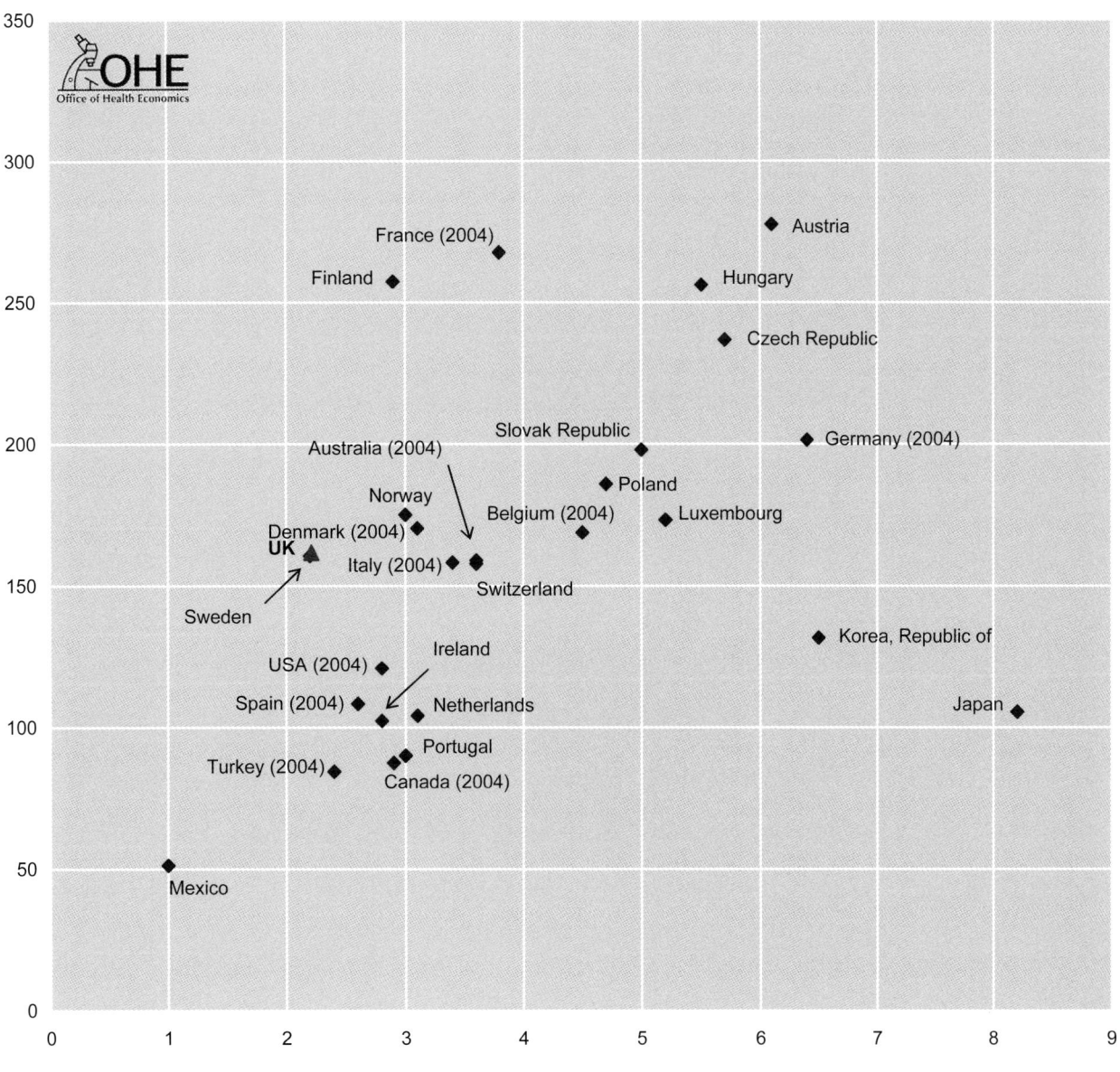

**Acute beds per 1,000 population**

*Notes:*      Year is 2005 unless stated otherwise.
              Cross-country comparison should be carried out with caution as figures may be based on different definitions.
*Sources:* OECD Health Database (OECD).
              Health and Personal Social Services Statistics for England (DH).
              Health Statistics Wales (NAW).
              Scottish Health Statistics (ISD).
              Hospital Episode Statistics (DH).
              Hospital Activity Statistics: England (DH).
              Hospital Statistics for Northern Ireland (DHSSPS).
              Population Projections Database (GAD).

Table 3.19   **Average inpatient length of stay in NHS hospitals, all specialties[1], UK, 1951 - 2005/06**

| | Average length of stay (days) | | | | Index (1951=100) | | | |
|---|---|---|---|---|---|---|---|---|
| Year | England and Wales | Scotland | Northern Ireland | United Kingdom | England and Wales | Scotland | Northern Ireland | United Kingdom |
| 1951 | 46.0 | 43.0 | 45.0 | 45.0 | 100 | 100 | 100 | 100 |
| 1955 | 43.0 | 41.0 | 42.0 | 42.0 | 93 | 95 | 93 | 93 |
| 1956 | 41.0 | 38.0 | 41.0 | 41.0 | 89 | 88 | 91 | 91 |
| 1957 | 40.0 | 38.0 | 40.0 | 40.0 | 87 | 88 | 89 | 89 |
| 1958 | 39.0 | 37.0 | 38.0 | 39.0 | 85 | 86 | 84 | 87 |
| 1959 | 38.0 | 35.0 | 35.0 | 37.0 | 83 | 81 | 78 | 82 |
| 1960 | 36.0 | 34.0 | 37.0 | 36.0 | 78 | 79 | 82 | 80 |
| 1961 | 35.0 | 33.0 | 35.0 | 34.0 | 76 | 77 | 78 | 76 |
| 1962 | 33.0 | 33.0 | 32.0 | 33.0 | 72 | 77 | 71 | 73 |
| 1963 | 32.0 | 32.0 | 31.0 | 32.0 | 70 | 74 | 69 | 71 |
| 1964 | 31.0 | 31.0 | 30.0 | 31.0 | 67 | 72 | 67 | 69 |
| 1965 | 30.0 | 31.0 | 29.0 | 30.0 | 65 | 72 | 64 | 67 |
| 1966 | 29.0 | 31.0 | 28.0 | 29.0 | 63 | 72 | 62 | 64 |
| 1967 | 28.0 | 30.0 | 27.0 | 29.0 | 61 | 70 | 60 | 64 |
| 1968 | 27.0 | 29.0 | 26.0 | 27.0 | 59 | 67 | 58 | 60 |
| 1969 | 26.0 | 29.0 | 26.0 | 27.0 | 57 | 67 | 58 | 60 |
| 1970 | 25.0 | 28.0 | 25.0 | 26.0 | 54 | 65 | 56 | 58 |
| 1971 | 24.0 | 27.0 | 24.0 | 25.0 | 52 | 63 | 53 | 56 |
| 1972 | 24.0 | 26.0 | 23.0 | 24.0 | 52 | 60 | 51 | 53 |
| 1973 | 23.0 | 27.0 | 23.0 | 24.0 | 50 | 63 | 51 | 53 |
| 1974 | 23.0 | 26.0 | 23.0 | 23.0 | 50 | 60 | 51 | 51 |
| 1975 | 23.0 | 26.0 | 23.0 | 23.0 | 50 | 60 | 51 | 51 |
| 1976 | 22.0 | 25.0 | 22.0 | 22.0 | 48 | 58 | 49 | 49 |
| 1977 | 21.0 | 25.0 | 22.0 | 21.0 | 46 | 58 | 49 | 47 |
| 1978 | 20.0 | 24.0 | 21.0 | 21.0 | 43 | 56 | 47 | 47 |
| 1979 | 20.0 | 24.0 | 21.0 | 20.0 | 43 | 56 | 47 | 44 |
| 1980 | 19.0 | 23.0 | 20.0 | 19.0 | 41 | 53 | 44 | 42 |
| 1981 | 18.0 | 22.0 | 20.0 | 19.0 | 39 | 51 | 44 | 42 |
| 1982 | 18.0 | 22.0 | 20.0 | 18.0 | 39 | 51 | 44 | 40 |
| 1983 | 17.0 | 22.0 | 19.0 | 17.0 | 37 | 51 | 42 | 38 |
| 1984 | 16.0 | 21.0 | 18.0 | 17.0 | 35 | 49 | 40 | 38 |
| 1985 | 15.0 | 21.0 | 17.0 | 16.0 | 33 | 49 | 38 | 36 |
| 1986 | 14.0 | 20.0 | 17.0 | 15.0 | 30 | 47 | 38 | 33 |
| 1987/88[1] | 13.0 | 19.0 | 17.0 | 14.0 | 28 | 44 | 38 | 31 |
| 1988/89 | 12.0 | 18.0 | 16.0 | 13.0 | 26 | 42 | 36 | 29 |
| 1989/90 | 11.0 | 18.0 | 15.0 | 12.0 | 24 | 42 | 33 | 27 |
| 1990/91 | 10.0 | 17.0 | 14.0 | 11.0 | 22 | 40 | 31 | 24 |
| 1991/92 | 9.0 | 16.0 | 13.0 | 10.0 | 20 | 37 | 29 | 22 |
| 1992/93 | 9.0 | 15.0 | 12.0 | 10.0 | 20 | 35 | 27 | 22 |
| 1993/94[1] | 8.3 | 9.0 | 7.4 | 8.3 | 18 | 21 | 16 | 18 |
| 1994/95 | 7.5 | 8.6 | 7.0 | 7.6 | 16 | 20 | 16 | 17 |
| 1995/96 | 7.4 | 8.2 | 6.7 | 7.4 | 16 | 19 | 15 | 16 |
| 1996/97 | 7.4 | 8.2 | 6.5 | 7.5 | 16 | 19 | 14 | 17 |
| 1997/98[2] | 5.3 | 7.8 | 6.3 | 5.6 | 11 | 18 | 14 | 12 |
| 1998/99 | 5.1 | 7.6 | 5.7 | 5.1 | 11 | 18 | 13 | 11 |
| 1999/00 | 5.0 | 7.5 | 5.6 | 5.0 | 11 | 17 | 13 | 11 |
| 2000/01 | 5.1 | 7.4 | 5.7 | 5.1 | 11 | 17 | 13 | 11 |
| 2001/02 | 5.1 | 7.3 | 5.8 | 5.1 | 11 | 17 | 13 | 11 |
| 2002/03 | 5.1 | 7.4 | 5.9 | 5.1 | 11 | 17 | 13 | 11 |
| 2003/04 | 5.0 | 7.0 | 5.9 | 5.0 | 11 | 16 | 13 | 11 |
| 2004/05 | 4.7 | 6.9 | 5.8 | 4.7 | 10 | 16 | 13 | 10 |
| 2005/06 | 4.4 | 6.5 | 5.6 | 4.4 | 10 | 15 | 12 | 10 |

*Notes:*   All figures relate to inpatients and from 1987/88 to financial years ending 31 March.

Figures relate to the average duration of a Finished Consultant Episode/Discharges and deaths and exclude day cases.

1 From 1987/88 in England and from 1993/94 in Scotland and N Ireland, figures are based on all specialties other than mental illness and learning disabilities.

2 The reduction in length of stay in England and Wales is largely due to a change in definition relating to bed days.

*Sources:*   Hospital Episodes Statistics (DH).

Health Statistics Wales (NAW).

Scottish Health Statistics (ISD).

Hospital Statistics for Northern Ireland (DHSSPS).

Figure 3.9  **Average inpatient length of stay in NHS acute hospitals, England, 1959 - 2005/06**

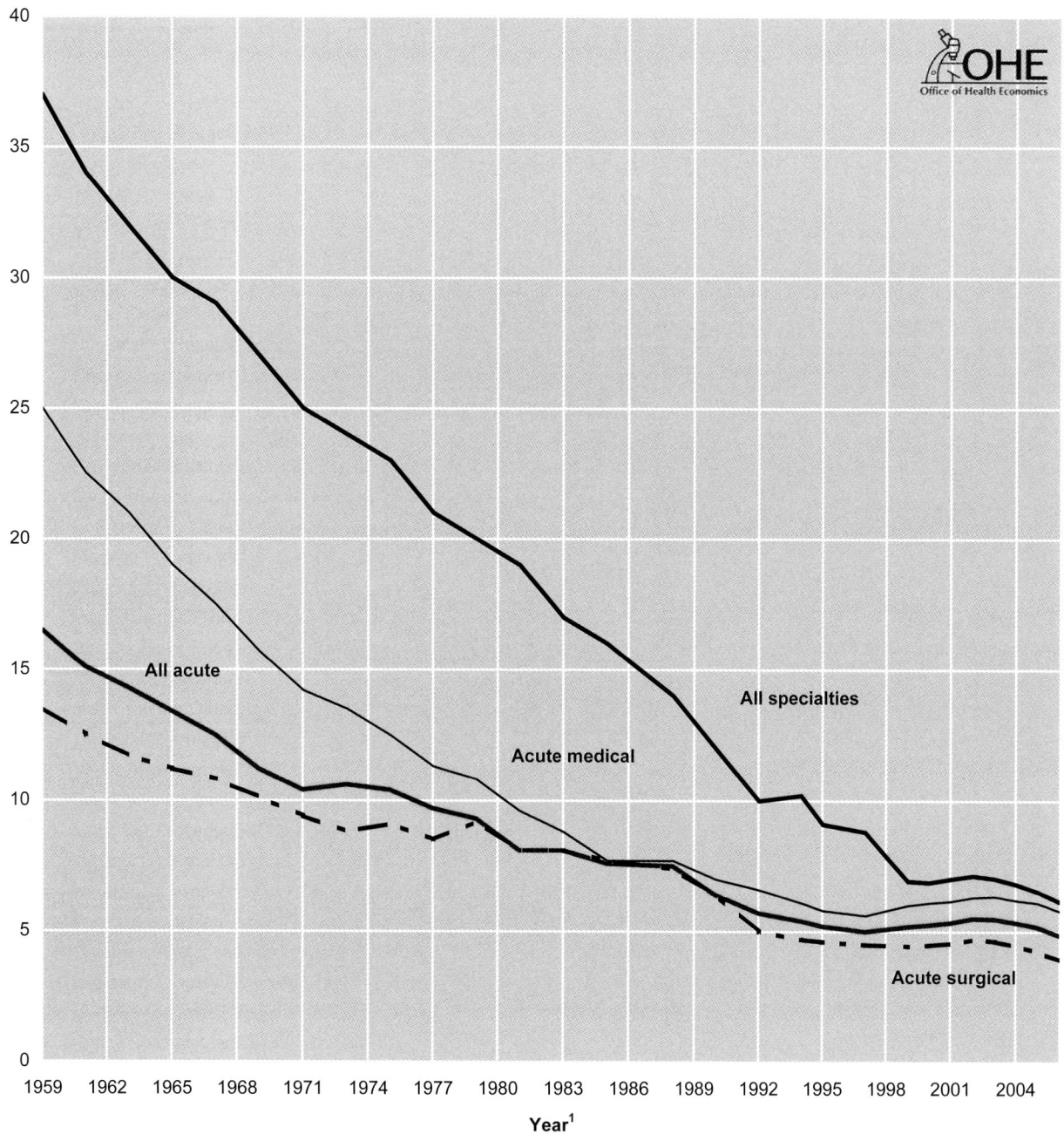

**Mean length of stay (days)**

All acute

All specialties

Acute medical

Acute surgical

Year[1]

*Notes:*   1 Figures from 1987 onwards relate to financial years ending 31 March (e.g. 1988 = 1987/88), prior to this figures relate to calendar year. Figures exclude day cases.  Figures from 1987 onwards relate to the average duration of a spell - a period of continuous admitted patient care within a particular NHS hospital trust.
*Source:*   Hospital Episode Statistics (IC).

Table 3.20 **Hospital finished consultant episodes[1] (FCEs) by primary diagnosis, England, 1995/96 - 2005/06**
Thousands

| ICD | Causes | Year | | | | | | | |
|---|---|---|---|---|---|---|---|---|---|
| | | 1995/96 | 1998/99 | 2000/01 | 2001/02 | 2002/03 | 2003/04 | 2004/05 | 2005/06 |
| | **All causes[2]** | **11,042** | **11,984** | **12,265** | **12,357** | **12,756** | **13,174** | **13,707** | **14,424** |
| | *per 1,000 population* | *228* | *242* | *249* | *250* | *257* | *264* | *273* | *285* |
| I | Infectious and parasitic diseases | 134 | 142 | 153 | 161 | 161 | 161 | 176 | 189 |
| II | Neoplasms | 1,032 | 1,279 | 1,354 | 1,348 | 1,379 | 1,390 | 1,423 | 1,521 |
| III | Blood and blood-forming organs | 126 | 153 | 168 | 180 | 188 | 197 | 208 | 223 |
| IV | Endocrine diseases[3] | 126 | 143 | 149 | 153 | 160 | 170 | 184 | 204 |
| V | Mental disorders | 289 | 243 | 221 | 221 | 225 | 217 | 225 | 219 |
| VI-VIII | Nervous system and sense organs | 628 | 686 | 715 | 724 | 756 | 793 | 811 | 831 |
| IX | Circulatory system | 957 | 1,057 | 1,072 | 1,086 | 1,149 | 1,169 | 1,195 | 1,244 |
| X | Respiratory system | 725 | 756 | 706 | 742 | 768 | 841 | 877 | 923 |
| XI | Digestive system | 1,154 | 1,265 | 1,302 | 1,298 | 1,345 | 1,354 | 1,416 | 1,534 |
| XII | Skin and subcutaneous tissue | 232 | 252 | 272 | 272 | 285 | 294 | 296 | 309 |
| XIII | Musculo-skeletal system | 588 | 636 | 658 | 662 | 722 | 767 | 813 | 881 |
| XIV | Genito-urinary system | 831 | 791 | 794 | 777 | 807 | 821 | 847 | 915 |
| XV | Pregnancy, childbirth etc.[3] | 1,162 | 1,182 | 1,153 | 1,169 | 1,205 | 1,225 | 1,278 | 1,339 |
| XVI | Conditions of the perinatal period[3] | 195 | 190 | 179 | 176 | 174 | 180 | 185 | 197 |
| XVII | Congenital anomalies | 107 | 99 | 97 | 98 | 102 | 104 | 106 | 111 |
| XVIII | Ill-defined conditions[3] | 948 | 1,317 | 1,526 | 1,530 | 1,516 | 1,633 | 1,732 | 1,743 |
| XIX | Injury and poisoning | 695 | 731 | 733 | 751 | 775 | 816 | 878 | 961 |
| XXI | Other[4] | 1,112 | 1,062 | 1,013 | 1,010 | 1,038 | 1,040 | 1,057 | 1,081 |

**Percentage distribution of FCEs**

| ICD | Causes | | | | | | | | |
|---|---|---|---|---|---|---|---|---|---|
| I | Infectious and parasitic diseases | 1.2 | 1.2 | 1.2 | 1.3 | 1.3 | 1.2 | 1.3 | 1.3 |
| II | Neoplasms | 9.3 | 10.7 | 11.0 | 10.9 | 10.8 | 10.6 | 10.4 | 10.5 |
| III | Blood and blood-forming organs | 1.1 | 1.3 | 1.4 | 1.5 | 1.5 | 1.5 | 1.5 | 1.5 |
| IV | Endocrine diseases[3] | 1.1 | 1.2 | 1.2 | 1.2 | 1.3 | 1.3 | 1.3 | 1.4 |
| V | Mental disorders | 2.6 | 2.0 | 1.8 | 1.8 | 1.8 | 1.6 | 1.6 | 1.5 |
| VI-VIII | Nervous system and sense organs | 5.7 | 5.7 | 5.8 | 5.9 | 5.9 | 6.0 | 5.9 | 5.8 |
| IX | Circulatory system | 8.7 | 8.8 | 8.7 | 8.8 | 9.0 | 8.9 | 8.7 | 8.6 |
| X | Respiratory system | 6.6 | 6.3 | 5.8 | 6.0 | 6.0 | 6.4 | 6.4 | 6.4 |
| XI | Digestive system | 10.5 | 10.6 | 10.6 | 10.5 | 10.5 | 10.3 | 10.3 | 10.6 |
| XII | Skin and subcutaneous tissue | 2.1 | 2.1 | 2.2 | 2.2 | 2.2 | 2.2 | 2.2 | 2.1 |
| XIII | Musculo-skeletal system | 5.3 | 5.3 | 5.4 | 5.4 | 5.7 | 5.8 | 5.9 | 6.1 |
| XIV | Genito-urinary system | 7.5 | 6.6 | 6.5 | 6.3 | 6.3 | 6.2 | 6.2 | 6.3 |
| XV | Pregnancy, childbirth etc.[3] | 10.5 | 9.9 | 9.4 | 9.5 | 9.4 | 9.3 | 9.3 | 9.3 |
| XVI | Conditions of the perinatal period[3] | 1.8 | 1.6 | 1.5 | 1.4 | 1.4 | 1.4 | 1.3 | 1.4 |
| XVII | Congenital anomalies | 1.0 | 0.8 | 0.8 | 0.8 | 0.8 | 0.8 | 0.8 | 0.8 |
| XVIII | Ill-defined conditions[3] | 8.6 | 11.0 | 12.4 | 12.4 | 11.9 | 12.4 | 12.6 | 12.1 |
| XIX | Injury and poisoning | 6.3 | 6.1 | 6.0 | 6.1 | 6.1 | 6.2 | 6.4 | 6.7 |
| XXI | Other[4] | 10.1 | 8.9 | 8.3 | 8.2 | 8.1 | 7.9 | 7.7 | 7.5 |

*Notes:* Finished consultant episode data for 2004/05 and 2005/06 have not been adjusted to take into account shortfalls in the number of records received or for missing/invalid clinical data.
Data for 1997/98 are not available.
1 Figures include ordinary admissions and day cases, in financial years ending 31 March. An ordinary admission is defined as an admission where the patient is expected to remain in hospital for at least one night.
2 From 1994/95, figures are based on all FCEs. Figures for previous years are based on a 25% sample of FCEs.
3 Headings have been abbreviated.
4 Figures include factors influencing health status and contact with health services.

*Sources:* Hospital Episode Statistics (IC).
Population Projections Database (GAD).

Table 3.21(a)   **Hospital finished consultant episodes[1] per 1,000 population by primary diagnosis, England, 1995/96 - 2005/06**

Per 1,000 population

| ICD | Causes | Year | | | | | | | |
|---|---|---|---|---|---|---|---|---|---|
| | | 1995/96 | 1998/99 | 2000/01 | 2001/02 | 2002/03 | 2003/04 | 2004/05 | 2005/06 |
| | **All causes[3]** | **228** | **245** | **249** | **250** | **257** | **264** | **273** | **285** |
| I | Infectious and parasitic diseases | 3 | 3 | 3 | 3 | 3 | 3 | 4 | 4 |
| II | Neoplasms | 21 | 26 | 27 | 27 | 28 | 28 | 28 | 30 |
| III | Blood and blood-forming organs | 3 | 3 | 3 | 4 | 4 | 4 | 4 | 4 |
| IV | Endocrine diseases[3] | 3 | 3 | 3 | 3 | 3 | 3 | 4 | 4 |
| V | Mental disorders | 6 | 5 | 4 | 4 | 5 | 4 | 4 | 4 |
| VI-VIII | Nervous system and sense organs | 13 | 14 | 15 | 15 | 15 | 16 | 16 | 16 |
| IX | Circulatory system | 20 | 22 | 22 | 22 | 23 | 23 | 24 | 25 |
| X | Respiratory system | 15 | 15 | 14 | 15 | 15 | 17 | 17 | 18 |
| XI | Digestive system | 24 | 26 | 26 | 26 | 27 | 27 | 28 | 30 |
| XII | Skin and subcutaneous tissue | 5 | 5 | 6 | 5 | 6 | 6 | 6 | 6 |
| XIII | Musculo-skeletal system | 12 | 13 | 13 | 13 | 15 | 15 | 16 | 17 |
| XIV | Genito-urinary system | 17 | 16 | 16 | 16 | 16 | 16 | 17 | 18 |
| XV | Pregnancy, childbirth etc.[3,4] | 115 | 116 | 113 | 114 | 117 | 118 | 123 | 127 |
| XVI | Conditions of the perinatal period[3] | 4 | 4 | 4 | 4 | 4 | 4 | 4 | 4 |
| XVII | Congenital anomalies | 2 | 2 | 2 | 2 | 2 | 2 | 2 | 2 |
| XVIII | Ill-defined conditions[3] | 20 | 27 | 31 | 31 | 31 | 33 | 35 | 34 |
| XIX | Injury and poisoning | 14 | 15 | 15 | 15 | 16 | 16 | 17 | 19 |
| XXI | Other[5] | 23 | 22 | 21 | 20 | 21 | 21 | 21 | 21 |

Table 3.21(b)   **Estimated[2] number of hospital finished consultant episodes[1], UK, 1995/96 - 2005/06**

Thousands

| ICD | Causes | 1995/96 | 1998/99 | 2000/01 | 2001/02 | 2002/03 | 2003/04 | 2004/05 | 2005/06 |
|---|---|---|---|---|---|---|---|---|---|
| | **All causes[3]** | **13,539** | **14,497** | **14,835** | **14,891** | **15,217** | **15,718** | **16,284** | **17,084** |
| I | Infectious and parasitic diseases | 161 | 170 | 183 | 192 | 192 | 193 | 210 | 225 |
| II | Neoplasms | 1,238 | 1,531 | 1,619 | 1,611 | 1,647 | 1,660 | 1,700 | 1,815 |
| III | Blood and blood-forming organs | 152 | 183 | 201 | 215 | 225 | 235 | 249 | 266 |
| IV | Endocrine diseases[3] | 151 | 171 | 178 | 183 | 192 | 203 | 220 | 244 |
| V | Mental disorders | 347 | 291 | 264 | 264 | 269 | 259 | 268 | 261 |
| VI-VIII | Nervous system and sense organs | 753 | 822 | 855 | 865 | 903 | 947 | 969 | 992 |
| IX | Circulatory system | 1,148 | 1,265 | 1,282 | 1,298 | 1,372 | 1,396 | 1,427 | 1,485 |
| X | Respiratory system | 869 | 906 | 844 | 887 | 918 | 1,005 | 1,048 | 1,102 |
| XI | Digestive system | 1,384 | 1,515 | 1,558 | 1,552 | 1,607 | 1,618 | 1,691 | 1,831 |
| XII | Skin and subcutaneous tissue | 278 | 302 | 325 | 325 | 341 | 351 | 353 | 369 |
| XIII | Musculo-skeletal system | 706 | 762 | 787 | 791 | 862 | 916 | 971 | 1,052 |
| XIV | Genito-urinary system | 996 | 947 | 949 | 929 | 964 | 981 | 1,011 | 1,092 |
| XV | Pregnancy, childbirth etc.[3,4] | 1,394 | 1,417 | 1,381 | 1,398 | 1,440 | 1,463 | 1,525 | 1,594 |
| XVI | Conditions of the perinatal period[3] | 234 | 227 | 214 | 210 | 208 | 215 | 220 | 235 |
| XVII | Congenital anomalies | 129 | 118 | 116 | 117 | 122 | 125 | 126 | 133 |
| XVIII | Ill-defined conditions[3] | 1,137 | 1,577 | 1,824 | 1,829 | 1,812 | 1,950 | 2,069 | 2,081 |
| XIX | Injury and poisoning | 833 | 876 | 877 | 898 | 926 | 975 | 1,048 | 1,147 |
| XXI | Other[5] | 1,333 | 1,272 | 1,211 | 1,207 | 1,240 | 1,242 | 1,262 | 1,290 |

*Notes:* Data for 1997/98 are not available.
Finished consultant episode data for 2004/05 and 2005/06 have not been adjusted to take into account shortfalls in the number of records received or for missing/invalid clinical data.
1 Figures include ordinary admissions and day cases, in financial years ending 31 March.
2 OHE estimate using a population grossing factor.
3 Headings have been abbreviated.
4 Per 1,000 female population aged 15-44.
5 Figures include factors influencing health status and contact with health services.

*Sources:* Hospital Episode Statistics (IC).
Population Projections Database (GAD).

Table 3.22  **Hospital ordinary admissions[1] (excluding day cases) by main cause, England, 1995/96 - 2005/06**

Thousands

| ICD | Causes | Year 1995/96 | 1998/99 | 2000/01 | 2001/02 | 2002/03 | 2003/04 | 2004/05 | 2005/06 |
|---|---|---|---|---|---|---|---|---|---|
| | All causes[2] | 8,302 | 8,563 | 8,645 | 8,764 | 9,042 | 9,417 | 9,859 | 10,310 |
| | *Admissions per 1,000 population* | *171* | *175* | *175* | *177* | *182* | *189* | *196* | *204* |
| I | Infectious and parasitic diseases | 120 | 127 | 138 | 146 | 146 | 146 | 160 | 174 |
| II | Neoplasms | 590 | 575 | 589 | 584 | 608 | 612 | 621 | 651 |
| III | Blood and blood-forming organs | 76 | 82 | 85 | 91 | 94 | 97 | 102 | 105 |
| IV | Endocrine diseases[3] | 89 | 94 | 101 | 107 | 114 | 120 | 129 | 141 |
| V | Mental disorders | 285 | 237 | 217 | 217 | 221 | 214 | 222 | 216 |
| VI-VIII | Nervous system and sense organs | 378 | 331 | 307 | 299 | 300 | 302 | 305 | 319 |
| IX | Circulatory system | 866 | 921 | 924 | 934 | 981 | 995 | 1,013 | 1,044 |
| X | Respiratory system | 690 | 720 | 671 | 707 | 732 | 805 | 838 | 878 |
| XI | Digestive system | 669 | 682 | 704 | 715 | 748 | 765 | 808 | 857 |
| XII | Skin and subcutaneous tissue | 121 | 133 | 149 | 151 | 160 | 171 | 176 | 185 |
| XIII | Musculo-skeletal system | 390 | 387 | 396 | 398 | 433 | 463 | 490 | 529 |
| XIV | Genito-urinary system | 509 | 457 | 447 | 444 | 462 | 490 | 509 | 549 |
| XV | Pregnancy, childbirth etc.[3] | 1,054 | 1,074 | 1,058 | 1,072 | 1,112 | 1,134 | 1,190 | 1,242 |
| XVI | Conditions of the perinatal period[3] | 194 | 188 | 178 | 174 | 173 | 178 | 183 | 195 |
| XVII | Congenital anomalies | 82 | 73 | 71 | 71 | 75 | 76 | 76 | 79 |
| XVIII | Ill-defined conditions[3] | 735 | 1,043 | 1,207 | 1,219 | 1,212 | 1,326 | 1,428 | 1,443 |
| XIX | Injury and poisoning | 663 | 701 | 703 | 720 | 743 | 784 | 843 | 923 |
| XXI | Other[4] | 791 | 737 | 701 | 714 | 731 | 740 | 767 | 780 |

**Percentage distribution of hospital ordinary admissions[1] (excluding day cases)**

| ICD | Causes | 1995/96 | 1998/99 | 2000/01 | 2001/02 | 2002/03 | 2003/04 | 2004/05 | 2005/06 |
|---|---|---|---|---|---|---|---|---|---|
| I | Infectious and parasitic diseases | 1.4 | 1.5 | 1.6 | 1.7 | 1.6 | 1.6 | 1.6 | 1.7 |
| II | Neoplasms | 7.1 | 6.7 | 6.8 | 6.7 | 6.7 | 6.5 | 6.3 | 6.3 |
| III | Blood and blood-forming organs | 0.9 | 1.0 | 1.0 | 1.0 | 1.0 | 1.0 | 1.0 | 1.0 |
| IV | Endocrine diseases[3] | 1.1 | 1.1 | 1.2 | 1.2 | 1.3 | 1.3 | 1.3 | 1.4 |
| V | Mental disorders | 3.4 | 2.8 | 2.5 | 2.5 | 2.4 | 2.3 | 2.3 | 2.1 |
| VI-VIII | Nervous system and sense organs | 4.6 | 3.9 | 3.6 | 3.4 | 3.3 | 3.2 | 3.1 | 3.1 |
| IX | Circulatory system | 10.4 | 10.8 | 10.7 | 10.7 | 10.8 | 10.6 | 10.3 | 10.1 |
| X | Respiratory system | 8.3 | 8.4 | 7.8 | 8.1 | 8.1 | 8.6 | 8.5 | 8.5 |
| XI | Digestive system | 8.1 | 8.0 | 8.1 | 8.2 | 8.3 | 8.1 | 8.2 | 8.3 |
| XII | Skin and subcutaneous tissue | 1.5 | 1.6 | 1.7 | 1.7 | 1.8 | 1.8 | 1.8 | 1.8 |
| XIII | Musculo-skeletal system | 4.7 | 4.5 | 4.6 | 4.5 | 4.8 | 4.9 | 5.0 | 5.1 |
| XIV | Genito-urinary system | 6.1 | 5.3 | 5.2 | 5.1 | 5.1 | 5.2 | 5.2 | 5.3 |
| XV | Pregnancy, childbirth etc.[3] | 12.7 | 12.5 | 12.2 | 12.2 | 12.3 | 12.0 | 12.1 | 12.0 |
| XVI | Conditions of the perinatal period[3] | 2.3 | 2.2 | 2.1 | 2.0 | 1.9 | 1.9 | 1.9 | 1.9 |
| XVII | Congenital anomalies | 1.0 | 0.9 | 0.8 | 0.8 | 0.8 | 0.8 | 0.8 | 0.8 |
| XVIII | Ill-defined conditions[3] | 8.9 | 12.2 | 14.0 | 13.9 | 13.4 | 14.1 | 14.5 | 14.0 |
| XIX | Injury and poisoning | 8.0 | 8.2 | 8.1 | 8.2 | 8.2 | 8.3 | 8.6 | 9.0 |
| XXI | Other[4] | 9.5 | 8.6 | 8.1 | 8.1 | 8.1 | 7.9 | 7.8 | 7.6 |

*Notes:*   Data for 1997/98 are not available.

Finished consultant episode data for 2004/05 and 2005/06 have not been adjusted to take into account shortfalls in the number of records received or for missing/invalid clinical data.

1 Figures relate to FCEs in financial years ending 31 March that were or resulted from ordinary admissions.  An ordinary admission is defined as an admission where the patient remains or is expected to remain in hospital for at least one night and includes patients in all NHS hospitals in England.

2 From 1994/95, figures are based on all FCEs. Figures for previous years are based on a 25% sample of FCEs.

3 Headings have been abbreviated.

4 Figures include factors influencing health status and contact with health services.

*Sources:*  Hospital Episode Statistics (IC).

Population Projections Database (GAD).

Table 3.23 **Mean length of stay of hospital ordinary admissions[1] and index (1995/96=100), by main cause, England, 1995/96 - 2005/06**
Days

| ICD | Causes | Year | | | | | | | |
|---|---|---|---|---|---|---|---|---|---|
| | | 1995/96 | 1998/99 | 2000/01 | 2001/02 | 2002/03 | 2003/04 | 2004/05 | 2005/06 |
| | All causes[2] | 8.1 | 8.0 | 8.2 | 8.1 | 7.9 | 7.4 | 7.1 | 6.6 |
| I | Infectious and parasitic diseases | 7.1 | 5.1 | 5.1 | 5.1 | 5.6 | 6.1 | 5.9 | 6.2 |
| II | Neoplasms | 7.7 | 8.4 | 8.6 | 8.8 | 8.6 | 8.4 | 8.4 | 8.0 |
| III | Blood and blood-forming organs | 5.8 | 6.6 | 6.6 | 6.7 | 6.7 | 6.3 | 6.0 | 5.7 |
| IV | Endocrine diseases[3] | 9.6 | 9.0 | 9.2 | 9.3 | 9.3 | 8.9 | 8.3 | 7.7 |
| V | Mental disorders | 68.6 | 50.0 | 50.1 | 49.4 | 47.9 | 49.0 | 48.7 | 46.0 |
| VI-VIII | Nervous system and sense organs | 7.7 | 7.5 | 8.1 | 8.6 | 8.1 | 8.2 | 7.6 | 7.2 |
| IX | Circulatory system | 9.4 | 10.1 | 10.4 | 10.8 | 11.1 | 10.7 | 10.5 | 9.9 |
| X | Respiratory system | 6.0 | 6.3 | 6.6 | 6.8 | 7.1 | 6.9 | 6.7 | 6.4 |
| XI | Digestive system | 4.8 | 5.8 | 6.0 | 6.3 | 6.4 | 6.1 | 6.0 | 5.7 |
| XII | Skin and subcutaneous tissue | 8.1 | 7.8 | 8.0 | 8.0 | 8.1 | 7.7 | 7.4 | 6.9 |
| XIII | Musculo-skeletal system | 7.4 | 7.0 | 6.7 | 6.6 | 6.6 | 6.0 | 5.8 | 5.3 |
| XIV | Genito-urinary system | 4.5 | 4.9 | 5.2 | 5.5 | 5.6 | 5.6 | 5.5 | 5.4 |
| XV | Pregnancy, childbirth etc.[3] | 2.4 | 2.1 | 1.9 | 1.9 | 1.8 | 1.8 | 1.8 | 1.6 |
| XVI | Conditions of the perinatal period[3] | 6.0 | 6.5 | 6.4 | 6.6 | 6.7 | 6.6 | 6.6 | 6.4 |
| XVII | Congenital anomalies | 5.9 | 4.9 | 4.5 | 4.5 | 4.4 | 4.2 | 4.8 | 4.3 |
| XVIII | Ill-defined conditions[3] | 4.6 | 7.6 | 7.5 | 7.2 | 6.8 | 6.6 | 5.8 | 5.2 |
| XIX | Injury and poisoning | 6.3 | 6.7 | 6.8 | 7.2 | 7.9 | 7.4 | 7.1 | 6.6 |
| XXI | Other[4] | 6.2 | 4.6 | 4.7 | 3.9 | 3.2 | 3.0 | 2.6 | 2.2 |

**Index of mean length of stay of hospital ordinary admissions[1] (1995/96=100)**

| ICD | Causes | 1995/96 | 1998/99 | 2000/01 | 2001/02 | 2002/03 | 2003/04 | 2004/05 | 2005/06 |
|---|---|---|---|---|---|---|---|---|---|
| | All causes | 100 | 98 | 101 | 100 | 97 | 91 | 87 | 81 |
| I | Infectious and parasitic diseases | 100 | 72 | 72 | 72 | 79 | 85 | 83 | 87 |
| II | Neoplasms | 100 | 109 | 112 | 115 | 113 | 110 | 109 | 104 |
| III | Blood and blood-forming organs | 100 | 113 | 115 | 116 | 115 | 109 | 103 | 99 |
| IV | Endocrine diseases[3] | 100 | 94 | 95 | 97 | 97 | 92 | 86 | 80 |
| V | Mental disorders | 100 | 73 | 73 | 72 | 70 | 71 | 71 | 67 |
| VI-VIII | Nervous system and sense organs | 100 | 98 | 105 | 113 | 106 | 107 | 99 | 95 |
| IX | Circulatory system | 100 | 108 | 111 | 115 | 119 | 114 | 112 | 105 |
| X | Respiratory system | 100 | 105 | 109 | 113 | 118 | 114 | 111 | 106 |
| XI | Digestive system | 100 | 120 | 124 | 130 | 132 | 127 | 125 | 118 |
| XII | Skin and subcutaneous tissue | 100 | 97 | 100 | 100 | 100 | 96 | 91 | 86 |
| XIII | Musculo-skeletal system | 100 | 94 | 90 | 89 | 88 | 81 | 77 | 71 |
| XIV | Genito-urinary system | 100 | 110 | 118 | 122 | 125 | 124 | 123 | 120 |
| XV | Pregnancy, childbirth etc.[3] | 100 | 88 | 81 | 81 | 77 | 77 | 73 | 69 |
| XVI | Conditions of the perinatal period[3] | 100 | 107 | 107 | 110 | 111 | 109 | 109 | 106 |
| XVII | Congenital anomalies | 100 | 83 | 77 | 76 | 75 | 72 | 82 | 74 |
| XVIII | Ill-defined conditions[3] | 100 | 164 | 164 | 156 | 148 | 143 | 125 | 113 |
| XIX | Injury and poisoning | 100 | 105 | 108 | 113 | 124 | 117 | 112 | 105 |
| XXI | Other[4] | 100 | 74 | 76 | 63 | 52 | 49 | 42 | 35 |

*Notes:* Data for 1997/98 are not available.
Finished consultant episode data for 2004/05 and 2005/06 have not been adjusted to take into account shortfalls in the number of records received or for missing/invalid clinical data.
1 Figures include ordinary admissions only, in financial years ending 31 March. An ordinary admission is defined as an admission where the patient remains or is expected to remain in hospital for at least one night and includes patients in all NHS hospitals in England.
2 From 1994/95, figures are based on all FCEs. Figures for previous years are based on a 25 % sample of FCEs.
3 Headings have been abbreviated.
4 Figures include factors influencing health status and contact with health services.
*Source:* Hospital Episode Statistics (IC).

Table 3.24　Number and percentage distribution of hospital bed days for ordinary admissions[1] by main cause
England, 1995/96 - 2005/06

Thousands

| ICD | Causes | Year | | | | | | | |
|---|---|---|---|---|---|---|---|---|---|
| | | 1995/96 | 1998/99 | 2000/01 | 2001/02 | 2002/03 | 2003/04 | 2004/05 | 2005/06 |
| | **All causes** | **67,461** | **50,752** | **50,893** | **51,564** | **52,347** | **54,620** | **54,555** | **52,920** |
| | *Bed days per 1,000 population* | *1,393* | *1,038* | *1,033* | *1,042* | *1,053* | *1,094* | *1,087* | *1,047* |
| I | Infectious and parasitic diseases | 852 | 565 | 598 | 632 | 672 | 721 | 790 | 861 |
| II | Neoplasms | 4,529 | 4,150 | 4,276 | 4,295 | 4,341 | 4,328 | 4,326 | 4,304 |
| III | Blood and blood-forming organs | 438 | 418 | 425 | 448 | 457 | 452 | 443 | 434 |
| IV | Endocrine diseases[2] | 855 | 681 | 717 | 756 | 787 | 814 | 809 | 820 |
| V | Mental disorders | 19,570 | 7,029 | 6,570 | 6,614 | 6,633 | 7,365 | 7,826 | 7,247 |
| VI-VIII | Nervous system and sense organs | 2,892 | 2,033 | 1,990 | 2,060 | 1,952 | 2,063 | 1,937 | 1,900 |
| IX | Circulatory system | 8,131 | 7,129 | 7,101 | 7,259 | 7,620 | 7,572 | 7,470 | 7,169 |
| X | Respiratory system | 4,159 | 3,775 | 3,532 | 3,790 | 3,890 | 4,257 | 4,217 | 4,210 |
| XI | Digestive system | 3,229 | 3,130 | 3,289 | 3,385 | 3,531 | 3,578 | 3,653 | 3,670 |
| XII | Skin and subcutaneous tissue | 975 | 888 | 990 | 1,004 | 1,039 | 1,098 | 1,065 | 1,041 |
| XIII | Musculo-skeletal system | 2,900 | 2,454 | 2,403 | 2,370 | 2,522 | 2,578 | 2,583 | 2,534 |
| XIV | Genito-urinary system | 2,274 | 2,013 | 2,040 | 2,102 | 2,206 | 2,297 | 2,371 | 2,446 |
| XV | Pregnancy, childbirth etc.[2] | 2,522 | 2,168 | 1,934 | 1,897 | 1,987 | 2,016 | 2,002 | 2,003 |
| XVI | Conditions of the perinatal period[2] | 1,170 | 1,034 | 935 | 932 | 972 | 1,022 | 1,047 | 1,075 |
| XVII | Congenital anomalies | 480 | 290 | 275 | 267 | 280 | 285 | 288 | 301 |
| XVIII | Ill-defined conditions[2] | 3,386 | 5,892 | 6,831 | 6,806 | 6,342 | 6,945 | 6,553 | 5,962 |
| XIX | Injury and poisoning | 4,210 | 4,123 | 4,260 | 4,499 | 4,948 | 5,138 | 5,246 | 5,299 |
| XXI | Other[3] | 4,888 | 2,979 | 2,727 | 2,447 | 2,168 | 2,092 | 1,929 | 1,643 |

**Percentage distribution of hospital bed days of ordinary admissions[1]**

| ICD | Causes | 1995/96 | 1998/99 | 2000/01 | 2001/02 | 2002/03 | 2003/04 | 2004/05 | 2005/06 |
|---|---|---|---|---|---|---|---|---|---|
| I | Infectious and parasitic diseases | 1.3 | 1.1 | 1.2 | 1.2 | 1.3 | 1.3 | 1.4 | 1.6 |
| II | Neoplasms | 6.7 | 8.2 | 8.4 | 8.3 | 8.3 | 7.9 | 7.9 | 8.1 |
| III | Blood and blood-forming organs | 0.6 | 0.8 | 0.8 | 0.9 | 0.9 | 0.8 | 0.8 | 0.8 |
| IV | Endocrine diseases[2] | 1.3 | 1.3 | 1.4 | 1.5 | 1.5 | 1.5 | 1.5 | 1.5 |
| V | Mental disorders | 29.0 | 13.9 | 12.9 | 12.8 | 12.7 | 13.5 | 14.3 | 13.7 |
| VI-VIII | Nervous system and sense organs | 4.3 | 4.0 | 3.9 | 4.0 | 3.7 | 3.8 | 3.5 | 3.6 |
| IX | Circulatory system | 12.1 | 14.0 | 14.0 | 14.1 | 14.6 | 13.9 | 13.7 | 13.5 |
| X | Respiratory system | 6.2 | 7.4 | 6.9 | 7.3 | 7.4 | 7.8 | 7.7 | 8.0 |
| XI | Digestive system | 4.8 | 6.2 | 6.5 | 6.6 | 6.7 | 6.6 | 6.7 | 6.9 |
| XII | Skin and subcutaneous tissue | 1.4 | 1.8 | 1.9 | 1.9 | 2.0 | 2.0 | 2.0 | 2.0 |
| XIII | Musculo-skeletal system | 4.3 | 4.8 | 4.7 | 4.6 | 4.8 | 4.7 | 4.7 | 4.8 |
| XIV | Genito-urinary system | 3.4 | 4.0 | 4.0 | 4.1 | 4.2 | 4.2 | 4.3 | 4.6 |
| XV | Pregnancy, childbirth etc.[2] | 3.7 | 4.3 | 3.8 | 3.7 | 3.8 | 3.7 | 3.7 | 3.8 |
| XVI | Conditions of the perinatal period[2] | 1.7 | 2.0 | 1.8 | 1.8 | 1.9 | 1.9 | 1.9 | 2.0 |
| XVII | Congenital anomalies | 0.7 | 0.6 | 0.5 | 0.5 | 0.5 | 0.5 | 0.5 | 0.6 |
| XVIII | Ill-defined conditions[2] | 5.0 | 11.6 | 13.4 | 13.2 | 12.1 | 12.7 | 12.0 | 11.3 |
| XIX | Injury and poisoning | 6.2 | 8.1 | 8.4 | 8.7 | 9.5 | 9.4 | 9.6 | 10.0 |
| XXI | Other[3] | 7.2 | 5.9 | 5.4 | 4.7 | 4.1 | 3.8 | 3.5 | 3.1 |

*Notes:*　Data for 1997/98 are not available.

Finished consultant episode data for 2004/05 and 2005/06 have not been adjusted to take into account shortfalls in the number of records received or for missing/invalid clinical data.

The reduction in the number of bed days since 1998/99 is due to change in definition.

1 Figures include ordinary admissions, in financial years ending 31 March. An ordinary admission is defined as an admission where the patient remains or is expected to remain in hospital for at least one night and includes patients in psychiatric hospitals.

2 Headings have been abbreviated.

3 Figures include factors influencing health status and contact with health services.

*Sources:*　Hospital Episode Statistics (IC).

Population Projections Database (GAD).

Table 3.25   **Estimated ordinary admissions by top major diagnostic group, England, 2000/01 - 2005/06**

| Major diagnosis (ICD10) | Estimated ordinary admissions per 10,000 population[1] | | | | As per cent of total ordinary admissions | | | |
|---|---|---|---|---|---|---|---|---|
| | 00/01 | 03/04 | 04/05 | 05/06 | 00/01 | 03/04 | 04/05 | 05/06 |
| Complications of labour and delivery (O10-O75, O85-O92, O95-O99)[2] | 799 | 872 | 914 | 970 | 11.6 | 11.5 | 11.6 | 11.9 |
| Health services in circumstances related to reproduction (Z30-Z39) | 85 | 100 | 113 | 118 | 5.9 | 6.4 | 6.9 | 7.0 |
| Delivery (O80-O84)[2] | 93 | 103 | 100 | 100 | 0.0 | 1.4 | 1.3 | 1.2 |
| Pregnancy with abortive outcome (O00-O08)[2] | 83 | 83 | 78 | 86 | 1.2 | 1.1 | 1.0 | 1.1 |
| Symptoms and signs involving the circulatory/respiratory system (R00-R09) | 48 | 57 | 64 | 67 | 3.3 | 3.6 | 3.9 | 4.0 |
| Symptoms and signs involving the digestive system and abdomen (R10-R19) | 46 | 47 | 53 | 56 | 3.2 | 3.0 | 3.2 | 3.3 |
| Ischaemic heart diseases (I20-I25) | 51 | 51 | 51 | 51 | 3.5 | 3.3 | 3.1 | 3.0 |
| Arthropathies (M00-M25) | 39 | 47 | 48 | 49 | 2.7 | 3.0 | 3.0 | 2.9 |
| General symptoms and signs (R50-R68) | 35 | 40 | 45 | 49 | 2.4 | 2.5 | 2.8 | 2.9 |
| Noninflammatory disorders of female genital tract (N80-N98)[3] | 49 | 46 | 45 | 46 | 1.7 | 1.5 | 1.4 | 1.4 |
| Other forms of heart disease (I30-I52) | 35 | 36 | 37 | 39 | 2.5 | 2.3 | 2.3 | 2.3 |
| Chronic lower respiratory diseases (J40-J47) | 32 | 36 | 38 | 36 | 2.2 | 2.3 | 2.3 | 2.1 |
| Other conditions originating in the perinatal period (P05-P96) | 27 | 29 | 31 | 32 | 1.9 | 1.9 | 1.9 | 1.9 |
| Other diseases of intestines (K55-K63) | 24 | 25 | 26 | 28 | 1.7 | 1.6 | 1.6 | 1.7 |
| Other diseases of the urinary system (N30-N39) | 18 | 22 | 25 | 27 | 1.3 | 1.4 | 1.5 | 1.6 |
| Injuries to the head (S00-S09) | 20 | 23 | 25 | 27 | 1.4 | 1.5 | 1.5 | 1.6 |
| Other infections and disorders of the skin (L00-L14, L55-L99) | 22 | 25 | 26 | 27 | 1.5 | 1.6 | 1.6 | 1.6 |
| Disorders of gall bladder, biliary tract and pancreas (K80-K87) | 20 | 23 | 23 | 24 | 1.4 | 1.5 | 1.4 | 1.4 |
| Diseases of male genital organs (N40-N51)[4] | 24 | 23 | 23 | 23 | 0.8 | 0.7 | 0.7 | 0.7 |
| Complications of surgical and medical care nec (T80-T88) | 19 | 21 | 22 | 23 | 1.3 | 1.3 | 1.3 | 1.4 |
| Unknown and unspecified causes of morbidity (R69) | 30 | 40 | 35 | 23 | 2.1 | 2.5 | 2.1 | 1.3 |
| Influenza and pneumonia (J10-J18) | 14 | 19 | 21 | 22 | 1.0 | 1.2 | 1.3 | 1.3 |
| Other acute lower respiratory infections (J20-J22) | 18 | 20 | 21 | 22 | 1.3 | 1.3 | 1.3 | 1.3 |
| Poisonings by drugs medicaments and biological substances (T36-T50) | 16 | 17 | 19 | 22 | 1.1 | 1.1 | 1.2 | 1.3 |
| Acute upper respiratory infections (J00-J06) | 15 | 18 | 16 | 21 | 1.1 | 1.1 | 1.0 | 1.2 |
| Soft tissue disorders (M60-M79) | 15 | 18 | 19 | 21 | 1.0 | 1.1 | 1.2 | 1.2 |
| Cerebrovascular diseases (I60-I69) | 18 | 20 | 21 | 21 | 1.3 | 1.3 | 1.3 | 1.2 |
| Malignant neoplasm of digestive organs (C15-C26) | 18 | 19 | 19 | 19 | 1.3 | 1.2 | 1.2 | 1.1 |
| Other diseases of upper respiratory tract (J30-J39) | 21 | 21 | 20 | 17 | 1.5 | 1.3 | 1.2 | 1.0 |
| In situ and benign neoplasms and others of uncertainty (D00-D48) | 17 | 17 | 16 | 17 | 1.2 | 1.1 | 1.0 | 1.0 |
| Noninfective enteritis and colitis (K50-K52) | 13 | 14 | 16 | 17 | 0.9 | 0.9 | 1.0 | 1.0 |
| Dorsopathies (M40-M54) | 12 | 13 | 15 | 17 | 0.8 | 0.8 | 0.9 | 1.0 |
| Injuries to the hip and thigh (S70-S79) | 14 | 15 | 16 | 17 | 0.9 | 1.0 | 1.0 | 1.0 |
| Epilepsy migraine and other episodic disorders (G40-G47) | 12 | 15 | 15 | 16 | 0.8 | 0.9 | 0.9 | 1.0 |
| Hernia (K40-K46) | 15 | 15 | 15 | 15 | 1.1 | 1.0 | 0.9 | 0.9 |
| Diseases of oesophagus, stomach and duodenum (K20-K31) | 13 | 13 | 13 | 14 | 0.9 | 0.8 | 0.8 | 0.8 |

*Notes*:   Figures exclude reproduction, pregnancy and childbirth diagnoses.
Data for 2004/05 and 2005/06 have not been adjusted to take into account shortfalls in the number of records received or for missing/invalid clinical data.
1 Estimated Ordinary admissions, excluding day cases.
2 Per 10,000 female population aged 15-44.
3 Per 10,000 female population.
4 Per 10,000 male population.
nec = not elsewhere classified.
*Sources*:   Hospital Episode Statistics (DH).
Population Projections Database (GAD).

Table 3.26   Inpatient[1] bed days and lengths of stay by top major diagnostic group, England, 2000/01 - 2005/06

| Major diagnosis (ICD10) | Bed days per 10,000 population | | | | Mean length of stay (days) | | | |
|---|---|---|---|---|---|---|---|---|
| | 00/01 | 03/04 | 04/05 | 05/06 | 00/01 | 03/04 | 04/05 | 05/06 |
| Complications of labour and delivery (O10-O75, O85-O92, O95-O99)[2] | 1,597 | 1,656 | 1,645 | 1,650 | 2.0 | 1.9 | 1.8 | 1.7 |
| Health services in circumstances related to reproduction (Z30-Z39) | 154 | 160 | 159 | 153 | 1.8 | 1.6 | 1.4 | 1.3 |
| Delivery (O80-O84)[2] | 196 | 195 | 180 | 170 | 2.1 | 1.9 | 1.8 | 1.7 |
| Pregnancy with abortive outcome (O00-O08)[2] | 92 | 91 | 93 | 86 | 1.1 | 1.1 | 1.2 | 1.0 |
| Symptoms and signs involving the circulatory/respiratory system (R00-R09) | 153 | 153 | 154 | 147 | 3.2 | 2.7 | 2.4 | 2.2 |
| Symptoms and signs involving the digestive system and abdomen (R10-R19) | 160 | 161 | 163 | 156 | 3.5 | 3.4 | 3.1 | 2.8 |
| Ischaemic heart diseases (I20-I25) | 346 | 369 | 365 | 334 | 6.8 | 7.2 | 7.1 | 6.6 |
| Arthropathies (M00-M25) | 287 | 309 | 303 | 291 | 7.4 | 6.6 | 6.3 | 5.9 |
| General symptoms and signs (R50-R68) | 236 | 263 | 261 | 250 | 6.8 | 6.6 | 5.8 | 5.1 |
| Noninflammatory disorders of female genital tract (N80-N98)[3] | 156 | 139 | 130 | 128 | 3.2 | 3.0 | 2.9 | 2.8 |
| Other forms of heart disease (I30-I52) | 351 | 349 | 346 | 332 | 9.9 | 9.6 | 9.3 | 8.6 |
| Chronic lower respiratory diseases (J40-J47) | 246 | 274 | 263 | 247 | 7.8 | 7.6 | 7.0 | 6.9 |
| Other conditions originating in the perinatal period (P05-P96) | 183 | 199 | 205 | 209 | 6.7 | 6.8 | 6.7 | 6.5 |
| Other diseases of intestines (K55-K63) | 164 | 180 | 184 | 184 | 6.8 | 7.1 | 7.0 | 6.5 |
| Other diseases of the urinary system (N30-N39) | 156 | 203 | 219 | 232 | 8.5 | 9.2 | 8.9 | 8.6 |
| Injuries to the head (S00-S09) | 65 | 85 | 85 | 86 | 3.2 | 3.7 | 3.4 | 3.2 |
| Other infections and disorders of the skin (L00-L14, L55-L99) | 176 | 198 | 192 | 188 | 8.1 | 7.8 | 7.5 | 7.1 |
| Disorders of gall bladder, biliary tract and pancreas (K80-K87) | 128 | 138 | 142 | 141 | 6.3 | 6.0 | 6.1 | 5.8 |
| Diseases of male genital organs (N40-N51)[4] | 83 | 76 | 71 | 66 | 3.5 | 3.3 | 3.1 | 2.8 |
| Complications of surgical and medical care nec (T80-T88) | 161 | 181 | 189 | 186 | 8.6 | 8.6 | 8.6 | 8.0 |
| Unknown and unspecified causes of morbidity (R69) | 623 | 638 | 558 | 464 | 20.9 | 16.1 | 16.0 | 20.5 |
| Influenza and pneumonia (J10-J18) | 181 | 250 | 253 | 259 | 13.2 | 12.9 | 12.3 | 11.5 |
| Other acute lower respiratory infections (J20-J22) | 147 | 164 | 155 | 154 | 8.0 | 8.2 | 7.4 | 6.9 |
| Poisonings by drugs medicaments and biological substances (T36-T50) | 29 | 31 | 31 | 33 | 1.8 | 1.8 | 1.6 | 1.5 |
| Acute upper respiratory infections (J00-J06) | 22 | 21 | 19 | 21 | 1.4 | 1.2 | 1.2 | 1.0 |
| Soft tissue disorders (M60-M79) | 44 | 47 | 46 | 46 | 2.9 | 2.6 | 2.4 | 2.2 |
| Cerebrovascular diseases (I60-I69) | 481 | 529 | 516 | 501 | 26.4 | 26.1 | 25.0 | 24.2 |
| Malignant neoplasm of digestive organs (C15-C26) | 212 | 212 | 211 | 210 | 11.6 | 11.3 | 11.2 | 10.8 |
| Other diseases of upper respiratory tract (J30-J39) | 30 | 29 | 28 | 24 | 1.4 | 1.4 | 1.4 | 1.4 |
| In situ and benign neoplasms and others of uncertainty (D00-D48) | 92 | 91 | 86 | 85 | 5.4 | 5.4 | 5.3 | 5.0 |
| Noninfective enteritis and colitis (K50-K52) | 80 | 91 | 97 | 99 | 6.4 | 6.4 | 6.0 | 5.8 |
| Dorsopathies (M40-M54) | 88 | 93 | 98 | 99 | 7.3 | 7.0 | 6.7 | 5.9 |
| Injuries to the hip and thigh (S70-S79) | 295 | 374 | 377 | 376 | 21.6 | 24.2 | 23.8 | 22.8 |
| Epilepsy migraine and other episodic disorders (G40-G47) | 72 | 70 | 68 | 68 | 6.0 | 4.8 | 4.5 | 4.2 |
| Hernia (K40-K46) | 49 | 51 | 49 | 46 | 3.2 | 3.3 | 3.3 | 3.1 |
| Diseases of oesophagus, stomach and duodenum (K20-K31) | 99 | 97 | 94 | 93 | 7.5 | 7.6 | 7.1 | 6.5 |
| Injuries to the wrist and hand (S60-S69) | 19 | 20 | 21 | 20 | 1.6 | 1.6 | 1.6 | 1.5 |
| Congenital malformations (Q00-Q89) | 53 | 55 | 55 | 57 | 4.4 | 4.1 | 4.7 | 4.2 |

*Notes:*   Figures exclude reproduction, pregnancy and childbirth diagnoses.
Finished consultant episode data for 2004/05 and 2005/06 have not been adjusted to take into account shortfalls in the number of records received or for missing/invalid clinical data.
The mean length of stay is the duration of the spell in days. Where the spell is a period of continuous admitted patient care within a particular NHS trust, calculated by subtracting the admission date from the discharge date.
1 Ordinary admission.
2 Per 10,000 female population aged 15-44.
3 Per 10,000 female population.
4 Per 10,000 male population.
nec = not elsewhere classified.
*Sources:*   Hospital Episode Statistics (IC).
Population Projections Database (GAD).

Table 3.27 **Number[1] and rate of surgical operations by main site, England, 1995/96 - 2005/06**

Thousands

| | Year | | | | | | | |
|---|---|---|---|---|---|---|---|---|
| | 1995/96 | 1998/99 | 2000/01 | 2001/02 | 2002/03 | 2003/04 | 2004/05 | 2005/06 |
| **Total operations** | **5,994** | **6,468** | **6,509** | **6,444** | **6,632** | **6,712** | **6,848** | **7,215** |
| Nervous system | 167 | 196 | 202 | 206 | 211 | 214 | 223 | 230 |
| Endocrine system and breast | 93 | 92 | 90 | 88 | 91 | 91 | 93 | 98 |
| Eye | 325 | 382 | 411 | 412 | 431 | 457 | 469 | 464 |
| Ear | 112 | 105 | 95 | 90 | 90 | 85 | 84 | 86 |
| Respiratory tract | 210 | 210 | 206 | 193 | 196 | 189 | 188 | 195 |
| Mouth | 288 | 272 | 235 | 235 | 244 | 241 | 245 | 263 |
| Upper digestive tract | 515 | 566 | 562 | 538 | 532 | 513 | 497 | 512 |
| Lower digestive tract | 356 | 439 | 474 | 462 | 481 | 484 | 500 | 557 |
| Other abdominal organs[2] | 92 | 95 | 97 | 99 | 103 | 106 | 106 | 113 |
| Heart | 151 | 175 | 195 | 210 | 228 | 248 | 265 | 283 |
| Arteries and veins | 187 | 191 | 183 | 178 | 182 | 180 | 177 | 186 |
| Urinary | 493 | 515 | 525 | 517 | 532 | 526 | 529 | 570 |
| Male genital organs | 124 | 110 | 97 | 94 | 97 | 94 | 88 | 88 |
| Lower female genital tract | 81 | 78 | 74 | 63 | 64 | 58 | 58 | 59 |
| Upper female genital tract | 524 | 480 | 434 | 407 | 399 | 385 | 370 | 393 |
| Female genital tract[3] | 594 | 558 | 527 | 532 | 544 | 567 | 582 | 597 |
| Skin | 300 | 316 | 316 | 308 | 318 | 315 | 314 | 331 |
| Soft tissue | 309 | 307 | 306 | 304 | 317 | 320 | 326 | 337 |
| Bones and joints of skull and spine | 65 | 71 | 72 | 74 | 80 | 82 | 87 | 99 |
| Other bones and joints | 499 | 524 | 536 | 543 | 573 | 592 | 612 | 648 |
| Miscellaneous operations | 508 | 787 | 872 | 890 | 922 | 964 | 1,036 | 1,104 |
| **Rate per 10,000 population** | | | | | | | | |
| **Total operations** | **1,238** | **1,307** | **1,321** | **1,302** | **1,334** | **1,344** | **1,364** | **1,428** |
| Nervous system | 35 | 40 | 41 | 42 | 43 | 43 | 44 | 46 |
| Endocrine system and breast | 19 | 19 | 18 | 18 | 18 | 18 | 18 | 19 |
| Eye | 67 | 77 | 83 | 83 | 87 | 92 | 93 | 92 |
| Ear | 23 | 21 | 19 | 18 | 18 | 17 | 17 | 17 |
| Respiratory tract | 43 | 42 | 42 | 39 | 39 | 38 | 37 | 38 |
| Mouth | 60 | 55 | 48 | 48 | 49 | 48 | 49 | 52 |
| Upper digestive tract | 106 | 114 | 114 | 109 | 107 | 103 | 99 | 101 |
| Lower digestive tract | 73 | 89 | 96 | 93 | 97 | 97 | 100 | 110 |
| Other abdominal organs[2] | 19 | 19 | 20 | 20 | 21 | 21 | 21 | 22 |
| Heart | 31 | 35 | 40 | 42 | 46 | 50 | 53 | 56 |
| Arteries and veins | 39 | 39 | 37 | 36 | 37 | 36 | 35 | 37 |
| Urinary | 102 | 104 | 107 | 104 | 107 | 105 | 105 | 113 |
| Male genital organs[4] | 53 | 45 | 40 | 39 | 40 | 38 | 36 | 36 |
| Lower female genital tract[5] | 33 | 31 | 29 | 25 | 25 | 23 | 23 | 23 |
| Upper female genital tract[5] | 211 | 191 | 172 | 161 | 157 | 151 | 145 | 153 |
| Female genital tract[3] | 586 | 547 | 514 | 517 | 526 | 547 | 558 | 568 |
| Skin | 62 | 64 | 64 | 62 | 64 | 63 | 63 | 65 |
| Soft tissue | 64 | 62 | 62 | 61 | 64 | 64 | 65 | 67 |
| Bones and joints of skull and spine | 13 | 14 | 15 | 15 | 16 | 17 | 17 | 20 |
| Other bones and joints | 103 | 106 | 109 | 110 | 115 | 119 | 122 | 128 |
| Miscellaneous operations | 105 | 159 | 177 | 180 | 185 | 193 | 206 | 218 |

*Notes:* All figures are based on OPCS 4th Revision operation codes and include ordinary admissions and day cases.
Data for 1997/98 are not available.
FCE data for 2004/05 and 2005/06 have not been adjusted to take into account shortfalls in the number of records received or for missing/invalid clinical data.
1 Relates to the number of episodes in which the procedure is recorded as the main operation (usually the most resources intensive operation performed during the episode).
2 Principally digestive.
3 Figures relate to operations associated with pregnancy, childbirth and puerperium. Rate is per 10,000 females aged 15-44.
4 Rates per 10,000 male population.
5 Rates per 10,000 female population.

*Sources:* Hospital Episode Statistics (IC).
Population Projections Database (GAD).

Table 3.28   **Number[1] and rate of NHS hospital surgical operations by site and age, England, 2005/06**
Thousands

| | Age group | | | | |
|---|---|---|---|---|---|
| | All ages[2] | 0-14 | 15-59 | 60-74 | >=75 |
| **All operations** | **7,215** | **449** | **3,684** | **1,774** | **1,287** |
| Nervous system | 230 | 18 | 134 | 51 | 28 |
| Endocrine system and breast | 98 | 1 | 65 | 24 | 8 |
| Eye | 464 | 17 | 89 | 144 | 215 |
| Ear | 86 | 41 | 30 | 9 | 6 |
| Respiratory tract | 195 | 18 | 92 | 53 | 32 |
| Mouth | 263 | 90 | 145 | 19 | 9 |
| Upper digestive tract | 512 | 12 | 219 | 156 | 125 |
| Lower digestive tract | 557 | 16 | 283 | 156 | 102 |
| Other abdominal organs[3] | 113 | 1 | 58 | 33 | 21 |
| Heart | 283 | 4 | 93 | 125 | 61 |
| Arteries and veins | 186 | 9 | 81 | 60 | 36 |
| Urinary | 570 | 9 | 174 | 204 | 183 |
| Male genital organs | 88 | 23 | 54 | 8 | 4 |
| Lower female genital tract | 59 | 1 | 36 | 15 | 6 |
| Upper female genital tract | 393 | 1 | 337 | 26 | 13 |
| Female genital tract[4] | 597 | - | 595 | - | - |
| Skin | 331 | 31 | 190 | 59 | 51 |
| Soft tissue | 337 | 21 | 181 | 85 | 50 |
| Bones and joints of skull and spine | 99 | 4 | 65 | 20 | 9 |
| Other bones and joints | 648 | 48 | 299 | 167 | 133 |
| Miscellaneous operations | 1,104 | 85 | 462 | 360 | 196 |

**Hospital surgical operations by site and age per 10,000 population, England, 2005/06**

| | All ages[2] | 0-14 | 15-59 | 60-74 | >=75 |
|---|---|---|---|---|---|
| **All operations** | **1,428** | **496** | **1,197** | **2,606** | **3,319** |
| Nervous system | 46 | 20 | 44 | 75 | 71 |
| Endocrine system and breast | 19 | 1 | 21 | 35 | 21 |
| Eye | 92 | 19 | 29 | 211 | 554 |
| Ear | 17 | 45 | 10 | 13 | 17 |
| Respiratory tract | 38 | 20 | 30 | 77 | 83 |
| Mouth | 52 | 99 | 47 | 28 | 22 |
| Upper digestive tract | 101 | 13 | 71 | 229 | 321 |
| Lower digestive tract | 110 | 17 | 92 | 230 | 264 |
| Other abdominal organs[3] | 22 | 1 | 19 | 49 | 53 |
| Heart | 56 | 5 | 30 | 184 | 157 |
| Arteries and veins | 37 | 10 | 26 | 88 | 93 |
| Urinary | 113 | 10 | 57 | 299 | 473 |
| Male genital organs[5] | 36 | 49 | 35 | 23 | 24 |
| Lower female genital tract[6] | 23 | 2 | 23 | 43 | 27 |
| Upper female genital tract[6] | 153 | 2 | 219 | 75 | 53 |
| Female genital tract[4] | 232 | - | 387 | | - |
| Skin | 65 | 34 | 62 | 87 | 131 |
| Soft tissue | 67 | 23 | 59 | 125 | 128 |
| Bones and joints of skull and spine | 20 | 4 | 21 | 30 | 24 |
| Other bones and joints | 128 | 53 | 97 | 246 | 343 |
| Miscellaneous operations | 218 | 94 | 150 | 529 | 505 |

*Notes:*   All figures are based on OPCS 4th Revision operation codes.
FCE data for 2004/05 and 2005/06 have not been adjusted to take into account shortfalls in the number of records received or for missing/invalid clinical data.
1 Relates to the number of episodes in which the procedure is recorded as the main operation (usually the most resources intensive operation performed during the episode).
2 Figures by age group may not add up to total due operation with unknown age.
3 Principally digestive.
4 Figures relate to operations associated with pregnancy, childbirth and puerperium.  These figures may differ from those shown in Table 3.27 due to differences in the denominator.
5 Rates per 10,000 male population.
6 Rates per 10,000 female population.                           - Not applicable.
*Sources:* Hospital Episode Statistics (IC).
Population Projections Database (GAD).

Table 3.29 **Number[1] and rate of most frequent surgical operations, England, 2000/01 - 2005/06**

| | Number of operations ('000's) | | | | Operations per 10,000 population | | | |
|---|---|---|---|---|---|---|---|---|
| | 00/01 | 03/04 | 04/05 | 05/06 | 00/01 | 03/04 | 04/05 | 05/06 |
| **All operations (OPCS-4)** | **6,509** | **6,721** | **6,848** | **7,215** | **1,321** | **1,346** | **1,364** | **1,428** |
| Endoscopic operations on upper gastrointestinal tract (G43-G45 | 503 | 458 | 441 | 453 | 102 | 92 | 88 | 90 |
| Endoscopic operations on colon (H20-H28) | 305 | 316 | 330 | 381 | 62 | 63 | 66 | 75 |
| Normal delivery (R24)[2] | 325 | 355 | 361 | 369 | 317 | 342 | 346 | 351 |
| Operations for the removal of cataract (C71-C72,C74,C75) | 238 | 298 | 306 | 287 | 48 | 60 | 61 | 57 |
| Endoscopic operations on bladder (M42-M45) | 273 | 263 | 260 | 282 | 55 | 53 | 52 | 56 |
| Extirpation of lesion of skin or subcutaneous tissue (S05-S11) | 176 | 179 | 175 | 185 | 36 | 36 | 35 | 37 |
| Reduction of fracture of bone (W19-W26) | 130 | 135 | 137 | 142 | 26 | 27 | 27 | 28 |
| Caesarean delivery (R17-R18)[2] | 112 | 128 | 132 | 139 | 109 | 123 | 126 | 132 |
| Endoscopic operations on joint (W82-W88) | 98 | 112 | 117 | 122 | 20 | 22 | 23 | 24 |
| Evacuation of contents of uterus (Q10-Q11)[3] | 128 | 103 | 97 | 95 | 51 | 40 | 38 | 37 |
| Operations on inguinal hernia (T19-T21) | 80 | 81 | 80 | 80 | 16 | 16 | 16 | 16 |
| Surgical removal of tooth (F09) | 69 | 65 | 67 | 73 | 14 | 13 | 13 | 14 |
| Compensation for renal failure (X40-X42) | 23 | 40 | 68 | 72 | 5 | 8 | 14 | 14 |
| Manipulative delivery (R19-R23)[2] | 61 | 63 | 66 | 68 | 59 | 60 | 64 | 65 |
| Simple extraction of tooth (F10) | 52 | 61 | 62 | 68 | 11 | 12 | 12 | 13 |
| Total prosthetic replacement of other joint (W40-W45) | 38 | 56 | 60 | 63 | 8 | 11 | 12 | 13 |
| Total prosthetic replacement of hip joint (W37-W39) | 48 | 58 | 59 | 61 | 10 | 12 | 12 | 12 |
| Excision of breast (B27-B28)[3] | 52 | 52 | 53 | 56 | 21 | 20 | 21 | 22 |
| Transluminal operations on coronary artery (K49-K51) | 25 | 41 | 50 | 55 | 5 | 8 | 10 | 11 |
| Heart operations (K49-K50) | 25 | 41 | 50 | 55 | 5 | 8 | 10 | 11 |
| Excision of gall bladder (J18) | 40 | 49 | 48 | 51 | 8 | 10 | 10 | 10 |
| Excision of tonsil (F34) | 46 | 51 | 51 | 51 | 9 | 10 | 10 | 10 |
| Release of entrapment of peripheral nerve at wrist (A65) | 38 | 47 | 50 | 50 | 8 | 9 | 10 | 10 |
| Endoscopic operations on bronchus (E48-E51) | 53 | 47 | 46 | 48 | 11 | 9 | 9 | 10 |
| Operations on cervix uteri (Q01-Q05)[3] | 56 | 39 | 35 | 39 | 22 | 15 | 14 | 15 |
| Excision of uterus (Q07-Q08)[3] | 47 | 40 | 38 | 39 | 19 | 16 | 15 | 15 |
| Operations on varicose vein of leg (L85-L87) | 45 | 42 | 38 | 37 | 9 | 9 | 8 | 7 |
| Operations on other abdominal hernia (T22-T27) | 28 | 33 | 33 | 36 | 6 | 7 | 7 | 7 |
| Endoscopic operations on peritoneum (T42-T43) | 43 | 38 | 37 | 35 | 9 | 8 | 7 | 7 |
| Drainage of middle ear (D15) | 44 | 36 | 34 | 35 | 9 | 7 | 7 | 7 |
| Endoscopic operations on bile and pancreatic ducts (J38-J45) | 34 | 31 | 32 | 34 | 7 | 6 | 6 | 7 |
| Incision of skin or subcutaneous tissue (S47) | 25 | 28 | 29 | 31 | 5 | 6 | 6 | 6 |
| Operations on prepuce (N30)[4] | 26 | 28 | 28 | 29 | 11 | 12 | 11 | 12 |
| Endoscopic operations on outlet of male bladder (M65-M67)[4] | 34 | 31 | 29 | 28 | 14 | 13 | 12 | 11 |
| Endoscopic operations on ureter (M26-M30) | 21 | 24 | 25 | 27 | 4 | 5 | 5 | 5 |
| Operations on haemorrhoid (H51-H53) | 26 | 24 | 23 | 25 | 5 | 5 | 5 | 5 |
| Prosthetic replacement of head of femur (W46-W48) | 23 | 24 | 24 | 24 | 5 | 5 | 5 | 5 |
| Operations on septum of nose (E03) | 26 | 24 | 23 | 23 | 5 | 5 | 5 | 5 |
| Repair of prolapse of vagina (P22-P23)[3] | 19 | 20 | 21 | 22 | 7 | 8 | 8 | 9 |
| Heart operations (K40-K46) | 23 | 23 | 23 | 21 | 5 | 5 | 5 | 4 |
| Suture of skin or subcutaneous tissue (S41-S42) | 12 | 16 | 18 | 21 | 3 | 3 | 4 | 4 |
| Excision of vas deferens (N17)[4] | 31 | 27 | 22 | 20 | 13 | 11 | 9 | 8 |
| Excision of colon (H04-H11) | 19 | 19 | 19 | 20 | 4 | 4 | 4 | 4 |
| Endoscopic operations on larynx (E34-E36) | 22 | 19 | 19 | 20 | 4 | 4 | 4 | 4 |
| Endoscopic occlusion of fallopian tube (Q35-Q36)[3] | 35 | 24 | 20 | 18 | 14 | 9 | 8 | 7 |
| Other bypass of coronary artery (K45-K46) | 11 | 15 | 17 | 17 | 2 | 3 | 3 | 3 |
| Excision of adnexa of uterus (Q22-Q24)[3] | 14 | 14 | 15 | 16 | 5 | 6 | 6 | 6 |

*Notes:* All figures are based on OPCS 4th Revision operation codes.
Operation groups are not mutually exclusive. As such the same operation may be included in more than one category.
FCE data for 2004/05 and 2005/06 have not been adjusted to take into account shortfalls in the number of records received or for missing/invalid clinical data.
1 Relates to the number of episodes in which the procedure is recorded as the main operation (usually the most resources intensive operation performed during the episode).
2 Rates per 10,000 female population aged 15-44.
3 Rates per 10,000 female population.
4 Rates per 10,000 male population.
*Sources:* Hospital Episode Statistics (IC).
Population Projections Database (GAD).

Table 3.30  **Patients waiting for elective admission, by selected specialties, England, 1997 - 2007**

**Ordinary admissions and day cases combined**

**Thousands waiting**

| 31st March | 1997 | 1998 | 1999 | 2000 | 2001 | 2002 | 2003 | 2004 | 2005 | 2006 | 2007 |
|---|---|---|---|---|---|---|---|---|---|---|---|
| **All specialties** | **1,158** | **1,298** | **1,073** | **1,037** | **1,007** | **1,035** | **992** | **906** | **822** | **785** | **701** |
| General surgery | 230 | 251 | 201 | 194 | 185 | 188 | 174 | 153 | 145 | 133 | 111 |
| Urology | 85 | 89 | 71 | 73 | 71 | 71 | 68 | 65 | 63 | 60 | 52 |
| Trauma and orthopaedics | 220 | 261 | 231 | 237 | 241 | 259 | 254 | 241 | 216 | 200 | 175 |
| ENT | 127 | 138 | 112 | 101 | 103 | 108 | 96 | 85 | 72 | 68 | 55 |
| Ophthalmology | 146 | 170 | 150 | 152 | 148 | 145 | 138 | 100 | 69 | 69 | 70 |
| Oral surgery | 59 | 62 | 46 | 38 | 33 | 35 | 38 | 41 | 43 | 40 | 39 |
| Plastic surgery | 47 | 49 | 40 | 40 | 40 | 44 | 42 | 37 | 36 | 33 | 26 |
| Gynaecology | 112 | 128 | 105 | 92 | 84 | 86 | 80 | 76 | 73 | 68 | 59 |
| Others | 132 | 151 | 120 | 112 | 102 | 99 | 101 | 108 | 106 | 113 | 113 |

**Per cent[1]** — **Ordinary admissions**

| | 1997 | 1998 | 1999 | 2000 | 2001 | 2002 | 2003 | 2004 | 2005 | 2006 | 2007 |
|---|---|---|---|---|---|---|---|---|---|---|---|
| **All specialties** | **49%** | **46%** | **47%** | **48%** | **48%** | **48%** | **46%** | **43%** | **43%** | **39%** | **35%** |
| General surgery | 49% | 46% | 48% | 50% | 51% | 51% | 49% | 46% | 45% | 41% | 37% |
| Urology | 45% | 42% | 44% | 48% | 49% | 49% | 46% | 43% | 42% | 38% | 38% |
| Trauma and orthopaedics | 60% | 60% | 62% | 64% | 64% | 63% | 61% | 59% | 57% | 53% | 51% |
| ENT | 78% | 75% | 76% | 76% | 76% | 74% | 73% | 69% | 65% | 61% | 50% |
| Ophthalmology | 33% | 24% | 19% | 14% | 10% | 8% | 7% | 6% | 7% | 6% | 5% |
| Oral surgery | 31% | 27% | 25% | 25% | 25% | 22% | 19% | 16% | 15% | 13% | 9% |
| Plastic surgery | 43% | 42% | 44% | 47% | 47% | 44% | 43% | 40% | 42% | 38% | 34% |
| Gynaecology | 45% | 42% | 46% | 47% | 47% | 49% | 48% | 44% | 44% | 42% | 40% |
| Others | 37% | 32% | 34% | 39% | 41% | 40% | 35% | 31% | 29% | 26% | 24% |

**Per cent[2]** — **Day cases**

| | 1997 | 1998 | 1999 | 2000 | 2001 | 2002 | 2003 | 2004 | 2005 | 2006 | 2007 |
|---|---|---|---|---|---|---|---|---|---|---|---|
| **All specialties** | **51%** | **54%** | **53%** | **52%** | **52%** | **52%** | **54%** | **57%** | **57%** | **61%** | **65%** |
| General surgery | 51% | 54% | 52% | 50% | 49% | 49% | 51% | 54% | 55% | 59% | 63% |
| Urology | 55% | 58% | 56% | 52% | 51% | 51% | 54% | 57% | 58% | 62% | 62% |
| Trauma and orthopaedics | 40% | 40% | 38% | 36% | 36% | 37% | 39% | 41% | 43% | 47% | 49% |
| ENT | 22% | 25% | 24% | 24% | 24% | 26% | 27% | 31% | 35% | 39% | 50% |
| Ophthalmology | 67% | 76% | 81% | 86% | 90% | 92% | 93% | 94% | 93% | 94% | 95% |
| Oral surgery | 69% | 73% | 75% | 75% | 75% | 78% | 81% | 84% | 85% | 87% | 91% |
| Plastic surgery | 57% | 58% | 56% | 53% | 53% | 56% | 57% | 60% | 58% | 62% | 66% |
| Gynaecology | 55% | 58% | 54% | 53% | 53% | 51% | 52% | 56% | 56% | 58% | 60% |
| Others | 63% | 68% | 66% | 61% | 59% | 60% | 65% | 69% | 71% | 74% | 76% |

*Notes:* Data relates to information on patients waiting to be admitted to NHS hospitals in England either as a day case or ordinary admission.  It does not include: patients admitted as emergency cases; outpatients; patients undergoing a planned programme of treatment e.g. a series of admissions for chemotherapy; expectant mothers booked for confinement; patients already in hospital; patients who are temporarily suspended from waiting lists for social reasons or because they are known to be not medically ready for treatment.
1 Relates to the percentage of people waiting for an ordinary admission.
2 Relates to the percentage of people waiting to be admitted as a day case.

*Source:* Elective admissions and patients waiting: England (DH).

Figure 3.10  **Patients waiting for elective admission, England, 1992 - 2007**

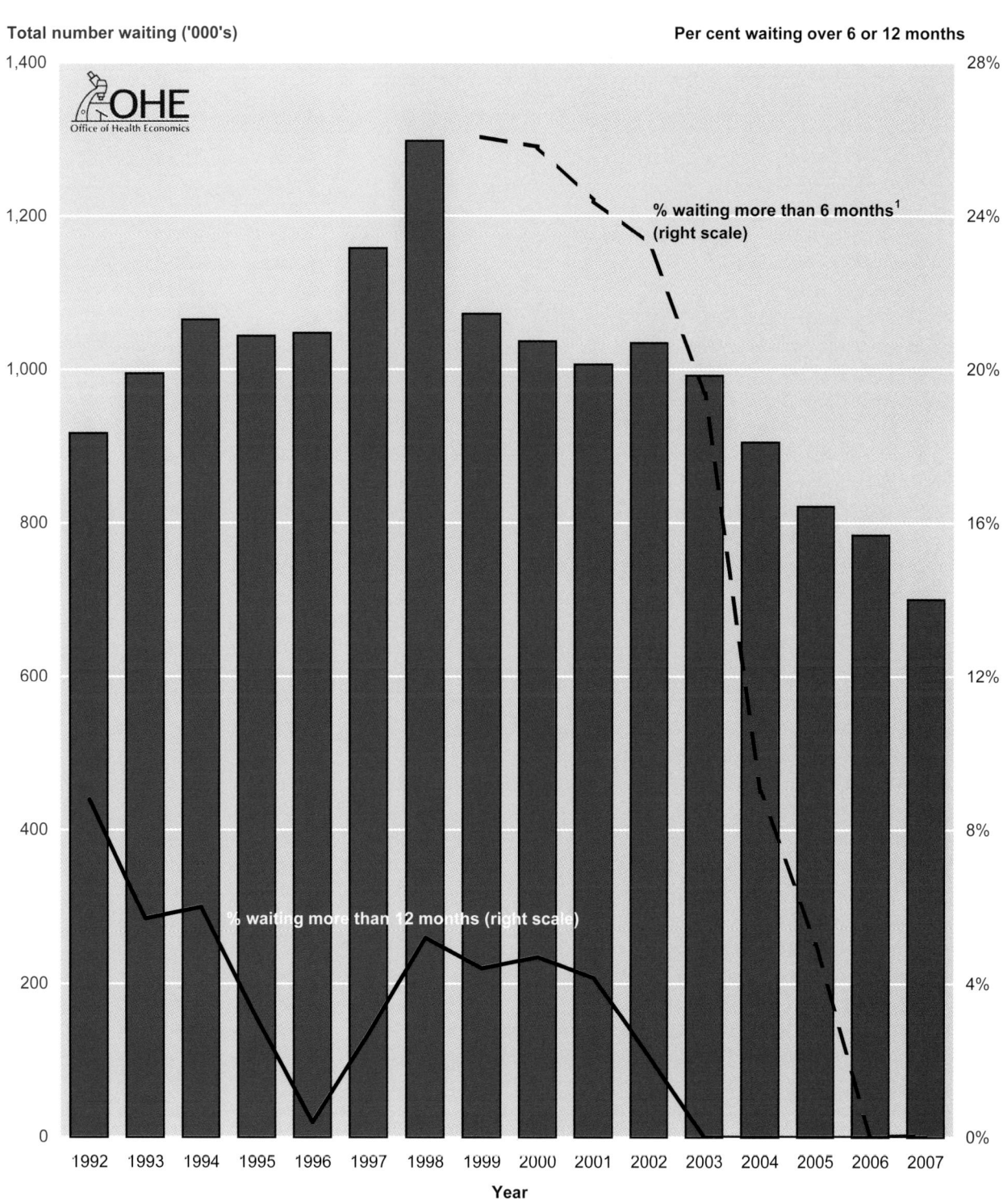

**Total number waiting ('000's)**

**Per cent waiting over 6 or 12 months**

% waiting more than 6 months[1]
(right scale)

% waiting more than 12 months (right scale)

*Notes:*   Figures relate to 31 March.
1 Data on 6 months waiting time were not available prior to 1999.
Total number waiting includes private patients waiting for NHS beds. Whereas per cent waiting 12+ months and 6+ months excludes private patients waiting for NHS beds (both from the numerator and denominator).
*Source:*   Elective admissions and patients waiting: England (DH).

Table 3.31   **Top 50 Healthcare Resource Groups (HRGs) with high mean waiting times, number of admissions and percentage admitted from waiting list, England, 2005/06**

| HRG code | Healthcare Resource Group | Admissions[1] | % Admitted from waiting list[2] | Mean waiting time (days)[3] |
|---|---|---|---|---|
| T05 | Mania without Section | 6,286 | 5% | 630 |
| T03 | Schizophreniform Psychoses without Section | 25,780 | 6% | 346 |
| D01 | Lung Transplant | 94 | 41% | 330 |
| E01 | Heart and Lung Transplant | 5 | 60% | 213 |
| H03 | Bilateral Primary Knee Replacement | 941 | 97% | 203 |
| H07 | Primary or Revisional Shoulder, Elbow, or Ankle Replacements | 3,846 | 94% | 181 |
| H04 | Primary Knee Replacement | 54,945 | 96% | 180 |
| H70 | Resurfacing of Hip | 3,235 | 97% | 178 |
| H12 | Foot Procedures - Category 2 | 20,940 | 96% | 176 |
| H01 | Bilateral Primary Hip Replacement | 323 | 95% | 172 |
| H08 | Joint Replacements or Revisions, Site Unspecified | 3,784 | 93% | 168 |
| H09 | Anterior Cruciate Ligament Reconstruction | 1,931 | 95% | 167 |
| R10 | Surgery for Scoliosis or Other Spinal Deformity | 1,147 | 79% | 167 |
| H80 | Primary Hip Replacement Cemented | 34,134 | 95% | 165 |
| H14 | Hand Procedures - Category 2 | 16,886 | 95% | 163 |
| H81 | Primary Hip Replacement Uncemented | 11,183 | 95% | 162 |
| J50 | Other Major Breast Surgery | 7,827 | 98% | 162 |
| L66 | Urethra Major Open Procedure - Paediatric | 2,459 | 69% | 158 |
| H18 | Soft Tissue or Other Bone Procedures - Category 2 >69 or w cc | 8,157 | 69% | 152 |
| H15 | Hand Procedures - Category 3 | 537 | 90% | 148 |
| J32 | Intermediate Skin Procedures | 3,220 | 86% | 148 |
| C32 | Major Nose Procedures | 19,344 | 87% | 147 |
| Q11 | Varicose Vein Procedures | 37,068 | 92% | 146 |
| H21 | Muscle, Tendon or Ligament Procedures - Category 2 | 8,846 | 81% | 145 |
| L26 | Bladder Neck Open Procedures Female | 1,161 | 96% | 144 |
| H71 | Revisional Procedures to Hips | 13,310 | 51% | 142 |
| C21 | Intermediate Ear Procedures | 5,884 | 94% | 141 |
| E02 | Heart Transplant | 84 | 52% | 140 |
| H11 | Foot Procedures - Category 1 | 8,182 | 96% | 140 |
| L37 | Penis Major or Intermediate Open Procedures | 1,935 | 89% | 139 |
| C31 | Major Ear Procedures | 18,848 | 95% | 135 |
| H19 | Soft Tissue or Other Bone Procedures - Category 2 <70 w/o cc | 43,852 | 51% | 135 |
| R03 | Decompression and Effusion for Degenerative Spinal Disorders | 12,417 | 83% | 135 |
| M03 | Lower Genital Tract Major Procedures | 33,128 | 98% | 134 |
| F14 | Stomach or Duodenum - Major Procedures <70 or w/o cc | 5,951 | 57% | 133 |
| E38 | Electrophysiological and Other Percutaneous Cardiac Procedures >18 | 12,817 | 66% | 131 |
| H10 | Arthroscopies | 118,570 | 95% | 131 |
| H17 | Soft Tissue or Other Bone Procedures - Category 1 <70 w/o cc | 38,335 | 89% | 131 |
| F72 | Abdominal Hernia Procedures <70 w/o cc | 10,053 | 91% | 128 |
| C22 | Intermediate Nose Procedures | 37,328 | 81% | 127 |
| T07 | Depression without Section | 34,609 | 6% | 126 |

*Notes:*   w/o cc = without complications and co-morbidity.
<70 = under 70 years of age.
FCE data for 2005/06 has not been adjusted to take into account shortfalls in the number of records received or for missing/invalid clinical data. Where the percentage admitted from a waiting list is less than 1%, the data is not shown.
cc = complications and co-morbidities.
1 Total admissions including emergency and elective inpatients and day cases.
2 The percentage admitted from the waiting list refers to elective admissions only, planned admissions are not included.
3 Waiting times relate to admissions from the waiting list, and correspond to the period between the date of the decision to admit and the date of actual admission.  Days of deferment and suspension are not taken into account.

*Source:*   Hospital Episode Statistics (IC).

Table 3.32 **Waiting time for first outpatient appointment by the top 30[1] specialties, England, 31 March 2007**

| Specialty | Number of GP written referral requests seen | Of those written referrals seen, the percentage who waited (in weeks)[2] | | | | Number of patients not yet seen, waiting (in weeks) | | | |
|---|---|---|---|---|---|---|---|---|---|
| | | 0 to <4 | 4 to <8 | 8 to <13 | 13 and over | 0 to <4 | 4 to <8 | 8 to <13 | 13 and over |
| *All specialties* | *1,950,098* | 40% | 30% | 29% | 1% | 580,896 | 309,858 | 77,389 | 1,396 |
| General surgery | 250,781 | 54% | 28% | 18% | 0% | 64,096 | 25,173 | 5,539 | 39 |
| Gynaecology | 188,720 | 52% | 28% | 20% | 1% | 48,128 | 21,321 | 4,396 | 22 |
| Trauma & orthopaedics | 186,538 | 27% | 32% | 39% | 2% | 59,514 | 35,712 | 9,997 | 477 |
| Ophthalmology | 176,376 | 31% | 31% | 36% | 1% | 56,643 | 34,412 | 8,630 | 40 |
| ENT | 169,176 | 31% | 32% | 35% | 1% | 57,410 | 33,388 | 7,949 | 16 |
| Dermatology | 150,621 | 41% | 29% | 29% | 1% | 43,004 | 21,839 | 4,891 | 124 |
| General medicine | 92,796 | 45% | 29% | 25% | 1% | 27,033 | 13,593 | 3,347 | 118 |
| Urology | 83,733 | 39% | 31% | 29% | 1% | 26,426 | 14,084 | 3,677 | 21 |
| Oral surgery | 82,181 | 22% | 30% | 45% | 3% | 30,703 | 21,993 | 6,604 | 41 |
| Cardiology | 77,300 | 46% | 27% | 26% | 1% | 21,124 | 11,408 | 2,807 | 18 |
| Obstetrics | 73,297 | 60% | 33% | 7% | 1% | 12,609 | 3,342 | 551 | - |
| Paediatrics | 67,882 | 44% | 36% | 20% | 0% | 20,995 | 10,006 | 1,950 | 5 |
| Neurology | 52,148 | 22% | 28% | 46% | 4% | 18,746 | 11,834 | 3,666 | 348 |
| Gastroenterology | 39,945 | 31% | 31% | 37% | 1% | 14,885 | 8,368 | 2,194 | 6 |
| Rheumatology | 45,870 | 32% | 37% | 30% | 1% | 14,598 | 7,386 | 1,637 | 5 |
| Thoracic medicine | 22,273 | 52% | 27% | 20% | 1% | 6,418 | 2,845 | 602 | 1 |
| Plastic surgery | 21,174 | 32% | 33% | 32% | 2% | 7,304 | 3,827 | 952 | 102 |
| Geriatric medicine | 19,166 | 68% | 24% | 8% | 0% | 4,166 | 1,148 | 199 | - |
| Orthodontics | 17,838 | 19% | 33% | 45% | 3% | 5,641 | 4,032 | 1,079 | 3 |
| Anaesthetics | 14,623 | 20% | 30% | 47% | 3% | 5,636 | 3,753 | 1,155 | 8 |
| Haematology (clinical) | 14,476 | 58% | 27% | 15% | 0% | 3,608 | 1,188 | 284 | - |
| Endocrinology | 11,431 | 29% | 34% | 35% | 1% | 4,024 | 2,269 | 554 | - |
| Nephrology | 10,595 | 20% | 32% | 46% | 2% | 3,520 | 2,303 | 649 | - |
| Mental illness | 7,844 | 46% | 36% | 18% | 0% | 2,316 | 1,187 | 259 | - |
| Restorative dentistry | 8,642 | 14% | 30% | 52% | 5% | 3,800 | 2,694 | 834 | - |
| Oral & maxillo facial surgery | 9,010 | 32% | 25% | 42% | 1% | 3,233 | 2,085 | 676 | - |
| Paediatric surgery | 6,953 | 34% | 36% | 29% | 1% | 2,312 | 1,190 | 296 | - |
| Old age psychiatry | 6,074 | 63% | 26% | 11% | 0% | 1,205 | 532 | 112 | - |
| Neurosurgery | 6,217 | 23% | 30% | 44% | 4% | 2,151 | 1,462 | 521 | 2 |
| Paediatric dentistry | 4,791 | 18% | 39% | 42% | 1% | 1,771 | 1,318 | 374 | - |

*Notes:* Figures relate to referral to NHS hospitals in England, they include private patients and patients referred from Scotland, Wales and Northern Ireland and overseas as well as NHS patients from England who were referred by a GP whether medical or dental. They exclude patients referred by consultants and other health professionals; self referrals and attendances at 'drop in' clinics; referrals resulting in ward attendances for nursing care; referrals initiated by the consultant in charge of the clinic.
Percentages >0% but <0.5% are displayed as 0%, where the percentage is 0 this is displayed as -.
1 Top 30 as defined by the number of GP written referrals.
2 Effective length of wait from receipt of GP written request to first outpatient appointment.

*Source:* Hospital Activity Statistics: England (DH).

Table 3.33 **Number of hospital day cases by main specialty[1], England, 2000/01 - 2005/06**

| | Numbers of day cases ('000) | | | | | Day cases as a % of FCEs[2] | | | | |
|---|---|---|---|---|---|---|---|---|---|---|
| | 00/01 | 02/03 | 03/04 | 04/05 | 05/06 | 00/01 | 02/03 | 03/04 | 04/05 | 05/06 |
| **All specialties** | **3,620** | **3,714** | **3,757** | **3,848** | **4,113** | **30** | **29** | **29** | **28** | **29** |
| All acute sector | 2,981 | 3,118 | 3,166 | 3,216 | 3,442 | 31 | 31 | 30 | 29 | 30 |
| Acute surgical | 1,848 | 1,924 | 1,935 | 1,941 | 2,066 | 42 | 42 | 41 | 40 | 40 |
| Acute medical | 1,133 | 1,194 | 1,230 | 1,275 | 1,376 | 22 | 21 | 21 | 21 | 21 |
| General surgery | 496 | 488 | 467 | 469 | 499 | 34 | 34 | 32 | 32 | 33 |
| Ophthalmology | 339 | 378 | 408 | 424 | 420 | 78 | 82 | 84 | 85 | 85 |
| Urology | 338 | 353 | 350 | 354 | 387 | 57 | 57 | 56 | 56 | 58 |
| General medicine | 370 | 351 | 350 | 343 | 349 | 17 | 15 | 14 | 13 | 13 |
| Obstetrics, gynaecology & general practice | 384 | 350 | 340 | 323 | 346 | 20 | 18 | 17 | 16 | 17 |
| Trauma and orthopaedics | 212 | 226 | 235 | 248 | 266 | 26 | 26 | 26 | 26 | 27 |
| Haematology (clinical) | 193 | 222 | 227 | 244 | 267 | 77 | 78 | 76 | 77 | 78 |
| Radiotherapy | 193 | 191 | 203 | 211 | 235 | 72 | 73 | 74 | 75 | 76 |
| Gastroenterology | 154 | 178 | 183 | 185 | 216 | 61 | 58 | 57 | 53 | 53 |
| Oral surgery | 138 | 142 | 141 | 131 | 141 | 70 | 72 | 71 | 72 | 73 |
| Medical oncology | 118 | 105 | 107 | 115 | 120 | 69 | 65 | 64 | 65 | 65 |
| Ear, nose and throat | 109 | 103 | 97 | 101 | 108 | 31 | 30 | 29 | 30 | 32 |
| Cardiology | 69 | 88 | 95 | 96 | 103 | 27 | 27 | 26 | 25 | 23 |
| Plastic surgery | 86 | 97 | 96 | 96 | 103 | 45 | 48 | 47 | 46 | 47 |
| Paediatrics | 53 | 60 | 60 | 65 | 67 | 5 | 5 | 5 | 6 | 5 |
| Anaesthetics | 55 | 52 | 47 | 61 | 74 | 70 | 66 | 65 | 75 | 80 |
| Rheumatology | 30 | 41 | 49 | 53 | 57 | 43 | 51 | 56 | 58 | 59 |
| Nephrology | 27 | 33 | 40 | 50 | 58 | 30 | 31 | 32 | 35 | 38 |
| Dermatology | 54 | 48 | 47 | 45 | 52 | 81 | 83 | 82 | 83 | 86 |
| Haematology | 33 | 34 | 31 | 28 | 28 | 72 | 74 | 78 | 81 | 83 |
| Neurology | 19 | 21 | 23 | 24 | 28 | 29 | 32 | 35 | 36 | 39 |
| Paediatric surgery | 18 | 18 | 19 | 20 | 20 | 32 | 33 | 34 | 35 | 36 |
| Thoracic medicine | 17 | 17 | 17 | 18 | 21 | 18 | 17 | 16 | 14 | 13 |
| Geriatric medicine | 13 | 13 | 13 | 12 | 12 | 2 | 2 | 2 | 2 | 2 |
| Endocrinology | 6 | 7 | 7 | 11 | 11 | 31 | 29 | 29 | 31 | 28 |
| Paediatric dentistry | 8 | 9 | 9 | 9 | 10 | 93 | 88 | 90 | 90 | 91 |
| Radiology | 9 | 8 | 8 | 9 | 6 | 76 | 71 | 64 | 62 | 56 |
| Neurosurgery | 4 | 5 | 6 | 7 | 8 | 8 | 10 | 11 | 11 | 12 |
| Accident and emergency | 5 | 4 | 3 | 4 | 4 | 6 | 5 | 2 | 1 | 1 |
| Clinical immunology and allergy | 2 | 2 | 2 | 4 | 5 | 89 | 89 | 89 | 90 | 91 |
| Restorative dentistry | 2 | 2 | 2 | 3 | 3 | 95 | 95 | 96 | 97 | 97 |
| Paediatric neurology | 3 | 3 | 3 | 3 | 3 | 34 | 37 | 35 | 35 | 38 |
| Immunopathology | 1 | 3 | 3 | 2 | 3 | 97 | 96 | 95 | 94 | 91 |
| Palliative medicine | 1 | 2 | 2 | 2 | 3 | 11 | 14 | 21 | 19 | 20 |
| Infectious diseases | 1 | 1 | 1 | 2 | 2 | 7 | 5 | 6 | 7 | 6 |
| Cardiothoracic surgery | 3 | 2 | 2 | 2 | 2 | 4 | 3 | 2 | 3 | 3 |

*Notes:*  All data relate to financial years ending 31 March.
A day case is defined as a patient attending a hospital ward for investigation, treatment or operation under clinical supervision on a planned non-resident basis and who occupies a bed.
FCE data for 2004/05 and 2005/06 have not been adjusted to take into account shortfalls in the number of records received or for missing/invalid clinical data.
Data for 1997/98 are not available.
1 Excluding specialties with one or no day cases in 2005/06.
2 FCEs = finished consultant episodes (ordinary admissions and day cases).

*Source:*  Hospital Episode Statistics (IC).

Table 3.34   **Reference costs per FCE and average length of stay of top 40 Healthcare Resource Groups (HRGs) ranked by total cost, NHS Trusts, elective inpatients, England, 2005/06**

| HRG code | Healthcare Resource Group (HRG) | No. of FCEs | Mean cost[1] (£) | Quartile range[1] (£) | | Average length of stay[2] (days) |
|---|---|---|---|---|---|---|
| | | | | 25% | 75% | |
| H04 | Primary Knee Replacement | 52,378 | 5,843 | 5,017 | 6,522 | 7.4 |
| H80 | Primary Hip Replacement Cemented | 31,247 | 5,521 | 4,475 | 6,484 | 7.9 |
| M07 | Upper Genital Tract Major Procedures | 47,970 | 2,870 | 2,223 | 3,404 | 4.7 |
| E04 | Coronary Bypass | 12,581 | 8,172 | 1,681 | 8,895 | 6.8 |
| C58 | Intermediate Mouth or Throat Procedures | 82,262 | 1,155 | 805 | 1,516 | 1.2 |
| E03 | Cardiac Valve Procedures | 7,009 | 10,612 | 4,644 | 11,777 | 8.9 |
| E15 | Percutaneous Coronary Intervention | 23,218 | 3,093 | 1,540 | 3,750 | 1.5 |
| F32 | Large Intestine - Very Major Procedures | 12,829 | 5,482 | 4,019 | 6,748 | 11.0 |
| M03 | Lower Genital Tract Major Procedures | 30,661 | 2,161 | 1,592 | 2,643 | 3.7 |
| H81 | Primary Hip Replacement Uncemented | 10,583 | 5,516 | 4,755 | 6,251 | 6.9 |
| G14 | Cholecystectomy <70 w/o cc | 28,896 | 1,999 | 1,471 | 2,515 | 2.0 |
| R03 | Decompression and Effusion for Degenerative Spinal Disorders | 10,227 | 5,308 | 3,103 | 6,152 | 5.7 |
| H10 | Arthroscopies | 36,877 | 1,459 | 1,002 | 1,799 | 1.4 |
| H71 | Revisional Procedures to Hips | 6,767 | 7,858 | 6,129 | 9,121 | 11.9 |
| F31 | Large Intestine - Complex Procedures | 7,629 | 6,185 | 4,857 | 7,483 | 11.7 |
| H19 | Soft Tissue or Other Bone Procedures - Category 2 <70 w/o cc | 16,993 | 2,382 | 1,348 | 2,572 | 2.4 |
| S22 | Planned Procedures Not Carried Out | 58,311 | 656 | 391 | 862 | 1.2 |
| L27 | Prostate Transurethral Resection Procedure >69 or w cc | 17,419 | 2,190 | 1,765 | 2,524 | 4.1 |
| C57 | Major Mouth or Throat Procedures | 13,747 | 2,693 | 1,402 | 2,815 | 2.7 |
| L17 | Bladder Major Endoscopic Procedure | 21,086 | 1,601 | 1,270 | 1,993 | 3.1 |
| H72 | Revisional Procedures to Knees | 4,639 | 7,245 | 5,154 | 8,348 | 9.3 |
| H17 | Soft Tissue or Other Bone Procedures - Category 1 <70 w/o cc | 17,545 | 1,829 | 1,164 | 2,252 | 1.9 |
| D02 | Complex Thoracic Procedures | 4,554 | 6,943 | 2,453 | 7,702 | 7.9 |
| J47 | Total Mastectomy w/o cc | 11,034 | 2,795 | 1,939 | 3,228 | 4.5 |
| R02 | Surgery for Prolapsed Intervertebral Disc | 8,696 | 3,381 | 2,202 | 3,774 | 3.9 |
| C31 | Major Ear Procedures | 14,620 | 1,984 | 1,354 | 2,489 | 1.3 |
| F73 | Inguinal Umbilical or Femoral Hernia Repairs >69 or w cc | 17,343 | 1,591 | 1,198 | 2,004 | 2.0 |
| F74 | Inguinal Umbilical or Femoral Hernia Repairs <70 w/o cc | 19,762 | 1,396 | 1,033 | 1,771 | 1.4 |
| E08 | Pacemaker Implant except for AMI, Heart Failure or Shock | 8,020 | 3,406 | 1,723 | 4,233 | 2.1 |
| E14 | Cardiac Catheterisation and Angiography w/o cc | 16,286 | 1,648 | 942 | 2,436 | 2.1 |
| C22 | Intermediate Nose Procedures | 21,400 | 1,249 | 979 | 1,585 | 1.2 |
| Q02 | Elective Abdominal Vascular Surgery | 4,337 | 6,126 | 2,782 | 6,700 | 8.1 |
| J49 | Partial/Subtotal Mastectomy w/o cc | 13,340 | 1,942 | 1,429 | 2,441 | 2.7 |
| A04 | Intracranial Procedures Except Trauma - Category 4 | 3,014 | 8,040 | 3,226 | 8,942 | 7.3 |
| H12 | Foot Procedures - Category 2 | 14,499 | 1,658 | 1,207 | 2,053 | 1.7 |
| L02 | Kidney Major Open Procedure >49 or w cc | 5,223 | 4,598 | 3,022 | 5,947 | 7.6 |
| S98 | Chemotherapy with a Haem., Inf. Dis., Pois, or N.S. Primary Diag.[3] | 9,884 | 2,364 | 797 | 2,709 | 5.5 |
| Q12 | Therapeutic Endovascular Procedures | 12,647 | 1,827 | 961 | 2,446 | 2.4 |
| M06 | Upper Genital Tract Intermediate Procedures | 18,304 | 1,231 | 987 | 1,685 | 1.4 |
| G13 | Malig. Dis. of the Lymphatic/Haematological Sys. with los >1 day[4] | 9,004 | 2,467 | 1,877 | 2,963 | 3.6 |

*Notes:*   w cc = with complications and co-morbidity; w/o cc = without complications and co-morbidity.
1 Mean cost corresponds to national average unit cost, calculated by the Department of Health, on a weighted basis, Whereas quartile range is based on individual data submissions for providers.
2 Average length of stay is derived by Department of Health using method of truncation by excluding bed days that fall outside nationally set lengths of stay.
3 Chemotherapy with a Haematology, Infectious Disease, Poisoning, or Non Specific Primary Diagnosis.
4 Malignant Disorder of the Lymphatic/ Haematological Systems with length of stay > 1 day.
<70 = under 70 years of age; >69 = Over 69 years of age.

*Source:*  The NHS Reference Costs (DH).

**Table 3.35  Reference costs per FCE and average length of stay of top 40 Healthcare Resource Groups (HRGs) ranked by total cost, NHS Trusts, non-elective inpatients, England, 2005/06**

| HRG code | Healthcare Resource Group (HRG) | No. of FCEs | Mean cost[1] (£) | Quartile range[1] (£) 25% | Quartile range[1] (£) 75% | Average length of stay[2] (days) |
|---|---|---|---|---|---|---|
| N12 | Antenatal Admissions not Related to Delivery Event | 618,564 | 587 | 446 | 815 | 1.2 |
| N07 | Normal Delivery w/o cc | 345,093 | 1,013 | 806 | 1,307 | 1.7 |
| N11 | Caesarean Section w/o cc | 113,585 | 2,309 | 1,807 | 2,755 | 3.8 |
| H99 | Complex Elderly with a Musculoskeletal System Primary Diagnosis | 32,560 | 5,184 | 1,874 | 5,527 | 17.5 |
| D99 | Complex Elderly with a Respiratory System Primary Diagnosis | 78,207 | 2,071 | 1,403 | 3,135 | 9.0 |
| A22 | Non-Transient Stroke or Cerebrovascular Accident >69 or w cc | 61,196 | 2,433 | 1,264 | 3,391 | 10.7 |
| L09 | Kidney or Urinary Tract Infections >69 or w cc | 73,423 | 1,726 | 1,042 | 2,277 | 7.3 |
| A99 | Complex Elderly with a Nervous System Primary Diagnosis | 35,870 | 3,325 | 1,425 | 4,331 | 15.3 |
| F46 | General Abdominal Disorders >69 or w cc | 76,907 | 1,242 | 809 | 1,721 | 3.8 |
| E99 | Complex Elderly with a Cardiac Primary Diagnosis | 45,347 | 2,088 | 1,419 | 3,018 | 8.8 |
| D41 | Unspecified Acute Lower Respiratory Infection | 72,077 | 1,287 | 968 | 2,139 | 5.2 |
| H37 | Closed Pelvis or Lower Limb Fractures <70 w/o cc | 38,103 | 2,380 | 771 | 2,339 | 4.4 |
| H36 | Closed Pelvis or Lower Limb Fractures >69 or w cc | 24,195 | 3,737 | 1,350 | 4,157 | 12.3 |
| N09 | Assisted Delivery w/o cc | 62,257 | 1,444 | 1,137 | 1,670 | 2.5 |
| E18 | Heart Failure or Shock >69 or w cc | 52,618 | 1,694 | 1,208 | 2,560 | 6.9 |
| F47 | General Abdominal Disorders <70 w/o cc | 104,213 | 825 | 534 | 1,107 | 2.1 |
| D40 | Chronic Obstructive Pulmonary Disease or Bronchitis w/o cc | 75,785 | 1,106 | 791 | 1,700 | 4.4 |
| F36 | Large Intestinal Disorders >69 or w cc | 47,434 | 1,760 | 1,092 | 2,278 | 6.0 |
| E15 | Percutaneous Coronary Intervention | 24,378 | 3,401 | 1,109 | 3,641 | 2.9 |
| E12 | Acute Myocardial Infarction w/o cc | 63,475 | 1,169 | 775 | 1,718 | 4.1 |
| F82 | Appendicectomy Procedures <70 w/o cc | 35,552 | 2,063 | 1,329 | 2,559 | 3.2 |
| D13 | Lobar, Atypical or Viral Pneumonia w cc | 36,016 | 1,980 | 1,404 | 3,134 | 8.2 |
| D25 | Respiratory Neoplasms | 33,500 | 2,072 | 1,280 | 2,998 | 7.9 |
| N10 | Caesarean Section w cc | 21,083 | 3,214 | 2,516 | 3,754 | 5.9 |
| E14 | Cardiac Catheterisation and Angiography w/o cc | 27,967 | 2,302 | 1,340 | 3,142 | 5.5 |
| S99 | Complex Elderly with Haem., Inf. Dis, Pois., or N.S. Primary Diag.[3] | 27,470 | 2,309 | 1,249 | 3,452 | 10.2 |
| E29 | Arrhythmia or Conduction Disorders >69 or w cc | 58,750 | 1,072 | 773 | 1,806 | 4.1 |
| D14 | Lobar, Atypical or Viral Pneumonia w/o cc | 48,041 | 1,199 | 936 | 2,058 | 4.6 |
| D39 | Chronic Obstructive Pulmonary Disease or Bronchitis w cc | 37,840 | 1,512 | 1,089 | 2,196 | 6.2 |
| P13 | Other Gastrointestinal or Metabolic Disorders | 73,374 | 740 | 468 | 956 | 1.5 |
| E22 | Ischaemic Heart Disease without intervention >69 or w cc | 52,951 | 1,005 | 711 | 1,620 | 3.6 |
| F32 | Large Intestine - Very Major Procedures | 8,915 | 5,933 | 2,726 | 6,731 | 13.2 |
| F17 | Stomach or Duodenum Disorders >69 or w cc | 38,489 | 1,369 | 889 | 2,026 | 5.0 |
| S19 | Complications of Procedures | 39,530 | 1,321 | 802 | 1,818 | 3.6 |
| J41 | Major Skin Infections >69 or w cc | 33,129 | 1,556 | 1,123 | 2,312 | 6.3 |
| Q15 | Amputations | 5,494 | 9,101 | 4,529 | 10,876 | 28.4 |
| S28 | Malig. Dis. of the Lymphatic/Haematological Sys. with los >1 day | 16,145 | 3,096 | 1,655 | 3,750 | 9.5 |
| H87 | Neck of Femur Fracture with Hip Replacement w/o cc | 8,387 | 5,890 | 4,121 | 6,910 | 13.8 |
| P03 | Upper Respiratory Tract Disorders | 79,288 | 615 | 426 | 863 | 1.2 |
| H39 | Closed Upper Limb Fractures or Dislocations >69 or w cc | 21,771 | 2,213 | 1,214 | 2,787 | 6.3 |
| L99 | Malig. Dis. of the Lymphatic/Haematological Sys. with los >1 day[4] | 19,342 | 2,446 | 1,408 | 3,225 | 10.8 |

Notes:  w cc = with complications and co-morbidity; w/o cc = without complications and co-morbidity.

Interquartile Ranges are based on the individual data submissions made by providers and not on a weighted basis and are therefore not comparable with the national average unit costs (mean cost).

1 Mean cost corresponds to national average unit cost, calculated by the Department of Health, on a weighted basis,  Whereas quartile range is based on individual data submissions for providers.

2 Average length of stay is derived by Department of Health using method of truncation by excluding bed days that fall outside nationally set lengths of stay.

3 Complex Elderly with a Haematology, Infectious Disease, Poisoning, or Non-specific Primary Diagnosis.

4 Malignant Disorder of the Lymphatic/ Haematological Systems with length of stay > 1 day.

<70 = under 70 years of age; >69 = Over 69 years of age.

Source:  The NHS Reference Costs (DH).

Table 3.36    **Reference costs per case of top 40 Healthcare Resource Groups (HRGs) ranked by total cost, NHS Trusts, day cases, England, 2005/06**

| HRG code | Healthcare Resource Group (HRG) | No. of day cases | Mean cost[1](£) | Quartile range[1] (£) | |
|---|---|---|---|---|---|
| | | | | **25%** | **75%** |
| B13 | Phakoemulsification Cataract Extraction and Insertion of Lens | 254,601 | 764 | 659 | 933 |
| F35 | Large Intestine - Endoscopic or Intermediate Procedures | 276,450 | 490 | 390 | 695 |
| F06 | Diagnostic Procedures, Oesophagus and Stomach | 322,983 | 418 | 347 | 728 |
| C58 | Intermediate Mouth or Throat Procedures | 163,614 | 663 | 457 | 875 |
| J37 | Minor Skin Procedures - Category 1 w/o cc | 156,482 | 605 | 467 | 847 |
| L21 | Bladder Minor Endoscopic Procedure w/o cc | 187,499 | 442 | 368 | 696 |
| H10 | Arthroscopies | 71,772 | 1,039 | 778 | 1,223 |
| E14 | Cardiac Catheterisation and Angiography without complications | 81,980 | 838 | 558 | 994 |
| A07 | Intermediate Pain Procedures | 100,326 | 576 | 398 | 763 |
| M05 | Upper Genital Tract Minor Procedures | 90,296 | 621 | 495 | 770 |
| S27 | Malignant Disorder of the Lymphatic/ Haematological  Systems with los <2 days | 122,214 | 426 | 266 | 546 |
| H13 | Hand Procedures - Category 1 | 54,347 | 780 | 552 | 914 |
| M06 | Upper Genital Tract Intermediate Procedures | 52,725 | 796 | 593 | 921 |
| S22 | Planned Procedures Not Carried Out | 97,222 | 393 | 259 | 564 |
| F74 | Inguinal Umbilical or Femoral Hernia Repairs <70 w/o cc | 35,363 | 984 | 668 | 1,169 |
| C55 | Minor Ear Procedures | 43,072 | 713 | 500 | 844 |
| B16 | Oculoplastic Low Complexity | 47,157 | 636 | 471 | 820 |
| F98 | Chemotherapy with a Digestive System Primary Diagnosis | 104,365 | 277 | 237 | 482 |
| S98 | Chemotherapy with a Haem., Inf. Dis., Pois, or N.S. Primary Diag.[2] | 69,105 | 408 | 259 | 532 |
| H22 | Minor Procedures to the Musculoskeletal System | 41,545 | 592 | 412 | 821 |
| J98 | Chemotherapy with a Skin, Breast or Burn Primary Diagnosis | 70,936 | 293 | 249 | 487 |
| Q11 | Varicose Vein Procedures | 22,031 | 934 | 529 | 1,083 |
| M10 | Surgical Termination of Pregnancy | 36,400 | 564 | 455 | 691 |
| M02 | Lower Genital Tract Intermediate Procedures | 32,736 | 620 | 490 | 799 |
| L20 | Bladder Minor Endoscopic Procedure w cc | 43,473 | 456 | 393 | 712 |
| F54 | Inflammatory Bowel Disease - Endoscopic or Intermediate Procedures <70 w/o cc | 40,336 | 474 | 394 | 731 |
| L39 | Penis Minor Open Procedure <70 w/o cc | 25,567 | 689 | 504 | 878 |
| S06 | Red Blood Cell Disorders <70 w/o cc | 39,222 | 427 | 245 | 522 |
| H17 | Soft Tissue or Other Bone Procedures - Category 1 <70 w/o cc | 16,632 | 957 | 551 | 1,047 |
| D07 | Fibreoptic Bronchoscopy | 28,089 | 555 | 367 | 864 |
| C56 | Minor Nose Procedures | 23,082 | 657 | 475 | 810 |
| H52 | Removal of Fixation Device <70 w/o cc | 13,912 | 968 | 684 | 1,145 |
| S33 | Examination, Follow up and Special Screening | 25,203 | 484 | 266 | 575 |
| L43 | Scrotum Testis or Vas Deferens Open Procedures <70 w/o cc | 14,171 | 852 | 539 | 969 |
| B29 | Surgical Retina Low Complexity | 21,151 | 561 | 472 | 903 |
| D98 | Chemotherapy with a Respiratory System Primary Diagnosis | 38,896 | 299 | 242 | 497 |
| H26 | Inflammatory Spine, Joint or Connective Tissue Disorders <70 w/o cc | 18,602 | 587 | 299 | 696 |
| J35 | Minor Skin Procedures - Category 2 w/o cc | 15,273 | 697 | 484 | 861 |
| C04 | Minor Mouth or Throat Procedures | 18,268 | 578 | 456 | 821 |
| L45 | Extracorporeal Lithotripsy | 16,622 | 625 | 385 | 672 |

*Notes:*    w cc = with complications and co-morbidity; w/o cc = without complications and co-morbidity.
1 Mean cost corresponds to national average unit cost, calculated by the Department of Health, on a weighted basis,  Whereas quartile range is based on individual data submissions for providers.
2 Chemotherapy with a Haematology, Infectious Disease, Poisoning, or Non Specific Primary Diagnosis.
<70 = under 70 years of age.

*Source:*  The NHS Reference Costs (DH).

Table 3.37  **Reference costs per FCE of top 40 Healthcare Resource Groups (HRGs) ranked by total cost, non-NHS providers[1], elective inpatients, England, 2005/06**

| HRG code | Healthcare Resource Group (HRG) | No. of FCEs | Mean cost[2] (£) | Average length of stay[3] (days) |
|---|---|---|---|---|
| H04 | Primary Knee Replacement | 4,354 | 6,928 | 5.4 |
| H80 | Primary Hip Replacement Cemented | 3,165 | 6,165 | 7.5 |
| E04 | Coronary Bypass | 996 | 6,641 | 4.0 |
| H81 | Primary Hip Replacement Uncemented | 749 | 6,825 | 5.3 |
| H10 | Arthroscopies | 2,741 | 1,649 | 1.3 |
| G14 | Cholecystectomy <70 w/o cc | 1,226 | 2,393 | 1.6 |
| E03 | Cardiac Valve Procedures | 306 | 8,010 | 2.4 |
| F74 | Inguinal Umbilical or Femoral Hernia Repairs <70 w/o cc | 1,353 | 1,495 | 1.3 |
| H17 | Soft Tissue or Other Bone Procedures - Category 1 <70 w/o cc | 1,078 | 1,792 | 1.4 |
| R03 | Decompression and Effusion for Degenerative Spinal Disorders | 253 | 7,195 | 5.6 |
| H12 | Foot Procedures - Category 2 | 900 | 1,987 | 1.4 |
| H21 | Muscle, Tendon or Ligament Procedures - Category 2 | 558 | 2,747 | 2.6 |
| F14 | Stomach or Duodenum - Major Procedures <70 or w/o cc | 275 | 5,568 | 1.8 |
| F12 | Stomach or Duodenum Very Major Procedures | 188 | 8,014 | 4.4 |
| H19 | Soft Tissue or Other Bone Procedures - Category 2 <70 w/o cc | 599 | 2,374 | 1.9 |
| H01 | Bilateral Primary Hip Replacement | 187 | 7,335 | 4.4 |
| C22 | Intermediate Nose Procedures | 819 | 1,436 | 1.3 |
| H03 | Bilateral Primary Knee Replacement | 134 | 8,396 | 6.0 |
| J37 | Minor Skin Procedures - Category 1 w/o cc | 887 | 1,238 | 1.6 |
| H13 | Hand Procedures - Category 1 | 910 | 1,201 | 1.3 |
| J50 | Other Major Breast Surgery | 203 | 5,348 | 1.7 |
| Q11 | Varicose Vein Procedures | 771 | 1,405 | 1.3 |
| C58 | Intermediate Mouth or Throat Procedures | 773 | 1,179 | 1.4 |
| E38 | Electrophysiological and other Percutaneous Cardiac Procedures >18 | 78 | 10,114 | 1.6 |
| H14 | Hand Procedures - Category 2 | 429 | 1,820 | 1.4 |
| E15 | Percutaneous Coronary Intervention | 185 | 4,195 | 1.8 |
| M07 | Upper Genital Tract Major Procedures | 244 | 3,054 | 2.7 |
| H71 | Revisional Procedures to Hips | 120 | 6,154 | 4.1 |
| S24 | Respite Care | 1,310 | 554 | 1.3 |
| R02 | Surgery for Prolapsed Intervertebral Disc | 139 | 5,178 | 2.8 |
| C32 | Major Nose Procedures | 337 | 2,107 | 1.3 |
| H72 | Revisional Procedures to Knees | 75 | 8,816 | 5.4 |
| M10 | Surgical Termination of Pregnancy | 1,616 | 399 | 1.0 |
| H07 | Primary or Revisional Shoulder, Elbow, or Ankle Replacements | 112 | 5,736 | 3.4 |
| H11 | Foot Procedures - Category 1 | 370 | 1,731 | 1.5 |
| J05 | Intermediate Breast Surgery w/o cc | 117 | 5,374 | 1.6 |
| M03 | Lower Genital Tract Major Procedures | 246 | 2,534 | 2.4 |
| F72 | Abdominal Hernia Procedures <70 w/o cc | 353 | 1,655 | 1.4 |
| H08 | Joint Replacements or Revisions, Site Unspecified | 104 | 5,227 | 4.1 |
| F35 | Large Intestine - Endoscopic or Intermediate Procedures | 649 | 728 | 1.0 |

*Notes:*  1 Independent sector providers of care to NHS funded patients.
2 Mean cost corresponds to national average unit cost, calculated by the Department of Health, on a weighted basis
3 Average length of stay is derived by Department of Health using method of truncation by excluding bed days that fall outside nationally set lengths of stay.
w cc = with complications and co-morbidity; w/o cc = without complications and co-morbidity.
<70 = under 70 years of age; >69 = Over 69 years of age.

*Source:*  The NHS Reference Costs (DH).

Table 3.38 **Reference costs per case of top 40 Healthcare Resource Groups (HRGs) ranked by total cost, non-NHS providers[1], day cases, England, 2005/06**

| HRG code | Healthcare Resource Group (HRG) | No. of day cases | Mean cost (£) |
|---|---|---|---|
| M10 | Surgical Termination of Pregnancy | 30,044 | 347 |
| B13 | Phakoemulsification Cataract Extraction and Insertion of Lens | 6,552 | 1,141 |
| H10 | Arthroscopies | 4,263 | 1,429 |
| H13 | Hand Procedures - Category 1 | 3,012 | 922 |
| H04 | Primary Knee Replacement | 314 | 7,978 |
| J37 | Minor Skin Procedures - Category 1 w/o cc | 4,804 | 390 |
| F74 | Inguinal Umbilical or Femoral Hernia Repairs <70 w/o cc | 1,219 | 1,508 |
| H80 | Primary Hip Replacement Cemented | 233 | 7,213 |
| L41 | Vasectomy Procedures | 7,548 | 204 |
| F06 | Diagnostic Procedures, Oesophagus and Stomach | 2,215 | 683 |
| F35 | Large Intestine - Endoscopic or Intermediate Procedures | 862 | 1,257 |
| M11 | Medical Termination of Pregnancy | 2,536 | 361 |
| H12 | Foot Procedures - Category 2 | 587 | 1,555 |
| H17 | Soft Tissue or Other Bone Procedures - Category 1 <70 w/o cc | 405 | 2,162 |
| E14 | Cardiac Catheterisation and Angiography w/o cc | 543 | 1,140 |
| H11 | Foot Procedures - Category 1 | 440 | 1,284 |
| C58 | Intermediate Mouth or Throat Procedures | 551 | 1,005 |
| H14 | Hand Procedures - Category 2 | 278 | 1,870 |
| H22 | Minor Procedures to the Musculoskeletal System | 649 | 741 |
| L21 | Bladder Minor Endoscopic Procedure w/o cc | 662 | 692 |
| F73 | Inguinal Umbilical or Femoral Hernia Repairs >69 or w cc | 276 | 1,510 |
| H19 | Soft Tissue or Other Bone Procedures - Category 2 <70 w/o cc | 105 | 3,765 |
| B14 | Non Phakoemulsification Cataract Surgery | 522 | 733 |
| B15 | Other Lens Surgery Low Complexity | 468 | 790 |
| H81 | Primary Hip Replacement Uncemented | 45 | 8,080 |
| B32 | Non Surgical Ophthalmology with los <2 days | 360 | 859 |
| G14 | Cholecystectomy <70 w/o cc | 157 | 1,954 |
| H20 | Muscle, Tendon or Ligament Procedures - Category 1 | 171 | 1,332 |
| S98 | Chemotherapy with a Haem., Inf. Dis., Pois, or N.S. Primary Diag.[2] | 240 | 948 |
| M08 | Upper Genital Tract Complex Major Procedures | 555 | 408 |
| Q11 | Varicose Vein Procedures | 152 | 1,373 |
| L19 | Bladder Intermediate Endoscopic Procedure w/o cc | 242 | 828 |
| F95 | Anus - Minor Procedures <70 w/o cc | 240 | 781 |
| A07 | Intermediate Pain Procedures | 191 | 926 |
| B16 | Oculoplastic Low Complexity | 150 | 1,162 |
| S33 | Examination, Follow up and Special Screening | 2,677 | 63 |
| B29 | Surgical Retina Low Complexity | 222 | 719 |
| J35 | Minor Skin Procedures - Category 2 w/o cc | 289 | 496 |
| H18 | Soft Tissue or Other Bone Procedures - Category 2 >69 or w cc | 33 | 3,935 |
| H21 | Muscle, Tendon or Ligament Procedures - Category 2 | 58 | 2,201 |

*Notes:* 1 Independent sector providers of care to NHS funded patients.
2 Chemotherapy with a Haematology, Infectious Disease, Poisoning, or Non Specific Primary Diagnosis.
w cc = with co-morbidity; w/o cc = without co-morbidity.
<70 = under 70 years of age; >69 = Over 69 years of age.

*Source:* The NHS Reference Costs (DH).

Table 3.39 **Hospital outpatient clinics: total attendances[1], by country, UK, 1952 - 2005/06**

| Year | Outpatient total attendances '000s | | | | Per 1,000 population | | | |
|---|---|---|---|---|---|---|---|---|
| | England and Wales[2] | Scotland[3] | Northern Ireland[4] | United Kingdom | England and Wales[2] | Scotland[3] | Northern Ireland[4] | United Kingdom |
| 1952 | 38,523 | 6,259 | 1,028 | 45,810 | 876 | 1,227 | 748 | 908 |
| 1955 | 39,584 | 7,120 | 1,193 | 47,897 | 891 | 1,393 | 856 | 940 |
| 1960 | 41,748 | 7,279 | 968 | 49,995 | 912 | 1,406 | 682 | 955 |
| 1965 | 44,869 | 7,983 | 1,121 | 53,973 | 941 | 1,532 | 764 | 993 |
| 1970 | 48,097 | 4,631 | 1,438 | 54,166 | 984 | 888 | 942 | 974 |
| 1971 | 48,707 | 4,743 | 1,451 | 54,901 | 991 | 906 | 642 | 982 |
| 1972 | 48,735 | 4,724 | 1,468 | 54,927 | 988 | 903 | 954 | 979 |
| 1973 | 49,034 | 4,770 | 1,543 | 55,347 | 991 | 911 | 1,008 | 984 |
| 1974 | 48,763 | 5,061 | 1,544 | 55,368 | 986 | 966 | 1,011 | 985 |
| 1975 | 50,141 | 5,000 | 1,518 | 56,659 | 1,014 | 956 | 996 | 1,008 |
| 1976 | 47,997 | 5,136 | 1,589 | 54,722 | 970 | 981 | 1,043 | 973 |
| 1977 | 49,027 | 5,128 | 1,590 | 55,745 | 992 | 981 | 1,044 | 992 |
| 1978 | 49,635 | 5,183 | 1,639 | 56,457 | 1,004 | 994 | 1,076 | 1,005 |
| 1979 | 49,921 | 5,203 | 1,670 | 56,794 | 1,008 | 1,000 | 1,093 | 1,010 |
| 1980 | 50,994 | 5,321 | 1,736 | 58,051 | 1,028 | 1,024 | 1,132 | 1,031 |
| 1981 | 51,656 | 5,434 | 1,746 | 58,836 | 1,041 | 1,049 | 1,135 | 1,044 |
| 1982 | 51,950 | 5,440 | 1,748 | 59,138 | 1,047 | 1,053 | 1,136 | 1,050 |
| 1983 | 53,068 | 5,422 | 1,893 | 60,383 | 1,069 | 1,053 | 1,227 | 1,072 |
| 1984 | 53,842 | 5,519 | 1,975 | 61,336 | 1,081 | 1,074 | 1,274 | 1,085 |
| 1985 | 54,324 | 5,593 | 2,028 | 61,945 | 1,087 | 1,088 | 1,300 | 1,093 |
| 1986 | 54,616 | 5,668 | 2,025 | 62,309 | 1,089 | 1,107 | 1,290 | 1,096 |
| 1987/88[5] | 54,716 | 5,693 | 2,049 | 62,458 | 1,088 | 1,128 | 1,305 | 1,097 |
| 1988/89 | 55,731 | 5,767 | 1,974 | 63,472 | 1,104 | 1,142 | 1,257 | 1,111 |
| 1989/90 | 56,198 | 5,815 | 1,989 | 64,002 | 1,109 | 1,164 | 1,248 | 1,118 |
| 1990/91 | 55,775 | 5,925 | 1,954 | 63,654 | 1,096 | 1,168 | 1,231 | 1,107 |
| 1991/92 | 55,596 | 5,971 | 1,963 | 63,530 | 1,088 | 1,175 | 1,226 | 1,100 |
| 1992/93 | 55,617 | 6,005 | 1,969 | 63,591 | 1,085 | 1,191 | 1,214 | 1,098 |
| 1993/94 | 55,971 | 6,086 | 1,967 | 64,024 | 1,086 | 1,199 | 1,193 | 1,099 |
| 1994/95 | 57,645 | 6,145 | 2,051 | 65,841 | 1,127 | 1,204 | 1,247 | 1,137 |
| 1995/96 | 58,929 | 6,241 | 2,087 | 67,257 | 1,149 | 1,224 | 1,263 | 1,158 |
| 1996/97 | 59,570 | 6,338 | 2,072 | 67,980 | 1,158 | 1,245 | 1,245 | 1,168 |
| 1997/98 | 60,674 | 6,333 | 2,083 | 69,091 | 1,176 | 1,246 | 1,245 | 1,184 |
| 1998/99 | 61,151 | 6,426 | 2,091 | 69,668 | 1,181 | 1,266 | 1,246 | 1,190 |
| 1999/00 | 62,476 | 6,453 | 2,106 | 71,034 | 1,202 | 1,273 | 1,254 | 1,209 |
| 2000/01 | 62,663 | 6,384 | 2,113 | 71,160 | 1,201 | 1,261 | 1,254 | 1,207 |
| 2001/02 | 62,913 | 6,256 | 2,131 | 71,300 | 1,200 | 1,236 | 1,260 | 1,205 |
| 2002/03 | 63,670 | 6,194 | 2,122 | 71,987 | 1,210 | 1,225 | 1,250 | 1,212 |
| 2003/04 | 65,541 | 6,149 | 2,161 | 73,851 | 1,240 | 1,215 | 1,268 | 1,238 |
| 2004/05 | 66,468 | 5,990 | 2,175 | 74,633 | 1,251 | 1,179 | 1,269 | 1,245 |
| 2005/06 | 72,741 | 6,071 | 2,221 | 81,033 | 1,360 | 1,190 | 1,285 | 1,343 |

*Notes:* 1 At consultant and general practitioner clinics and accident and emergency departments.

2 Information on general practitioner maternity clinics is not collected separately in England but is included for Wales.

3 Prior to 1969, figures relate to casualty and ancillary departments.

4 Figures relate to casualty and ancillary departments.

5 Figures from 1987/88 for England and Scotland, from 1983/84 for Wales and for 1988/89 for Northern Ireland relate to financial years.

Information on general practitioner maternity clinics is not collected separately in England but is included for Wales.

*Sources:* Annual Abstract of Statistics (ONS).

Health Statistics Wales (NAW).

Scottish Health Statistics (ISD).

Health and Personal Social Services Statistics for England (DH).

Hospital Episode Statistics (IC).

Hospital Activity Statistics (DH).

Population Projections Database (GAD).

Table 3.40   **Hospital outpatient clinics[1]: new cases, by country, UK, 1952 - 2005/06**

| Year | New outpatient cases '000s | | | | New cases per 1,000 population | | | |
|------|---------------------|-----------|---------------------|-----------|----------------------|-----------|---------------------|-----------|
|      | England and Wales[2] | Scotland[3] | Northern Ireland[4] | United Kingdom | England and Wales[2] | Scotland[3] | Northern Ireland[4] | United Kingdom |
| 1952 | - | - | 321 | - | - | - | 233 | - |
| 1953 | 11,307 | - | 322 | 11,629 | 256 | - | 233 | 256 |
| 1954 | 11,366 | 2,022 | 348 | 13,736 | 257 | 396 | 251 | 271 |
| 1955 | 11,636 | 2,131 | 386 | 14,153 | 262 | 417 | 277 | 278 |
| 1960 | 12,768 | 2,238 | 341 | 15,347 | 279 | 432 | 240 | 293 |
| 1965 | 14,588 | 2,593 | 385 | 17,566 | 306 | 498 | 262 | 323 |
| 1970 | 16,391 | 1,673 | 515 | 18,579 | 335 | 321 | 337 | 334 |
| 1971 | 16,682 | 1,707 | 519 | 18,908 | 339 | 326 | 337 | 338 |
| 1972 | 16,825 | 1,730 | 529 | 19,084 | 341 | 331 | 344 | 340 |
| 1973 | 17,205 | 1,782 | 556 | 19,543 | 348 | 340 | 363 | 348 |
| 1974 | 16,994 | 1,819 | 559 | 19,372 | 344 | 347 | 366 | 344 |
| 1975 | 16,179 | 1,812 | 563 | 18,554 | 327 | 346 | 369 | 330 |
| 1976 | 17,224 | 1,882 | 589 | 19,695 | 348 | 360 | 386 | 350 |
| 1977 | 17,455 | 1,920 | 592 | 19,967 | 353 | 367 | 389 | 355 |
| 1978 | 17,769 | 1,961 | 608 | 20,338 | 359 | 376 | 399 | 362 |
| 1979 | 17,873 | 1,961 | 618 | 20,452 | 361 | 377 | 404 | 364 |
| 1980 | 18,146 | 1,999 | 628 | 20,773 | 366 | 385 | 410 | 369 |
| 1981 | 18,489 | 2,033 | 637 | 21,159 | 373 | 392 | 414 | 375 |
| 1982 | 18,782 | 2,047 | 647 | 21,476 | 379 | 396 | 421 | 381 |
| 1983 | 19,324 | 2,042 | 685 | 22,051 | 389 | 397 | 444 | 391 |
| 1984 | 19,813 | 2,083 | 720 | 22,616 | 398 | 405 | 465 | 400 |
| 1985 | 20,193 | 2,144 | 739 | 23,076 | 404 | 417 | 474 | 407 |
| 1986 | 20,424 | 2,196 | 756 | 23,376 | 407 | 429 | 482 | 411 |
| 1987/88 [5] | 20,568 | 2,233 | 770 | 23,571 | 409 | 445 | 489 | 414 |
| 1988/89 | 20,557 | 2,275 | 761 | 23,593 | 407 | 456 | 482 | 414 |
| 1989/90 | 20,982 | 2,325 | 780 | 24,087 | 414 | 468 | 493 | 421 |
| 1990/91 | 20,950 | 2,381 | 782 | 24,113 | 412 | 471 | 493 | 419 |
| 1991/92 | 21,231 | 2,403 | 799 | 24,433 | 415 | 475 | 501 | 423 |
| 1992/93 | 21,589 | 2,426 | 819 | 24,834 | 420 | 481 | 505 | 426 |
| 1993/94 | 22,462 | 2,457 | 836 | 25,755 | 435 | 488 | 503 | 442 |
| 1994/95 | 23,742 | 2,503 | 873 | 27,118 | 464 | 491 | 531 | 468 |
| 1995/96 | 24,856 | 2,577 | 937 | 28,370 | 484 | 505 | 567 | 489 |
| 1996/97 | 25,203 | 2,666 | 933 | 28,802 | 490 | 524 | 561 | 495 |
| 1997/98 | 25,843 | 2,716 | 952 | 29,511 | 501 | 534 | 569 | 506 |
| 1998/99 | 26,111 | 2,735 | 962 | 29,808 | 504 | 539 | 573 | 509 |
| 1999/00 | 26,866 | 2,767 | 980 | 30,613 | 517 | 546 | 583 | 521 |
| 2000/01 | 26,972 | 2,749 | 994 | 30,715 | 517 | 543 | 590 | 521 |
| 2001/02 | 27,142 | 2,729 | 997 | 30,868 | 518 | 539 | 590 | 522 |
| 2002/03 | 27,603 | 2,731 | 992 | 31,326 | 524 | 540 | 584 | 528 |
| 2003/04 | 30,400 | 2,751 | 1,014 | 34,165 | 575 | 543 | 595 | 573 |
| 2004/05 | 31,761 | 2,720 | 1,027 | 35,508 | 598 | 535 | 599 | 592 |
| 2005/06 | 34,412 | 2,738 | 1,043 | 38,193 | 643 | 537 | 603 | 633 |

*Notes:*   1 At consultant and general practitioner clinics and accident and emergency departments.
2 Information on general practitioner maternity clinics is not collected separately in England but is included for Wales.
3 Prior to 1969, figures relate to casualty and ancillary departments.
4 Figures relate to casualty and ancillary departments.
5 Figures from 1987/88 for England and Scotland, from 1983/84 for Wales and for 1988/89 for Northern Ireland relate to financial years.
Information on general practitioner maternity clinics is not collected separately in England but is included for Wales.
- Figures not available.

*Sources:*   Annual Abstract of Statistics (ONS).
Health Statistics Wales (NAW).
Scottish Health Statistics (ISD).
Health and Personal Social Services Statistics for England (DH).
Hospital Episode Statistics (IC).
Hospital Activity Statistics (DH).
Population Projections database (GAD).

Table 3.41(a)  **Percentage of population attending[1] NHS hospital outpatient departments[2] by age group in 3 months prior to survey interview, Great Britain, 1985/86 - 2005**

| | Year | | | | | | | | |
| | 1985/86 | 1995/96 | 1998/99 | 2000/01 | 2001/02 | 2002/03 | 2003/04 | 2004/05 | 2005 |
|---|---|---|---|---|---|---|---|---|---|
| **All Males** | **13** | **14** | **16** | **15** | **14** | **14** | **14** | **14** | **14** |
| 0-4 | 13 | 12 | 16 | 14 | 16 | 17 | 13 | 14 | 15 |
| 5-15 | 12 | 11 | 12 | 11 | 10 | 11 | 10 | 11 | 10 |
| 16-44 | 12 | 12 | 13 | 12 | 11 | 11 | 11 | 10 | 10 |
| 45-64 | 16 | 16 | 17 | 16 | 16 | 15 | 16 | 17 | 16 |
| 65-74 | 16 | 21 | 25 | 24 | 22 | 24 | 21 | 24 | 22 |
| over 74 | 15 | 26 | 29 | 26 | 31 | 26 | 24 | 26 | 26 |
| **All Females** | **13** | **14** | **16** | **15** | **14** | **14** | **15** | **15** | **15** |
| 0-4 | 11 | 12 | 13 | 10 | 11 | 12 | 11 | 11 | 12 |
| 5-15 | 9 | 9 | 11 | 8 | 8 | 9 | 9 | 8 | 9 |
| 16-44 | 12 | 12 | 13 | 13 | 12 | 12 | 13 | 12 | 12 |
| 45-64 | 15 | 17 | 18 | 16 | 18 | 16 | 18 | 18 | 16 |
| 65-74 | 17 | 21 | 21 | 21 | 21 | 20 | 20 | 21 | 21 |
| over 74 | 17 | 22 | 26 | 24 | 23 | 25 | 22 | 22 | 24 |
| **All Persons** | **13** | **14** | **16** | **15** | **14** | **14** | **14** | **14** | **14** |
| 0-4 | 12 | 12 | 14 | 12 | 13 | 14 | 12 | 13 | 13 |
| 5-15 | 10 | 10 | 11 | 10 | 9 | 10 | 10 | 10 | 9 |
| 16-44 | 12 | 12 | 13 | 13 | 12 | 12 | 12 | 11 | 11 |
| 45-64 | 15 | 16 | 18 | 16 | 17 | 15 | 17 | 18 | 16 |
| 65-74 | 17 | 21 | 23 | 22 | 21 | 22 | 21 | 22 | 21 |
| over 74 | 16 | 24 | 27 | 25 | 26 | 25 | 23 | 24 | 25 |

Table 3.41(b)  **Estimated number[3] of annual NHS hospital outpatient department[2] attendances[1] by age group, UK, 1985/86 - 2005**

Thousands

| | Year | | | | | | | | |
| | 1985/86 | 1995/96 | 1998/99 | 2000/01 | 2001/02 | 2002/03 | 2003/04 | 2004/05 | 2005 |
|---|---|---|---|---|---|---|---|---|---|
| **All Males** | **32,222** | **33,942** | **37,455** | **36,166** | **33,543** | **31,578** | **30,009** | **33,220** | **32,401** |
| 0-4 | 1,495 | 1,541 | 1,718 | 1,619 | 1,908 | 1,888 | 1,144 | 1,319 | 1,387 |
| 5-15 | 3,243 | 2,523 | 3,172 | 3,019 | 2,656 | 2,493 | 2,898 | 2,645 | 2,574 |
| 16-44 | 13,062 | 13,852 | 13,093 | 12,929 | 10,796 | 10,103 | 9,286 | 9,703 | 8,771 |
| 45-64 | 10,013 | 9,226 | 10,163 | 9,834 | 10,002 | 9,334 | 8,652 | 10,183 | 10,752 |
| 65-74 | 2,561 | 4,173 | 5,642 | 5,345 | 4,015 | 4,469 | 4,543 | 5,318 | 4,707 |
| over 74 | 1,848 | 2,628 | 3,667 | 3,420 | 4,165 | 3,292 | 3,485 | 4,052 | 4,210 |
| **All Females** | **32,816** | **37,658** | **39,851** | **35,728** | **38,318** | **35,598** | **34,532** | **37,437** | **35,289** |
| 0-4 | 1,108 | 1,134 | 1,313 | 1,109 | 917 | 1,133 | 1,386 | 1,174 | 986 |
| 5-15 | 2,231 | 1,975 | 3,024 | 2,090 | 1,971 | 1,890 | 2,206 | 1,823 | 1,978 |
| 16-44 | 12,710 | 14,116 | 14,383 | 12,880 | 13,175 | 13,326 | 11,877 | 12,535 | 12,982 |
| 45-64 | 7,985 | 10,480 | 10,444 | 9,848 | 10,802 | 8,770 | 10,840 | 11,717 | 9,117 |
| 65-74 | 3,812 | 4,908 | 4,996 | 4,260 | 5,227 | 4,252 | 3,738 | 4,387 | 4,760 |
| over 74 | 4,971 | 5,044 | 5,692 | 5,541 | 6,226 | 6,226 | 4,486 | 5,802 | 5,464 |
| **All Persons** | **65,038** | **71,600** | **77,306** | **71,893** | **71,861** | **67,176** | **64,541** | **70,657** | **67,689** |
| 0-4 | 2,603 | 2,675 | 3,032 | 2,728 | 2,825 | 3,021 | 2,530 | 2,493 | 2,373 |
| 5-15 | 5,474 | 4,499 | 6,195 | 5,109 | 4,627 | 4,383 | 5,105 | 4,467 | 4,552 |
| 16-44 | 25,771 | 27,967 | 27,476 | 25,809 | 23,972 | 23,430 | 21,163 | 22,238 | 21,753 |
| 45-64 | 17,998 | 19,706 | 20,608 | 19,682 | 20,804 | 18,103 | 19,492 | 21,900 | 19,870 |
| 65-74 | 6,373 | 9,081 | 10,637 | 9,605 | 9,242 | 8,721 | 8,281 | 9,705 | 9,467 |
| over 74 | 6,819 | 7,672 | 9,359 | 8,961 | 10,391 | 9,518 | 7,971 | 9,854 | 9,674 |

*Notes:*  1 Figures relate to 3 months before survey interview.
2 Including casualty departments.
3 Based on Great Britain rates applied to the UK population.
From 1988 to 2004 the General Household Survey was on a financial year basis with interviews taking place from April to the following March.
1997/98 and 1999/00 data are not available.

*Sources:*  Living in Britain: Results from the General Household Survey (ONS).
Population Projections Database (GAD).

# Family Health Services (FHS)

## Main Points

- The gross cost of UK Family Health Services was £22.5 billion in 2005/06, representing 23.1% of total NHS costs in that year.

- The number of GPs in the UK increased only slightly over the previous year, standing at 43,021 in 2006.

- Between 1996 and 2006, while the number of GPs in the UK grew 20%, the number of patient consultations GPs fell slightly.

- The total UK NHS medicines bill in 2006 (at manufacturers' prices) is estimated at £10.7 billion, representing 10.5% of total NHS spending or £177 per head of the population.

- The UK spends less of its national income on medicines (including over-the-counter medicines) than any other major industrialised countries: 1.1% of GDP in 2005 compared with 1.6% in Germany and 1.8% in France.

UK Family Health Services (FHS) include the General Pharmaceutical (GPS), General Medical (GMS), General Dental (GDS) and General Ophthalmic (GOS) services. The FHS are provided in the community by family practitioners: general medial practitioners (GPs), dentists, pharmacists and opticians. In England, under the Personal Medical Services (PMS) and Personal Dental Services (PDS) schemes, a number of GPs and dentists have become salaried in recent years.

There have been significant changes in key areas of Family Health Services in recent years, including the introduction of the new GMS contract throughout the UK on 1st April 2004, amendments to this contract in 2006/07 and an overhaul of dental charges in England and Wales.

Box 1 **Real[1] decadal growth (per cent) of FHS expenditure, UK**

| | FHS | Hospital | All NHS |
|---|---|---|---|
| 1965/66 – 1975/76 | 56 | 100 | 97 |
| 1975/76 – 1985/86 | 21 | -2 | 5 |
| 1985/86 – 1995/96 | 50 | 37 | 51 |
| 1995/96 – 2005/06 | 69 | 54 | 77 |

Notes: All figures include patient charges and capital spending.
All NHS includes more than FHS and hospital, such as central health and miscellaneous services.
1 As adjusted by the GDP deflator at market prices.
Sources: Health and Personal Social Services Statistics for England (DH).
Health Statistics Wales (NAW).
Scottish Health Statistics (ISD).
Annual Statistical Report (Northern Ireland CSA).
Annual Abstract of Statistics (ONS).
Department of Health Departmental Report (DH).
NHS Board Operating Costs and Capital Expenditure (ISD Scotland).
Public Expenditure Statistical Analyses (HM Treasury).

Since the early 1960s, expenditure on FHS has gradually increased (**Table 4.1**). In 2005/06 the cost of FHS rose to £22.5 billion, 6 times in real terms the cost

in 1949/50, the first full year after the NHS was established.

Expenditure in the hospital sector has grown even faster over the life of the NHS (**Figure 4.3**). However, over the past 30 years, growth in FHS spending has exceeded that of the hospital sector (**Box 1**). In 2005/06, £744 per capita was spent on the hospital sector in the UK, while FHS expenditure was half that at just £373 per capita, (**Box 2, Table 4.3**).

Box 2 **FHS gross expenditure per capita at 2005/06 prices[1], UK**

| | FHS £ | Hospital £ | All NHS £ |
|---|---|---|---|
| 1950/51 | 74 | 125 | 226 |
| 1960/61 | 74 | 156 | 262 |
| 1970/71 | 102 | 260 | 383 |
| 1980/81 | 127 | 354 | 576 |
| 1990/91 | 184 | 413 | 770 |
| 2000/01 | 275 | 554 | 1,127 |
| 2001/02 | 287 | 582 | 1,212 |
| 2002/03 | 299 | 617 | 1,303 |
| 2003/04 | 316 | 650 | 1,430 |
| 2004/05 | 360 | 698 | 1,501 |
| 2005/06 | 373 | 744 | 1,612 |

Notes: All figures include charges paid by patients.
1 As adjusted by the GDP deflator at market prices.
Sources: Health and Personal Social Services Statistics for England (DH).
Health Statistics Wales (NAW).
Scottish Health Statistics (ISD).
Annual Statistical Report (Northern Ireland CSA).
Annual Abstract of Statistics (ONS).
Department of Health Departmental Report (DH).
NHS Board Operating Costs and Capital Expenditure (ISD Scotland).
Public Expenditure Statistical Analyses (HM Treasury).
Population Projections Database (GAD).

Expenditure on FHS in England has been consistently lower than that in the rest of the UK. In 2005/06 per capita FHS expenditure was £369 in England, compared to £398 in Northern Ireland, £394 in Scotland and £382 in Wales. However, expenditure in all constituent countries of the UK has more than trebled over the past 30 years (**Box 3** and **Table 4.4**).

The FHS share of total NHS expenditure was 23% in 2005/06, compared to 36% when the NHS was first established (**Figure 4.1** and **Table 4.2**). Compared to some high income countries, including Sweden and the USA the UK spends a relatively small proportion of total health care expenditure, on primary health care (**Figure 4.2**). However, international comparisons should be made with care owing to possible variation in definitions of primary care.

Pharmaceutical services spending has consistently accounted for the greatest portion of the FHS spend over the past 40 years. In 2005/06, 46% of all FHS spending in the UK was for pharmaceutical services (**Table 4.2**). In contrast, 40% of the FHS budget went on General Medical Services (£150 per capita – **Table 4.3**).

# Family Health Services (FHS)

Dental and ophthalmic services account for just 12% and 2% respectively (**Table 4.2**).

Box 3  **Annual average real[1] growth (per cent) in per capita FHS expenditure**

|  | England | Wales | Scotland | Northern Ireland | UK |
|---|---|---|---|---|---|
| 1985/86 - 1990/91 | 2.7 | 2.2 | 3.2 | 3.4 | 2.7 |
| 1990/91 - 1995/96 | 4.6 | 5.0 | 5.0 | 6.3 | 4.7 |
| 1995/96 - 2000/01 | 3.6 | 4.4 | 4.7 | 3.6 | 3.7 |
| 2000/01 - 2005/06 | 6.6 | 4.6 | 5.6 | 5.0 | 6.3 |

*Notes:* All figures include charges paid by patients.
All NHS includes more than FHS and hospital, such as central health and miscellaneous services.
1 As adjusted by the GDP deflator at market prices.
*Sources:* Health and Personal Social Services Statistics for England (DH).
Health Statistics Wales (NAW).
Scottish Health Statistics (ISD).
Annual Statistical Report (Northern Ireland CSA).
Annual Abstract of Statistics (ONS).
Department of Health Departmental Report (DH).
NHS Board Operating Costs and Capital Expenditure (ISD Scotland).
Public Expenditure Statistical Analyses (HM Treasury).
Population Projections Database (GAD).

Expenditure per capita on both the pharmaceutical services and General Medical Services is considerably higher than 50 years earlier (**Table 4.3**). In contrast, NHS expenditure on General Ophthalmic Services has declined by 75% since the NHS was first established and is now just £7.36 per capita in 2005/06. **Box 4** shows the substantial growth in real terms in all areas of FHS expenditure during the past decade, and the decrease in expenditure on ophthalmic services during the 1980s.

Box 4  **Real[1] decadal growth (per cent) in FHS expenditure by service, UK**

|  | Pharma-ceutical Services | Medical Services | Dental Services | Ophthalmic Services |
|---|---|---|---|---|
| 1965/66 - 1975/76 | 28 | 35 | 40 | 42 |
| 1975/76 - 1985/86 | 56 | 40 | 20 | -17 |
| 1985/86 - 1995/96 | 60 | 60 | 26 | 1 |
| 1995/96 - 2005/06 | 56 | 114 | 32 | 26 |

*Notes:* All figures include charges paid by patients.
1 As adjusted by the GDP deflator at market prices.
*Sources:* Health and Personal Social Services Statistics for England (DH).
Health Statistics Wales (NAW).
Scottish Health Statistics (ISD).
Annual Statistical Report (Northern Ireland CSA).
Annual Abstract of Statistics (ONS).
Department of Health Departmental Report (DH).
NHS Board Operating Costs and Capital Expenditure (ISD Scotland).
Public Expenditure Statistical Analyses (HM Treasury).

Table 4.1 **Cost of Family Health Services (FHS) at 2005/06 prices[1], UK, 1949/50 - 2005/06**

| Year | Pharma-ceutical £m | General Medical £m | General Dental £m | General Ophthalmic £m | Total FHS £m | Index 1949=100[1] | | |
|---|---|---|---|---|---|---|---|---|
| | | | | | | FHS | Hospital | NHS |
| 1949/50 | 868 | 1,142 | 1,169 | 583 | 3,762 | 100 | 100 | 100 |
| 1950/51 | 958 | 1,157 | 1,102 | 530 | 3,747 | 100 | 114 | 108 |
| 1955/56 | 973 | 1,201 | 619 | 170 | 2,963 | 79 | 121 | 106 |
| 1960/61 | 1,300 | 1,611 | 775 | 181 | 3,866 | 103 | 148 | 130 |
| 1965/66 | 2,076 | 1,393 | 937 | 295 | 4,701 | 125 | 196 | 165 |
| 1970/71 | 2,317 | 1,889 | 1,148 | 324 | 5,678 | 151 | 261 | 202 |
| 1971/72 | 2,384 | 1,877 | 1,168 | 268 | 5,698 | 151 | 278 | 211 |
| 1972/73 | 2,517 | 1,872 | 1,166 | 274 | 5,828 | 155 | 297 | 224 |
| 1973/74 | 2,583 | 1,882 | 1,213 | 289 | 5,967 | 159 | 326 | 247 |
| 1974/75 | 3,036 | 1,829 | 1,408 | 352 | 6,624 | 176 | 345 | 271 |
| 1975/76 | 2,667 | 1,875 | 1,314 | 418 | 6,275 | 167 | 335 | 278 |
| 1976/77 | 2,994 | 1,861 | 1,284 | 383 | 6,522 | 173 | 338 | 285 |
| 1977/78 | 3,177 | 1,731 | 1,164 | 341 | 6,413 | 170 | 330 | 280 |
| 1978/79 | 3,378 | 1,777 | 1,267 | 346 | 6,768 | 180 | 335 | 287 |
| 1979/80 | 3,239 | 1,872 | 1,297 | 358 | 6,766 | 180 | 346 | 293 |
| 1980/81 | 3,371 | 2,096 | 1,373 | 342 | 7,182 | 191 | 360 | 306 |
| 1981/82 | 3,537 | 2,197 | 1,426 | 376 | 7,535 | 200 | 377 | 317 |
| 1982/83 | 3,789 | 2,305 | 1,490 | 564 | 8,148 | 217 | 383 | 321 |
| 1983/84 | 4,001 | 2,375 | 1,542 | 432 | 8,350 | 222 | 374 | 328 |
| 1984/85 | 4,128 | 2,564 | 1,607 | 443 | 8,742 | 232 | 376 | 332 |
| 1985/86 | 4,163 | 2,633 | 1,583 | 347 | 8,725 | 232 | 378 | 337 |
| 1986/87 | 4,415 | 2,712 | 1,732 | 306 | 9,166 | 244 | 392 | 355 |
| 1987/88 | 4,599 | 2,832 | 1,818 | 344 | 9,593 | 255 | 402 | 385 |
| 1988/89 | 4,890 | 2,967 | 1,968 | 357 | 10,181 | 271 | 412 | 400 |
| 1989/90 | 4,901 | 3,095 | 1,839 | 221 | 10,057 | 267 | 418 | 403 |
| 1990/91 | 4,919 | 3,548 | 1,865 | 206 | 10,539 | 280 | 428 | 417 |
| 1991/92 | 5,172 | 3,846 | 2,135 | 247 | 11,400 | 303 | 451 | 445 |
| 1992/93 | 5,614 | 4,048 | 2,158 | 289 | 12,110 | 322 | 476 | 472 |
| 1993/94 | 6,045 | 4,112 | 1,969 | 316 | 12,443 | 331 | 512 | 477 |
| 1994/95 | 6,390 | 4,172 | 2,024 | 344 | 12,931 | 344 | 508 | 506 |
| 1995/96 | 6,675 | 4,223 | 1,991 | 352 | 13,241 | 352 | 523 | 514 |
| 1996/97 | 7,025 | 4,316 | 1,976 | 363 | 13,680 | 364 | 489 | 516 |
| 1997/98 | 7,320 | 4,431 | 1,959 | 361 | 14,071 | 374 | 500 | 528 |
| 1998/99 | 7,533 | 4,491 | 2,050 | 351 | 14,425 | 383 | 516 | 543 |
| 1999/00 | 8,141 | 4,752 | 2,074 | 398 | 15,365 | 408 | 547 | 583 |
| 2000/01 | 8,538 | 5,085 | 2,155 | 408 | 16,187 | 430 | 590 | 627 |
| 2001/02 | 9,126 | 5,217 | 2,243 | 412 | 16,998 | 452 | 622 | 677 |
| 2002/03 | 9,754 | 5,313 | 2,278 | 404 | 17,749 | 472 | 662 | 730 |
| 2003/04 | 10,322 | 5,838 | 2,292 | 413 | 18,865 | 502 | 700 | 805 |
| 2004/05[2] | 10,504 | 8,270 | 2,390 | 427 | 21,590 | 574 | *756* | 849 |
| 2005/06 | 10,391 | 9,032 | 2,621 | 444 | 22,488 | 598 | 810 | 918 |

*Notes:* All General Medical figures for England, reported up to and including 2003/04 were based on a former statement of financial allowance (SFA). New GMS arrangements are wholly discretionary and are not "comparable against or reconcilable to" the figures shown up to 2003/04 (Departmental Report DH).

All figures include charges paid by patients. Except Welsh pharmaceutical and dental figures which are net of patient charges.

1 At constant prices, as adjusted by the Gross Domestic Product (GDP) deflator at market prices.

2 Figure in italics includes available data from Scotland and Wales for 2004/05 and OHE estimates based on trend for England and Northern Ireland using data pre and post 2004/05.

*Sources:* Health and Personal Social Services Statistics for England (DH).
Health Statistics Wales (NAW).
Scottish Health Statistics (ISD).
Annual Statistical Report (Northern Ireland CSA).
Annual Abstract of Statistics (ONS).
Department of Health Departmental Report (DH).
Economic Trends (ONS).
NHS Board Operating Costs and Capital Expenditure, (ISD Scotland).
Public Expenditure Statistical Analyses (HM Treasury).

Figure 4.1  **Family Health Services (FHS) expenditure as a percentage of gross NHS cost, UK, 1949/50 - 2005/06**

**FHS as % of NHS**

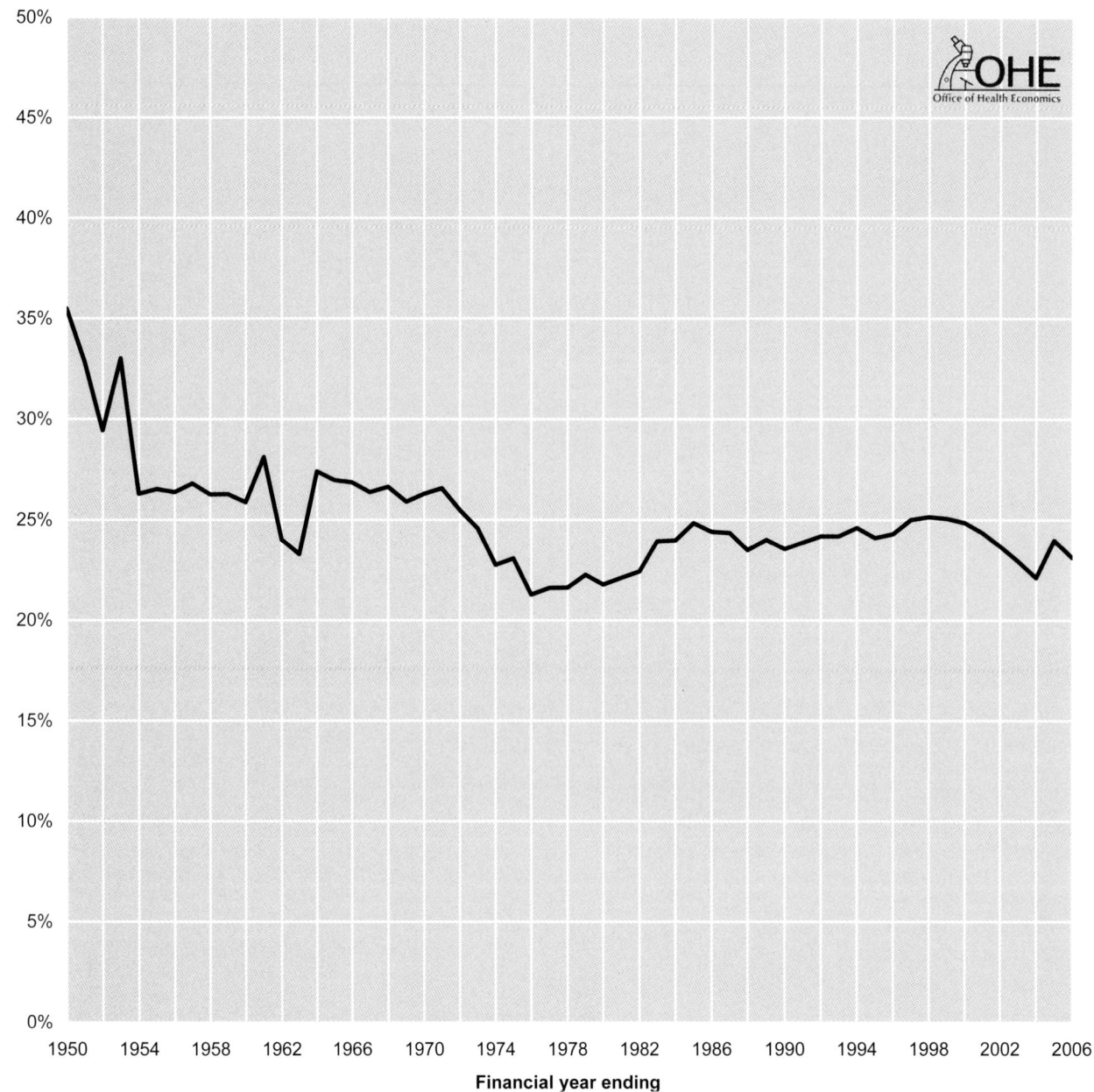

**Financial year ending**

*Notes:*   All General Medical figures for England, reported up to and including 2003/04 were based on a former statement of financial allowance (SFA). New GMS arrangements are wholly discretionary and are not comparable against or reconcilable to" the figures shown up to 2003/04 (Departmental Report DH).
All figures include charges paid by patients.  Except Welsh pharmaceutical and dental figures which are net of patient charges.
Figures are for financial year ending 31 March e.g. 2000 = 1999/2000.

*Sources:*   Health and Personal Social Services Statistics for England (DH).
Health Statistics Wales (NAW).
Scottish Health Statistics (ISD).
Annual Statistical Report (Northern Ireland CSA).
Annual Abstract of Statistics (ONS).
Economic Trends (ONS).
Department of Health Departmental Report (DH).
NHS Board Operating Costs and Capital Expenditure (ISD Scotland).
Public Expenditure Statistical Analyses (HM Treasury).

# Family Health Services (FHS)

Table 4.2  **Family Health Services (FHS) expenditure distribution by service, UK, 1949/50 - 2005/06**

| Year | Pharma-ceutical % | General Medical % | General Dental % | General Ophthalmic % | Total FHS cost: Cash £m | Total FHS cost: Real index[1] 1949=100 | Total FHS as a % of NHS cost |
|---|---|---|---|---|---|---|---|
| 1949/50 | 23.1 | 30.4 | 31.1 | 15.5 | 159 | 100 | 35.5 |
| 1950/51 | 25.6 | 30.9 | 29.4 | 14.1 | 158 | 98 | 32.9 |
| 1955/56 | 32.8 | 40.5 | 20.9 | 5.7 | 157 | 77 | 26.4 |
| 1960/61 | 33.6 | 41.7 | 20.0 | 4.7 | 248 | 101 | 28.1 |
| 1965/66 | 44.2 | 29.6 | 19.9 | 6.3 | 351 | 122 | 26.9 |
| 1966/67 | 43.1 | 29.6 | 21.2 | 6.1 | 378 | 126 | 26.4 |
| 1967/68 | 43.1 | 31.3 | 19.8 | 5.8 | 415 | 135 | 26.7 |
| 1968/69 | 42.9 | 31.8 | 19.6 | 5.8 | 434 | 135 | 25.9 |
| 1969/70 | 43.2 | 31.4 | 19.5 | 5.9 | 472 | 139 | 26.3 |
| 1970/71 | 40.8 | 33.3 | 20.2 | 5.7 | 544 | 148 | 26.6 |
| 1971/72 | 41.8 | 32.9 | 20.5 | 4.7 | 595 | 148 | 25.5 |
| 1972/73 | 43.2 | 32.1 | 20.0 | 4.7 | 660 | 152 | 24.6 |
| 1973/74 | 43.3 | 31.5 | 20.3 | 4.8 | 723 | 155 | 22.8 |
| 1974/75 | 45.8 | 27.6 | 21.3 | 5.3 | 960 | 172 | 23.1 |
| 1975/76 | 42.5 | 29.9 | 20.9 | 6.7 | 1,141 | 163 | 21.3 |
| 1976/77 | 45.9 | 28.5 | 19.7 | 5.9 | 1,346 | 170 | 21.6 |
| 1977/78 | 49.5 | 27.0 | 18.2 | 5.3 | 1,504 | 167 | 21.6 |
| 1978/79 | 49.9 | 26.3 | 18.7 | 5.1 | 1,763 | 176 | 22.3 |
| 1979/80 | 47.9 | 27.7 | 19.2 | 5.3 | 2,060 | 176 | 21.8 |
| 1980/81 | 46.9 | 29.2 | 19.1 | 4.8 | 2,584 | 187 | 22.1 |
| 1981/82 | 46.9 | 29.2 | 18.9 | 5.0 | 2,970 | 196 | 22.5 |
| 1982/83 | 46.5 | 28.3 | 18.3 | 6.9 | 3,439 | 212 | 23.9 |
| 1983/84 | 47.9 | 28.4 | 18.5 | 5.2 | 3,688 | 217 | 24.0 |
| 1984/85 | 47.2 | 29.3 | 18.4 | 5.1 | 4,064 | 228 | 24.9 |
| 1985/86 | 47.7 | 30.2 | 18.1 | 4.0 | 4,278 | 227 | 24.4 |
| 1986/87 | 48.2 | 29.6 | 18.9 | 3.3 | 4,640 | 239 | 24.4 |
| 1987/88 | 47.9 | 29.5 | 19.0 | 3.6 | 5,129 | 250 | 23.5 |
| 1988/89 | 48.0 | 29.1 | 19.3 | 3.5 | 5,824 | 265 | 24.0 |
| 1989/90 | 48.7 | 30.8 | 18.3 | 2.2 | 6,165 | 262 | 23.6 |
| 1990/91 | 46.7 | 33.7 | 17.7 | 2.0 | 6,968 | 274 | 23.9 |
| 1991/92 | 45.4 | 33.7 | 18.7 | 2.2 | 7,996 | 297 | 24.2 |
| 1992/93 | 46.4 | 33.4 | 17.8 | 2.4 | 8,769 | 315 | 24.2 |
| 1993/94 | 48.6 | 33.0 | 15.8 | 2.5 | 9,245 | 324 | 24.6 |
| 1994/95 | 49.4 | 32.3 | 15.7 | 2.7 | 9,753 | 337 | 24.1 |
| 1995/96 | 50.4 | 31.9 | 15.0 | 2.7 | 10,290 | 345 | 24.3 |
| 1996/97 | 51.3 | 31.6 | 14.4 | 2.7 | 10,989 | 356 | 25.0 |
| 1997/98 | 52.0 | 31.5 | 13.9 | 2.6 | 11,634 | 366 | 25.2 |
| 1998/99 | 52.2 | 31.1 | 14.2 | 2.4 | 12,229 | 376 | 25.1 |
| 1999/00 | 53.0 | 30.9 | 13.5 | 2.6 | 13,288 | 400 | 24.9 |
| 2000/01 | 52.7 | 31.4 | 13.3 | 2.5 | 14,199 | 421 | 24.4 |
| 2001/02 | 53.7 | 30.7 | 13.2 | 2.4 | 15,268 | 443 | 23.7 |
| 2002/03 | 55.0 | 29.9 | 12.8 | 2.3 | 16,440 | 462 | 22.9 |
| 2003/04 | 54.7 | 30.9 | 12.2 | 2.2 | 17,980 | 491 | 22.1 |
| 2004/05 | 48.7 | 38.3 | 11.1 | 2.0 | 21,146 | 562 | 24.0 |
| 2005/06 | 46.2 | 40.2 | 11.7 | 2.0 | 22,488 | 586 | 23.1 |

*Notes:*  All General Medical figures for England, reported up to and including 2003/04 were based on a former statement of financial allowance (SFA). New GMS arrangements are wholly discretionary and are not "comparable against or reconcilable to" the figures shown up to 2003/04 (Departmental Report DH).
All figures include charges paid by patients.   Except Welsh pharmaceutical and dental figures which are net of patient charges.
1 At constant prices, as adjusted by the Gross Domestic Product (GDP) deflator at market prices.

*Sources:*  Health and Personal Social Services Statistics for England (DH).
Health Statistics Wales (NAW).
Scottish Health Statistics (ISD).
Annual Statistical Report (Northern Ireland CSA).
Annual Abstract of Statistics (ONS).
Department of Health Departmental Report (DH).
Economic Trends (ONS).
NHS Board Operating Costs and Capital Expenditure, (ISD Scotland).
Public Expenditure Statistical Analyses (HM Treasury).

Figure 4.2 **Primary health care as a percentage of total health expenditure[1] in selected OECD countries, circa 2005**

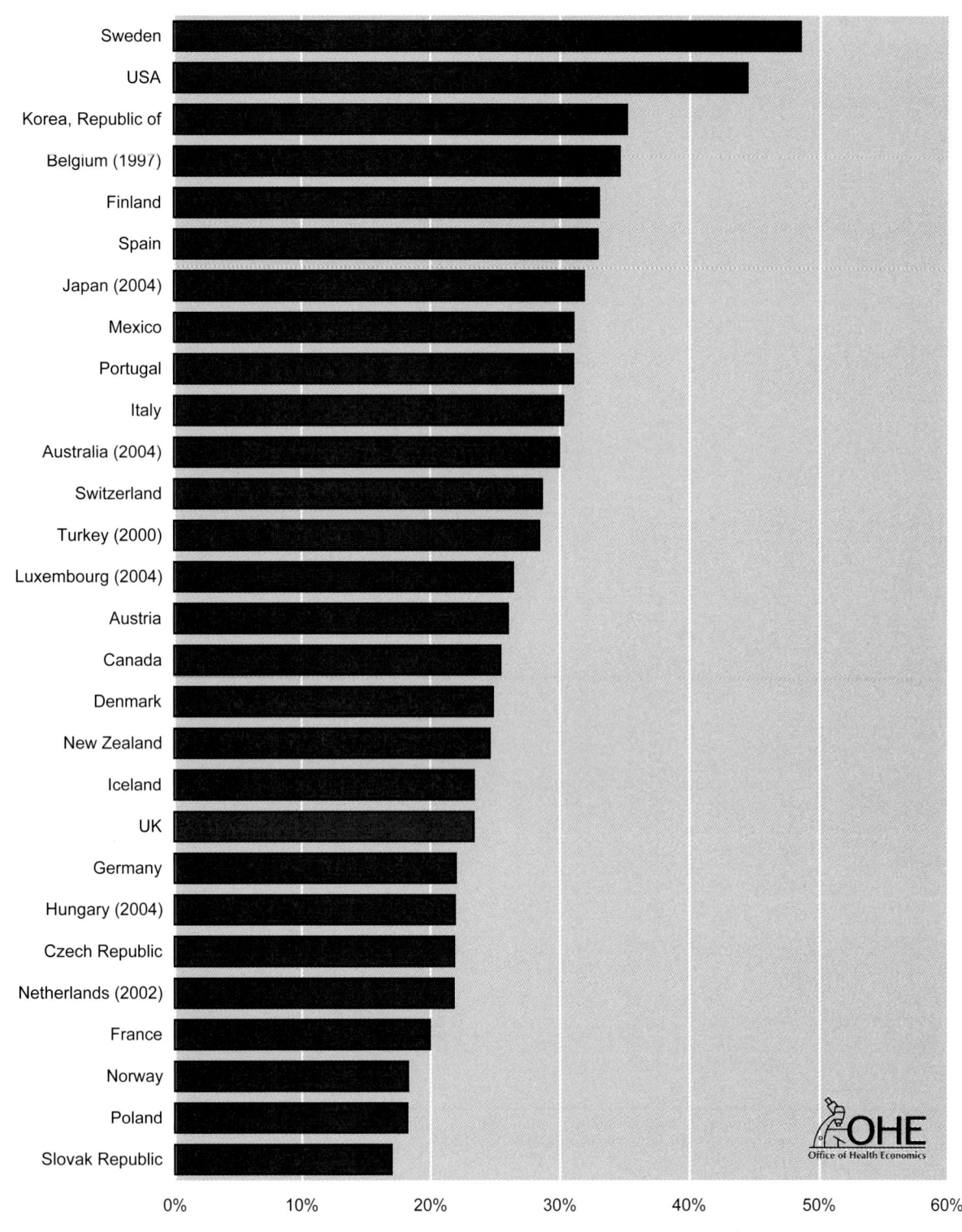

**Primary health care as % of total health care expenditure[1]**

Notes:   Year is 2005 unless stated otherwise.
1 Figures relate to both public and private health expenditure.
Figure for UK relates to NHS expenditure only.
Sources: OECD Health Database.
World Health Organisation National Health Accounts Series (WHO).
For UK, see Table 4.1.

Figure 4.3  **Real[1] growth in expenditure on Family Health Services (FHS) and hospital services, UK, 1949/50 - 2005/06**

**Index 1949/50=100**

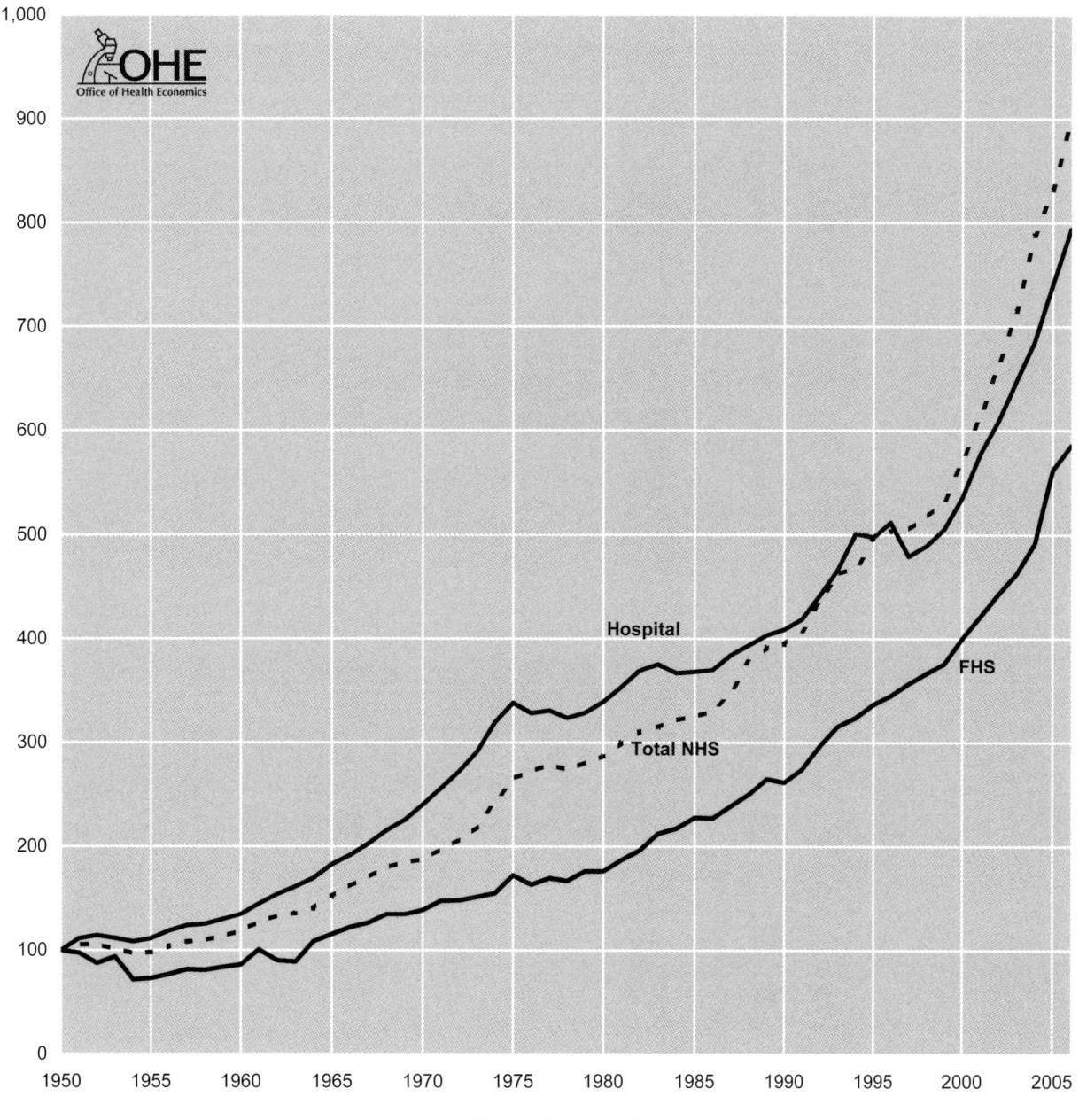

**Financial year ending**

Notes:   All figures include charges paid by patients.  Except Welsh pharmaceutical and dental figures which are net of patient charges.
Figures relate to financial year ending 31 March (e.g. 2000 = 1999/2000).
1 As adjusted by the Gross Domestic Product (GDP) deflator at market prices.

Sources: Health and Personal Social Services Statistics for England (DH).
Health Statistics Wales (NAW).
Scottish Health Statistics (ISD).
Annual Statistical Report (Northern Ireland CSA).
Annual Abstract of Statistics (ONS).
Economic Trends (ONS).
Department of Health Departmental Report (DH).
NHS Board Operating Costs and Capital Expenditure (ISD Scotland).
Public Expenditure Statistical Analyses (HM Treasury).

Table 4.3 **Real[1] cost of Family Health Services (FHS) per capita, UK, 1949/50 - 2005/06**

At 2005/06 prices[1]

| Year | Pharma-ceutical £ | General Medical £ | General Dental £ | General Ophthalmic £ | Total FHS cost per capita[1] | | Hospital cost per capita |
|---|---|---|---|---|---|---|---|
| | | | | | £ | Index (1949=100) | (1949=100) |
| 1949/50 | 17.58 | 23.15 | 23.68 | 11.82 | 76 | 100 | 100 |
| 1950/51 | 18.97 | 22.90 | 21.83 | 10.49 | 74 | 97 | 111 |
| 1955/56 | 19.08 | 23.55 | 12.13 | 3.33 | 58 | 76 | 117 |
| 1960/61 | 24.76 | 30.69 | 14.77 | 3.44 | 74 | 97 | 139 |
| 1965/66 | 38.14 | 25.59 | 17.22 | 5.41 | 86 | 113 | 178 |
| 1966/67 | 38.27 | 26.29 | 18.78 | 5.40 | 89 | 116 | 187 |
| 1967/68 | 40.63 | 29.51 | 18.61 | 5.45 | 94 | 124 | 197 |
| 1968/69 | 40.11 | 29.76 | 18.33 | 5.39 | 94 | 123 | 206 |
| 1969/70 | 41.56 | 30.15 | 18.74 | 5.70 | 96 | 126 | 218 |
| 1970/71 | 41.59 | 33.91 | 20.61 | 5.81 | 102 | 134 | 232 |
| 1971/72 | 42.60 | 33.53 | 20.87 | 4.79 | 102 | 134 | 246 |
| 1972/73 | 44.84 | 33.35 | 20.77 | 4.88 | 104 | 136 | 261 |
| 1973/74 | 45.94 | 33.46 | 21.58 | 5.14 | 106 | 139 | 286 |
| 1974/75 | 53.99 | 32.52 | 25.03 | 6.26 | 118 | 155 | 303 |
| 1975/76 | 47.44 | 33.35 | 23.38 | 7.43 | 112 | 146 | 294 |
| 1976/77 | 53.27 | 33.10 | 22.84 | 6.81 | 116 | 152 | 296 |
| 1977/78 | 56.54 | 30.81 | 20.72 | 6.07 | 114 | 150 | 290 |
| 1978/79 | 60.12 | 31.63 | 22.54 | 6.15 | 120 | 158 | 294 |
| 1979/80 | 57.56 | 33.28 | 23.06 | 6.36 | 120 | 158 | 304 |
| 1980/81 | 59.84 | 37.20 | 24.37 | 6.07 | 127 | 167 | 316 |
| 1981/82 | 62.78 | 39.00 | 25.31 | 6.67 | 134 | 175 | 330 |
| 1982/83 | 67.30 | 40.95 | 26.47 | 10.02 | 145 | 190 | 336 |
| 1983/84 | 71.01 | 42.16 | 27.37 | 7.68 | 148 | 194 | 328 |
| 1984/85 | 73.13 | 45.42 | 28.47 | 7.85 | 155 | 203 | 328 |
| 1985/86 | 73.56 | 46.53 | 27.97 | 6.13 | 154 | 202 | 329 |
| 1986/87 | 77.84 | 47.82 | 30.55 | 5.40 | 162 | 212 | 341 |
| 1987/88 | 80.93 | 49.83 | 31.99 | 6.06 | 169 | 221 | 349 |
| 1988/89 | 85.85 | 52.09 | 34.56 | 6.26 | 179 | 234 | 357 |
| 1989/90 | 85.81 | 54.19 | 32.20 | 3.87 | 176 | 231 | 361 |
| 1990/91 | 85.87 | 61.94 | 32.56 | 3.60 | 184 | 241 | 368 |
| 1991/92 | 89.99 | 66.92 | 37.15 | 4.29 | 198 | 260 | 387 |
| 1992/93 | 97.43 | 70.26 | 37.46 | 5.02 | 210 | 276 | 407 |
| 1993/94 | 104.68 | 71.20 | 34.10 | 5.48 | 215 | 283 | 437 |
| 1994/95 | 110.37 | 72.05 | 34.96 | 5.94 | 223 | 293 | 433 |
| 1995/96 | 114.97 | 72.73 | 34.30 | 6.06 | 228 | 299 | 444 |
| 1996/97 | 120.69 | 74.16 | 33.95 | 6.24 | 235 | 308 | 415 |
| 1997/98 | 125.43 | 75.93 | 33.58 | 6.19 | 241 | 316 | 422 |
| 1998/99 | 128.70 | 76.73 | 35.03 | 6.00 | 246 | 323 | 435 |
| 1999/00 | 138.61 | 80.90 | 35.30 | 6.78 | 262 | 343 | 460 |
| 2000/01 | 144.85 | 86.28 | 36.57 | 6.93 | 275 | 360 | 494 |
| 2001/02 | 154.24 | 88.18 | 37.92 | 6.96 | 287 | 377 | 519 |
| 2002/03 | 164.25 | 89.47 | 38.37 | 6.80 | 299 | 392 | 550 |
| 2003/04 | 173.10 | 97.90 | 38.44 | 6.93 | 316 | 415 | 579 |
| 2004/05[2] | 175.23 | 137.96 | 39.86 | 7.12 | 360 | 472 | 622 |
| 2005/06 | 172.24 | 149.72 | 43.45 | 7.36 | 373 | 489 | 663 |

*Notes:* All General Medical figures for England, reported up to and including 2003/04 were based on a former statement of financial allowance (SFA). New GMS arrangements are wholly discretionary and are not "comparable against or reconcilable to" the figures shown up to 2003/04 (Departmental Report DH).
All figures include charges paid by patients. Except welsh pharmaceutical and dental figures which are net of patient charges.
1 At constant prices, as adjusted by the Gross Domestic Product (GDP) deflator at market prices.
2 Figure in italics includes available data from Scotland and Wales for 2004/05 and OHE estimates based on trend for England and Northern Ireland using data pre and post 2004/05.

*Sources:* Health and Personal Social Services Statistics for England (DH).
Health Statistics Wales (NAW).
Scottish Health Statistics (ISD).
Annual Statistical Report (Northern Ireland CSA).
Annual Abstract of Statistics (ONS).
Department of Health Departmental Report (DH).
Economic Trends (ONS).
NHS Board Operating Costs and Capital Expenditure, (ISD Scotland).
Public Expenditure Statistical Analyses (HM Treasury).

Table 4.4   Family Health Services (FHS) gross expenditure (revenue and capital) per capita and per household, UK, 1975/76 - 2005/06

| Year | England | Wales | Scotland | Northern Ireland | UK | England | Wales | Scotland | Northern Ireland | UK |
|---|---|---|---|---|---|---|---|---|---|---|
| | | | | | FHS expenditure per capita (£ cash) | | | | | |
| | | | (£ cash) | | | At constant prices[1] (Index 1975/76=100) | | | | |
| 1975/76 | 20 | 22 | 21 | 21 | 20 | 100 | 100 | 100 | 100 | 100 |
| 1980/81 | 46 | 50 | 47 | 49 | 46 | 116 | 115 | 113 | 118 | 116 |
| 1985/86 | 76 | 84 | 77 | 79 | 77 | 141 | 142 | 136 | 140 | 141 |
| 1986/87 | 81 | 90 | 85 | 84 | 82 | 145 | 147 | 145 | 144 | 146 |
| 1987/88 | 89 | 99 | 94 | 94 | 90 | 151 | 153 | 152 | 152 | 152 |
| 1988/89 | 100 | 110 | 106 | 104 | 101 | 159 | 159 | 160 | 157 | 159 |
| 1989/90 | 107 | 113 | 111 | 115 | 108 | 159 | 152 | 157 | 162 | 158 |
| 1990/91 | 120 | 131 | 125 | 129 | 122 | 166 | 164 | 163 | 170 | 165 |
| 1991/92 | 137 | 155 | 143 | 150 | 139 | 178 | 182 | 176 | 186 | 178 |
| 1992/93 | 151 | 162 | 155 | 167 | 152 | 189 | 185 | 185 | 200 | 189 |
| 1993/94 | 158 | 171 | 163 | 178 | 160 | 194 | 191 | 190 | 208 | 194 |
| 1994/95 | 167 | 178 | 172 | 188 | 168 | 201 | 195 | 198 | 216 | 201 |
| 1995/96 | 174 | 193 | 186 | 206 | 177 | 204 | 205 | 207 | 229 | 205 |
| 1996/97 | 185 | 203 | 205 | 223 | 189 | 210 | 209 | 221 | 241 | 211 |
| 1997/98 | 195 | 217 | 219 | 236 | 199 | 214 | 217 | 229 | 247 | 217 |
| 1998/99 | 204 | 228 | 232 | 246 | 209 | 219 | 222 | 237 | 252 | 222 |
| 1999/00 | 221 | 252 | 249 | 265 | 226 | 232 | 241 | 249 | 265 | 235 |
| 2000/01 | 236 | 269 | 263 | 272 | 241 | 245 | 254 | 259 | 269 | 247 |
| 2001/02 | 252 | 287 | 287 | 291 | 258 | 255 | 264 | 277 | 280 | 258 |
| 2002/03 | 270 | 310 | 316 | 316 | 277 | 265 | 277 | 295 | 295 | 269 |
| 2003/04 | 294 | 333 | 341 | 350 | 302 | 281 | 289 | 309 | 318 | 285 |
| 2004/05 | 349 | 366 | 371 | 378 | 353 | 324 | 309 | 328 | 334 | 324 |
| 2005/06 | 369 | 382 | 394 | 398 | 373 | 336 | 316 | 341 | 345 | 335 |
| | | | | | FHS expenditure per household (£ cash) | | | | | |
| | | | (£ cash) | | | At constant prices[1] (Index 1975/76=100) | | | | |
| 1975/76 | 57 | 64 | 62 | 66 | 58 | 100 | 100 | 100 | 100 | 100 |
| 1980/81 | 126 | 140 | 133 | 147 | 128 | 112 | 111 | 107 | 112 | 112 |
| 1985/86 | 199 | 224 | 203 | 238 | 202 | 130 | 130 | 121 | 133 | 130 |
| 1986/87 | 211 | 238 | 221 | 252 | 215 | 134 | 134 | 127 | 137 | 133 |
| 1987/88 | 230 | 259 | 242 | 281 | 234 | 138 | 138 | 132 | 144 | 138 |
| 1988/89 | 256 | 285 | 270 | 310 | 261 | 143 | 142 | 137 | 149 | 143 |
| 1989/90 | 271 | 289 | 281 | 340 | 275 | 142 | 134 | 133 | 152 | 141 |
| 1990/91 | 303 | 334 | 312 | 378 | 307 | 147 | 144 | 137 | 156 | 146 |
| 1991/92 | 343 | 391 | 356 | 439 | 349 | 157 | 159 | 148 | 171 | 157 |
| 1992/93 | 376 | 408 | 382 | 478 | 380 | 166 | 161 | 154 | 181 | 165 |
| 1993/94 | 393 | 429 | 401 | 508 | 399 | 170 | 164 | 157 | 187 | 169 |
| 1994/95 | 413 | 444 | 420 | 519 | 418 | 175 | 167 | 162 | 188 | 174 |
| 1995/96 | 431 | 477 | 449 | 572 | 438 | 178 | 175 | 168 | 202 | 177 |
| 1996/97 | 456 | 501 | 490 | 608 | 465 | 182 | 178 | 178 | 207 | 182 |
| 1997/98 | 479 | 533 | 520 | 684 | 491 | 186 | 183 | 183 | 227 | 187 |
| 1998/99 | 501 | 558 | 547 | 694 | 513 | 189 | 187 | 188 | 224 | 190 |
| 1999/00 | 541 | 616 | 582 | 729 | 553 | 201 | 203 | 196 | 231 | 201 |
| 2000/01 | 575 | 655 | 611 | 736 | 586 | 210 | 212 | 203 | 230 | 210 |
| 2001/02 | 608 | 691 | 662 | 782 | 622 | 217 | 219 | 215 | 239 | 218 |
| 2002/03 | 647 | 740 | 723 | 841 | 663 | 224 | 228 | 227 | 249 | 225 |
| 2003/04 | 702 | 791 | 774 | 924 | 719 | 236 | 236 | 237 | 266 | 237 |
| 2004/05 | 832 | 865 | 840 | 993 | 839 | 272 | 251 | 250 | 278 | 269 |
| 2005/06 | 876 | 898 | 884 | 1041 | 882 | 281 | 256 | 258 | 285 | 278 |

Notes:   All figures include charges paid by patients and relate to financial years ending 31 March.
1 At constant prices, as adjusted by the Gross Domestic Product (GDP) deflator at market prices.

Sources:   The Government's Expenditure Plans (DH).
Health and Personal Social Services Statistics for England (DH).
Scottish Health Statistics (ISD).
Health Statistics Wales (NAW).
Annual Abstract of Statistics (ONS).
Economic Data (HM Treasury).

For most people seeking medical treatment, a General Medical Practitioner (GP) is the first point of contact with the NHS. Visits to the GP surgery are free. The large majority of the UK population are registered with a GP. In the UK in 2006 there were 43,021 GPs, providing medical care under the NHS (**Table 4.7**). According to the Royal College of General Practitioners there were 10,352 practices in 2005, this represents a year on year decrease over the previous 5 years, corresponding to a shift towards multi-GP practices.

## Cost of the General Medical Services

Approximately 9.3% of NHS spend in 2005/06 was on GMS, a slightly lower percentage than for 1949/50, the first full year after the NHS was established, but considerably less than the peak of 17% observed in the early 1950s (**Figure 4.4**).

The total cost of General Medical Services (GMS) in the UK rose to £9bn in 2005/06, a massive increase of 77.6% in real terms over the previous five years alone (**Figure 4.4** and **Table 4.1**), and almost eight times higher than the cost in 1949 in real terms. **Box 5** shows the considerable increases in GMS expenditure over the past 40 years and in particular for the past two decades.

| Box 5 **Real[1] decadal growth (per cent) of GMS expenditure, UK** | | |
|---|---|---|
| | **Total GMS\*** | **GMS per capita[1]** |
| 1965/66 - 1975/76 | 35 | 30 |
| 1975/76 - 1985/86 | 40 | 40 |
| 1985/86 - 1995/96 | 60 | 56 |
| 1995/96 - 2005/06 | 114 | 106 |

*Note:* 1 At constant prices, as adjusted by the GDP deflator at market prices.
*Sources:* Health and Personal Social Services Statistics for England (DH).
Health Statistics Wales (NAW).
Scottish Health Statistics (ISD).
Annual Statistical Report (Northern Ireland CSA).
Annual Abstract of Statistics (ONS).
Department of Health Departmental Report (DH).
NHS Board Operating Costs and Capital Expenditure (ISD Scotland).
Public Expenditure Statistical Analyses (HM Treasury) .
Population Projections Database (GAD).

Expenditure on GMS per capita stood at £150 in the UK in 2005/06, more than double the level just a decade earlier in real terms (**Table 4.5**). In recent years all countries within the UK have seen considerable increases in per capita GMS spend but it is highest in England and lowest in Northern Ireland.

## GMS workforce and list characteristics

There are various types of general medical practitioners (GPs) working in general practice. The classification of GPs is based on their qualifications and the type of contract that practitioners have with the NHS. Under the new GMS contact from 1 April 2004, GPs working in general practice are categorised as registrars, retainers and medical practitioners. A GP registrar is a fully registered practitioner who is being trained for general practice, while a GP retainer is one who is employed by the general practice to provide approximately half a day each week. All practitioners, contracted or salaried, excluding registrars and retainers, are collectively termed medical practitioners. Due to this new categorisation of medical practitioners working in general practice, comparisons over time and between countries in the UK should be treated with caution.

In 2006 there were over 143,000 medical staff working in the NHS in the UK, including 43,000 GPs, over 98,000 hospital medical staff and almost 2,000 community medical staff (**Table 4.6**). In recent years the number of support staff working in general practice, as well as the number of GPs, has seen a considerable increase (**Box 6).**

| Box 6 **Staff (full-time equivalents) employed in GP practices, England** | | | |
|---|---|---|---|
| | **1996** | **2001** | **2006** |
| Total staff | 59,318 | 64,998 | 76,977 |
| Practice nurses | 9,821 | 11,163 | 14,616 |
| Direct patient care | 1,486 | 2,090 | 5,170 |
| Admin and clerical | 47,637 | 51,390 | 55,116 |
| Other | 374 | 355 | 2,075 |

*Note:* All figures relate to 30 September.
*Source:* General and Personal Medical Services in England (Statistical Bulletin) (DH).

In 2006 the NHS contracted with 43,021 GPs (including registrars), an increase of almost 20% on 1996 (**Table 4.7**), and almost double the number of GPs reported 50 years earlier (**Table 4.6**). Although the numbers of medical practitioners have risen in all constituent countries of the UK over the past decade, England and Wales saw the greatest growth at 18.2% more GPs between 1996 and 2006, compared to an increase of 9.8% in Northern Ireland (**Box 7**).

# FHS: General Medical Services

**Box 7 Decadal change (per cent) in the numbers of medical practitioners (excluding registrars and retainers), UK**

| | England and Wales | Scotland | Northern Ireland | UK |
|---|---|---|---|---|
| 1966 - 1976 | 10.1 | 9.7 | -3.1 | 9.6 |
| 1976 - 1986 | 19.1 | 16.0 | 24.6 | 18.9 |
| 1986 - 1996 | 13.7 | 11.1 | 11.6 | 13.4 |
| 1996 - 2006[1] | 18.2 | 14.2 | 9.8 | 17.6 |

*Notes:* 1 Figures from 1994 have been revised to allow for changes following the new GMS contract (2004). Medical practitioners include all contracted and salaried GPs but exclude registrars and retainers. Prior to 2004 these medical practitioners were known as unrestricted principals.
Figures exclude GP locums.
*Sources:* Annual Abstract of Statistics (ONS).
General and Personal Medical Services Statistics (DH).
General Medical Practitioners by type – StatWales (NAW).
GP Statistics (ISD Scotland).
General Medical Practitioners (Northern Ireland CSA).

In the UK there were 66 medical practitioners (excluding trainees and retainers) in general practice for every 100,000 population in 2006. However, this ratio was highly variable across the UK, with over 81 per 100,000 population in Scotland, compared to just 65 in England, 64 in Northern Ireland, and 63 in Wales (**Table 4.8**).

Over the past 50 years there has been a decrease in the number of patients per medical practitioner (excluding GP registrars and retainers) in general practice in total and for all age groups bar the 75 and over age group (**Tables 4.12** and **4.13**).

Average list size per medical practitioner has decreased 13% in the last 10 years in the UK, (**Figure 4.6** and **Table 4.11**). The average list size was considerably lower in Scotland than in the rest of the UK in 2006, an estimated 1,309. In comparison, the average list sizes in the other constituent countries were all over 1,600 in 2006 (**Table 4.11** and **Figure 4.6**).

In recent years the trend towards GP consolidation into larger multi-partner practices in has accelerated somewhat. The majority of medical practitioners in the UK were in partnerships of five or more in 2005: 60% compared to 43% ten years earlier (**Table 4.15**). In contrast, 5% of GPs were single handed in 2005 compared to 10% a decade earlier. **Figure 4.7** clearly shows the increased number of medical practitioners in practices with 5 and 6 or more doctors in England and Wales and the decreased number of single handed practices which has continued into 2006. The shift towards larger practice sizes has been consistent throughout all countries in the UK (**Tables 4.16a, b** and **c**).

The age and sex profile of GPs has changed somewhat over the past 20 years, with considerable increases in the number of female practitioners and decreases in the proportion of GPs aged under 40. In 2006, 42% of GPs were female, double the proportion observed 20 years earlier (**Table 4.14**). The proportion of GPs aged under 40 declined from 40% in 1985 to 31% in 2005.

## GP consultations

The 2005 *General Household Survey* revealed that on average each member of the population consults a GP four times per year. **Box 8** shows that, at an average cost of about £30 per consultation in England in 2005, the total annual per capita cost of GP consultations in the UK is about £138 per person, almost double in real terms to the per capita cost of 10 years earlier.

**Box 8 Average cost of a GP consultation, UK (2005 prices)**

| Year | Cost (£) per consultation | Annual cost (£) of GP consultations per capita |
|---|---|---|
| 1989 | 10.92 | 50 |
| 1990 | 10.43 | 53 |
| 1991 | 13.50 | 61 |
| 1992 | 13.57 | 66 |
| 1993 | 14.05 | 69 |
| 1994 | 13.98 | 71 |
| 1995 | 14.02 | 71 |
| 1996 | 14.10 | 71 |
| 1997 | 15.17 | 73 |
| 1998 | 16.31 | 75 |
| 1999 | 16.94 | 77 |
| 2000 | 18.19 | 82 |
| 2001 | 19.35 | 86 |
| 2002 | 17.61 | 87 |
| 2003 | 20.59 | 90 |
| 2004 | 23.63 | 106 |
| 2005 | 30.45 | 138 |

*Notes:* All figures are in 2005 prices and are survey based, hence subject to sampling error.
From 1988 to 2004 the General Household Survey was on a financial year basis with interviews taking place from April to the following March.
*Sources:* The Government's Expenditure Plans (DH).
General Household Survey (ONS).
Population Projections Database (GAD).

The number of NHS GP consultations was estimated at 274 million in 2005, slightly above the 2000 level, but slightly below the 1990 level (**Table 4.17**), based on data from the *General Household Survey*. Although there has been an increase in the number of individuals visiting NHS GPs, the average number of NHS consultations per GP has decreased, to 6,884 per GP in 2005 (**Table 4.18**).

The number of GP consultations remains greater for women than for men. The difference is mainly due to the 16 to 44 age group, for which women have a GP consultation rate nearly twice that of men. Part of this difference can be attributed to pregnancy and family planning consultations.

While the number of consultations for those 75 years and over has increased (**Table 4.17**), there has been a considerable shift in the way they access services, with approximately 78% of consultations taking place in the GP's surgery in 2005 compared to just 36% in 1975 (**Box 9**). Considering all ages combined, just 13 percent of consultations took place outside the surgery in 2005. Data from the *General Household Survey* indicate that along with the fall in home visits and increased number of consultations in the surgery, there has been an increase in the number of consultations taking place over the telephone.

Box 9 **Per cent of NHS GP consultations taking place in surgery, Great Britain**

|      | All ages | 75 and over |
|------|----------|-------------|
| 1975 | 78       | 36          |
| 1980 | 78       | 46          |
| 1985 | 79       | 47          |
| 1990 | 78       | 48          |
| 1991 | 81       | 56          |
| 1992 | 83       | 60          |
| 1993 | 84       | 56          |
| 1994 | 83       | 66          |
| 1996 | 84       | 68          |
| 1998 | 84       | 71          |
| 2000 | 86       | 71          |
| 2001 | 85       | 73          |
| 2002 | 86       | 75          |
| 2003 | 86       | 82          |
| 2004 | 87       | 79          |
| 2005 | 87       | 78          |

*Notes:* Some of the fluctuations in these time series are due to sampling error.
Figures from 1998 onwards are weighted.
Figures for 75 and over may overestimate the proportion of consultations at surgery, due to consultations taking place at more than one site.
From 1988 to 2004 the General Household Survey was on a financial year basis with interviews taking place from April to the following March.
Data for 1995, 1997 and 1999 are not available.
*Source:* Living In Britain: Results from the General Household Survey (ONS).

## Dispensing doctors

Although most NHS prescriptions are dispensed by pharmacies, a small and slowly growing proportion is dispensed by GPs in their surgeries. In rural areas a doctor may dispense medicines to patients who would have difficulties in obtaining them from a pharmacist because of distance.

In 2005 over 60 million prescriptions were dispensed by dispensing doctors in the UK (**Table 4.19**), an increase of 64% on the past decade alone. This is despite the number of dispensing doctors having declined in recent years, standing at 3,869 in 2005.

# FHS: General Medical Services

Table 4.5   Cost of General Medical Services (GMS) per capita and per household, UK, 1975/76 - 2005/06

| Year | England | Wales | Scotland | Northern Ireland | UK | England | Wales | Scotland | Northern Ireland | UK |
|------|---------|-------|----------|------------------|-----|---------|-------|----------|------------------|-----|
| | | | | | GMS expenditure per capita | | | | | |
| | | | (£ cash) | | | At constant prices[1] (Index 1975/76=100) | | | | |
| 1975/76 | 6 | 6 | 6 | 6 | 6 | 100 | 100 | 100 | 100 | 100 |
| 1980/81 | 13 | 13 | 15 | 13 | 13 | 110 | 110 | 126 | 110 | 110 |
| 1985/86 | 23 | 23 | 25 | 22 | 23 | 142 | 142 | 155 | 136 | 142 |
| 1987/88 | 26 | 27 | 29 | 25 | 27 | 147 | 153 | 164 | 142 | 153 |
| 1988/89 | 29 | 30 | 32 | 27 | 30 | 154 | 159 | 170 | 143 | 159 |
| 1989/90 | 33 | 34 | 36 | 31 | 33 | 163 | 166 | 178 | 152 | 164 |
| 1990/91 | 41 | 41 | 44 | 37 | 41 | 187 | 186 | 200 | 171 | 188 |
| 1991/92 | 47 | 46 | 49 | 38 | 47 | 203 | 201 | 210 | 164 | 203 |
| 1992/93 | 51 | 49 | 52 | 44 | 51 | 214 | 207 | 217 | 183 | 213 |
| 1993/94 | 53 | 52 | 54 | 46 | 53 | 217 | 212 | 220 | 186 | 216 |
| 1994/95 | 54 | 51 | 57 | 50 | 54 | 219 | 206 | 230 | 200 | 218 |
| 1995/96 | 56 | 57 | 61 | 51 | 57 | 219 | 224 | 238 | 200 | 220 |
| 1996/97 | 59 | 59 | 65 | 54 | 60 | 223 | 223 | 247 | 205 | 225 |
| 1997/98 | 62 | 62 | 70 | 56 | 63 | 228 | 228 | 257 | 206 | 230 |
| 1998/99 | 65 | 64 | 72 | 58 | 65 | 231 | 229 | 258 | 207 | 233 |
| 1999/00 | 70 | 70 | 74 | 64 | 70 | 244 | 247 | 261 | 225 | 245 |
| 2000/01 | 76 | 74 | 80 | 63 | 76 | 262 | 256 | 276 | 219 | 261 |
| 2001/02 | 79 | 78 | 85 | 66 | 79 | 267 | 262 | 286 | 221 | 267 |
| 2002/03 | 82 | 82 | 92 | 76 | 83 | 269 | 269 | 303 | 249 | 271 |
| 2003/04 | 93 | 92 | 103 | 90 | 93 | 294 | 291 | 326 | 286 | 297 |
| 2004/05 | 137 | 132 | 124 | 107 | 135 | 425 | 407 | 383 | 332 | 418 |
| 2005/06 | 152 | 142 | 137 | 123 | 150 | 462 | 429 | 417 | 372 | 454 |
| | | | | | GMS expenditure per household | | | | | |
| | | | (£ cash) | | | At constant prices[1] (Index 1975/76=100) | | | | |
| 1975/76 | 17 | 17 | 18 | 19 | 17 | 100 | 100 | 100 | 100 | 100 |
| 1980/81 | 35 | 36 | 42 | 41 | 36 | 106 | 105 | 120 | 111 | 105 |
| 1985/86 | 60 | 61 | 66 | 66 | 60 | 131 | 130 | 137 | 132 | 131 |
| 1987/88 | 67 | 70 | 75 | 76 | 70 | 134 | 138 | 142 | 138 | 139 |
| 1988/89 | 74 | 78 | 81 | 83 | 77 | 138 | 142 | 145 | 143 | 143 |
| 1989/90 | 83 | 86 | 91 | 91 | 84 | 145 | 147 | 151 | 145 | 146 |
| 1990/91 | 102 | 103 | 109 | 109 | 103 | 166 | 163 | 169 | 161 | 166 |
| 1991/92 | 118 | 117 | 121 | 110 | 118 | 179 | 175 | 176 | 154 | 178 |
| 1992/93 | 127 | 124 | 128 | 125 | 127 | 188 | 179 | 180 | 169 | 186 |
| 1993/94 | 132 | 130 | 132 | 129 | 131 | 190 | 183 | 182 | 170 | 188 |
| 1994/95 | 134 | 128 | 139 | 137 | 135 | 191 | 177 | 188 | 178 | 189 |
| 1995/96 | 138 | 142 | 147 | 142 | 139 | 191 | 191 | 194 | 178 | 191 |
| 1996/97 | 145 | 146 | 157 | 150 | 147 | 194 | 190 | 199 | 183 | 194 |
| 1997/98 | 153 | 152 | 166 | 162 | 154 | 198 | 193 | 206 | 192 | 198 |
| 1998/99 | 158 | 157 | 170 | 162 | 159 | 200 | 194 | 205 | 187 | 200 |
| 1999/00 | 170 | 172 | 174 | 176 | 171 | 211 | 208 | 206 | 199 | 210 |
| 2000/01 | 184 | 180 | 185 | 171 | 184 | 224 | 214 | 216 | 190 | 222 |
| 2001/02 | 190 | 187 | 195 | 176 | 190 | 227 | 218 | 222 | 192 | 225 |
| 2002/03 | 197 | 196 | 211 | 202 | 198 | 227 | 222 | 233 | 213 | 227 |
| 2003/04 | 221 | 217 | 232 | 237 | 222 | 248 | 238 | 249 | 243 | 247 |
| 2004/05 | 327 | 310 | 279 | 281 | 320 | 357 | 331 | 291 | 280 | 347 |
| 2005/06 | 361 | 332 | 308 | 320 | 354 | 386 | 347 | 315 | 314 | 375 |

*Notes:*   All figures include salaries, fees, allowances, superannuation, directly reimbursed expenses (e.g. rent and rates) and other expenses, in financial years ending 31 March.

Figures from 2004/05 for England based on new GMS contract figures.

All General Medical figures for England, reported up to and including 2003/04 were based on a former statement of financial allowance (SFA). New GMS arrangements are wholly discretionary and are not "comparable against or reconcilable to" the figures shown up to 2003/04 (Departmental Report DH).

1 At constant prices, as adjusted by the Gross Domestic Product (GDP) deflator at market prices.

*Sources:*   The Government's Expenditure Plans (DH).
Health and Personal Social Services Statistics for England (DH).
Scottish Health Statistics (ISD).
Health Statistics Wales (NAW).
Annual Abstract of Statistics (ONS).
Economic Data (HM Treasury).

Figure 4.4  **Cost of General Medical Services (GMS) at 2005/06 prices[1], UK, 1949/50 - 2005/06**

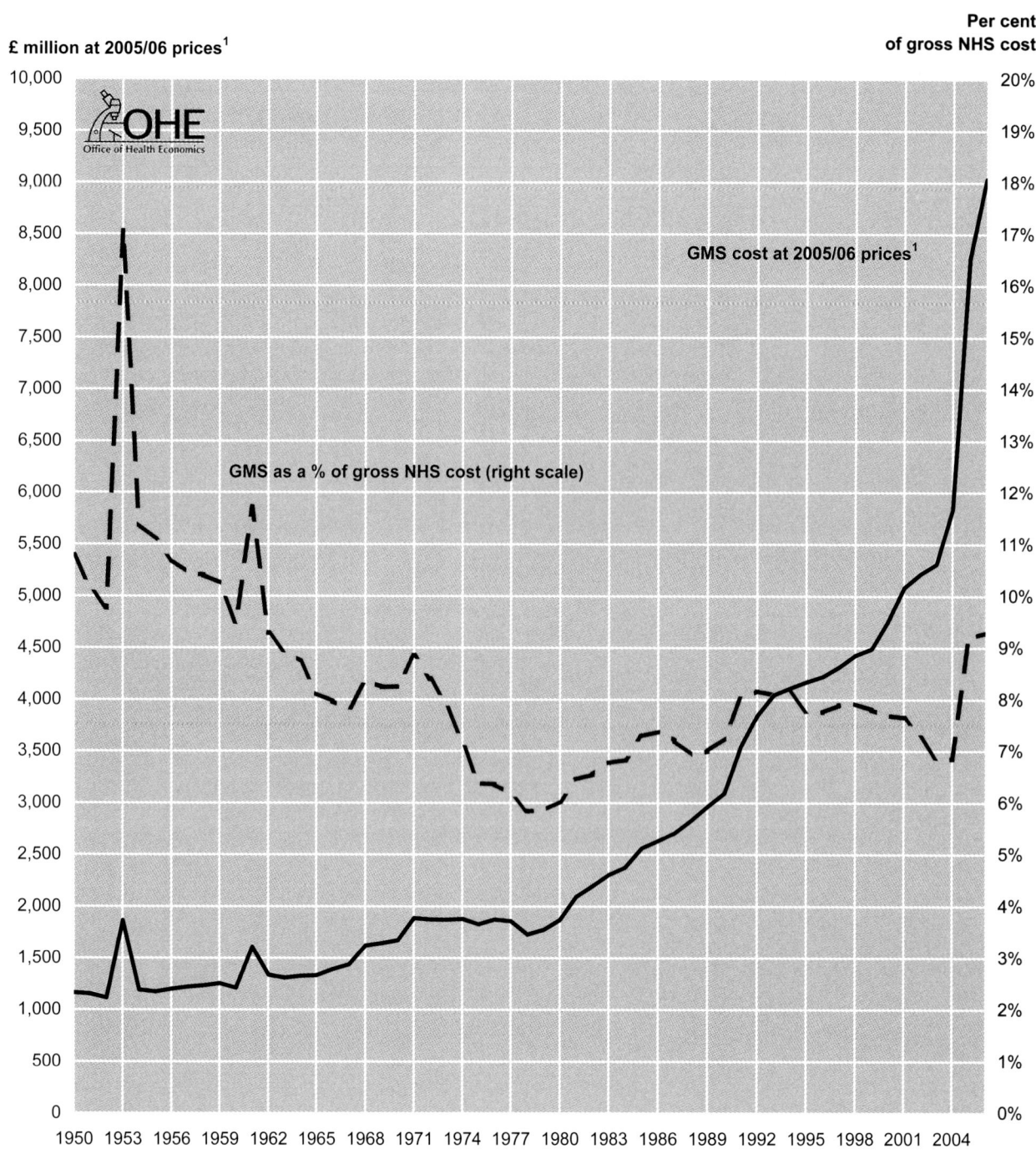

**£ million at 2005/06 prices[1]**

**Per cent of gross NHS cost**

GMS cost at 2005/06 prices[1]

GMS as a % of gross NHS cost (right scale)

**Financial year ending**

*Notes:*   Figures for 1952 and 1953 reflect payments of arrears awarded for the period from 1948 to 1952.
Figures relate to financial year ending 31 March (e.g. 2000 = 1999/2000).
1 As adjusted by the Gross Domestic Product (GDP) deflator at market prices.

*Sources:*  Health and Personal Social Services Statistics for England (DH).
Health Statistics Wales (NAW).
Scottish Health Statistics (ISD).
Annual Statistical Report (Northern Ireland CSA).
Annual Abstract of Statistics (ONS).
Economic Trends (ONS).
Department of Health Departmental Report (DH).
NHS Board Operating Costs and Capital Expenditure, ISD Scotland.
Public Expenditure Statistical Analyses (HM Treasury).

Table 4.6 **NHS medical workforce (GPs, hospital and community medical staff), UK, 1951 - 2006**

| Year | All GPs[1] | Hospital medical staff[2] | Community medical staff[3] | Total UK medical staff | Per 100,000 population | | | |
|---|---|---|---|---|---|---|---|---|
| | | | | | All GPs[1] | Hospital medical staff[2] | Community medical staff[3] | Total UK medical staff |
| | Number | FTE | FTE | | | | | |
| 1951 | 22,478 | 14,393 | - | 36,871 | 45 | 29 | - | 73 |
| 1955 | 22,771 | 16,033 | - | 38,804 | 45 | 31 | - | 76 |
| 1960 | 23,408 | 19,337 | 959 | 43,704 | 45 | 37 | 2 | 83 |
| 1965 | 24,292 | 22,338 | 1,037 | 47,667 | 45 | 41 | 2 | 88 |
| 1966 | 24,423 | 22,991 | 2,293 | 49,708 | 45 | 42 | 4 | 91 |
| 1967 | 24,565 | 24,010 | 2,296 | 50,871 | 45 | 44 | 4 | 93 |
| 1968 | 24,679 | 25,011 | 2,354 | 52,044 | 45 | 45 | 4 | 94 |
| 1969 | 24,789 | 25,912 | 2,343 | 53,044 | 45 | 47 | 4 | 96 |
| 1970 | 24,865 | 26,684 | 2,415 | 53,964 | 45 | 48 | 4 | 97 |
| 1971 | 24,998 | 28,102 | 2,430 | 55,530 | 45 | 50 | 4 | 99 |
| 1972 | 25,073 | 29,574 | 2,493 | 57,140 | 45 | 53 | 4 | 102 |
| 1973 | 25,130 | 30,847 | 2,642 | 58,618 | 45 | 55 | 5 | 104 |
| 1974 | 25,135 | 32,258 | 2,523 | 59,916 | 45 | 57 | 4 | 107 |
| 1975 | 26,942 | 33,922 | 3,295 | 64,159 | 48 | 60 | 6 | 114 |
| 1976 | 27,255 | 34,829 | 3,433 | 65,517 | 48 | 62 | 6 | 117 |
| 1977 | 27,657 | 35,839 | 3,498 | 66,994 | 49 | 64 | 6 | 119 |
| 1978 | 28,067 | 36,994 | 3,537 | 68,599 | 50 | 66 | 6 | 122 |
| 1979 | 28,565 | 38,399 | 3,566 | 70,530 | 51 | 68 | 6 | 125 |
| 1980 | 29,336 | 39,562 | 3,593 | 72,491 | 52 | 70 | 6 | 129 |
| 1981 | 30,182 | 40,386 | 3,654 | 74,222 | 54 | 72 | 6 | 132 |
| 1982 | 30,727 | 43,003 | 3,642 | 77,372 | 55 | 76 | 6 | 137 |
| 1983 | 31,314 | 43,812 | 3,659 | 78,786 | 56 | 78 | 6 | 140 |
| 1984 | 31,886 | 44,177 | 3,623 | 79,686 | 57 | 78 | 6 | 141 |
| 1985 | 32,436 | 44,757 | 3,678 | 80,871 | 57 | 79 | 7 | 143 |
| 1986 | 32,843 | 45,156 | 3,674 | 81,673 | 58 | 80 | 6 | 144 |
| 1987 | 33,430 | 45,512 | 3,483 | 82,425 | 59 | 80 | 6 | 145 |
| 1988 | 33,900 | 46,716 | 3,538 | 84,154 | 60 | 82 | 6 | 148 |
| 1989 | 34,331 | 48,265 | 3,483 | 86,079 | 60 | 85 | 6 | 151 |
| 1990 | 34,083 | 49,314 | 3,457 | 86,854 | 60 | 86 | 6 | 152 |
| 1991 | 34,498 | 51,060 | 3,494 | 89,052 | 60 | 89 | 6 | 155 |
| 1992 | 34,880 | 52,206 | 3,487 | 90,573 | 61 | 91 | 6 | 157 |
| 1993 | 35,184 | 54,685 | 3,479 | 92,480 | 61 | 96 | 6 | 160 |
| 1994 | 35,435 | 56,145 | 3,230 | 94,810 | 61 | 98 | 5 | 164 |
| 1995 | 35,619 | 59,352 | 3,113 | 98,093 | 61 | 104 | 5 | 171 |
| 1996 | 35,868 | 62,793 | 2,717 | 101,378 | 62 | 108 | 5 | 174 |
| 1997 | 36,266 | 64,223 | 2,464 | 102,953 | 62 | 110 | 4 | 177 |
| 1998 | 36,677 | 67,447 | 2,401 | 106,525 | 63 | 115 | 4 | 182 |
| 1999 | 37,033 | 69,241 | 2,358 | 108,632 | 63 | 118 | 4 | 185 |
| 2000 | 37,314 | 71,235 | 2,248 | 110,797 | 63 | 121 | 4 | 188 |
| 2001 | 37,852 | 73,645 | 2,173 | 113,670 | 64 | 125 | 4 | 192 |
| 2002 | 38,388 | 78,737 | 1,966 | 119,091 | 65 | 133 | 3 | 201 |
| 2003 | 39,878 | 83,318 | 1,815 | 125,012 | 67 | 140 | 3 | 210 |
| 2004 | 41,388 | 90,625 | 1,869 | 133,882 | 69 | 151 | 3 | 224 |
| 2005 | 42,773 | *94,601* | *1,897* | 139,270 | 71 | *157* | *3* | 231 |
| 2006 | 43,021 | *98,534* | *1,947* | 143,502 | 71 | *163* | *3* | 237 |

*Notes:* Figures in italics are OHE estimates based on the total HCHS staff and the trend in the split between hospital and community staff over time. Figures for the UK are aggregates of England, Wales, Scotland and Northern Ireland, which are not all based precisely on the same definition or timing. Also, community medical staff in Northern Ireland have been estimated.

FTE = Full-time equivalents.

1 Including all medical practitioners and trainee GPs but excluding retainers.

2 Prior to 1958, figures include some community medical staff. Also Northern Ireland figures include dental staff.

3 From 1958 to 1965, figures relate to medical staff of school health services. From 1966 to 1973, figures include school health services and local health authority medical staff. From 1995 figures for Great Britain relate to Public Health Medicine and Community Health Services medical staff.

*Sources:* Health and Personal Social Services Statistics for England (DH).
Scottish Health Statistics (ISD).
Health Statistics Wales (NAW).
Annual Abstract of Statistics (ONS).
HPSS Workforce Census (DHSSPS in Northern Ireland).
Community Statistics (DHSSPS in Northern Ireland).
Population Projections Database (GAD).

Figure 4.5 **Number of GPs[1] per 1,000 population in selected OECD and EU countries, circa 2005**

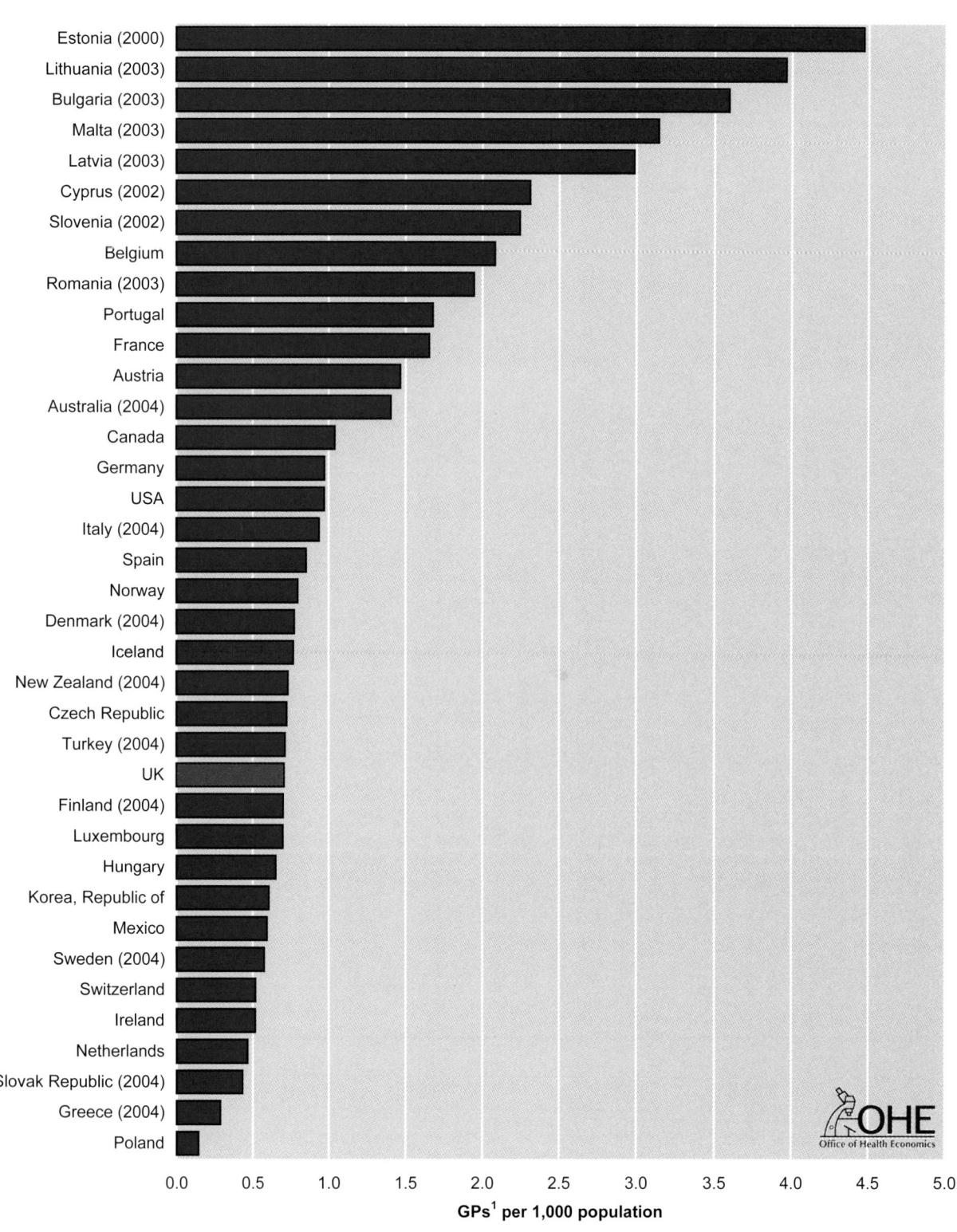

GPs[1] per 1,000 population

Notes: 1 Active doctors working in primary health care services.
Year is 2005 unless otherwise stated.
Differences in figures could be due to varying proportions of part time staff between countries or definitional differences.
Sources: OECD Health Database.
For UK figure, see Table 4.7.
World Health Statistics (WHO).
World Health Organisation National Health Accounts Series (WHO).

Table 4.7    **Number of general medical practitioners[1] (GPs including registrars) in general practice, and per 100,000 population, by country, UK, 1985 - 2006**

30th September[2]

| Year | Number of medical practitioners[1] | | | | | Per 100,000 population | | | | |
|---|---|---|---|---|---|---|---|---|---|---|
| | England[3] | Wales | Scotland | Northern Ireland | UK | England[3] | Wales | Scotland | Northern Ireland | UK |
| 1985 | 27,482 | - | 3,539 | 933 | 31,954 | 58 | - | 69 | 60 | 57 |
| 1986 | 27,823 | - | 3,575 | 956 | 32,354 | 59 | - | 70 | 61 | 57 |
| 1987 | 28,385 | - | 3,614 | 956 | 32,955 | 60 | - | 71 | 60 | 58 |
| 1988 | 28,771 | - | 3,671 | 972 | 33,414 | 61 | - | 72 | 61 | 59 |
| 1989 | 29,139 | - | 3,730 | 984 | 33,853 | 61 | - | 73 | 62 | 59 |
| 1990 | 28,967 | - | 3,689 | 969 | 33,625 | 61 | - | 73 | 61 | 59 |
| 1991 | 29,110 | - | 3,705 | 959 | 33,774 | 61 | - | 73 | 60 | 59 |
| 1992 | 29,390 | - | 3,742 | 978 | 34,110 | 61 | - | 74 | 60 | 59 |
| 1993 | 29,644 | - | 3,759 | 988 | 34,391 | 62 | - | 74 | 60 | 60 |
| 1994 | 28,735 | 1,850 | 3,836 | 1,018 | 35,439 | 60 | 64 | 75 | 62 | 61 |
| 1995 | 28,869 | 1,845 | 3,872 | 1,033 | 35,619 | 60 | 64 | 76 | 63 | 61 |
| 1996 | 29,116 | 1,832 | 3,869 | 1,051 | 35,868 | 60 | 63 | 76 | 63 | 62 |
| 1997 | 29,389 | 1,874 | 3,935 | 1,068 | 36,266 | 60 | 65 | 77 | 64 | 62 |
| 1998 | 29,697 | 1,888 | 4,019 | 1,073 | 36,677 | 61 | 65 | 79 | 64 | 63 |
| 1999 | 29,987 | 1,891 | 4,068 | 1,087 | 37,033 | 61 | 65 | 80 | 65 | 63 |
| 2000 | 30,252 | 1,903 | 4,067 | 1,092 | 37,314 | 61 | 65 | 80 | 65 | 63 |
| 2001 | 30,685 | 1,919 | 4,148 | 1,100 | 37,852 | 62 | 66 | 82 | 65 | 64 |
| 2002 | 31,182 | 1,930 | 4,163 | 1,113 | 38,388 | 63 | 66 | 82 | 66 | 65 |
| 2003 | 32,593 | 1,932 | 4,237 | 1,116 | 39,878 | 65 | 66 | 84 | 66 | 67 |
| 2004 | 34,085 | 1,931 | 4,252 | 1,120 | 41,388 | 68 | 66 | 84 | 65 | 69 |
| 2005 | 35,302 | 1,952 | 4,395 | 1,124 | 42,773 | 70 | 66 | 86 | 65 | 71 |
| 2006 | 35,369 | 2,034 | 4,460 | 1,158 | 43,021 | 70 | 69 | 87 | 66 | 71 |

*Notes:*    1 Comprising all medical practitioners in general practice, including GP registrars (trainees) but excluding GP retainers.
2 Data for England, Wales and Scotland are as at 1st October before 2000 and for Northern Ireland from 1996 to 2002 are as at 1 January, and from 2003 onwards are as at 1 October.
3 Figures from 1985 to 1993 are for England and Wales combined.

*Sources:*    Health and Personal Social Services Statistics for England (DH).
Health Statistics Wales (NAW).
Scottish Health Statistics (ISD).
Annual Statistical Report (Northern Ireland CSA).
General and Personal Medical Services Statistics: England and Wales (DH).
Population Projections Database (GAD).

Table 4.8  **Number of medical practitioners (excluding registrars and retainers) in general practice, UK, 1951 - 2006**

30th September[2]

| Year | Number of medical practitioners[1] | | | | | Per 100,000 population | | | | |
|------|----------|-------|----------|---------|--------|----------|-------|----------|---------|------|
| | England[3] | Wales | Scotland | Northern Ireland | UK | England[3] | Wales | Scotland | Northern Ireland | UK |
| 1951 | 17,135 | - | 2,331 | 713 | 20,179 | 39.1 | - | 45.7 | 52.0 | 40.1 |
| 1955 | 18,832 | - | 2,532 | 733 | 22,097 | 42.4 | - | 49.5 | 52.6 | 43.4 |
| 1960 | 19,905 | - | 2,632 | 746 | 23,283 | 43.5 | - | 50.8 | 52.5 | 44.5 |
| 1965 | 20,014 | - | 2,594 | 747 | 23,355 | 42.0 | - | 49.8 | 50.9 | 43.0 |
| 1966 | 19,832 | - | 2,570 | 750 | 23,152 | 41.3 | - | 49.4 | 50.8 | 42.4 |
| 1967 | 19,837 | - | 2,584 | 753 | 23,174 | 41.1 | - | 49.7 | 50.6 | 42.2 |
| 1968 | 19,957 | - | 2,572 | 746 | 23,275 | 41.4 | - | 49.5 | 49.6 | 42.4 |
| 1969 | 20,133 | - | 2,593 | 745 | 23,471 | 41.3 | - | 49.8 | 49.2 | 42.3 |
| 1970 | 20,357 | - | 2,604 | 744 | 23,705 | 41.6 | - | 49.9 | 48.7 | 42.6 |
| 1971 | 20,633 | - | 2,619 | 754 | 24,006 | 42.0 | - | 50.0 | 49.0 | 42.9 |
| 1972 | 21,044 | - | 2,677 | 746 | 24,467 | 42.7 | - | 51.2 | 48.5 | 43.6 |
| 1973 | 21,266 | - | 2,699 | 742 | 24,707 | 43.0 | - | 51.6 | 48.5 | 43.9 |
| 1974 | 21,510 | - | 2,745 | 739 | 24,994 | 43.5 | - | 52.4 | 48.4 | 44.4 |
| 1975 | 21,667 | - | 2,797 | 737 | 25,201 | 43.8 | - | 53.5 | 48.4 | 44.8 |
| 1976 | 21,837 | - | 2,820 | 727 | 25,384 | 44.2 | - | 53.9 | 47.7 | 45.2 |
| 1977 | 22,100 | - | 2,839 | 729 | 25,668 | 44.7 | - | 54.3 | 47.9 | 45.7 |
| 1978 | 22,362 | - | 2,884 | 722 | 25,968 | 45.2 | - | 55.3 | 47.4 | 46.2 |
| 1979 | 22,696 | - | 2,921 | 735 | 26,352 | 45.8 | - | 56.1 | 48.0 | 46.9 |
| 1980 | 23,184 | - | 2,959 | 762 | 26,905 | 46.7 | - | 57.0 | 49.7 | 47.8 |
| 1981 | 23,701 | - | 3,001 | 788 | 27,490 | 47.8 | - | 57.9 | 51.2 | 48.8 |
| 1982 | 24,217 | - | 3,040 | 813 | 28,069 | 48.8 | - | 58.8 | 52.9 | 49.8 |
| 1983 | 24,719 | - | 3,106 | 832 | 28,657 | 49.8 | - | 60.3 | 53.9 | 50.8 |
| 1984 | 25,132 | - | 3,169 | 845 | 29,146 | 50.5 | - | 61.6 | 54.5 | 51.6 |
| 1985 | 25,558 | - | 3,223 | 881 | 29,662 | 51.2 | - | 62.8 | 56.6 | 52.3 |
| 1986 | 26,009 | - | 3,272 | 906 | 30,187 | 51.9 | - | 63.9 | 57.8 | 53.1 |
| 1987 | 26,509 | - | 3,305 | 905 | 30,719 | 52.8 | - | 64.7 | 57.5 | 53.9 |
| 1988 | 26,921 | - | 3,355 | 921 | 31,197 | 53.4 | - | 65.9 | 58.4 | 54.6 |
| 1989 | 27,239 | - | 3,391 | 933 | 31,563 | 53.9 | - | 66.6 | 58.9 | 55.0 |
| 1990 | 27,257 | - | 3,359 | 924 | 31,540 | 53.7 | - | 65.9 | 58.2 | 54.8 |
| 1991 | 27,333 | - | 3,380 | 917 | 31,630 | 53.5 | - | 66.2 | 57.3 | 54.7 |
| 1992 | 27,644 | - | 3,421 | 937 | 32,002 | 53.9 | - | 67.0 | 57.9 | 55.2 |
| 1993 | 27,991 | - | 3,456 | 950 | 32,397 | 54.4 | - | 67.5 | 58.2 | 55.7 |
| 1994 | 27,290 | 1,732 | 3,558 | 979 | 33,559 | 56.6 | 60.0 | 68.0 | 59.6 | 56.1 |
| 1995 | 27,465 | 1,741 | 3,590 | 994 | 33,790 | 56.8 | 60.3 | 68.6 | 60.3 | 56.2 |
| 1996 | 27,811 | 1,766 | 3,635 | 1,011 | 34,223 | 57.3 | 61.1 | 71.4 | 60.8 | 58.8 |
| 1997 | 28,046 | 1,779 | 3,695 | 1,026 | 34,546 | 57.6 | 61.5 | 72.7 | 61.4 | 59.2 |
| 1998 | 28,251 | 1,778 | 3,745 | 1,033 | 34,807 | 57.9 | 61.3 | 73.8 | 61.6 | 59.5 |
| 1999 | 28,467 | 1,792 | 3,784 | 1,039 | 35,082 | 58.1 | 61.8 | 74.6 | 61.9 | 59.8 |
| 2000 | 28,593 | 1,795 | 3,806 | 1,049 | 35,243 | 58.1 | 61.7 | 75.2 | 62.3 | 59.8 |
| 2001 | 28,802 | 1,807 | 3,865 | 1,054 | 35,528 | 58.2 | 62.1 | 76.3 | 62.4 | 60.1 |
| 2002 | 29,202 | 1,808 | 3,879 | 1,064 | 35,953 | 58.8 | 61.9 | 76.7 | 62.7 | 60.6 |
| 2003 | 30,358 | 1,822 | 3,956 | 1,076 | 37,212 | 60.9 | 62.2 | 78.2 | 63.2 | 62.5 |
| 2004 | 31,523 | 1,816 | 3,970 | 1,078 | 38,387 | 62.9 | 61.6 | 78.2 | 63.0 | 64.1 |
| 2005 | 32,738 | 1,849 | 4,087 | 1,084 | 39,758 | 64.9 | 62.6 | 80.2 | 62.9 | 66.0 |
| 2006 | 33,091 | 1,882 | 4,151 | 1,110 | 40,234 | 65.2 | 63.5 | 81.1 | 63.7 | 66.4 |

Notes: 1 Due to the introduction of the new GMS contract (1st April 2004), some of the definitions and groupings used to represent the GP workforce have changed. Figures presented from 1994 have been revised in light of the new GP contract and correspond to medical practitioners, including all contracted and salaried GPs but excluding registrars and retainers. Prior to 1994 figures relate to unrestricted principals (UPE), the category of UPE is no longer identified apart from in Northern Ireland.

2 Data for England and Wales are as at 1st October before 2000 and for Northern Ireland from 1996 to 2002 are as at 1 January, and from 2003 onwards are as at 1 October. Data for Scotland are as at 1 October.

3 Data prior to 1994 relates to England and Wales.

Sources: General and Personal Medical Services Statistics: England and Wales (DH).
Health Statistics Wales (NAW).
Annual Abstract of Statistics (ONS).
Scottish Health Statistics (ISD).
Northern Ireland Annual Abstract of Statistics (Northern Ireland Department of Finance and Personnel).
Information Unit, Family Practitioner Services (CSA).

Table 4.9(a)   **Number of GP registrars by country, UK, 1996 - 2006**

30th September

| | Year | | | | | | | | | |
|---|---|---|---|---|---|---|---|---|---|---|
| | **1996** | **1998** | **1999** | **2000** | **2001** | **2002** | **2003** | **2004** | **2005** | **2006** |
| **United Kingdom** | 1,645 | 1,870 | 1,951 | 2,071 | 2,324 | 2,435 | 2,666 | 3,001 | 3,015 | 2,787 |
| **England** | 1,305 | 1,446 | 1,520 | 1,659 | 1,883 | 1,980 | 2,235 | 2,562 | 2,564 | 2,278 |
| **Wales** | 66 | 110 | 99 | 108 | 112 | 122 | 110 | 115 | 103 | 152 |
| **Scotland** | 234 | 274 | 284 | 261 | 283 | 284 | 281 | 282 | 308 | 309 |
| **Northern Ireland** | 40 | 40 | 48 | 43 | 46 | 49 | 40 | 42 | 40 | 48 |

Table 4.9(b)   **Number of medical practitioners in general practice (excluding GP retainers) per GP registrar, by country, UK, 1996 - 2006**

30th September

| | Year | | | | | | | | | |
|---|---|---|---|---|---|---|---|---|---|---|
| | **1996** | **1998** | **1999** | **2000** | **2001** | **2002** | **2003** | **2004** | **2005** | **2006** |
| **United Kingdom** | 21 | 19 | 18 | 17 | 15 | 15 | 14 | 13 | 13 | 14 |
| **England** | 21 | 20 | 19 | 17 | 15 | 15 | 14 | 12 | 13 | 15 |
| **Wales** | 27 | 16 | 18 | 17 | 16 | 15 | 17 | 16 | 18 | 12 |
| **Scotland** | 16 | 14 | 13 | 15 | 14 | 14 | 14 | 14 | 13 | 13 |
| **Northern Ireland** | 25 | 26 | 22 | 24 | 23 | 22 | 27 | 26 | 27 | 23 |

*Notes:*   Data for England and Wales are as at 1st October before 2000 and for Northern Ireland from 1996 to 2002 are as at 1 January, and from 2003 onwards are as at 1 October.  Data for Scotland are as at 1 October.

*Sources:*   Health and Personal Social Services Statistics for England (DH).
Scottish Health Statistics (ISD).
Health Statistics Wales (NAW).
Annual Statistical Report (Northern Ireland CSA).
General and Personal Medical Services Statistics: England and Wales (DH).

Table 4.10 **Resident population per medical practitioner (excluding GP registrars and retainers) in general practice, UK, 1951 - 2006**

30th September[1]

| Year | Population per medical practitioner[2] | | | | Index (1951=100) | | | |
|------|------------------|----------|---------------------|-------|---------------------|----------|---------------------|-------|
| | England and Wales | Scotland | Northern Ireland | UK | England and Wales | Scotland | Northern Ireland | UK |
| 1951 | 2,557 | 2,189 | 1,926 | 2,492 | 100 | 100 | 100 | 100 |
| 1955 | 2,360 | 2,019 | 1,902 | 2,306 | 92 | 92 | 99 | 93 |
| 1960 | 2,300 | 1,967 | 1,903 | 2,249 | 90 | 90 | 99 | 90 |
| 1965 | 2,382 | 2,008 | 1,965 | 2,327 | 93 | 92 | 102 | 93 |
| 1966 | 2,419 | 2,023 | 1,968 | 2,360 | 95 | 92 | 102 | 95 |
| 1967 | 2,433 | 2,012 | 1,977 | 2,372 | 95 | 92 | 103 | 95 |
| 1968 | 2,431 | 2,022 | 2,015 | 2,372 | 95 | 92 | 105 | 95 |
| 1969 | 2,421 | 2,009 | 2,034 | 2,363 | 95 | 92 | 106 | 95 |
| 1970 | 2,402 | 2,002 | 2,054 | 2,347 | 94 | 91 | 107 | 94 |
| 1971 | 2,382 | 1,999 | 2,044 | 2,330 | 93 | 91 | 106 | 93 |
| 1972 | 2,344 | 1,954 | 2,064 | 2,293 | 92 | 89 | 107 | 92 |
| 1973 | 2,326 | 1,939 | 2,062 | 2,276 | 91 | 89 | 107 | 91 |
| 1974 | 2,300 | 1,909 | 2,066 | 2,250 | 90 | 87 | 107 | 90 |
| 1975 | 2,283 | 1,871 | 2,066 | 2,231 | 89 | 85 | 107 | 90 |
| 1976 | 2,265 | 1,856 | 2,096 | 2,215 | 89 | 85 | 109 | 89 |
| 1977 | 2,237 | 1,841 | 2,089 | 2,189 | 87 | 84 | 108 | 88 |
| 1978 | 2,211 | 1,808 | 2,111 | 2,163 | 86 | 83 | 110 | 87 |
| 1979 | 2,181 | 1,782 | 2,079 | 2,134 | 85 | 81 | 108 | 86 |
| 1980 | 2,140 | 1,755 | 2,012 | 2,094 | 84 | 80 | 104 | 84 |
| 1981 | 2,094 | 1,726 | 1,951 | 2,050 | 82 | 79 | 101 | 82 |
| 1982 | 2,047 | 1,699 | 1,900 | 2,005 | 80 | 78 | 99 | 80 |
| 1983 | 2,007 | 1,657 | 1,864 | 1,965 | 78 | 76 | 97 | 79 |
| 1984 | 1,978 | 1,622 | 1,843 | 1,935 | 77 | 74 | 96 | 78 |
| 1985 | 1,951 | 1,591 | 1,777 | 1,907 | 76 | 73 | 92 | 77 |
| 1986 | 1,922 | 1,562 | 1,737 | 1,878 | 75 | 71 | 90 | 75 |
| 1987 | 1,891 | 1,543 | 1,748 | 1,849 | 74 | 70 | 91 | 74 |
| 1988 | 1,867 | 1,513 | 1,721 | 1,824 | 73 | 69 | 89 | 73 |
| 1989 | 1,851 | 1,498 | 1,705 | 1,808 | 72 | 68 | 89 | 73 |
| 1990 | 1,855 | 1,513 | 1,727 | 1,815 | 73 | 69 | 90 | 73 |
| 1991 | 1,857 | 1,504 | 1,753 | 1,816 | 73 | 69 | 91 | 73 |
| 1992 | 1,840 | 1,487 | 1,732 | 1,799 | 72 | 68 | 90 | 72 |
| 1993 | 1,822 | 1,473 | 1,722 | 1,781 | 71 | 67 | 89 | 71 |
| 1994 | 1,761 | 1,434 | 1,679 | 1,724 | 69 | 66 | 87 | 69 |
| 1995 | 1,756 | 1,422 | 1,659 | 1,717 | 69 | 65 | 86 | 69 |
| 1996 | 1,738 | 1,401 | 1,644 | 1,700 | 68 | 64 | 85 | 68 |
| 1997 | 1,729 | 1,376 | 1,629 | 1,688 | 68 | 63 | 85 | 68 |
| 1998 | 1,722 | 1,356 | 1,624 | 1,680 | 67 | 62 | 84 | 67 |
| 1999 | 1,716 | 1,340 | 1,616 | 1,673 | 67 | 61 | 84 | 67 |
| 2000 | 1,716 | 1,330 | 1,604 | 1,671 | 67 | 61 | 83 | 67 |
| 2001 | 1,711 | 1,310 | 1,603 | 1,664 | 67 | 60 | 83 | 67 |
| 2002 | 1,695 | 1,303 | 1,595 | 1,650 | 66 | 60 | 83 | 66 |
| 2003 | 1,641 | 1,278 | 1,582 | 1,600 | 64 | 58 | 82 | 64 |
| 2004 | 1,591 | 1,279 | 1,587 | 1,559 | 62 | 58 | 82 | 63 |
| 2005 | 1,544 | 1,247 | 1,591 | 1,515 | 60 | 57 | 83 | 61 |
| 2006 | 1,536 | 1,233 | 1,569 | 1,506 | 60 | 56 | 81 | 60 |

*Notes:* 1 Data for England and Wales are as at 1st October before 2000. Data for Northern Ireland from 1996 to 2002 are as at 1 January, and from 2003 onwards are as at 1 October. Data for Scotland are as at 1 October.

2 Due to the introduction of the new GMS contract (1st April 2004), some of the definitions and groupings used to represent the GP workforce have changed. Figures presented from 1994 have been revised in light of the new GP contract and correspond to medical practitioners, including all contracted and salaried GPs but excluding registrars and retainers. Prior to 1994 figures relate to unrestricted principals (UPE), the category of UPE is no longer identified apart from in Northern Ireland.

*Sources:* Health and Personal Social Services Statistics for England (DH).
Scottish Health Statistics (ISD).
Health Statistics Wales (NAW).
Annual Abstract of Statistics (ONS).
Annual Statistical Report (Northern Ireland CSA).

## FHS: General Medical Services

**Table 4.11  Average list size of medical practitioners[1] (excluding GP registrars and retainers) in general practice, by country, UK, 1964 - 2006**

30th September[2]

| Year | Average list size | | | | |
|------|---------|-------|----------|------------------|-----|
|      | England | Wales | Scotland | Northern Ireland | UK |
| 1964 | 2,379 | 2,136 | 2,013 | 1982 | - |
| 1965 | 2,423 | 2,192 | 2,066 | 2001 | - |
| 1966 | 2,470 | 2,219 | 2,089 | 2014 | - |
| 1967 | 2,490 | 2,229 | 2,086 | 2027 | - |
| 1968 | 2,494 | 2,231 | 2,106 | 2069 | - |
| 1969 | 2,495 | 2,232 | 2,102 | 2083 | - |
| 1970 | 2,478 | 2,192 | 2,045 | 2091 | - |
| 1971 | 2,460 | 2,203 | 2,061 | 2071 | - |
| 1972 | 2,421 | 2,197 | 2,024 | 2095 | - |
| 1973 | 2,398 | 2,207 | 2,020 | 2102 | - |
| 1974 | 2,384 | 2,189 | 1,973 | 2107 | - |
| 1975 | 2,365 | 2,193 | 1,939 | 2105 | - |
| 1976 | 2,351 | 2,199 | 1,928 | 2140 | - |
| 1977 | 2,331 | 2,175 | 1,905 | 2163 | - |
| 1978 | 2,312 | 2,148 | 1,875 | 2189 | - |
| 1979 | 2,286 | 2,133 | 1,856 | 2165 | - |
| 1980 | 2,247 | 2,086 | 1,832 | 2097 | - |
| 1981 | 2,201 | 2,057 | 1,804 | 2032 | - |
| 1982 | 2,155 | 2,013 | 1,778 | 1981 | - |
| 1983 | 2,116 | 1,975 | 1,739 | 1951 | - |
| 1984 | 2,089 | 1,946 | 1,704 | 1924 | - |
| 1985 | 2,068 | 1,914 | 1,668 | 1,865 | 2,016 |
| 1986 | 2,042 | 1,881 | 1,653 | 1,825 | 1,990 |
| 1987 | 2,010 | 1,946 | 1,630 | 1,835 | 1,961 |
| 1988 | 1,999 | 1,914 | 1,665 | 1,808 | 1,953 |
| 1989 | 1,971 | 1,819 | 1,590 | 1,792 | 1,917 |
| 1990 | 1,942 | 1,813 | 1,592 | 1,811 | 1,894 |
| 1991 | 1,938 | 1,794 | 1,580 | 1,835 | 1,892 |
| 1992 | 1,922 | 1,743 | 1,555 | 1,808 | 1,870 |
| 1993 | 1,904 | 1,736 | 1,542 | 1,794 | 1,853 |
| 1994 | 1,900 | 1,717 | 1,524 | 1,741 | 1,847 |
| 1995 | 1,835 | 1,708 | 1,506 | 1,714 | 1,833 |
| 1996 | 1,820 | 1,694 | 1,488 | 1,700 | 1,818 |
| 1997 | 1,815 | 1,681 | 1,468 | 1,690 | 1,810 |
| 1998 | 1,809 | 1,685 | 1,450 | 1,693 | 1,801 |
| 1999 | 1,788 | 1,665 | 1,441 | 1,679 | 1,778 |
| 2000 | 1,795 | 1,676 | 1,425 | 1,686 | 1,779 |
| 2001 | 1,780 | 1,665 | 1,409 | 1,670 | 1,768 |
| 2002 | 1,764 | 1,679 | 1,392 | 1,652 | 1,716 |
| 2003 | 1,736 | 1,659 | 1,380 | 1,658 | 1,692 |
| 2004 | 1,666 | 1,674 | 1,343 | 1,663 | 1,633 |
| 2005 | 1,613 | 1,650 | *1,321* | 1,655 | 1,586 |
| 2006 | 1,610 | 1,643 | *1,309* | 1,631 | 1,581 |

*Notes:*  Figures for the UK are weighted averages.
1 Due to the introduction of the new GMS contract (1st April 2004), some of the definitions and groupings used to represent the GP workforce have changed. Figures presented from 1994 have been revised in light of the new GP contract and correspond to medical practitioners, including all contracted and salaried GPs but excluding registrars and retainers. Prior to 1994 figures relate to unrestricted principals (UPE), the category of UPE is no longer identified apart from in Northern Ireland.
2 Data for England and Wales are as at 1st October before 2000. Data for Northern Ireland from 1996 to 2002 are as at 1 January, and from 2003 onwards are as at 1 October. Data for Scotland are as at 1 October.
Figures in italics for Scotland for 2005 and 2006 are OHE estimates based on the average practice list size, the number of practices and the number of medical practitioners (excluding GP registrars and retainers) in Scotland.
- UK figures are not available prior to 1985.

*Sources:*  Health and Personal Social Services Statistics for England (DH).
Scottish Health Statistics (ISD).
Health Statistics Wales (NAW).
Annual Statistical Report (Northern Ireland CSA).
Annual Abstract of Statistics (ONS).
NHS Staff (IC).
General and Personal Medical Services Statistics: England and Wales (DH).
General Medical Practitioners - StatWales (NAW).
General Medical Services Statistics (Northern Ireland CSA).

Figure 4.6  **Average list size of medical practitioners (excluding GP registrars and retainers) in general practice, by country, UK, 1964 - 2006**

**Average list size**

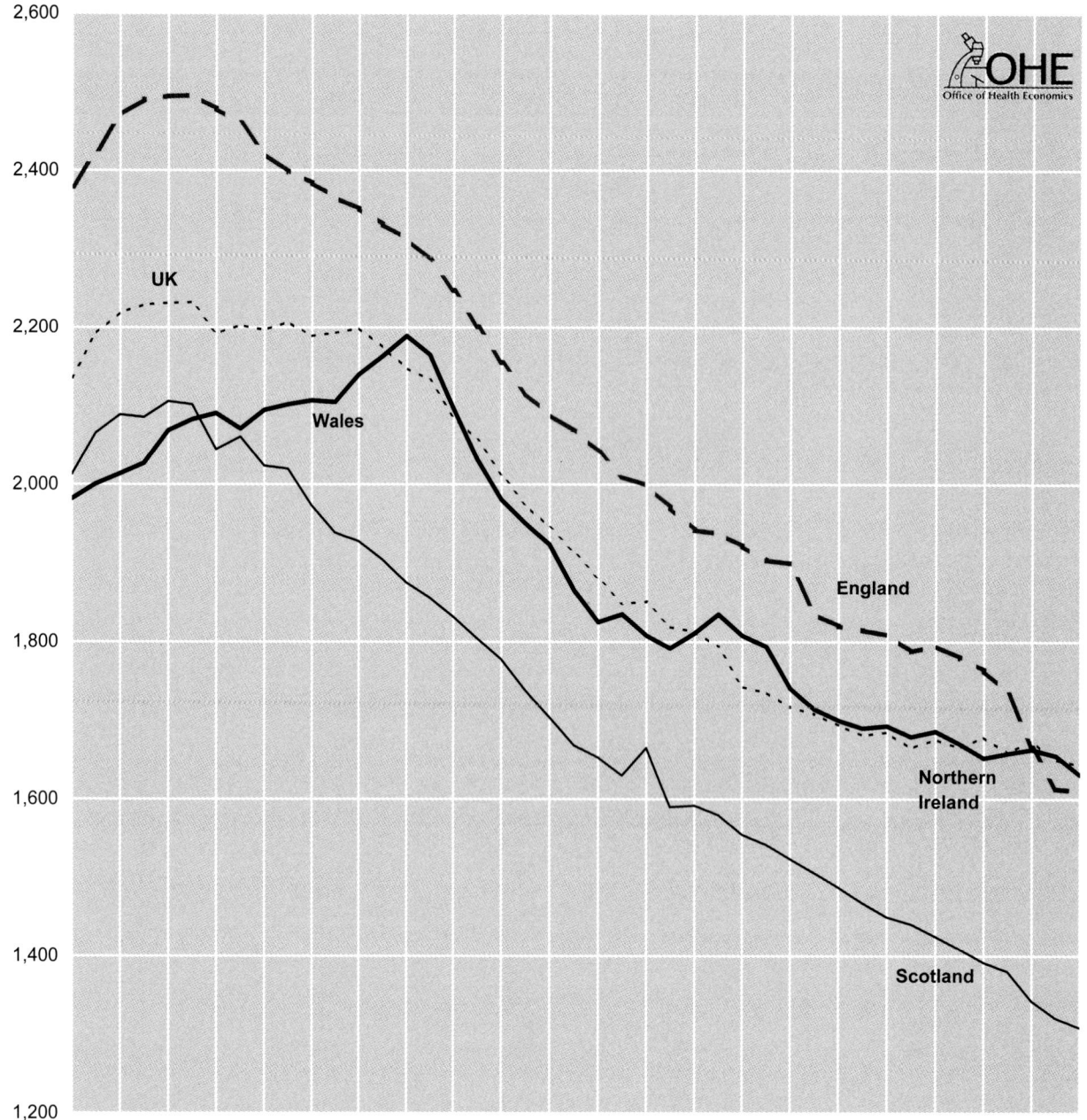

**Year**

Note:    Figure for Scotland from 2005 onwards are an OHE estimates based on the average practice list size, the number of practices and the number of medical  practitioners (excluding GP registrars and retainers) in Scotland.

Sources:  Health and Personal Social Services Statistics for England (DH).
Scottish Health Statistics (ISD).
Health Statistics Wales (NAW).
Annual Statistical Report (Northern Ireland CSA).
Annual Abstract of Statistics (ONS).
NHS Staff (IC).
General and Personal Medical Services Statistics: England and Wales (DH).
General Medical Practitioners - StatWales (NAW).
General Medical Services Statistics (Northern Ireland CSA).

# FHS: General Medical Services

Table 4.12 **Number of patients[1] per medical practitioner (excluding GP registrars and retainers) in general practice, by patient age group, UK, 1951 - 2006**

30th September

| Year | Age group | | | | | | | | |
|------|-----|------|-------|-------|-------|-------|------|------|----------|
|      | <5  | <15  | 15-29 | 30-44 | 45-64 | 65-74 | >=75 | >=85 | All ages |
| 1951 | 215 | 565 | 522 | 554 | 594 | 183 | 88 | 11 | 2,506 |
| 1955 | 174 | 529 | 458 | 497 | 573 | 171 | 90 | 12 | 2,318 |
| 1960 | 179 | 525 | 442 | 453 | 573 | 169 | 95 | 14 | 2,257 |
| 1961 | 181 | 524 | 443 | 447 | 568 | 169 | 94 | 15 | 2,245 |
| 1962 | 186 | 520 | 456 | 448 | 565 | 169 | 95 | 15 | 2,253 |
| 1963 | 191 | 522 | 466 | 450 | 561 | 171 | 95 | 15 | 2,265 |
| 1964 | 197 | 529 | 476 | 452 | 562 | 174 | 98 | 16 | 2,291 |
| 1965 | 204 | 542 | 488 | 451 | 573 | 179 | 101 | 17 | 2,334 |
| 1966 | 208 | 554 | 497 | 447 | 583 | 184 | 103 | 17 | 2,367 |
| 1967 | 208 | 561 | 499 | 440 | 585 | 188 | 105 | 18 | 2,378 |
| 1968 | 206 | 566 | 500 | 435 | 582 | 191 | 106 | 18 | 2,380 |
| 1969 | 202 | 567 | 499 | 429 | 576 | 193 | 107 | 18 | 2,371 |
| 1970 | 193 | 564 | 488 | 415 | 567 | 196 | 108 | 19 | 2,338 |
| 1971 | 188 | 559 | 488 | 406 | 558 | 197 | 109 | 20 | 2,317 |
| 1972 | 180 | 549 | 485 | 397 | 544 | 197 | 108 | 20 | 2,280 |
| 1973 | 174 | 542 | 484 | 395 | 535 | 199 | 109 | 20 | 2,263 |
| 1974 | 165 | 533 | 485 | 395 | 526 | 201 | 110 | 21 | 2,250 |
| 1975 | 156 | 521 | 485 | 393 | 518 | 201 | 112 | 21 | 2,231 |
| 1976 | 147 | 508 | 488 | 394 | 511 | 201 | 113 | 21 | 2,215 |
| 1977 | 137 | 491 | 481 | 401 | 505 | 200 | 115 | 21 | 2,189 |
| 1978 | 131 | 474 | 477 | 405 | 496 | 199 | 117 | 22 | 2,163 |
| 1979 | 128 | 458 | 476 | 407 | 484 | 198 | 118 | 22 | 2,134 |
| 1980 | 127 | 440 | 472 | 404 | 469 | 194 | 119 | 22 | 2,094 |
| 1981 | 126 | 422 | 468 | 399 | 456 | 189 | 119 | 22 | 2,050 |
| 1982 | 125 | 405 | 463 | 393 | 445 | 182 | 120 | 22 | 2,006 |
| 1983 | 125 | 390 | 458 | 388 | 436 | 173 | 120 | 22 | 1,967 |
| 1984 | 123 | 377 | 455 | 385 | 431 | 166 | 121 | 23 | 1,939 |
| 1985 | 122 | 367 | 452 | 382 | 419 | 167 | 122 | 23 | 1,911 |
| 1986 | 121 | 358 | 447 | 381 | 407 | 166 | 122 | 23 | 1,883 |
| 1987 | 120 | 350 | 441 | 379 | 397 | 164 | 123 | 25 | 1,856 |
| 1988 | 120 | 345 | 432 | 377 | 391 | 161 | 124 | 26 | 1,832 |
| 1989 | 121 | 343 | 423 | 376 | 389 | 159 | 125 | 26 | 1,817 |
| 1990 | 122 | 346 | 419 | 380 | 391 | 159 | 126 | 27 | 1,825 |
| 1991 | 123 | 350 | 410 | 385 | 392 | 161 | 127 | 28 | 1,828 |
| 1992 | 122 | 350 | 400 | 382 | 397 | 160 | 126 | 29 | 1,813 |
| 1993 | 121 | 349 | 388 | 382 | 397 | 157 | 126 | 30 | 1,797 |
| 1994 | 115 | 336 | 359 | 366 | 390 | 156 | 117 | 29 | 1,724 |
| 1995 | 113 | 334 | 352 | 368 | 391 | 152 | 120 | 30 | 1,717 |
| 1996 | 109 | 330 | 342 | 369 | 390 | 148 | 121 | 30 | 1,700 |
| 1997 | 107 | 327 | 333 | 371 | 390 | 145 | 122 | 30 | 1,688 |
| 1998 | 105 | 324 | 326 | 372 | 391 | 143 | 123 | 31 | 1,680 |
| 1999 | 103 | 322 | 321 | 374 | 392 | 141 | 123 | 31 | 1,673 |
| 2000 | 101 | 318 | 318 | 377 | 395 | 140 | 124 | 32 | 1,671 |
| 2001 | 98 | 313 | 315 | 377 | 396 | 139 | 125 | 32 | 1,664 |
| 2002 | 95 | 306 | 311 | 375 | 395 | 138 | 124 | 31 | 1,650 |
| 2003 | 91 | 294 | 302 | 363 | 386 | 134 | 121 | 30 | 1,600 |
| 2004 | 88 | 283 | 297 | 351 | 379 | 131 | 118 | 29 | 1,559 |
| 2005 | 86 | 272 | 293 | 338 | 370 | 127 | 116 | 30 | 1,515 |
| 2006 | 87 | 267 | 295 | 331 | 372 | 125 | 116 | 31 | 1,506 |

*Notes:* See Table 4.8.

1 Figures are based on the UK population size in each age category as opposed to the number of registered patients.

*Sources:* Health and Personal Social Services Statistics for England (DH).
Scottish Health Statistics (ISD).
Health Statistics Wales (NAW).
Annual Statistical Report (Northern Ireland CSA).
Annual Abstract of Statistics (ONS).
Population Projections Database (GAD).

Table 4.13(a)   **People aged 65 and over per medical practitioner (excluding GP registrars and retainers) in general practice, by country, UK, 1996 - 2006**

30th September[1]

|  | Year | | | | | | | | | | |
|---|---|---|---|---|---|---|---|---|---|---|---|
|  | **1996** | **1997** | **1998** | **1999** | **2000** | **2001** | **2002** | **2003** | **2004** | **2005** | **2006** |
| **United Kingdom** | 270 | 268 | 266 | 264 | 264 | 264 | 263 | 255 | 249 | 242 | 241 |
| **England** | 278 | 276 | 274 | 273 | 272 | 272 | 270 | 262 | 254 | 246 | 244 |
| **Wales** | 285 | 283 | 284 | 281 | 281 | 280 | 282 | 282 | 285 | 282 | 279 |
| **Scotland** | 216 | 214 | 212 | 210 | 210 | 209 | 210 | 207 | 208 | 204 | 202 |
| **Northern Ireland** | 214 | 212 | 212 | 212 | 211 | 213 | 214 | 214 | 216 | 218 | 216 |

Table 4.13(b)   **People aged 75 and over per medical practitioner (excluding GP registrars and retainers) in general practice, by country, UK, 1996 - 2006**

30th September[1]

|  | Year | | | | | | | | | | |
|---|---|---|---|---|---|---|---|---|---|---|---|
|  | **1996** | **1997** | **1998** | **1999** | **2000** | **2001** | **2002** | **2003** | **2004** | **2005** | **2006** |
| **United Kingdom** | 121 | 122 | 123 | 123 | 124 | 125 | 124 | 121 | 118 | 116 | 116 |
| **England** | 126 | 127 | 128 | 128 | 129 | 129 | 129 | 125 | 121 | 118 | 118 |
| **Wales** | 127 | 129 | 131 | 131 | 133 | 134 | 135 | 135 | 136 | 135 | 134 |
| **Scotland** | 93 | 93 | 93 | 93 | 93 | 93 | 94 | 93 | 94 | 92 | 92 |
| **Northern Ireland** | 93 | 93 | 94 | 94 | 94 | 95 | 97 | 97 | 98 | 100 | 99 |

*Notes:*   1 Data for England and Wales are as at 1st October before 2000. Data for Northern Ireland from 1996 to 2002 are as at 1 January, and from 2003 onwards are as at 1 October.  Data for Scotland are as at 1 October.

*Sources:*   Health and Personal Social Services Statistics for England (DH).
Scottish Health Statistics (ISD).
Health Statistics Wales (NAW).
Annual Statistical Report (Northern Ireland CSA).
Annual Abstract of Statistics (ONS).
Population Projections Database (GAD).

Table 4.14    **Number of all general medical practitioners (excluding GP retainers) in general practice by age and sex, England, 1996 - 2006**

30th September

|  | 1996 | 1997 | 1998 | 1999 | 2000 | 2001 | 2002 | 2003 | 2004 | 2005[1] | 2006[1,2] |
|---|---|---|---|---|---|---|---|---|---|---|---|
| **Number of all GPs** | | | | | | | | | | | |
| **Total** | **29,116** | **29,389** | **29,697** | **29,987** | **30,252** | **30,685** | **31,182** | **32,593** | **34,085** | **35,302** | **35,369** |
| <30 years | 1,158 | 1,133 | 1,162 | 1,174 | 1,221 | 1,295 | 1,372 | 1,506 | 1,534 | 1,514 | 1,516 |
| 30-34 | 4,181 | 4,015 | 3,700 | 3,456 | 3,198 | 3,229 | 3,341 | 3,640 | 4,081 | 4,344 | 4,324 |
| 35-39 | 5,674 | 5,733 | 5,767 | 5,660 | 5,451 | 5,189 | 4,999 | 4,927 | 4,954 | 4,939 | 4,837 |
| 40-44 | 5,055 | 5,255 | 5,454 | 5,667 | 5,771 | 5,989 | 6,062 | 6,239 | 6,355 | 6,361 | 6,116 |
| 45-49 | 4,819 | 4,826 | 4,826 | 4,831 | 5,015 | 5,152 | 5,330 | 5,612 | 5,906 | 6,155 | 6,362 |
| 50-54 | 3,758 | 4,056 | 4,329 | 4,433 | 4,598 | 4,653 | 4,638 | 4,726 | 4,800 | 4,992 | 5,144 |
| 55-59 | 2,483 | 2,539 | 2,654 | 2,889 | 3,060 | 3,236 | 3,437 | 3,763 | 3,918 | 4,164 | 4,155 |
| 60-64 | 1,307 | 1,353 | 1,335 | 1,388 | 1,399 | 1,396 | 1,423 | 1,544 | 1,791 | 1,949 | 1,974 |
| 65-69 | 399 | 434 | 426 | 452 | 480 | 486 | 521 | 561 | 614 | 701 | 719 |
| >=70 years | 103 | 45 | 44 | 37 | 59 | 59 | 59 | 75 | 132 | 178 | 220 |
| **Male** | | | | | | | | | | | |
| Medical practitioners in general practice as a percentage of total | | | | | | | | | | | |
|  | **68** | **68** | **67** | **66** | **65** | **64** | **63** | **61** | **60** | **58** | **58** |
| Those in each age group as a percentage of male medical practitioners in general practice | | | | | | | | | | | |
| <30 years | 2 | 2 | 2 | 2 | 2 | 2 | 2 | 2 | 2 | 2 | 2 |
| 30-34 | 11 | 10 | 9 | 9 | 8 | 8 | 8 | 7 | 8 | 8 | 8 |
| 35-39 | 18 | 18 | 17 | 17 | 16 | 15 | 14 | 14 | 12 | 11 | 11 |
| 40-44 | 18 | 18 | 18 | 19 | 19 | 19 | 19 | 19 | 18 | 17 | 16 |
| 45-49 | 18 | 18 | 18 | 17 | 17 | 18 | 18 | 18 | 19 | 19 | 19 |
| 50-54 | 15 | 16 | 17 | 17 | 18 | 18 | 17 | 17 | 16 | 16 | 17 |
| 55-59 | 10 | 10 | 11 | 12 | 12 | 13 | 14 | 13 | 15 | 15 | 15 |
| 60-64 | 6 | 6 | 6 | 6 | 6 | 6 | 6 | 6 | 7 | 8 | 8 |
| 65-69 | 2 | 2 | 2 | 2 | 2 | 2 | 2 | 2 | 2 | 3 | 3 |
| >=70 years | 0 | 0 | 0 | 0 | 0 | 0 | 0 | 0 | 0 | 1 | 1 |
| **Female** | | | | | | | | | | | |
| Medical practitioners in general practice as a percentage of total | | | | | | | | | | | |
|  | **31** | **32** | **33** | **34** | **35** | **36** | **37** | **39** | **40** | **42** | **42** |
| Those in each age group as a percentage of female medical practitioners in general practice | | | | | | | | | | | |
| <30 years | 8 | 7 | 7 | 7 | 8 | 8 | 8 | 7 | 8 | 7 | 7 |
| 30-34 | 22 | 21 | 19 | 17 | 16 | 15 | 16 | 15 | 18 | 18 | 18 |
| 35-39 | 23 | 23 | 23 | 23 | 22 | 21 | 20 | 18 | 18 | 18 | 17 |
| 40-44 | 17 | 18 | 19 | 19 | 19 | 20 | 20 | 18 | 20 | 20 | 19 |
| 45-49 | 13 | 13 | 14 | 14 | 15 | 15 | 15 | 14 | 16 | 16 | 17 |
| 50-54 | 9 | 9 | 10 | 10 | 11 | 11 | 11 | 10 | 11 | 11 | 11 |
| 55-59 | 5 | 5 | 6 | 6 | 6 | 6 | 7 | 6 | 7 | 7 | 7 |
| 60-64 | 2 | 2 | 2 | 2 | 3 | 2 | 2 | 2 | 2 | 3 | 3 |
| 65-69 | 0 | 0 | 0 | 0 | 0 | 0 | 0 | 0 | 0 | 0 | 0 |
| >=70 years | 0 | 0 | 0 | 0 | 0 | 0 | 0 | 0 | 0 | 0 | 0 |

*Notes:*    All GPs: all medical practitioners including GP registrars but excluding GP retainers.
Data are as at 1 October before 2000.
Percentages may not sum to total due to rounding.
Percentages less than 0.5% are displayed as 0.
1 Total for 2005 includes 5 of unknown age.  Total for 2006 includes 2 of unknown age.

*Sources:*    Health and Personal Social Services Statistics for England (DH).
General and Personal Medical Services Statistics (DH).

Table 4.15    **Distribution of medical practitioners (excluding GP registrars and retainers) in general practice by size of practice, UK, 1975 - 2005**

Percentage

| Year | Single handed | In partnerships of: | | | | | All GPs[2] |
|---|---|---|---|---|---|---|---|
| | | 2 | 3 | 4 | 5[1] | >=6 | |
| 1975 | 17% | 21% | 25% | 18% | 10% | 9% | 25,191 |
| 1980 | 14% | 18% | 24% | 20% | 12% | 12% | 26,907 |
| 1985 | 12% | 16% | 21% | 19% | 15% | 17% | 29,662 |
| 1990 | 11% | 15% | 18% | 18% | 16% | 21% | 31,541 |
| 1991 | 11% | 14% | 18% | 19% | 16% | 22% | 31,630 |
| 1992 | 10% | 14% | 17% | 19% | 16% | 23% | 32,003 |
| 1993 | 10% | 14% | 17% | 18% | 16% | 24% | 32,397 |
| 1994 | 10% | 13% | 17% | 18% | 16% | 26% | 33,559 |
| 1995 | 10% | 13% | 16% | 18% | 17% | 26% | 33,790 |
| 1996 | 9% | 13% | 15% | 17% | 16% | 27% | 34,223 |
| 1997 | 9% | 13% | 14% | 17% | 16% | 30% | 34,546 |
| 1998 | 9% | 12% | 14% | 17% | 16% | 32% | 34,807 |
| 1999 | 8% | 12% | 14% | 16% | 16% | 33% | 35,082 |
| 2000 | 8% | 12% | 14% | 17% | 17% | 33% | 35,243 |
| 2001 | 8% | 12% | 13% | 17% | 17% | 34% | 35,528 |
| 2002 | 8% | 11% | 13% | 16% | 17% | 35% | 35,953 |
| 2003 | 8% | 11% | 12% | 15% | 16% | 39% | 37,212 |
| 2004 | 6% | 10% | 12% | 14% | 16% | 42% | 38,387 |
| 2005 | 5% | 10% | 11% | 13% | 15% | 45% | 39,758 |

*Notes:*    Figures for Northern Ireland are as at 1st April and for Scotland are as at 1st October.  Figures for England and Wales are as at 30th September.
Figures in previous years relate to various points of the year and may differ between the constituent countries of the UK.
1 Figures include practices of more than five principals in Northern Ireland.
2 Totals in some years differ from those shown in Table 4.8 due to the inclusion of some restricted principals in Northern Ireland and a few assistants and vacancies in Scotland.
Data for 2006 are not yet available for Northern Ireland or Scotland.

*Sources:*    Health and Personal Social Services Statistics for England (DH).
General and Personal Medical Services Statistics: England and Wales (DH).
Scottish Health Statistics (ISD).
Health Statistics Wales (NAW).
Annual Statistical Report (Northern Ireland CSA).

Table 4.16(a)    **Number of medical practitioners (excluding GP registrars and retainers) in general practice by size of practice, England and Wales, 1975 - 2006**

Number

| Year | Single handed | In partnerships of: | | | | | All GPs |
|---|---|---|---|---|---|---|---|
| | | 2 | 3 | 4 | 5 | >=6 | |
| 1975 | 3,746 | 4,548 | 5,322 | 3,988 | 2,170 | 1,874 | 21,667 |
| 1980 | 3,218 | 4,270 | 5,526 | 4,552 | 2,864 | 2,754 | 23,184 |
| 1985 | 3,048 | 4,130 | 5,322 | 4,740 | 3,845 | 4,473 | 25,558 |
| 1990 | 3,124 | 4,101 | 4,893 | 4,907 | 4,392 | 5,840 | 27,257 |
| 1991 | 3,058 | 3,945 | 4,803 | 5,039 | 4,375 | 6,113 | 27,333 |
| 1992 | 2,992 | 3,910 | 4,707 | 5,152 | 4,339 | 6,544 | 27,644 |
| 1993 | 3,017 | 3,860 | 4,674 | 5,080 | 4,455 | 6,905 | 27,991 |
| 1994 | 3,003 | 3,790 | 4,566 | 5,176 | 4,490 | 7,069 | 29,022 |
| 1995 | 2,924 | 3,796 | 4,323 | 5,140 | 4,660 | 7,570 | 29,206 |
| 1996 | 2,863 | 3,752 | 4,269 | 5,028 | 4,665 | 9,000 | 29,577 |
| 1997 | 2,847 | 3,768 | 4,131 | 5,052 | 4,765 | 9,262 | 29,825 |
| 1998 | 2,769 | 3,674 | 4,083 | 5,036 | 4,680 | 9,787 | 30,029 |
| 1999 | 2,659 | 3,564 | 4,038 | 4,900 | 4,670 | 10,428 | 30,259 |
| 2000 | 2,709 | 3,580 | 4,011 | 5,040 | 4,880 | 10,168 | 30,388 |
| 2001 | 2,647 | 3,564 | 3,852 | 5,012 | 4,900 | 10,634 | 30,609 |
| 2002 | 2,598 | 3,456 | 3,933 | 4,836 | 4,940 | 11,247 | 31,010 |
| 2003 | 2,609 | 3,412 | 3,765 | 4,800 | 4,770 | 12,824 | 32,180 |
| 2004 | 2,045 | 3,418 | 3,819 | 4,616 | 5,015 | 14,426 | 33,339 |
| 2005 | 1,924 | 3,282 | 3,618 | 4,532 | 5,015 | 16,216 | 34,587 |
| 2006 | 1,717 | 2,876 | 3,363 | 4,292 | 4,650 | 18,075 | 34,973 |

*Notes:*    Figures are as at 30th September.
Figures exclude PCT employed GPs.

*Sources:*    Health and Personal Social Services Statistics for England (DH).
General and Personal Medical Services Statistics: England and Wales (DH).

Table 4.16(b)    **Number of medical practitioners (excluding GP registrars and retainers) in general practice by size of practice, Scotland, 1975 - 2005**

Number

| Year | Single handed | In partnerships of: | | | | | All GPs[1] |
|------|------|------|------|------|------|------|------|
| | | 2 | 3 | 4 | 5 | >=6 | |
| 1975 | 428 | 568 | 759 | 508 | 260 | 274 | 2,797 |
| 1980 | 354 | 485 | 709 | 619 | 387 | 405 | 2,959 |
| 1985 | 322 | 490 | 611 | 703 | 476 | 652 | 3,254 |
| 1990 | 258 | 442 | 618 | 700 | 570 | 796 | 3,384 |
| 1991 | 237 | 452 | 639 | 656 | 610 | 814 | 3,408 |
| 1992 | 227 | 430 | 648 | 652 | 625 | 862 | 3,444 |
| 1993 | 221 | 426 | 630 | 652 | 645 | 901 | 3,475 |
| 1994 | 216 | 438 | 609 | 668 | 640 | 942 | 3,558 |
| 1995 | 213 | 398 | 648 | 664 | 650 | 980 | 3,590 |
| 1996 | 213 | 400 | 600 | 696 | 605 | 1,068 | 3,635 |
| 1997 | 200 | 380 | 573 | 696 | 645 | 1201 | 3,695 |
| 1998 | 198 | 366 | 594 | 672 | 680 | 1235 | 3,745 |
| 1999 | 192 | 360 | 609 | 640 | 705 | 1278 | 3,784 |
| 2000 | 184 | 366 | 591 | 668 | 665 | 1332 | 3,806 |
| 2001 | 186 | 352 | 594 | 656 | 685 | 1392 | 3,865 |
| 2002 | 184 | 342 | 564 | 640 | 700 | 1449 | 3,879 |
| 2003 | 175 | 346 | 591 | 600 | 700 | 1544 | 3,956 |
| 2004 | 158 | 336 | 573 | 569 | 715 | 1619 | 3,970 |
| 2005 | 125 | 396 | 585 | 580 | 710 | 1691 | 4,087 |

Notes:    1 Totals may not agree with those shown elsewhere because of the inclusion of vacancies.
Figures are as at 1st October.
Source:    Scottish Health Statistics (ISD).

Table 4.16(c)    **Number of medical practitioners (excluding GP registrars and retainers) in general practice by size of practice, Northern Ireland[1], 1975 - 2005**

Number

| Year | Single handed | In partnerships of: | | | | All GPs |
|------|------|------|------|------|------|------|
| | | 2 | 3 | 4 | >=5 | |
| 1975 | 188 | 228 | 183 | 88 | 59 | 746 |
| 1980 | 157 | 186 | 207 | 120 | 94 | 762 |
| 1985 | 112 | 156 | 276 | 156 | 181 | 881 |
| 1990 | 88 | 177 | 229 | 197 | 211 | 924 |
| 1991 | 89 | 181 | 251 | 189 | 207 | 917 |
| 1992 | 85 | 188 | 245 | 211 | 208 | 937 |
| 1993 | 87 | 183 | 260 | 170 | 250 | 950 |
| 1994 | 78 | 186 | 253 | 179 | 283 | 979 |
| 1995 | 75 | 184 | 258 | 198 | 279 | 994 |
| 1996 | 73 | 192 | 258 | 200 | 291 | 1,011 |
| 1997 | 77 | 180 | 255 | 224 | 290 | 1,026 |
| 1998 | 79 | 180 | 246 | 212 | 316 | 1,033 |
| 1999 | 80 | 188 | 246 | 224 | 301 | 1,039 |
| 2000 | 76 | 192 | 246 | 236 | 299 | 1,049 |
| 2001 | 73 | 192 | 261 | 216 | 312 | 1,054 |
| 2002 | 66 | 196 | 273 | 192 | 337 | 1,064 |
| 2003 | 67 | 206 | 267 | 172 | 364 | 1,076 |
| 2004 | 72 | 206 | 261 | 184 | 355 | 1,078 |
| 2005 | 70 | 190 | 258 | 200 | 366 | 1,084 |

Note:    1 Figures for Northern Ireland from 1996 onwards are at 1st January, apart from 2005 where figures are as at 1 April.
Source:    Annual Statistical Report (Northern Ireland CSA).

Figure 4.7  **Index (1959=100) of number of medical practitioners (excluding GP registrars and retainers) in general practice, by size of practice, England and Wales, 1959 - 2006**

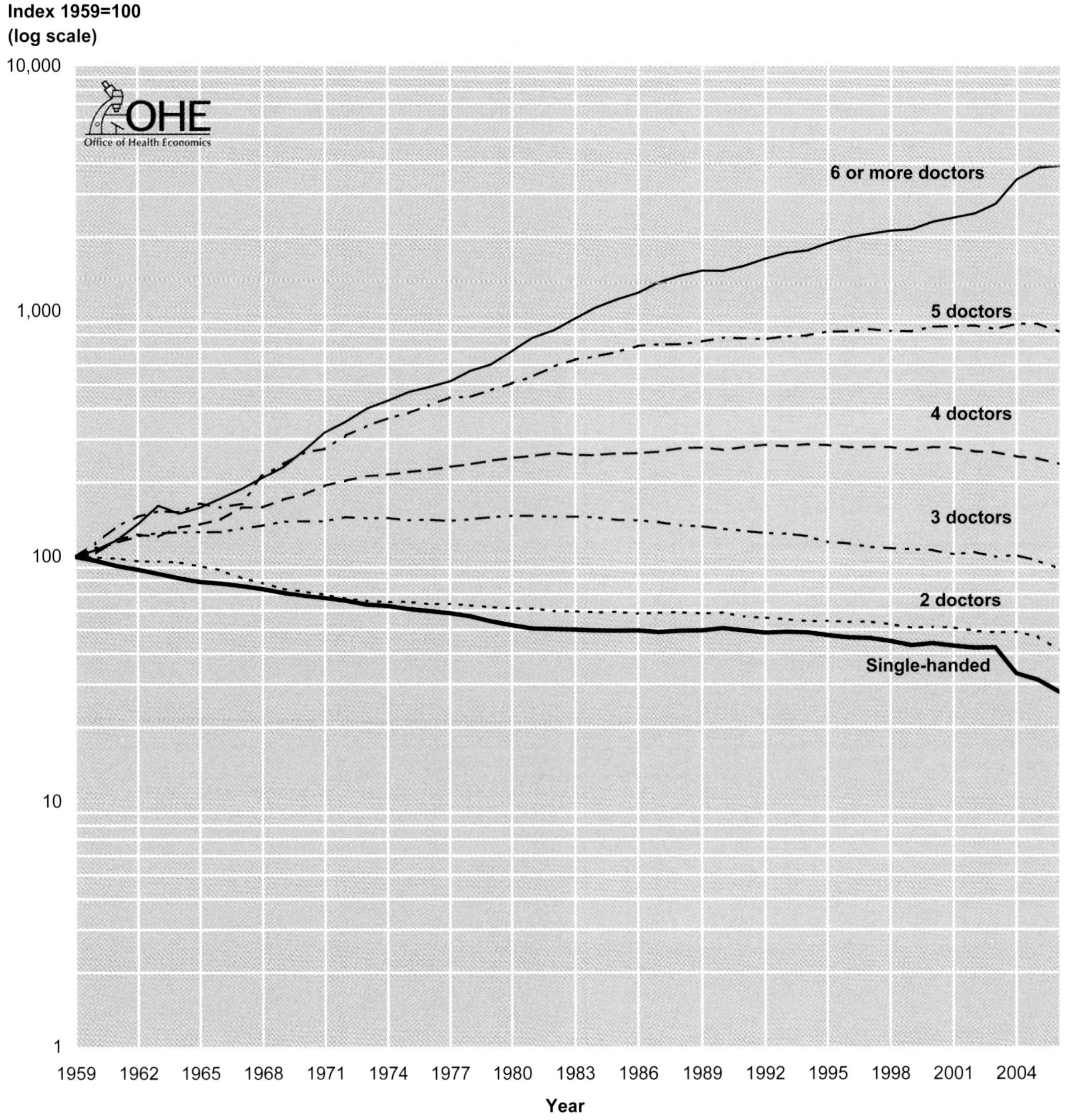

**Index 1959=100**
**(log scale)**

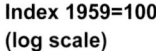

*Note:*      Figures are as at 1st October before 2000 and are as at 30th September thereafter.
*Source:*   General and Personal Medical Services Statistics (DH).

# FHS: General Medical Services

Table 4.17  **Estimated number and index (1975=100) of NHS GP consultations by age group, UK, 1975 - 2005**

Millions

| | Year | | | | | | | | | | |
|---|---|---|---|---|---|---|---|---|---|---|---|
| | 1975 | 1980 | 1985 | 1990 | 1995 | 2000 | 2001 | 2002 | 2003 | 2004 | 2005 |
| **All Males** | **83** | **99** | **91** | **117** | **111** | **113** | **106** | **124** | **110** | **106** | **107** |
| 0-4 | 8 | 11 | 13 | 18 | 14 | 11 | 11 | 12 | 10 | 9 | 9 |
| 5-15[1] | 10 | 14 | 11 | 11 | 11 | 8 | 8 | 12 | 8 | 8 | 8 |
| 16-44[1] | 27 | 31 | 25 | 38 | 36 | 37 | 37 | 37 | 37 | 37 | 38 |
| 45-64 | 23 | 23 | 24 | 30 | 26 | 34 | 28 | 35 | 28 | 29 | 29 |
| 65-74 | 8 | 13 | 11 | 11 | 12 | 14 | 12 | 16 | 14 | 12 | 12 |
| 75 and over | 6 | 7 | 7 | 9 | 11 | 10 | 11 | 12 | 12 | 12 | 12 |
| **All Females** | **113** | **143** | **147** | **174** | **172** | **153** | **156** | **168** | **149** | **162** | **166** |
| 0-4 | 7 | 9 | 12 | 13 | 13 | 7 | 10 | 7 | 8 | 10 | 8 |
| 5-15[1] | 9 | 13 | 11 | 14 | 15 | 11 | 11 | 7 | 7 | 7 | 7 |
| 16-44[1] | 46 | 63 | 61 | 75 | 73 | 61 | 62 | 74 | 62 | 62 | 75 |
| 45-64 | 25 | 28 | 32 | 37 | 33 | 35 | 43 | 36 | 36 | 44 | 37 |
| 65-74 | 15 | 17 | 14 | 17 | 20 | 19 | 13 | 18 | 19 | 19 | 19 |
| 75 and over | 11 | 14 | 17 | 18 | 19 | 19 | 17 | 25 | 17 | 20 | 20 |
| **Total** | **196** | **241** | **238** | **291** | **283** | **266** | **262** | **292** | **259** | **268** | **274** |
| 0-4 | 15 | 20 | 25 | 31 | 27 | 18 | 21 | 19 | 19 | 19 | 17 |
| 5-15[1] | 20 | 27 | 22 | 25 | 26 | 19 | 19 | 19 | 15 | 15 | 15 |
| 16-44[1] | 73 | 94 | 86 | 113 | 109 | 98 | 98 | 111 | 99 | 99 | 113 |
| 45-64 | 48 | 51 | 56 | 68 | 60 | 70 | 70 | 71 | 65 | 73 | 66 |
| 65-74 | 23 | 29 | 25 | 28 | 31 | 32 | 25 | 35 | 33 | 30 | 31 |
| 75 and over | 17 | 21 | 24 | 28 | 30 | 29 | 28 | 37 | 29 | 32 | 32 |

## Index (1975=100)

| | Year | | | | | | | | | | |
|---|---|---|---|---|---|---|---|---|---|---|---|
| | 1975 | 1980 | 1985 | 1990 | 1995 | 2000 | 2001 | 2002 | 2003 | 2004 | 2005 |
| **All Males** | **100** | **119** | **110** | **141** | **133** | **136** | **128** | **149** | **132** | **128** | **129** |
| 0-4 | 100 | 139 | 161 | 220 | 171 | 136 | 134 | 153 | 130 | 109 | 110 |
| 5-15[1] | 100 | 134 | 112 | 108 | 115 | 78 | 78 | 117 | 77 | 77 | 76 |
| 16-44[1] | 100 | 115 | 92 | 140 | 135 | 136 | 136 | 137 | 138 | 138 | 140 |
| 45-64 | 100 | 99 | 106 | 132 | 114 | 149 | 121 | 152 | 123 | 125 | 126 |
| 65-74 | 100 | 156 | 136 | 141 | 146 | 172 | 144 | 203 | 176 | 148 | 149 |
| 75 and over | 100 | 113 | 120 | 157 | 187 | 158 | 189 | 193 | 196 | 200 | 204 |
| **All Females** | **100** | **126** | **130** | **154** | **152** | **135** | **138** | **149** | **132** | **143** | **147** |
| 0-4 | 100 | 116 | 176 | 187 | 186 | 99 | 146 | 95 | 118 | 142 | 120 |
| 5-15[1] | 100 | 134 | 118 | 153 | 163 | 124 | 124 | 82 | 82 | 81 | 80 |
| 16-44[1] | 100 | 137 | 133 | 163 | 159 | 133 | 134 | 161 | 134 | 135 | 163 |
| 45-64 | 100 | 113 | 127 | 150 | 134 | 141 | 171 | 144 | 145 | 177 | 149 |
| 65-74 | 100 | 111 | 93 | 112 | 131 | 123 | 88 | 123 | 124 | 124 | 124 |
| 75 and over | 100 | 130 | 154 | 167 | 169 | 177 | 153 | 230 | 154 | 180 | 181 |
| **Total** | **100** | **123** | **121** | **149** | **144** | **136** | **133** | **149** | **132** | **137** | **140** |
| 0-4 | 100 | 128 | 168 | 205 | 178 | 119 | 139 | 126 | 124 | 124 | 114 |
| 5-15[1] | 100 | 134 | 109 | 123 | 131 | 95 | 95 | 96 | 75 | 75 | 74 |
| 16-44[1] | 100 | 129 | 118 | 154 | 150 | 134 | 135 | 152 | 136 | 136 | 154 |
| 45-64 | 100 | 107 | 117 | 141 | 124 | 145 | 147 | 148 | 135 | 152 | 138 |
| 65-74 | 100 | 127 | 108 | 122 | 136 | 140 | 108 | 151 | 142 | 132 | 133 |
| 75 and over | 100 | 123 | 142 | 163 | 175 | 171 | 166 | 217 | 169 | 187 | 189 |

*Notes:*  All figures are subject to rounding and sampling errors.
Data shown for 1998 onwards are based on data weighted to compensate for differential non-response.
From 1988 to 2004 the General Household Survey was on a financial year basis with interviews taking place from April to the following March.
1 In 1975, figures relate to age groups 5-14 and 15-44, respectively.

*Sources:* Living in Britain: Results from the General Household Survey (ONS).
Population Projections database (GAD).

Table 4.18 **Estimated number and index (1975=100) of NHS consultations per medical practitioner (excluding GP registrars and retainers), in general practice, by age, UK, 1975 - 2005**

| | Year | | | | | | | | | | |
| --- | --- | --- | --- | --- | --- | --- | --- | --- | --- | --- | --- |
| | 1975 | 1980 | 1985 | 1990 | 1995 | 2000 | 2001 | 2002 | 2003 | 2004 | 2005 |
| **All Males** | **3,285** | **3,668** | **3,083** | **3,717** | **3,274** | **3,206** | **2,983** | **3,444** | **2,943** | **2,767** | **2,698** |
| 0-4 | 314 | 409 | 436 | 558 | 404 | 310 | 301 | 340 | 279 | 226 | 221 |
| 5-15[1] | 409 | 515 | 377 | 343 | 339 | 222 | 220 | 325 | 208 | 200 | 190 |
| 16-44[1] | 1,068 | 1,153 | 839 | 1,196 | 1,079 | 1,038 | 1,036 | 1,029 | 999 | 974 | 948 |
| 45-64 | 926 | 862 | 823 | 964 | 775 | 976 | 782 | 975 | 762 | 747 | 731 |
| 65-74 | 317 | 465 | 366 | 357 | 345 | 391 | 325 | 453 | 378 | 308 | 299 |
| 75 and over | 250 | 264 | 243 | 298 | 333 | 270 | 319 | 322 | 316 | 312 | 308 |
| **All Females** | **4,495** | **5,306** | **4,943** | **5,520** | **5,098** | **4,331** | **4,379** | **4,670** | **4,013** | **4,218** | **4,187** |
| 0-4 | 295 | 320 | 415 | 415 | 385 | 197 | 287 | 186 | 222 | 258 | 210 |
| 5-15[1] | 376 | 472 | 358 | 437 | 433 | 318 | 314 | 206 | 198 | 190 | 181 |
| 16-44[1] | 1,820 | 2,333 | 2,060 | 2,371 | 2,161 | 1,740 | 1,733 | 2,058 | 1,662 | 1,617 | 1,887 |
| 45-64 | 990 | 1,050 | 1,068 | 1,186 | 988 | 998 | 1,200 | 1,000 | 977 | 1,151 | 939 |
| 65-74 | 590 | 615 | 469 | 531 | 581 | 526 | 371 | 514 | 499 | 485 | 469 |
| 75 and over | 424 | 515 | 572 | 581 | 550 | 553 | 474 | 705 | 455 | 516 | 501 |
| **Total** | **7,780** | **8,975** | **8,026** | **9,237** | **8,372** | **7,537** | **7,362** | **8,113** | **6,956** | **6,985** | **6,884** |
| 0-4 | 609 | 729 | 851 | 973 | 789 | 506 | 588 | 526 | 501 | 485 | 431 |
| 5-15[1] | 785 | 987 | 735 | 780 | 772 | 540 | 534 | 531 | 406 | 389 | 371 |
| 16-44[1] | 2,889 | 3,486 | 2,899 | 3,567 | 3,240 | 2,779 | 2,769 | 3,088 | 2,661 | 2,591 | 2,835 |
| 45-64 | 1,916 | 1,913 | 1,892 | 2,150 | 1,762 | 1,974 | 1,982 | 1,975 | 1,739 | 1,898 | 1,670 |
| 65-74 | 907 | 1,080 | 835 | 888 | 926 | 916 | 696 | 967 | 878 | 794 | 769 |
| 75 and over | 674 | 780 | 815 | 879 | 883 | 823 | 793 | 1,027 | 771 | 828 | 809 |

### Index (1975=100)

| | Year | | | | | | | | | | |
| --- | --- | --- | --- | --- | --- | --- | --- | --- | --- | --- | --- |
| | 1975 | 1980 | 1985 | 1990 | 1995 | 2000 | 2001 | 2002 | 2003 | 2004 | 2005 |
| **All Males** | **100** | **110** | **94** | **113** | **100** | **98** | **91** | **105** | **90** | **84** | **82** |
| 0-4 | 100 | 125 | 139 | 178 | 129 | 99 | 96 | 108 | 89 | 72 | 70 |
| 5-15[1] | 100 | 83 | 92 | 84 | 83 | 54 | 54 | 80 | 51 | 49 | 47 |
| 16-44[1] | 100 | 126 | 79 | 112 | 101 | 97 | 97 | 96 | 94 | 91 | 89 |
| 45-64 | 100 | 101 | 89 | 104 | 84 | 105 | 84 | 105 | 82 | 81 | 79 |
| 65-74 | 100 | 135 | 115 | 113 | 109 | 123 | 102 | 143 | 119 | 97 | 94 |
| 75 and over | 100 | 76 | 97 | 119 | 133 | 108 | 128 | 129 | 127 | 125 | 123 |
| **All Females** | **100** | **115** | **110** | **123** | **113** | **96** | **97** | **104** | **89** | **94** | **93** |
| 0-4 | 100 | 106 | 141 | 141 | 131 | 67 | 97 | 63 | 75 | 88 | 71 |
| 5-15[1] | 100 | 128 | 95 | 116 | 115 | 84 | 84 | 55 | 53 | 50 | 48 |
| 16-44[1] | 100 | 119 | 113 | 130 | 119 | 96 | 95 | 113 | 91 | 89 | 104 |
| 45-64 | 100 | 99 | 108 | 120 | 100 | 101 | 121 | 101 | 99 | 116 | 95 |
| 65-74 | 100 | 95 | 79 | 90 | 98 | 89 | 63 | 87 | 85 | 82 | 80 |
| 75 and over | 100 | 151 | 135 | 137 | 130 | 130 | 112 | 166 | 107 | 122 | 118 |
| **Total** | **100** | **113** | **103** | **119** | **108** | **97** | **95** | **104** | **89** | **90** | **88** |
| 0-4 | 100 | 116 | 140 | 160 | 130 | 83 | 97 | 86 | 82 | 80 | 71 |
| 5-15[1] | 100 | 105 | 94 | 99 | 98 | 69 | 68 | 68 | 52 | 50 | 47 |
| 16-44[1] | 100 | 122 | 100 | 123 | 112 | 96 | 96 | 107 | 92 | 90 | 98 |
| 45-64 | 100 | 100 | 99 | 112 | 92 | 103 | 103 | 103 | 91 | 99 | 87 |
| 65-74 | 100 | 109 | 92 | 98 | 102 | 101 | 77 | 107 | 97 | 87 | 85 |
| 75 and over | 100 | 123 | 121 | 130 | 131 | 122 | 118 | 152 | 114 | 123 | 120 |

*Notes:* All figures are subject to rounding and sampling errors.
Data shown for 1998 onwards are based on data weighted to compensate for differential non-response.
From 1988 to 2004 the General Household Survey was on a financial year basis with interviews taking place from April to the following March.
For timing of data see Table 4.8.
1 In 1975, figures relate to age groups 5-14 and 15-44, respectively.

*Sources:* Living in Britain: Results from the General Household Survey (ONS).
Population Projections Database (GAD).

Table 4.19(a)   **Number of dispensing doctors by country, UK, 1995 - 2005**

30th September

| | Year | | | | | | | | | |
|---|---|---|---|---|---|---|---|---|---|---|
| | **1995** | **1996** | **1998** | **1999** | **2000** | **2001** | **2002** | **2003** | **2004** | **2005** |
| **United Kingdom** | 4,729 | 4,783 | 4,783 | 4,933 | 4,973 | 4,707 | 4,483 | 4,034 | 4,213 | 3,869 |
| **England** | 4,122 | 4,187 | 4,171 | 4,321 | 4,356 | 4,084 | 3,858 | 3,409 | 3,588 | 3,290 |
| **Wales** | 289 | 292 | 299 | 305 | 318 | 328 | 331 | 327 | 327 | 285 |
| **Scotland** | 258 | 265 | 268 | 263 | 277 | 274 | 269 | 276 | 281 | 276 |
| **Northern Ireland** | 71 | 71 | 61 | 44 | 22 | 21 | 25 | 22 | 17 | 18 |

*Note:*    Data for England and Wales are as at 1 October before 2000. Data for Northern Ireland from 1996 to 2002 are as at 1 January, and from 2003 onwards are as at 1 October.  Data for Scotland are as at 1 October.

*Sources:*  Prescription Pricing Authority Annual Reports (PPA).
Health and Personal Social Services Statistics for England (DH).
Scottish Health Statistics (ISD).
Health Statistics Wales (NAW).
Annual Statistical Report (Northern Ireland CSA).
General and Personal Medical Services Statistics: Detailed Results (DH).

Table 4.19(b)   **Number of NHS prescription items dispensed by dispensing doctors by country, UK, 1995 - 2005**

Millions

| | Year | | | | | | | | | |
|---|---|---|---|---|---|---|---|---|---|---|
| | **1995** | **1996** | **1998** | **1999** | **2000** | **2001** | **2002** | **2003** | **2004** | **2005** |
| **United Kingdom** | 36.6 | 37.6 | 40.6 | 42.1 | 44.3 | 47.1 | 49.9 | 53.0 | 56.6 | 60.2 |
| **England** | 32.1 | 33.0 | 35.7 | 37.1 | 39.0 | 41.6 | 44.2 | 47.1 | 50.4 | 53.6 |
| **Wales** | 2.0 | 2.1 | 2.3 | 2.3 | 2.5 | 2.6 | 2.8 | 2.9 | 3.1 | 3.3 |
| **Scotland** | 1.9 | 1.9 | 2.1 | 2.2 | 2.4 | 2.6 | 2.6 | 2.7 | 2.8 | 3.0 |
| **Northern Ireland** | 0.6 | 0.6 | 0.6 | 0.5 | 0.4 | 0.3 | 0.3 | 0.3 | 0.3 | 0.2 |

*Sources:*  Prescription Pricing Authority Annual Reports (PPA).
Health and Personal Social Services Statistics for England (DH).
Scottish Health Statistics (ISD).
Health Statistics Wales (NAW).
Annual Statistical Report (Northern Ireland CSA).
General and Personal Medical Services Statistics: Detailed Results (DH).

# FHS: General Pharmaceutical Services

In 2005/06, 891 million NHS prescription items were dispensed by the UK FHS, (i.e. outside hospitals) (**Table 4.24**). Prescriptions are written mainly by GPs, although small proportions are written by dentists, hospital doctors and nurses. Ninety three per cent of FHS prescriptions are dispensed by chemists and appliance contractors of the General Pharmaceutical Services. The remainder are dispensed directly by dispensing doctors (see General Medical Services). Together with medicines issued and dispensed by hospitals, these sources constitute the NHS medicines supply system.

## Community pharmacies and appliance contractors

In this section of the Compendium, the term "Pharmacies and appliance contractors" refers to Community pharmacies and appliance suppliers who are contracted to the NHS unless otherwise specified. Appliance contractors provide such things as contraceptive devices, elastic hosiery, dressings and orthopaedic equipment. These items, some of which are also provided by retail chemist outlets, are included in figures for the total number of prescriptions dispensed. Throughout this section of the Compendium, the terms 'chemists' and 'pharmacies' are used interchangeably to refer to dispensing chemists and appliance contractors.

A prescription form, issued by a doctor to a patient, may contain one or more items of medicines or appliances. All prescription items are supposed to attract a professional fee. Prescription statistics obtained from the Prescription Pricing Authority (PPA) for England are prescription fee based while those from PPA for Wales, Scotland and Northern Ireland are based on items. There are minor differences of about 1% between the two counting systems. In the volume statistics shown throughout the Compendium, the term 'prescriptions' refers to the number of fees or items dispensed by chemists and appliance contractors. The same applies to medicines provided by dispensing doctors under the General Medical Services. *Prescription Cost Analysis for England* published by the Department of Health (DH) in England since 1991, however, is items based.

Community pharmacies are required by their terms of service to supply medicines and certain appliances ordered on NHS prescription forms. Dispensing must be performed by a registered pharmacist and medicines must be of the quality specified. Medicines and appliances will normally be supplied from stock purchased by the retail pharmacies from a wholesaler, or in some cases directly from the manufacturer. Remuneration of, and reimbursement to, community pharmacies are financed directly by the Department of Health (or its Scotland, Wales and Northern Ireland counterparts). In England payments to chemists are administered by the Prescription Pricing Authority (PPA). Similar bodies exist in the other countries of the UK.

In 2006 there were 12,407 pharmacies under contract to the NHS in the UK, a slight increase in numbers on 2005, after several years of gradual decline (**Table 4.21**). The number of pharmacies per capita in the UK has therefore also declined slightly over the same period, standing at just over 20 per 100,000 population in 2006. There are large variations between the countries of the UK. The highest provision is in Northern Ireland, where there were 50% more pharmacies per capita than in England in 2006 (**Table 4.21**). **Figure 4.11** shows that the UK ranks in the middle among OECD countries for the number of practising pharmacists per population.

## Prescribing in the community

According to the *General Household Survey 2005*, about 66% of patients who consulted an NHS GP obtained a prescription, compared with 74% in 1984. **Box 10** shows that although older patients are more likely to obtain a prescription than younger people, they were, in 2005, less likely to be prescribed medicine than they were in 1984.

| Box 10 | **Proportion (%) of patients consulting a NHS GP who obtained a prescription, Great Britain** | | | | |
|---|---|---|---|---|---|
| Age group | 1984 | 1994 | 2000 | 2004 | 2005 |
| All ages | 74 | 71 | 66 | 67 | 66 |
| 0-15 years | 72 | 70 | 59 | 58 | 61 |
| 16-44 years | 67 | 68 | 62 | 66 | 63 |
| 45-64 years | 80 | 73 | 70 | 68 | 69 |
| over 65 years | 82 | 75 | 72 | 71 | 71 |

*Notes:* From 2000 figures are based on weighted data.
From 1988 to 2004 the General Household Survey was on a financial year basis with interviews taking place from April to the following March. Data was not available for 1985 or 1995.

*Source:* Living in Britain: Results from the General Household Survey (ONS).

The number of prescriptions dispensed in the UK by community pharmacies and dispensing doctors grew to 927 million in 2006 (**Table 4.23**), with increases of approximately 50% occurring during each of the past two decades (**Box 11**).

In 2006, the number of prescription items per pharmacy was over 70,000, having grown steadily by an annual average of 4.6% over the previous decade (**Table 4.22**).

In 2005/06 14.8 prescription items were dispensed per capita in the UK, compared to 10 per capita in 1995/96 (**Table 4.24**). Although all countries in the UK have experienced growth, there are large variations between them in both the number of prescriptions issued to patients and the growth rates, with 14.4 items per capita on average in England but 19.3 items in Wales in 2005/06. Among the countries of the UK, Scotland had the largest growth in the number of prescription items dispensed per capita over the last ten years, although Wales still has the highest rate per capita (**Table 4.24**).

**Box 11 Change (%) in number of prescriptions dispensed, UK**

| | Total | Per capita |
|---|---|---|
| 1956 - 1966 | 16 | 9 |
| 1966 - 1976 | 20 | 17 |
| 1976 - 1986 | 10 | 9 |
| 1986 - 1996 | 50 | 47 |
| 1996 - 2006 | 55 | 49 |

Sources: Prescription Pricing Authority England.
Health of Wales information Services.
Information Services Division of the NHS in Scotland.
Central Services Agency, Northern Ireland.
Health and Personal Social Services Statistics for England (DH).
Scottish Health Statistics (ISD).
Health Statistics Wales (NAW).
Annual Statistical Report (Northern Ireland CSA).
Annual Abstract of Statistics (ONS).

**Box 12 Charges on non-exempt prescriptions, UK[1]**

| Year (1st April) | Charge per item (£ cash) | Charge per item (£ at 2007 prices[2]) | Index[2] 1956=100 |
|---|---|---|---|
| 1956 | 0.05 | 0.91 | 100 |
| 1961 | 0.10 | 1.58 | 174 |
| 1971 | 0.20 | 1.99 | 220 |
| 1981 | 1.00 | 2.64 | 292 |
| 1991 | 3.40 | 5.15 | 568 |
| 1992 | 3.75 | 5.47 | 604 |
| 1993 | 4.25 | 6.03 | 666 |
| 1994 | 4.75 | 6.64 | 733 |
| 1995 | 5.25 | 7.15 | 789 |
| 1996 | 5.50 | 7.22 | 797 |
| 1997 | 5.65 | 7.23 | 798 |
| 1998 | 5.80 | 7.24 | 800 |
| 1999 | 5.90 | 7.24 | 800 |
| 2000 | 6.00 | 7.28 | 804 |
| 2001 | 6.10 | 7.20 | 795 |
| 2002 | 6.20 | 7.07 | 781 |
| 2003 | 6.30 | 6.96 | 769 |
| 2004 | 6.40 | 6.89 | 761 |
| 2005 | 6.50 | 6.85 | 756 |
| 2006 | 6.65 | 6.84 | 755 |
| 2007 | 6.85 | 6.85 | 756 |

Notes: 1 In Wales, prescription charges were frozen at £6 in April 2000, reduced to £4 on 1st April 2005, reduced to £3 on 1st April 2006 and subsequently were free from 1st April 2007.
2 At constant prices, as adjusted by the GDP deflator at market prices.
Sources: Prescription Pricing Authority, England.
Health of Wales Information Services.
Information Services Division of the NHS in Scotland.
Central Services Agency, Northern Ireland.
Health and Personal Social Services Statistics for England (DH).
Scottish Health Statistics (ISD).
Health Statistics Wales (NAW).
Annual Statistical Report (Northern Ireland CSA).
Annual Abstract of Statistics (ONS).
Economic Trends (ONS).

There are many factors contributing to the rise in UK prescribing levels over the past four decades. These include increases in the overall population and shifts in its demographic structure, particularly the rising proportion of elderly people (see **Section 1**). Adding to this is the number of new medicines that have become available. Increasing public expectations may have also had an effect.

Of all prescription items dispensed in 2006, over 441 million, 59%, were for the elderly, up from 44% just a decade earlier (**Figure 4.13**). The number of prescription items dispensed decreased over the same 10 year period for those under 16 years, from 5 per person to 4.4 (**Table 4.25**).

## Prescription charges

Since 1952 - except for the period between February 1965 and June 1968 - patients requiring NHS medicines via prescriptions have been subject to a charge. There have been numerous increases in the charges, the latest taking effect on 1 April 2007 (except in Wales). The charge has increased in every year since 1979 (with the exception of Wales since 2000, where prescriptions were free from 1 April 2007) (**Box 12** and **Figure 4.15**). After allowing for general inflation, prescription charges have fallen somewhat below their peak level in 2000 (**Box 12**).

In 2006, 90.2 million of the total number of prescription items dispensed were chargeable, representing just 12% of the total (**Table 4.25**). In 2006 charges contributed 5% of total prescription costs (**Figure 4.16**).

When the prescription charge was reintroduced in June 1968, an exemption scheme was instituted. Additional exemption categories were added in later years. The current list of the groups of people not required to pay prescription charges is shown in **Box 13**. The number

of people entitled to free prescriptions increased from about 22 million in 1969 to about half the UK population today. Exempt prescriptions rose from 71% of the total number dispensed in 1986, to 88% in 2006 (**Figure 4.18**).

Box 13 **Prescription charge exemption categories**

Providing that the appropriate declaration is received, a charge is not payable to the contractor or dispensing doctor for drugs or appliances, including elastic hosiery, supplied for:

Children under 16 (except for Wales where prescriptions are free as of 1 April 2007).

Students aged 16, 17 or 18 in full-time education.

Men and women aged 60 and over.

People holding Health Authority exemption certificates, which are issued to:

- Expectant mothers;
- Women who have borne a child in the last 12 months;
- People suffering from the following specified conditions:
  - Permanent fistula (including Caecostomy, Colostomy, Ileostomy or Laryngostomy) requiring continuous surgical dressing or an appliance;
  - Forms of hypoadrenalism (including Addison's disease) for which specific substitution therapy is essential;
  - Diabetes insipidus and other forms of hypopituitarism;
  - Diabetes Mellitus except where treatment is by diet alone;
  - Hypoparathyroidism;
  - Myasthenia gravis;
  - Myxoedema (hypothroidism);
  - Epilepsy requiring continuous anti-convulsive therapy;
  - A continuing physical disability which prevents the patient leaving his residence except with the help of another person (this does not mean a temporary disability even if it is likely to last for a few months).

War and service pensioners (for prescriptions needed for treating their accepted disablement).

NHS Low Income Scheme Charge Remission.

No charge is payable for contraceptive substances and listed contraceptive appliances for women prescribed on FP10 or any of its variants.

*Note:* As of 1 April 2007 Prescriptions were free in Wales.

*Source:* Charges for drugs and appliances payable under Regulations made under Section 77(1) of the NHS Act 1977.

## Cost of General Pharmaceutical Services

General Pharmaceutical Services costs consist of the cost of medicines; pharmacists' remuneration in the form of dispensing fees; container costs; and on-cost allowances.

In 2005/06 the General Pharmaceutical Services represented 10.7% of all NHS spending in the UK, having fallen slightly as a share in recent years (**Figure 4.8**). The total cost of NHS prescriptions dispensed in the UK by NHS chemists and appliance contractors and dispensing doctors was £10.8 billion in 2006, (**Table 4.26**), 55% higher in real terms than the figure 10 years earlier (**Box 14**).

Box 14 **Decadal change (percentage) in the real[1] total cost of prescriptions dispensed[2], UK**

| Decade | Total cost | Cost per capita |
|---|---|---|
| 1966 - 1976 | 34 | 30 |
| 1976 - 1986 | 48 | 47 |
| 1986 - 1996 | 71 | 66 |
| 1996 - 2006 | 55 | 48 |

*Notes:* Total cost includes ingredient cost, dispensing fees, allowances etc.
1 As adjusted by the GDP deflator at market prices.
2 Figures relate to prescriptions dispensed by chemists and appliance suppliers and dispensing doctors.

*Sources:* Prescription Pricing Authority, England.
Health of Wales Information Services.
Information Services Division of the NHS in Scotland.
Central Services Agency, Northern Ireland.
Health and Personal Social Services Statistics for England (DH).
Scottish Health Statistics (ISD).
Health Statistics Wales (NAW).
Annual Statistical Report (Northern Ireland CSA).

The average cost per prescriptions fell again in 2006 (**Figure 4.14**). Relative to England, the per capita cost of prescriptions in 2006 was 34% higher in Northern Ireland, 21% higher in Wales and 16% higher in Scotland (**Table 4.26**).

UK outlay on pharmaceuticals (including medicines bought over the counter) at 1.1% of GDP is modest by OECD standards (**Figure 4.9**). **Figure 4.10** shows that expenditure per head on pharmaceuticals in the UK was £233 in 2005, considerably lower than that reported for France and Germany amongst other countries.

The proportion of the gross cost of pharmaceutical services that is pharmacists' income rose between 2004 and 2005, following a steady downward trend over the previous decade to stand at 13% in 2005 (**Box 15**).

Box 15 **Total dispensing cost as a % of the gross cost of pharmaceutical services, UK**

| | Income (%) |
|---|---|
| 1995 | 15.4 |
| 1996 | 14.7 |
| 1997 | 14.5 |
| 1998 | 14.1 |
| 1999 | 13.1 |
| 2000 | 12.7 |
| 2001 | 12.3 |
| 2002 | 11.5 |
| 2003 | 10.9 |
| 2004 | 10.8 |
| 2005 | 12.8 |

*Sources:* Prescription Pricing Authority, England.
Health of Wales Information Services.
Information Services Division of the NHS in Scotland.
Central Services Agency, Northern Ireland.
Health and Personal Social Services Statistics for England (DH).
Scottish Health Statistics (ISD).
Health Statistics Wales (NAW).
Annual Statistical Report (Northern Ireland CSA).

## Net ingredient cost

Since 1957, the prices of pharmaceutical products sold to the NHS, excluding unbranded generic medicines from 1986 onwards, have been regulated by negotiation between the pharmaceutical industry and the Department of Health, through the Pharmaceutical Price Regulation Scheme (PPRS). The scheme applies to all companies supplying branded medicines to the NHS. The outcome of the latest PPRS settlement, which came into force on 1st January 2005, included an agreement to a general price reduction of 7% on all branded preparations. These prices are known as NHS Basic Prices or Net Ingredient Cost (NIC) and, together with the *Drug Tariff* for generic preparations, constitute the basis on which the Prescription Pricing Authority costs NHS prescriptions. The NIC, however, does not represent the total amount spent by the NHS on medicines, as it is before discounts and other reimbursement deductions.

The aggregate NIC of NHS prescriptions was £9.8 billion in 2006, a slight increase on the NIC in 2005 (**Table 4.27** and **Box 16**).

| Box 16  **Decadal change (percentage) in real[1] NIC, UK** | | | |
|---|---|---|---|
| | **Total NIC** | **NIC per capita** | **NIC per item** |
| 1966 - 1976 | 38 | 34 | 14 |
| 1976 - 1986 | 61 | 60 | 46 |
| 1986 - 1996 | 71 | 67 | 14 |
| 1996 - 2006 | 60 | 53 | 3 |

*Notes:*  Net Ingredient Cost (NIC) is the basic price before discount, dressings and appliances, (including dispensing doctors).
1 As adjusted by the GDP deflator, at market prices.
*Sources:* Prescription Pricing Authority, England.
Health of Wales Information Services.
Information Services Division of the NHS in Scotland.
Central Services Agency, Northern Ireland.
Health and Personal Social Services Statistics for England (DH).
Scottish Health Statistics (ISD).
Health Statistics Wales (NAW).
Annual Statistical Report (Northern Ireland CSA).
Populations Projections Database (GAD).

The NIC of prescriptions per person was £162 in the UK in 2006, with a real terms AGR of 4.3% over the past decade (**Box 17**). However this was not consistent across the UK. Relative to England, outlay on NHS medicines per capita in 2006 was 36% higher in Northern Ireland, 20% higher in Wales and 7% higher in Scotland (**Table 4.29**).

The NIC per prescription in the UK increased year on year between 1996 and 2004, then fell back to £10.62 in 2006 (**Table 4.28**). Much of the change in total NIC was due to the NIC of prescriptions for older people (**Table 4.30** and **Figure 4.19**). Despite a decrease between 2004 and 2005, per capita spending on medicines for the older age group was still over 2 times higher in real terms in 2006 than a decade earlier.

NHS prescriptions (including dressings, appliances and other drugs) can be categorised into 16 broad therapeutic groups as defined in the *British National Formulary* (BNF). Each group relates to a particular function of the human body or to some aspect of medical care. Each group is further divided into a number of sub-groups which give a finer level of classification.

| Box 17 **Total NIC and NIC per capita of NHS prescriptions, UK, 1996-2006** | | | | | | |
|---|---|---|---|---|---|---|
| | **Total NIC of NHS prescriptions (£millions 2006 prices)[1]** | | | **Total NIC of NHS prescriptions per capita (£ 2006 prices)[1]** | | |
| | **1996** | **2006** | **AGR % 1996-2006** | **1996** | **2006** | **AGR % 1996-2006** |
| **United Kingdom** | 6,181 | 9,844 | 4.8 | 106 | 162 | 4.3 |
| **England** | 5,001 | 8,037 | 4.9 | 103 | 158 | 4.4 |
| **Wales** | 361 | 564 | 4.6 | 125 | 190 | 4.3 |
| **Scotland** | 571 | 869 | 4.3 | 112 | 170 | 4.2 |
| **Northern Ireland** | 249 | 374 | 4.2 | 150 | 215 | 3.7 |

*Note:*  1 At 2006 prices as adjusted by GDP deflator
*Sources:*  Prescription Pricing Authority, England.
Health of Wales Information Service.
Information Services Division of the NHS in Scotland.
Central Services Agency, Northern Ireland.
Population Projections Database (GAD).
Economic Trends (ONS).

**Tables 4.31, 4.32, 4.33, 4.34** and **4.35** show the number of prescriptions and NIC by therapeutic group from 1996 to 2006 for the UK and the four constituent countries. **Tables 4.36, 4.37, 4.38, 4.39** and **4.40** present the percentage distribution of prescriptions and NIC across the 16 broad therapeutic groups (also known as BNF chapters) and selected sub-groups within each chapter (BNF sections) for the UK and each constituent country. Among the BNF groups, the most frequently prescribed medicines were for the cardiovascular system, which accounted for 31% of all prescriptions items dispensed in the UK in 2006 and 23% of total NIC (**Table 4.36**). **Box 18** shows that the top eight broad therapeutic groups accounted for 86% of all the items and 79% of the NIC of all NHS prescriptions in the UK in 2006.

**Figure 4.20** charts the trends in prescribing per capita in the eight major therapeutic groups since 1995 in the UK. Prescriptions for preparations acting on the cardiovascular system showed the greatest increase, reflecting in part the growing prevalence of heart disease in the community and the Government's National Service Framework for dealing with this. The drop in cardiovascular NIC in 2006 reflects major price cuts in some commonly prescribed medicines in this area following patent expiry. In NIC per capita terms, the central nervous system and endocrine categories have also seen rapid rises in recent years (**Figure 4.21**).

**Box 18  Share of the top eight broad therapeutic groups, (by number of prescriptions and NIC) UK 2006**

| Therapeutic group (BNF) | Share of total items (%) | Share of total NIC (%) |
|---|---|---|
| Total of eight major groups | 85.6% | 78.9% |
| Cardiovascular system | 30.9% | 22.9% |
| Central nervous system | 17.7% | 19.8% |
| Endocrine system | 8.2% | 10.6% |
| Respiratory system | 7.0% | 10.3% |
| Gastro-intestinal system | 7.7% | 7.1% |
| Infections | 5.7% | 2.8% |
| Skin | 4.7% | 2.7% |
| Musculo-skeletal and joint disease | 3.8% | 2.7% |

*Sources:* Prescription Cost Analysis, England (DH).
Prescription Cost Analysis, Wales (HOWIS).
Prescription Cost Analysis, Scotland (ISD).
Prescription Cost Analysis, Northern Ireland (CSA).

Comparisons of average costs of prescription items can be misleading even within a specific drug category, as relative cost reflects not only price but also the quantity of each medicine dispensed. Such figures can also conceal the impact of innovative drugs on medical treatment, many of which offer new approaches to disease management. Although new medicines may be relatively expensive, they may also be more cost effective than rival treatments, delivering more health care benefit, with fewer side-effects, per pound spent (**Tables 4.41, 4.42, 4.43, 4.44** and **4.45**).

## Generic prescribing

It has been Government policy for many years to promote generic prescribing. PACT reports sent to GPs include information on the availability of generic medicines and cost comparisons with branded drugs. NHS medical and pharmacy advisors also promote the use of generic medicines. In 2006 generics accounted for 60% of the total number of prescriptions dispensed by chemists in England, compared with fewer than one in six as recently as 1982 (**Figure 4.22**).

The level of generic dispensing is considerably lower than the percentage of items prescribed generically for most chapters (**Figure 4.23**). **Box 19** shows that prescriptions for branded products are on average four times as expensive as those for generics.

**Box 19  Cost per item[1] comparison of generic and branded prescriptions dispensed in England**

| Year | Generic (£) | Branded (£) | Ratio[2] |
|---|---|---|---|
| 1996 | 3.03 | 16.08 | 5.30 |
| 1997 | 3.42 | 16.84 | 4.92 |
| 1998 | 3.49 | 17.55 | 5.03 |
| 1999 | 4.40 | 18.40 | 4.18 |
| 2000 | 4.85 | 18.94 | 3.90 |
| 2001 | 3.99 | 20.04 | 5.02 |
| 2002 | 4.52 | 20.46 | 4.53 |
| 2003 | 5.19 | 20.75 | 3.99 |
| 2004 | 5.48 | 20.98 | 3.83 |
| 2005 | 4.87 | 19.79 | 4.06 |
| 2006 | 4.76 | 19.35 | 4.06 |

*Notes:* 1 NIC cost per item at 2006 prices, as adjusted by the GDP deflator, at market prices.
2 Ratio – relates to the ratio of Branded to Generic cost per item.
Prices are averages for both generic and branded prescriptions.
*Source:* OHE calculations based on data from Prescriptions Dispensed in the Community Statistics: England (DH Statistical Bulletin).

## Total NHS medicines bill

In addition to expenditure on the General Pharmaceutical Services, the total NHS medicines bill includes expenditure on medicines in the Hospital and Community Health Services and by dispensing GPs. Over the years the distribution of spending between these three elements of the NHS medicines bill has remained stable, with the General Pharmaceutical Services accounting for 71% in 2006, hospital purchases 24% and dispensing GPs less than 5%. **Table 4.46** gives a breakdown of the UK NHS medicines bill at manufacturers' prices, by sector, from 1969 to 2006. It shows that over this period, total medicines spending in the UK NHS at manufacturers' prices has grown from £144 million in 1969 to £10.7 billion (in money of the day terms) in 2006, which is equivalent to an average of £177 per person. The NHS medicines bill represented 10.5% of total NHS spending in 2006; down from a peak of 12.5 in 1999 (**Figure 4.24**).

# FHS: General Pharmaceutical Services

Table 4.20 **Cost of General Pharmaceutical Services (GPS) per capita and per household, UK, 1989/90 - 2005/06**

| Year | England | Wales | Scotland | Northern Ireland | UK | England | Wales | Scotland | Northern Ireland | UK |
|---|---|---|---|---|---|---|---|---|---|---|
| | | | | | **GPS expenditure per capita (£ cash)** | | | | | |
| | | | **(£ cash)** | | | **At constant prices[1] (Index 1989/90=100)** | | | | |
| 1989/90 | 52 | 58 | 53 | 61 | 53 | 100 | 100 | 100 | 100 | 100 |
| 1990/91 | 56 | 68 | 59 | 68 | 57 | 99 | 107 | 102 | 102 | 100 |
| 1991/92 | 61 | 81 | 65 | 80 | 63 | 103 | 121 | 107 | 113 | 105 |
| 1992/93 | 69 | 83 | 73 | 90 | 71 | 112 | 120 | 116 | 125 | 114 |
| 1993/94 | 76 | 91 | 80 | 101 | 78 | 121 | 129 | 124 | 136 | 122 |
| 1994/95 | 81 | 97 | 85 | 105 | 83 | 128 | 135 | 130 | 139 | 129 |
| 1995/96 | 87 | 105 | 93 | 120 | 89 | 132 | 142 | 138 | 154 | 134 |
| 1996/97 | 94 | 113 | 107 | 132 | 97 | 138 | 147 | 153 | 164 | 141 |
| 1997/98 | 100 | 122 | 116 | 142 | 104 | 143 | 154 | 161 | 171 | 146 |
| 1998/99 | 105 | 129 | 124 | 148 | 109 | 146 | 159 | 168 | 175 | 150 |
| 1999/00 | 115 | 145 | 137 | 159 | 120 | 157 | 176 | 182 | 183 | 162 |
| 2000/01 | 122 | 157 | 144 | 165 | 127 | 165 | 187 | 190 | 188 | 169 |
| 2001/02 | 133 | 169 | 160 | 179 | 139 | 175 | 197 | 205 | 200 | 180 |
| 2002/03 | 146 | 186 | 178 | 193 | 152 | 186 | 211 | 222 | 208 | 191 |
| 2003/04 | 159 | 199 | 192 | 213 | 165 | 197 | 219 | 232 | 223 | 202 |
| 2004/05 | 166 | 191 | 197 | 223 | 172 | 200 | 204 | 232 | 228 | 204 |
| 2005/06 | 166 | 196 | 201 | 226 | 172 | 196 | 206 | 231 | 226 | 201 |
| | | | | | **GPS expenditure per household (£ cash)** | | | | | |
| | | | **(£ cash)** | | | **At constant prices[1] (Index 1989/90=100)** | | | | |
| 1989/90 | 131 | 150 | 134 | 180 | 133 | 100 | 100 | 100 | 100 | 100 |
| 1990/91 | 139 | 172 | 147 | 197 | 143 | 99 | 107 | 102 | 101 | 99 |
| 1991/92 | 153 | 203 | 161 | 231 | 158 | 102 | 119 | 105 | 112 | 104 |
| 1992/93 | 171 | 208 | 179 | 258 | 176 | 111 | 118 | 114 | 121 | 112 |
| 1993/94 | 188 | 228 | 195 | 286 | 193 | 118 | 126 | 120 | 131 | 119 |
| 1994/95 | 201 | 242 | 207 | 291 | 206 | 125 | 131 | 126 | 131 | 125 |
| 1995/96 | 214 | 260 | 224 | 331 | 221 | 129 | 137 | 132 | 145 | 130 |
| 1996/97 | 231 | 277 | 255 | 365 | 239 | 134 | 141 | 146 | 154 | 136 |
| 1997/98 | 246 | 298 | 275 | 407 | 255 | 139 | 148 | 152 | 167 | 142 |
| 1998/99 | 257 | 315 | 291 | 415 | 267 | 142 | 152 | 157 | 166 | 145 |
| 1999/00 | 282 | 354 | 320 | 435 | 293 | 152 | 167 | 169 | 171 | 155 |
| 2000/01 | 297 | 380 | 335 | 446 | 308 | 158 | 177 | 175 | 173 | 161 |
| 2001/02 | 320 | 406 | 368 | 481 | 333 | 167 | 185 | 188 | 182 | 170 |
| 2002/03 | 350 | 443 | 406 | 512 | 364 | 177 | 196 | 201 | 188 | 180 |
| 2003/04 | 378 | 471 | 434 | 560 | 393 | 186 | 202 | 209 | 200 | 189 |
| 2004/05 | 395 | 450 | 444 | 584 | 407 | 188 | 188 | 208 | 203 | 191 |
| 2005/06 | 393 | 459 | 449 | 590 | 407 | 184 | 188 | 206 | 200 | 187 |

*Notes:* All figures include salaries, fees, allowances, superannuation, directly reimbursed expenses (e.g. rent and rates) and other expenses, in financial years ending 31 March.
1 At constant prices, as adjusted by the Gross Domestic Product (GDP) deflator at market prices.

*Sources:* The Government's Expenditure Plans (DH).
Health and Personal Social Services Statistics for England (DH).
Scottish Health Statistics (ISD).
Health Statistics Wales (NAW).
Annual Abstract of Statistics (ONS).
Economic Data (HM Treasury).

Figure 4.8 **Gross[1] cost of General Pharmaceutical Services (GPS), UK, 1951/52 - 2005/06**

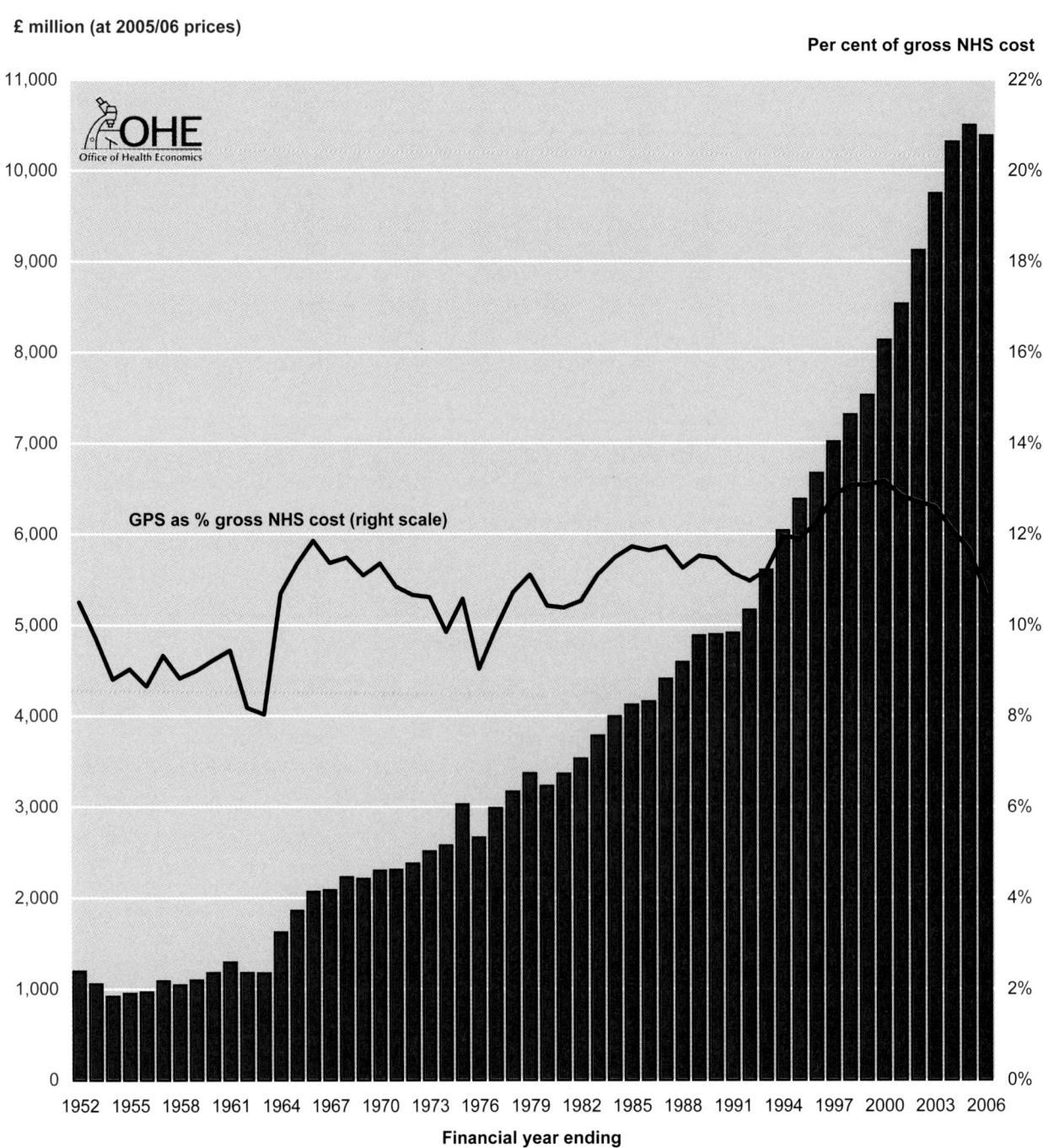

£ million (at 2005/06 prices)

Per cent of gross NHS cost

GPS as % gross NHS cost (right scale)

Financial year ending

*Notes:* Figures relate to 31st March year ending, i.e. 2006 =2005/06.

1 Figures include dispensing fees, allowances and prescription charges, at 2005/06 prices, as adjusted by the Gross Domestic Product (GDP).

deflator at market prices.

*Sources:* The Government's Expenditure Plans (DH).

Health and Personal Social Services Statistics for England (DH).

Scottish Health Statistics (ISD).

Health Statistics Wales (NAW).

Annual Statistical Report (Northern Ireland CSA).

Annual Abstract of Statistics (ONS).

Figure 4.9  **Pharmaceutical expenditure[1] as per cent of GDP in selected OECD countries, circa 2005**

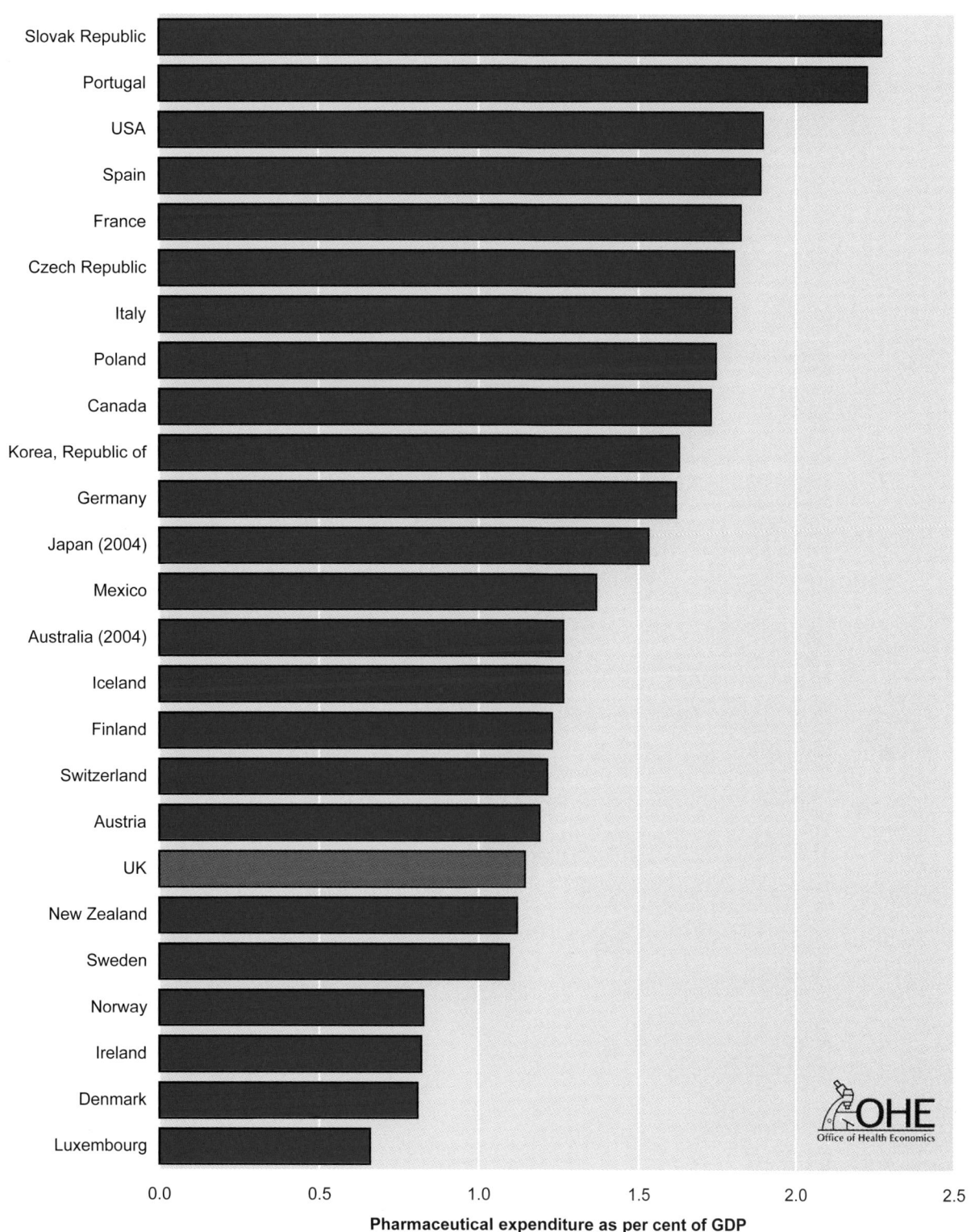

**Pharmaceutical expenditure as per cent of GDP**

Notes:    1 All prescription and over-the-counter medicines at ex-factory prices.  This includes sales through all retail outlets, hospitals and government agencies.
          GDP = Gross Domestic Product.
          Year is 2005 unless stated otherwise.
Sources:  OECD Health Database.
          Consumer Trends (ONS).
          See Table 4.46 for further UK sources.

Figure 4.10 **Pharmaceutical expenditure[1] per capita in selected OECD countries, circa 2005**

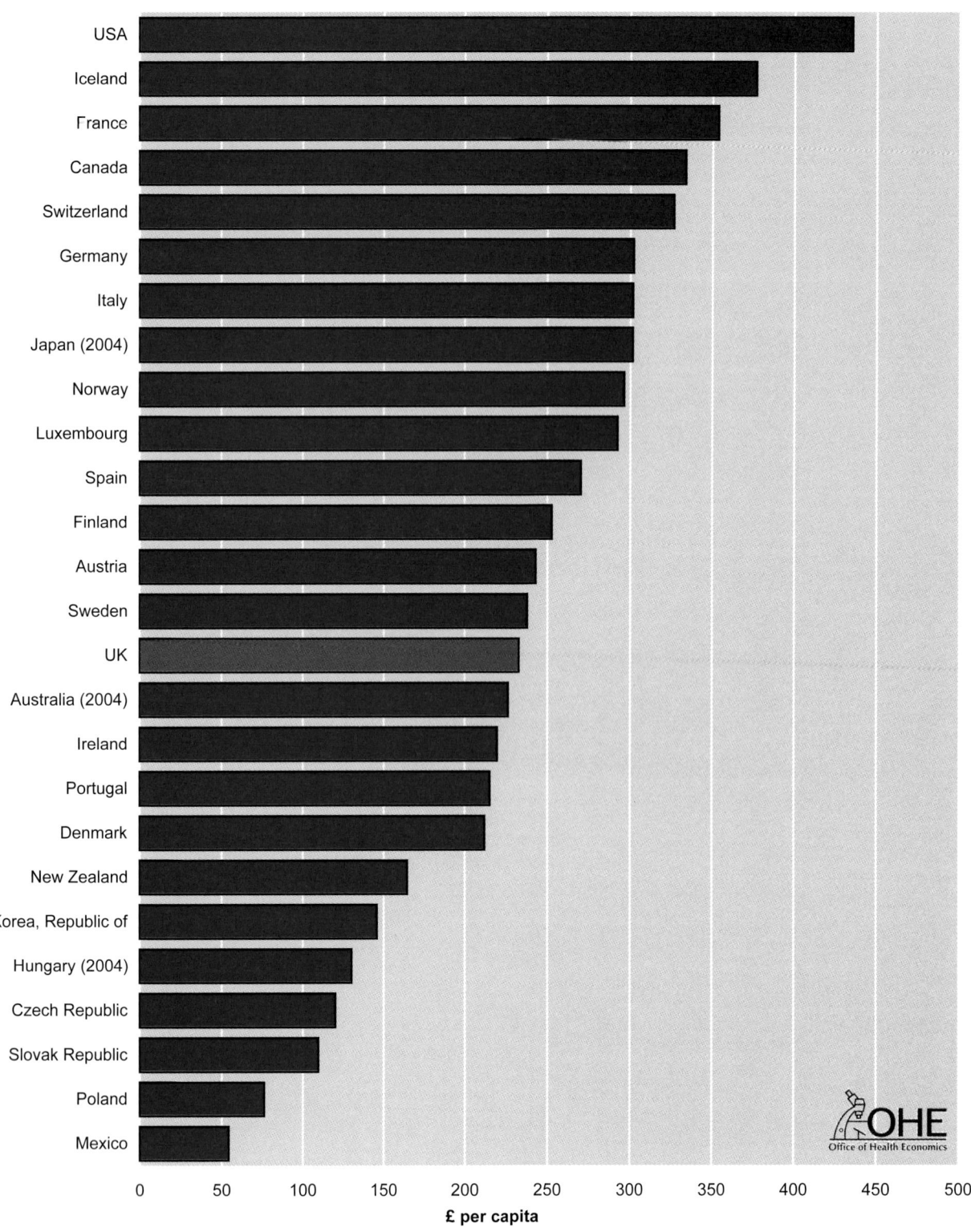

£ per capita

*Notes:* 1 All prescription and over-the-counter medicines at ex-factory prices. This includes sales through all retail outlets, hospitals and government agencies.

Year is 2005 unless stated otherwise.

*Sources:* OECD Health Database.

Consumer Trends.

Population Projections Database (GAD).

See Table 4.46 for further UK sources.

# FHS: General Pharmaceutical Services

Table 4.21  **Number of community pharmacies and appliance contractors and number per 100,000 population by country, UK, 1996 - 2006**

## Number of chemists and appliance contractors

| | Year | | | | | | | | | | |
|---|---|---|---|---|---|---|---|---|---|---|---|
| | **1996** | **1997** | **1998** | **1999** | **2000** | **2001** | **2002** | **2003** | **2004** | **2005** | **2006** |
| **United Kingdom** | 12,392 | 12,348 | 12,339 | 12,337 | 12,302 | 12,293 | 12,276 | 12,284 | 12,277 | 12,247 | 12,407 |
| **England** | 10,023 | 9,968 | 9,963 | 9,968 | 9,935 | 9,924 | 9,910 | 9,910 | 9,905 | 9,870 | 10,011 |
| **Wales** | 723 | 727 | 724 | 717 | 713 | 712 | 712 | 711 | 710 | 710 | 713 |
| **Scotland** | 1,142 | 1,143 | 1,145 | 1,145 | 1,144 | 1,145 | 1,143 | 1,151 | 1,148 | 1,154 | 1,170 |
| **Northern Ireland** | 507 | 511 | 509 | 507 | 510 | 512 | 511 | 512 | 514 | 513 | 513 |

## Number of community pharmacies and appliance contractors per 100,000 population

| | Year | | | | | | | | | | |
|---|---|---|---|---|---|---|---|---|---|---|---|
| | **1996** | **1997** | **1998** | **1999** | **2000** | **2001** | **2002** | **2003** | **2004** | **2005** | **2006** |
| **United Kingdom** | 21.3 | 21.2 | 21.1 | 21.0 | 20.9 | 20.8 | 20.7 | 20.6 | 20.5 | 20.3 | 20.5 |
| **England** | 20.7 | 20.5 | 20.4 | 20.3 | 20.2 | 20.1 | 20.0 | 19.9 | 19.8 | 19.6 | 19.7 |
| **Wales** | 25.0 | 25.1 | 25.0 | 24.7 | 24.5 | 24.5 | 24.4 | 24.3 | 24.1 | 24.0 | 24.0 |
| **Scotland** | 22.4 | 22.5 | 22.5 | 22.6 | 22.6 | 22.6 | 22.6 | 22.8 | 22.6 | 22.7 | 22.9 |
| **Northern Ireland** | 30.5 | 30.6 | 30.3 | 30.2 | 30.3 | 30.3 | 30.1 | 30.1 | 30.1 | 29.7 | 29.5 |

*Notes:*   Pharmacies relate to the number of community pharmacies and appliance suppliers who are contracted to the NHS.
From 2002 figures for England and Wales relate to 31 March, from 1996 to 2001 figures relate to 30 September.
Figures for Northern Ireland from 1995 to 2005 relate to October, and to 31 March for 2006.
Figures for Scotland relate to financial year ending 31st March.

*Sources:*   Community Pharmacies in England and Wales (DH Statistical Bulletin).
Prescription Pricing Authority Annual Report (PPA).
Health and Personal Social Services Statistics for England (DH).
Scottish Health Statistics (ISD).
Health Statistics Wales (NAW).
Annual Statistical Report (Northern Ireland CSA).
Population Projections Database (GAD).

Figure 4.11 **Practising pharmacists per 1,000 population in selected OECD and EU countries, circa 2005**

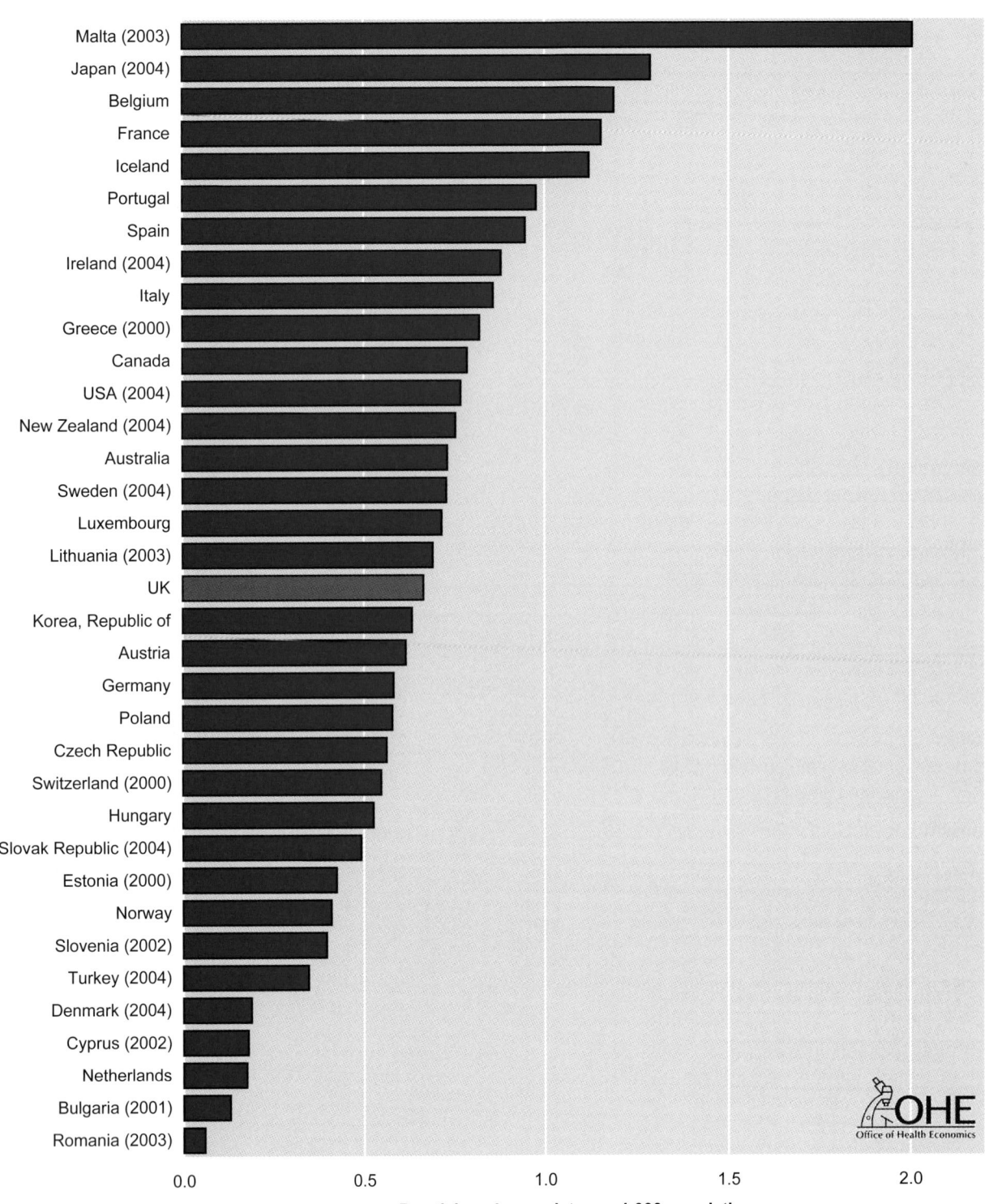

**Practising pharmacists per 1,000 population**

*Note:* Year is 2005 unless stated otherwise.
*Sources:* OECD Health Database.
UK figure is from the Royal Pharmaceutical Society Annual Workforce Census.
World Health Statistics (WHO).

# FHS: General Pharmaceutical Services

Table 4.22   **Number and index (1996=100) of prescription items dispensed per community pharmacy by country, UK, 1996 - 2006**

**Number of prescription items dispensed per pharmacy**

| | Year | | | | | | | | | | |
|---|---|---|---|---|---|---|---|---|---|---|---|
| | **1996** | **1997** | **1998** | **1999** | **2000** | **2001** | **2002** | **2003** | **2004** | **2005** | **2006** |
| **United Kingdom** | 45,166 | 46,787 | 48,152 | 49,697 | 51,805 | 55,048 | 58,012 | 60,961 | 64,288 | 67,427 | 69,666 |
| **England** | 45,026 | 46,665 | 47,988 | 49,477 | 51,578 | 55,021 | 57,991 | 61,110 | 64,558 | 67,975 | 70,299 |
| **Wales** | 48,824 | 50,527 | 52,210 | 54,547 | 56,949 | 61,070 | 64,863 | 68,013 | 72,256 | 75,725 | 78,569 |
| **Scotland** | 46,181 | 47,799 | 49,298 | 50,751 | 53,349 | 54,985 | 57,873 | 59,742 | 62,237 | 63,589 | 64,626 |
| **Northern Ireland** | 40,434 | 41,579 | 43,026 | 44,777 | 45,581 | 47,336 | 49,169 | 51,009 | 52,641 | 54,035 | 56,429 |

**Index (1996=100)**

| | Year | | | | | | | | | | |
|---|---|---|---|---|---|---|---|---|---|---|---|
| | **1996** | **1997** | **1998** | **1999** | **2000** | **2001** | **2002** | **2003** | **2004** | **2005** | **2006** |
| **United Kingdom** | 100 | 104 | 107 | 110 | 115 | 122 | 128 | 135 | 142 | 149 | 154 |
| **England** | 100 | 104 | 107 | 110 | 115 | 122 | 129 | 136 | 143 | 151 | 156 |
| **Wales** | 100 | 103 | 107 | 112 | 117 | 125 | 133 | 139 | 148 | 155 | 161 |
| **Scotland** | 100 | 104 | 107 | 110 | 116 | 119 | 125 | 129 | 135 | 138 | 140 |
| **Northern Ireland** | 100 | 103 | 106 | 111 | 113 | 117 | 122 | 126 | 130 | 134 | 140 |

Notes:  Figures relate to the number of community pharmacies and appliance suppliers who are contracted to the NHS.
These figures do not take into account those prescriptions dispensed by dispensing doctors.
Sources:  Health and Personal Social Services Statistics for England (DH).
Scottish Health Statistics (ISD).
Health Statistics Wales (NAW).
Annual Statistical Report (Northern Ireland CSA).

# FHS: General Pharmaceutical Services

Table 4.23   Number of NHS prescriptions (R$_x$s) (based on fees)[1] dispensed by community pharmacists and appliance contractors, UK, 1948 - 2006

| Year | England (millions) | Wales (millions) | Scotland (millions) | Northern Ireland (millions) | United Kingdom (millions) | England Per head | Wales Per head | Scotland Per head | Northern Ireland Per head | United Kingdom Per head |
|---|---|---|---|---|---|---|---|---|---|---|
| 1948[2] | 83.7[3] | - | 6.6 | 2.3 | 92.6 | - | - | - | - | - |
| 1950 | 217.1[3] | - | 19.5 | 6.6 | 243.2 | 5.0 | - | 3.8 | 4.8 | 4.8 |
| 1955 | 226.1[3] | - | 21.2 | 7.3 | 254.6 | 5.1 | - | 4.1 | 5.2 | 5.0 |
| 1960 | 218.7[3] | - | 22.0 | 7.2 | 247.9 | 4.7 | - | 4.2 | 5.1 | 4.7 |
| 1965 | 244.3[3] | - | 25.6 | 9.0 | 278.9 | 5.1 | - | 4.9 | 6.1 | 5.1 |
| 1966 | 243.4 | 18.6 | 27.5 | 10.1 | 299.6 | 5.4 | 6.9 | 5.3 | 6.8 | 5.5 |
| 1967 | 251.9 | 19.3 | 28.2 | 10.3 | 309.7 | 5.5 | 7.1 | 5.4 | 6.9 | 5.6 |
| 1968 | 248.4 | 18.9 | 28.5 | 10.5 | 306.3 | 5.4 | 7.0 | 5.5 | 7.0 | 5.5 |
| 1969 | 245.5 | 18.6 | 28.2 | 10.2 | 302.5 | 5.3 | 6.8 | 5.4 | 6.7 | 5.5 |
| 1970 | 247.7 | 18.9 | 28.9 | 10.5 | 306.0 | 5.4 | 6.9 | 5.5 | 6.9 | 5.5 |
| 1971 | 247.5 | 19.0 | 27.9 | 10.1 | 304.5 | 5.3 | 6.9 | 5.3 | 6.6 | 5.4 |
| 1972 | 256.3 | 19.6 | 29.1 | 10.5 | 315.5 | 5.5 | 7.1 | 5.6 | 6.8 | 5.6 |
| 1973 | 263.9 | 20.3 | 29.7 | 10.8 | 324.7 | 5.7 | 7.3 | 5.7 | 7.1 | 5.8 |
| 1974 | 274.0 | 21.1 | 30.6 | 11.2 | 336.9 | 5.9 | 7.6 | 5.8 | 7.3 | 6.0 |
| 1975 | 281.8 | 21.8 | 31.2 | 11.4 | 346.2 | 6.0 | 7.8 | 6.0 | 7.5 | 6.2 |
| 1976 | 292.9 | 22.5 | 33.5 | 12.0 | 360.9 | 6.3 | 8.0 | 6.4 | 7.9 | 6.4 |
| 1977 | 295.7 | 22.8 | 32.9 | 12.2 | 363.6 | 6.3 | 8.1 | 6.3 | 8.0 | 6.5 |
| 1978 | 307.1 | 23.9 | 34.5 | 12.6 | 378.1 | 6.6 | 8.5 | 6.6 | 8.3 | 6.7 |
| 1979 | 304.6 | 23.6 | 34.3 | 12.6 | 375.1 | 6.5 | 8.4 | 6.6 | 8.2 | 6.7 |
| 1980 | 303.3 | 23.7 | 34.3 | 12.7 | 374.0 | 6.5 | 8.4 | 6.6 | 8.3 | 6.6 |
| 1981 | 299.9 | 23.4 | 33.9 | 12.7 | 369.9 | 6.4 | 8.3 | 6.5 | 8.3 | 6.6 |
| 1982 | 311.3 | 24.0 | 35.0 | 13.1 | 383.3 | 6.7 | 8.6 | 6.8 | 8.5 | 6.8 |
| 1983 | 315.3 | 24.6 | 35.7 | 13.6 | 389.1 | 6.7 | 8.8 | 6.9 | 8.8 | 6.9 |
| 1984 | 320.5 | 25.0 | 36.4 | 13.7 | 395.6 | 6.8 | 8.9 | 7.1 | 8.8 | 7.0 |
| 1985 | 318.7 | 24.7 | 36.4 | 13.3 | 393.1 | 6.8 | 8.8 | 7.1 | 8.5 | 7.0 |
| 1986 | 322.6 | 25.1 | 36.8 | 13.2 | 397.6 | 6.8 | 8.9 | 7.2 | 8.4 | 7.0 |
| 1987 | 335.3 | 26.1 | 38.3 | 13.9 | 413.6 | 7.1 | 9.2 | 7.5 | 8.8 | 7.3 |
| 1988 | 346.5 | 27.1 | 39.5 | 14.6 | 427.7 | 7.3 | 9.5 | 7.8 | 9.2 | 7.5 |
| 1989 | 351.9 | 27.8 | 41.0 | 15.1 | 435.8 | 7.4 | 9.7 | 8.1 | 9.5 | 7.6 |
| 1990 | 360.5 | 28.3 | 42.4 | 15.4 | 446.6 | 7.6 | 9.9 | 8.3 | 9.7 | 7.8 |
| 1991 | 377.5 | 29.7 | 44.3 | 16.2 | 467.7 | 7.9 | 10.3 | 8.7 | 10.1 | 8.1 |
| 1992 | 394.2 | 31.0 | 46.1 | 16.9 | 488.2 | 8.2 | 10.8 | 9.1 | 10.4 | 8.5 |
| 1993 | 413.3 | 32.4 | 48.2 | 18.0 | 511.9 | 8.6 | 11.2 | 9.5 | 11.0 | 8.9 |
| 1994 | 454.7 | 35.2 | 51.2 | 19.2 | 560.3 | 9.4 | 12.2 | 10.0 | 11.7 | 9.7 |
| 1995 | 472.5 | 36.6 | 53.0 | 20.3 | 582.4 | 9.8 | 12.7 | 10.4 | 12.3 | 10.0 |
| 1996 | 485.3 | 37.4 | 54.5 | 21.1 | 598.4 | 10.0 | 13.0 | 10.7 | 12.7 | 10.3 |
| 1997 | 500.1 | 38.9 | 56.4 | 21.9 | 617.3 | 10.3 | 13.5 | 11.1 | 13.1 | 10.6 |
| 1998 | 513.8 | 40.1 | 58.5 | 22.5 | 634.9 | 10.5 | 13.8 | 11.5 | 13.4 | 10.9 |
| 1999 | 530.3 | 41.5 | 60.3 | 23.2 | 655.3 | 10.8 | 14.3 | 11.9 | 13.8 | 11.2 |
| 2000 | 551.5 | 43.1 | 63.4 | 23.7 | 681.6 | 11.2 | 14.8 | 12.5 | 14.1 | 11.6 |
| 2001 | 587.7 | 46.1 | 65.5 | 24.6 | 723.9 | 11.9 | 15.8 | 12.9 | 14.5 | 12.2 |
| 2002 | 619.1 | 49.0 | 68.8 | 25.4 | 762.2 | 12.5 | 16.8 | 13.6 | 15.0 | 12.8 |
| 2003 | 652.7 | 51.3 | 71.5 | 26.4 | 801.8 | 13.1 | 17.5 | 14.1 | 15.5 | 13.5 |
| 2004 | 689.9 | 54.4 | 74.3 | 27.3 | 845.8 | 13.8 | 18.5 | 14.6 | 16.0 | 14.1 |
| 2005 | 724.6 | 56.7 | 76.4 | 28.0 | 885.6 | 14.4 | 19.2 | 15.0 | 16.2 | 14.7 |
| 2006 | 760.1 | 59.5 | 78.7 | 29.2 | 927.4 | 15.0 | 20.1 | 15.4 | 16.8 | 15.3 |

*Notes:*   Figures relate to community pharmacists and applance suppliers who are contracted to the NHS.  Figures for 1994 onwards include prescriptions dispensed by dispensing doctors.

1 Figures in this table differ from those shown in Table 4.24 as the above data are taken from prescription reports from the various agencies dealing with prescription information in the constituent countries of the UK and relate to the number of prescriptions (number of fees), as opposed to total count of items written and dispensed as in Table 4.24.

2 From July to December.

3 Figures relate to England and Wales.

*Sources:* Prescription Pricing Authority, England.
Health of Wales Information Service.
Information Services Division of the NHS in Scotland.
Central Services Agency, Northern Ireland.
Health and Personal Social Services Statistics for England (DH).
Scottish Health Statistics (ISD).
Health Statistics Wales (NAW).
Annual Statistical Report (Northern Ireland CSA).
Annual Abstract of Statistics (ONS).

# FHS: General Pharmaceutical Services

Figure 4.12   **Index of number of prescriptions (Rxs) (based on fees) dispensed by community pharmacies and appliance contractors, by country, UK, 1949 - 2006**

**Index 1949=100**

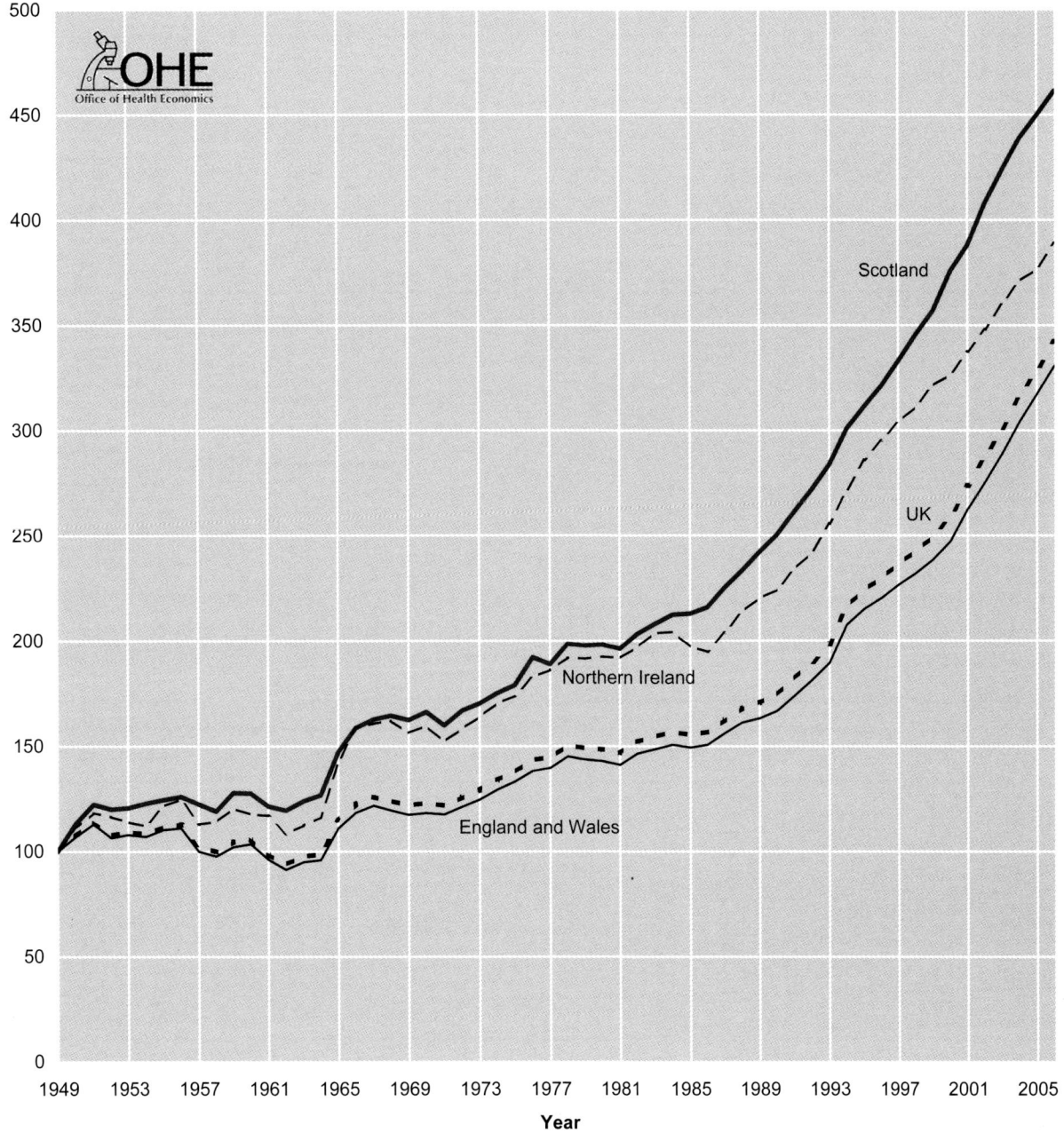

**Year**

*Notes:*   Figures relate to the number of community pharmacies and applicance suppliers who are contracted to the NHS. Figures for 1994 onwards include prescriptions dispensed by dispensing doctors.

Figures in this graph differ from those shown in Table 4.24 as the above data are taken from prescription reports from the various agencies dealing with prescription information in the constituent countries of the UK ad relate to the number of prescriptions (number of fees), as opposed to total count of items written and dispensed as in Table 4.24.

*Sources:*   Prescription Pricing Authority, England.
Health of Wales Information Service (HOWIS).
Information Services Division of the NHS in Scotland (ISD).
Central Services Agency, Northern Ireland (CSA).
Scottish Health Statistics (ISD).
Health Statistics Wales (NAW).
Annual Statistical Report (Northern Ireland CSA).
Annual Abstract of Statistics (ONS).

Table 4.24    Total[1] number of NHS prescriptions (based on items) dispensed by country, UK, 1995/96 - 2005/6

Millions

| | Year | | | | | | | | | |
|---|---|---|---|---|---|---|---|---|---|---|
| | 1995/96 | 1997/98 | 1998/99 | 1999/00 | 2000/01 | 2001/02 | 2002/03 | 2003/04 | 2004/05 | 2005/06 |
| United Kingdom | 581.9 | 622.9 | 638.9 | 660.4 | 690.5 | 729.1 | 755.6 | 796.1 | 834.4 | 890.9 |
| England | 473.8 | 504.6 | 516.9 | 534.7 | 561.2 | 592.9 | 611.9 | 646.3 | 678.4 | 728.2 |
| Wales | 37.1 | 39.6 | 40.7 | 42.1 | 43.0 | 46.0 | 49.0 | 51.0 | 54.0 | 57.0 |
| Scotland | 51.1 | 56.6 | 58.5 | 60.4 | 62.3 | 65.6 | 69.1 | 72.2 | 74.7 | 77.3 |
| Northern Ireland | 19.9 | 22.0 | 22.8 | 23.2 | 24.0 | 24.7 | 25.5 | 26.7 | 27.4 | 28.4 |

Number[1] of NHS prescriptions (based on items) dispensed per capita by country, UK, 1995/96 - 2005/06

| | Year | | | | | | | | | |
|---|---|---|---|---|---|---|---|---|---|---|
| | 1995/96 | 1997/98 | 1998/99 | 1999/00 | 2000/01 | 2001/02 | 2002/03 | 2003/04 | 2004/05 | 2005/06 |
| United Kingdom | 10.0 | 10.7 | 10.9 | 11.2 | 11.7 | 12.3 | 12.7 | 13.4 | 13.9 | 14.8 |
| England | 9.8 | 10.4 | 10.6 | 10.9 | 11.4 | 12.0 | 12.3 | 12.9 | 13.5 | 14.4 |
| Wales | 12.8 | 13.7 | 14.0 | 14.5 | 14.8 | 15.8 | 16.8 | 17.4 | 18.3 | 19.3 |
| Scotland | 10.0 | 11.1 | 11.5 | 11.9 | 12.3 | 13.0 | 13.7 | 14.3 | 14.7 | 15.2 |
| Northern Ireland | 12.0 | 13.2 | 13.6 | 13.8 | 14.2 | 14.6 | 15.0 | 15.6 | 16.0 | 16.4 |

Notes:    1 Figures relate to all prescription items dispensed by community pharmacists, appliance contractors who are contracted to the NHS and dispensing doctors.
Figures in this table differ from those in Table 4.23, as the above data from 2002/03 are taken from the Prescription Pricing Authority Annual Report and relate to the total count of items written and dispensed. Data for England for 2005/06 are from the Information Centre.

Sources:    Prescription Pricing Authority Annual Reports (PPA).
Health and Personal Social Services Statistics for England (DH).
Statistics of Prescriptions Dispensed in the Community: England (IC).
Annual Abstract of Statistics (ONS).
Scottish Health Statistics (ISD).
Health Statistics Wales (NAW).
Annual Statistical Report (Northern Ireland CSA).

# FHS: General Pharmaceutical Services

Table 4.25   **Number of prescription items dispensed, and per capita, by age group, England, 1978 - 2006**

| Year | Number of prescription items (millions) | | | | As a percentage of total | | |
|------|-------|-----------|----------|-------------|-----------|----------|------------|
| | Total | Under 16[3] | Elderly[4] | Chargeable[5] | Under 16[3] | Elderly[4] | Chargeable |
| 1978 | 307.1 | 37.0 | 98.3 | 114.0 | 12 | 32 | 37 |
| 1980 | 303.3 | 37.0 | 108.8 | 90.9 | 12 | 36 | 30 |
| 1985 | 318.7 | 38.3 | 125.7 | 63.2 | 12 | 39 | 20 |
| 1986 | 322.5 | 36.6 | 129.6 | 60.3 | 11 | 40 | 19 |
| 1987 | 335.3 | 38.3 | 135.7 | 60.6 | 11 | 41 | 18 |
| 1988 | 346.5 | 40.6 | 142.6 | 61.6 | 12 | 41 | 18 |
| 1989 | 351.9 | 40.5 | 147.3 | 61.4 | 12 | 42 | 17 |
| 1990 | 360.5 | 40.0 | 153.2 | 60.1 | 11 | 42 | 17 |
| 1991[1] | 370.7 | 41.8 | 159.7 | 56.1 | 11 | 43 | 15 |
| 1992 | 386.8 | 43.4 | 167.8 | 55.0 | 11 | 43 | 14 |
| 1993 | 405.1 | 47.5 | 176.5 | 52.7 | 12 | 44 | 13 |
| 1994 | 414.1 | 47.0 | 184.2 | 50.2 | 11 | 45 | 12 |
| 1995 | 430.6 | 51.0 | 193.9 | 48.2 | 11 | 41 | 15 |
| 1996 | 484.9 | 50.0 | 212.9 | 63.4 | 10 | 44 | 13 |
| 1997 | 500.2 | 49.4 | 223.9 | 66.1 | 10 | 45 | 13 |
| 1998 | 513.2 | 46.7 | 234.0 | 68.0 | 9 | 46 | 13 |
| 1999 | 529.8 | 43.7 | 252.2 | 71.5 | 8 | 48 | 13 |
| 2000 | 551.8 | 41.6 | 270.2 | 74.6 | 8 | 49 | 14 |
| 2001[2] | 587.0 | 44.2 | 317.5 | 85.5 | 8 | 54 | 15 |
| 2002 | 617.0 | 42.8 | 339.7 | 88.4 | 7 | 55 | 14 |
| 2003 | 649.7 | 42.4 | 363.5 | 89.5 | 7 | 56 | 14 |
| 2004 | 686.1 | 41.1 | 391.4 | 90.0 | 6 | 57 | 13 |
| 2005 | 720.3 | 42.5 | 409.5 | 89.6 | 6 | 57 | 12 |
| 2006 | 751.9 | 42.7 | 440.8 | 90.2 | 6 | 59 | 12 |

**Per capita prescription items dispensed**

| Year | Prescription items per capita | | | Index 1978=100 | | |
|------|-------|-----------|----------|-------|-----------|----------|
| | Total | Under 16[3] | Elderly[4] | Total | Under 16[3] | Elderly[4] |
| 1978 | 6.6 | 3.4 | 12.2 | 100 | 100 | 100 |
| 1979 | 6.6 | 3.2 | 12.5 | 100 | 94 | 102 |
| 1980 | 6.5 | 3.5 | 13.2 | 98 | 104 | 108 |
| 1981 | 6.4 | 3.5 | 13.3 | 97 | 102 | 109 |
| 1982 | 6.7 | 6.7 | 13.3 | 101 | 117 | 109 |
| 1983 | 6.7 | 6.7 | 13.8 | 102 | 116 | 114 |
| 1984 | 7.3 | 7.3 | 14.3 | 111 | 117 | 117 |
| 1985 | 7.3 | 4.0 | 14.7 | 110 | 117 | 120 |
| 1986 | 7.3 | 3.8 | 15.0 | 111 | 112 | 123 |
| 1987 | 7.6 | 4.0 | 15.6 | 116 | 118 | 128 |
| 1988 | 7.9 | 4.3 | 16.3 | 120 | 126 | 134 |
| 1989 | 8.1 | 4.3 | 16.8 | 122 | 125 | 138 |
| 1990 | 8.3 | 4.2 | 17.4 | 125 | 123 | 143 |
| 1991[1] | 8.5 | 4.3 | 18.1 | 129 | 127 | 148 |
| 1992 | 8.9 | 4.4 | 19.0 | 134 | 131 | 155 |
| 1993 | 9.3 | 4.8 | 19.9 | 140 | 142 | 163 |
| 1994 | 9.5 | 4.7 | 20.8 | 143 | 139 | 170 |
| 1995 | 9.8 | 5.1 | 21.8 | 148 | 150 | 179 |
| 1996 | 10.0 | 5.0 | 21.2 | 151 | 147 | 174 |
| 1997 | 10.3 | 4.9 | 22.3 | 156 | 145 | 183 |
| 1998 | 10.5 | 4.7 | 23.2 | 159 | 137 | 190 |
| 1999 | 10.8 | 4.4 | 24.8 | 164 | 128 | 204 |
| 2000 | 11.2 | 4.2 | 26.5 | 170 | 123 | 217 |
| 2001[2] | 11.9 | 4.5 | 31.0 | 180 | 131 | 254 |
| 2002 | 12.4 | 4.3 | 33.0 | 188 | 128 | 271 |
| 2003 | 13.0 | 4.3 | 35.0 | 197 | 127 | 287 |
| 2004 | 13.7 | 4.2 | 37.3 | 207 | 124 | 306 |
| 2005 | 14.3 | 4.4 | 38.5 | 216 | 129 | 316 |
| 2006 | 14.8 | 4.4 | 40.9 | 224 | 130 | 335 |

*Notes:*   1 Figures for 1991 and after are not strictly comparable with previous years and may differ from those shown elsewhere in the Compendium.
Since 1991, figures relate to the total count of items written and dispensed, whereas earlier figures relate to the aggregate prescription fees.
2 Prior to 2001 figures are based on a sample of 1 in 20 prescriptions dispensed by community pharmacists and appliance suppliers who are contracted to the NHS only.
From 2001 all figures also include prescriptions dispensed by dispensing doctors and personally administered prescriptions.
3 Figures relate to children aged under 16 and others aged under 19 and receiving full-time education.
4 Prior to 20th October 1995 "elderly people" includes men aged 65 years and over and women aged 60 and over.  After this date "elderly people" includes men and women aged 60 years and over.
5 From 1984 onwards figures for chargeable prescriptions include pre-payment certificates.

*Sources:* Prescriptions Dispensed in the Community Statistics: England (DH Statistical Bulletin).
Population Projections Database (GAD).

# FHS: General Pharmaceutical Services

Figure 4.13  **Prescription items dispensed per capita among elderly people[1], England, 1978 - 2006**

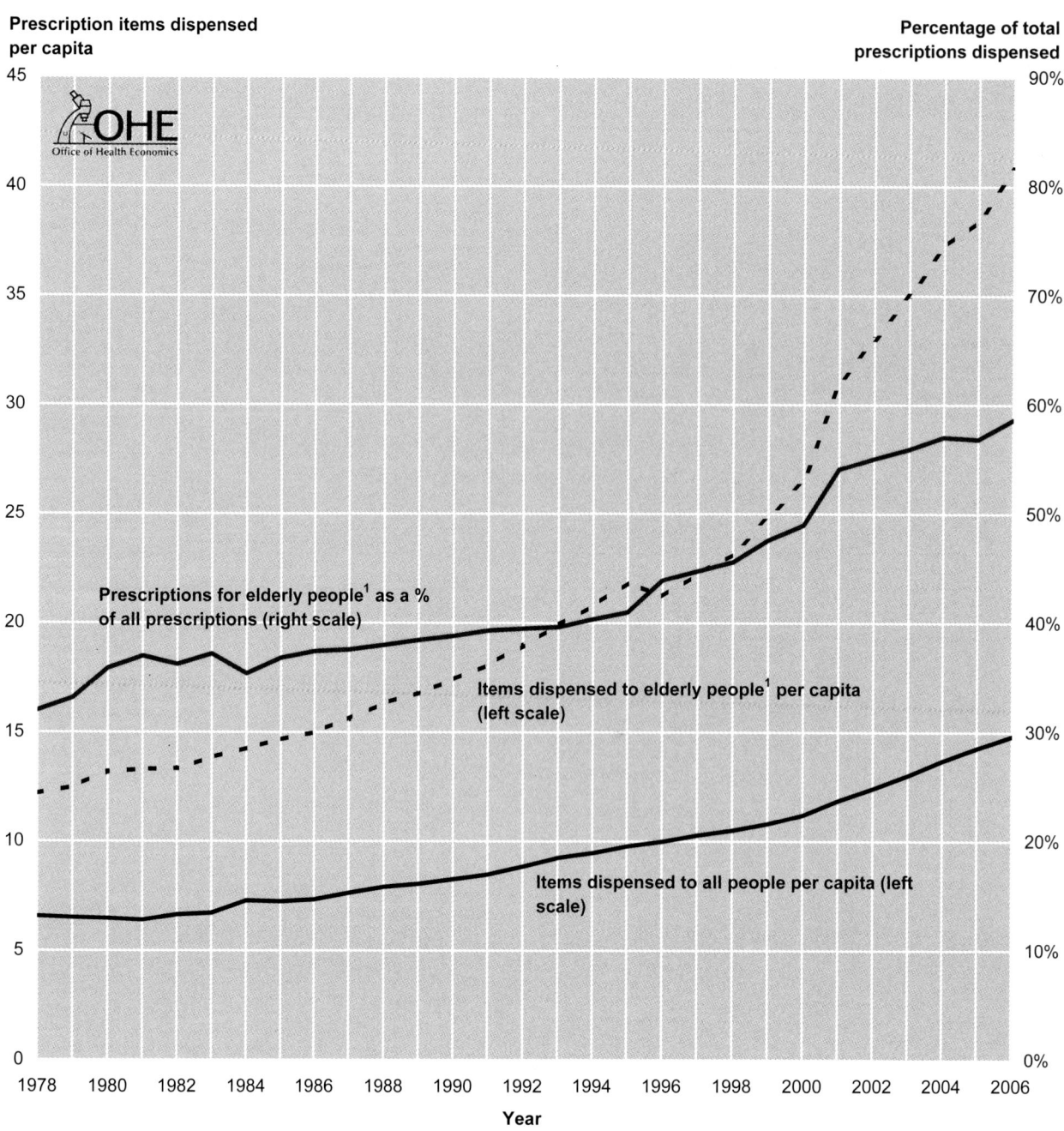

**Prescription items dispensed per capita**

**Percentage of total prescriptions dispensed**

Prescriptions for elderly people[1] as a % of all prescriptions (right scale)

Items dispensed to elderly people[1] per capita (left scale)

Items dispensed to all people per capita (left scale)

Year

*Note:*  1 Prior to 20th October 1995 "elderly people" includes men aged 65 years and over and women aged 60 and over. After this date "elderly people" includes men and women aged 60 years and over.

*Sources:*  Prescriptions Dispensed in the Community Statistics: England (DH Statistical Bulletin).
Prescriptions Dispensed in the Community Statistics: England (IC).
Population Projections Database (GAD).

# FHS: General Pharmaceutical Services

Table 4.26  **Total cost of NHS prescriptions ($R_x$s) dispensed[1], UK, 1948 - 2006**

| Year | £m | | | | | £ per capita | | | | |
|---|---|---|---|---|---|---|---|---|---|---|
| | England | Wales | Scotland | Northern Ireland | United Kingdom | England | Wales | Scotland | Northern Ireland | United Kingdom |
| 1948[2] | 11[3] | - | 2 | - | 13 | - | - | - | - | - |
| 1950 | 35[3] | - | 4 | 1 | 41 | 0.80[3] | - | 0.77 | 0.72 | 0.81 |
| 1955 | 49[3] | - | 6 | 2 | 57 | 1.10[3] | - | 1.17 | 1.43 | 1.11 |
| 1960 | 79[3] | - | 9 | 3 | 91 | 1.73[3] | - | 1.74 | 2.11 | 1.74 |
| 1965 | 126[3] | - | 14 | 5 | 145 | 2.64[3] | - | 2.69 | 3.41 | 2.67 |
| 1970 | 167 | 13 | 21 | 8 | 209 | 3.62 | 4.76 | 4.03 | 5.24 | 3.76 |
| 1971 | 187 | 15 | 23 | 9 | 234 | 4.03 | 5.47 | 4.39 | 5.84 | 4.18 |
| 1972 | 211 | 17 | 26 | 10 | 263 | 4.53 | 6.17 | 4.97 | 6.49 | 4.69 |
| 1973 | 233 | 18 | 28 | 11 | 290 | 4.99 | 6.49 | 5.35 | 7.19 | 5.16 |
| 1974 | 272 | 22 | 34 | 13 | 340 | 5.83 | 7.90 | 6.49 | 8.51 | 6.04 |
| 1975 | 360 | 28 | 44 | 16 | 448 | 7.71 | 10.02 | 8.41 | 10.51 | 7.96 |
| 1976 | 451 | 35 | 57 | 21 | 563 | 9.67 | 12.50 | 10.89 | 13.78 | 10.01 |
| 1977 | 554 | 43 | 63 | 25 | 684 | 11.88 | 15.35 | 12.06 | 16.41 | 12.18 |
| 1978 | 658 | 51 | 81 | 29 | 819 | 14.11 | 18.19 | 15.54 | 19.03 | 14.57 |
| 1979 | 739 | 57 | 90 | 33 | 919 | 15.83 | 20.28 | 17.29 | 21.60 | 16.34 |
| 1980 | 898 | 69 | 111 | 41 | 1,119 | 19.19 | 24.50 | 21.37 | 26.74 | 19.86 |
| 1981 | 1,026 | 77 | 127 | 48 | 1,278 | 21.91 | 27.37 | 24.52 | 31.23 | 22.68 |
| 1982 | 1,181 | 88 | 144 | 55 | 1,469 | 25.25 | 31.38 | 27.88 | 35.61 | 26.08 |
| 1983 | 1,308 | 97 | 161 | 62 | 1,627 | 27.94 | 34.60 | 31.27 | 39.98 | 28.88 |
| 1984 | 1,409 | 105 | 170 | 64 | 1,748 | 30.03 | 37.49 | 33.08 | 41.10 | 30.96 |
| 1985 | 1,518 | 112 | 180 | 66 | 1,876 | 32.26 | 39.95 | 35.10 | 42.16 | 33.17 |
| 1986 | 1,643 | 120 | 197 | 71 | 2,031 | 34.82 | 42.69 | 38.54 | 45.12 | 35.83 |
| 1987 | 1,831 | 134 | 218 | 80 | 2,263 | 38.71 | 47.47 | 42.75 | 50.57 | 39.84 |
| 1988 | 2,046 | 149 | 244 | 89 | 2,528 | 43.15 | 52.44 | 48.06 | 56.14 | 44.42 |
| 1989 | 2,198 | 162 | 270 | 98 | 2,728 | 46.22 | 56.74 | 53.17 | 61.62 | 47.80 |
| 1990 | 2,402 | 176 | 298 | 108 | 2,984 | 50.36 | 61.51 | 58.65 | 67.69 | 52.13 |
| 1991 | 2,689 | 199 | 330 | 124 | 3,342 | 56.17 | 69.27 | 64.92 | 77.15 | 58.18 |
| 1992 | 2,995 | 221 | 370 | 142 | 3,728 | 62.40 | 76.80 | 72.75 | 87.48 | 64.74 |
| 1993 | 3,283 | 242 | 406 | 160 | 4,091 | 68.25 | 83.92 | 79.73 | 97.83 | 70.88 |
| 1994 | 3,799 | 276 | 453 | 179 | 4,707 | 78.77 | 95.52 | 88.78 | 108.73 | 81.34 |
| 1995 | 4,081 | 299 | 493 | 199 | 5,071 | 84.34 | 103.36 | 96.57 | 120.71 | 87.39 |
| 1996 | 4,412 | 320 | 533 | 218 | 5,484 | 90.94 | 110.83 | 104.76 | 130.96 | 94.28 |
| 1997 | 4,711 | 344 | 578 | 233 | 5,866 | 96.81 | 118.79 | 113.72 | 139.32 | 100.59 |
| 1998 | 5,007 | 364 | 616 | 246 | 6,233 | 102.55 | 125.49 | 121.35 | 146.53 | 106.59 |
| 1999 | 5,473 | 395 | 681 | 263 | 6,812 | 111.61 | 136.32 | 134.34 | 156.45 | 116.08 |
| 2000 | 5,799 | 424 | 732 | 274 | 7,229 | 117.79 | 145.96 | 144.55 | 162.68 | 122.76 |
| 2001 | 6,317 | 461 | 775 | 296 | 7,849 | 127.75 | 158.25 | 153.11 | 174.99 | 132.78 |
| 2002 | 6,984 | 510 | 852 | 324 | 8,671 | 140.67 | 174.74 | 168.60 | 190.75 | 146.16 |
| 2003 | 7,628 | 551 | 925 | 354 | 9,458 | 152.97 | 187.82 | 182.83 | 208.12 | 158.80 |
| 2004 | 8,222 | 590 | 971 | 381 | 10,164 | 164.07 | 200.41 | 191.12 | 222.77 | 169.83 |
| 2005 | 8,374 | 592 | 972 | 383 | 10,321 | 165.93 | 200.36 | 190.75 | 222.19 | 171.33 |
| 2006 | 8,760 | 619 | 1,026 | 403 | 10,808 | 172.56 | 208.68 | 200.49 | 231.51 | 178.38 |

*Notes:*  For the years 1948-1963, total cost for England and Wales consists of net ingredient cost, less discount, plus on-cost, dispensing fee, container allowance and oxygen delivery allowances.  From 1964 total cost includes net ingredient cost, less discount, plus dispensing fee, container and on-cost allowances, oxygen payments and from 1973 value added tax for appliances.  Total cost shown includes charges paid by patients.

The above data are taken from prescription reports from the various agencies dealing with prescription information in the constituent countries of the UK and relate to the number of prescriptions (number of fees).

1 Figures from 1994 onwards relate to prescriptions dispensed by community pharmacists and appliance suppliers who are contracted to the NHS and dispensing doctors, prior to this they relate to community pharmacists and appliance contractors only.

2 From July to December.

3 Figures relate to England and Wales.

- Not available.

*Sources:*  Prescription Pricing Authority, England.
Health of Wales Information Services.
Information Services Division of NHS in Scotland.
Central Services Agency, Northern Ireland.
Health and Personal Social Services Statistics for England (DH).
Health Statistics Wales (NAW).
Scottish Health Statistics (ISD).
Annual Statistical Report (Northern Ireland CSA).
Annual Abstract of Statistics (ONS).

# FHS: General Pharmaceutical Services

Figure 4.14  **Total costs of NHS prescription ($R_x$s) dispensed[1], as a percentage of total NHS cost and total cost per prescription, UK, 1949 - 2006**

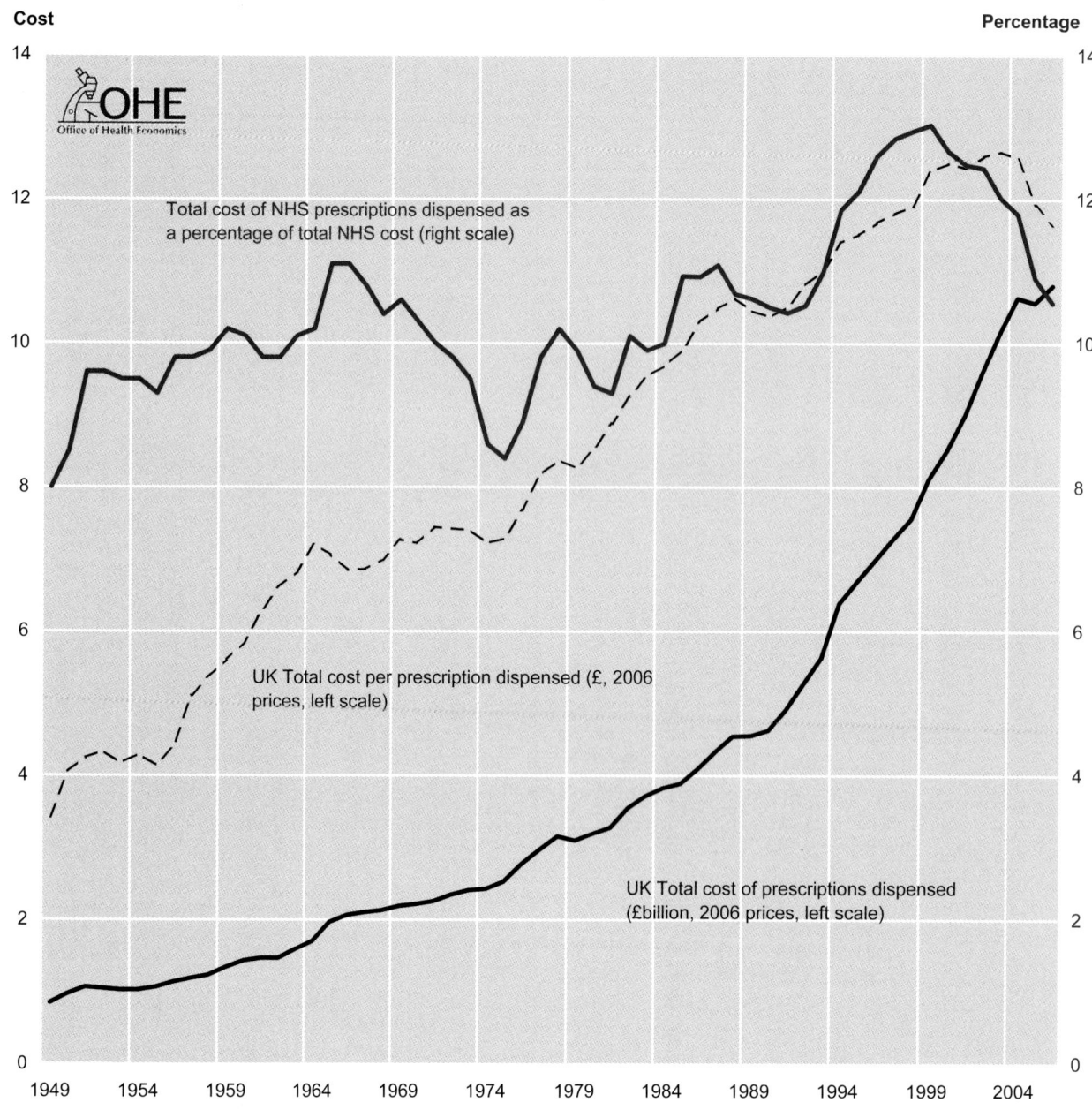

*Notes:*   The above data are taken from prescription reports from the various agencies dealing with prescription information in the  constituent
          countries of the UK and relate to the number of prescriptions (number of fees). Total cost shown includes charges paid by patients.
          For the years 1949-1963, total cost for the English and Welsh component of the UK consists of net ingredient cost, less discount,
          plus on-cost, dispensing fee, container allowance and oxygen delivery allowances.  From 1964 total cost includes net ingredient cost,
          less discount, plus dispensing fee, container and on-cost allowances, oxygen payments and from 1973 value added tax for
          appliances.
          1 From 1994 onwards figures relate to prescriptions dispensed by community pharmacists and appliance suppliers who are contracted to the
          NHS and dispensing doctors.
*Sources:*  Prescription Pricing Authority, England.
          Health of Wales Information Services.
          Information Services Division of NHS in Scotland.
          Central Services Agency, Northern Ireland.
          Health and Personal Social Services Statistics for England (DH).
          Health Statistics Wales (NAW).
          Scottish Health Statistics (ICD).
          Annual Statistical Report (Northern Ireland CSA).
          Annual Abstract of Statistics (ONS).

Figure 4.15  **NHS prescription charges[1] and items dispensed by community pharmacists and appliance contractors, UK, 1949 - 2006**

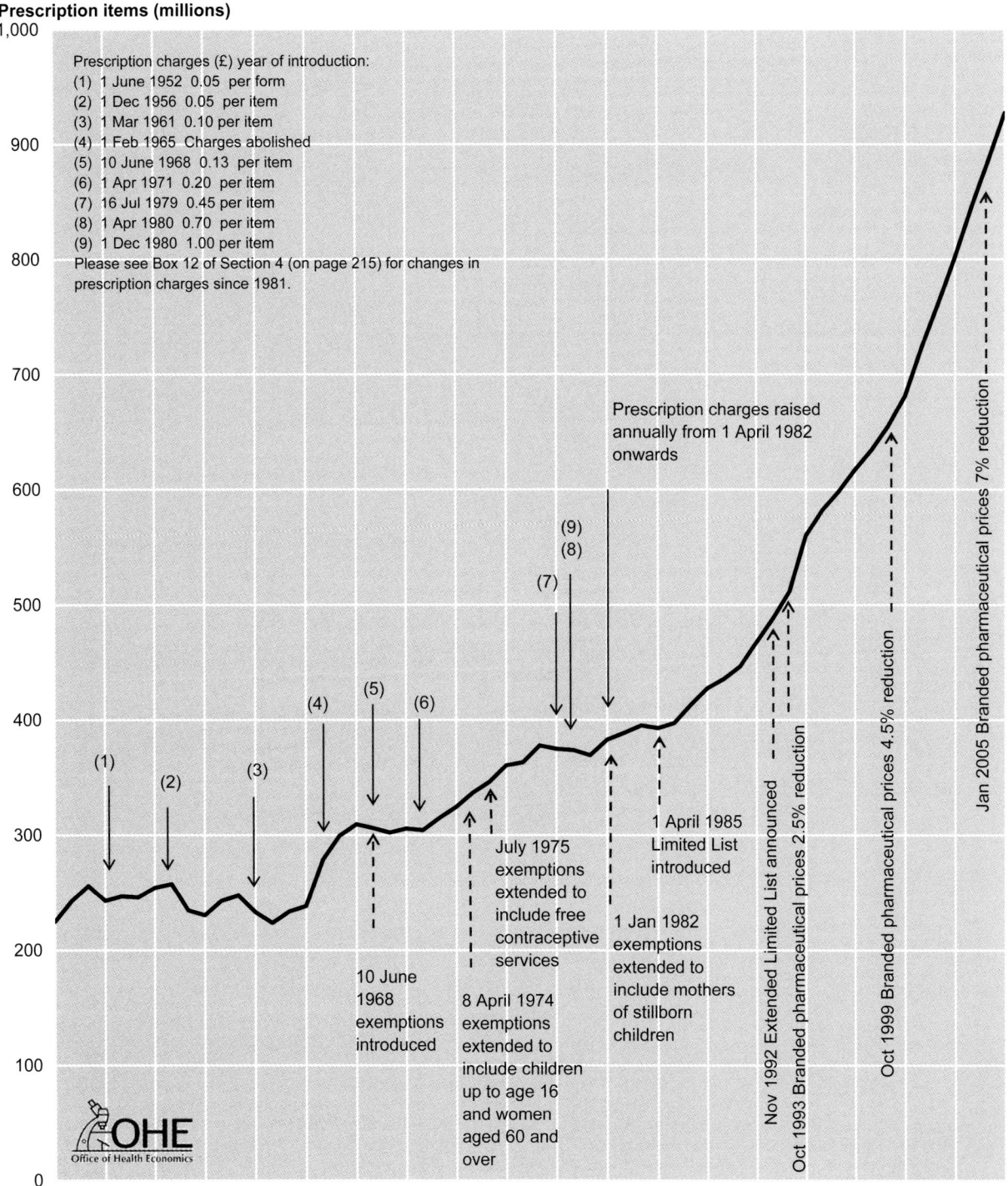

**Prescription items (millions)**

Prescription charges (£) year of introduction:
(1) 1 June 1952  0.05  per form
(2) 1 Dec 1956  0.05  per item
(3) 1 Mar 1961  0.10 per item
(4) 1 Feb 1965  Charges abolished
(5) 10 June 1968  0.13  per item
(6) 1 Apr 1971  0.20  per item
(7) 16 Jul 1979  0.45  per item
(8) 1 Apr 1980  0.70  per item
(9) 1 Dec 1980  1.00 per item
Please see Box 12 of Section 4 (on page 215) for changes in
prescription charges since 1981.

Prescription charges raised
annually from 1 April 1982
onwards

July 1975
exemptions
extended to
include free
contraceptive
services

10 June
1968
exemptions
introduced

8 April 1974
exemptions
extended to
include children
up to age 16
and women
aged 60 and
over

1 Jan 1982
exemptions
extended to
include mothers
of stillborn
children

1 April 1985
Limited List
introduced

Nov 1992 Extended Limited List announced

Oct 1993 Branded pharmaceutical prices 2.5% reduction

Oct 1999 Branded pharmaceutical prices 4.5% reduction

Jan 2005 Branded pharmaceutical prices 7% reduction

**Year**

*Notes:*  1 The same prescription charge applied in all parts of the UK until March 2000.  Charges in Wales were frozen at £6.00 in April 2000, reduced to
£4.00 on 1st April 2005 and then made free on 1st April 2007.  The age limit for free prescriptions for younger people is 16 everywhere except
Wales.  From 1994 onwards figures relate to prescriptions dispensed by community pharmacists and appliance contractors who are contracted
to the NHS and dispensing doctors.
Information on pre-payment certificates is not included.
*Sources:*  Prescriptions Dispensed in the Community Statistics: England (DH).
Prescriptions Dispensed in the Community: England (Information Centre IC).
PPA Annual Reports.

Figure 4.16  **Basic rate of prescription charges at constant prices and as a percentage of total prescription costs, UK, 1978 - 2006**

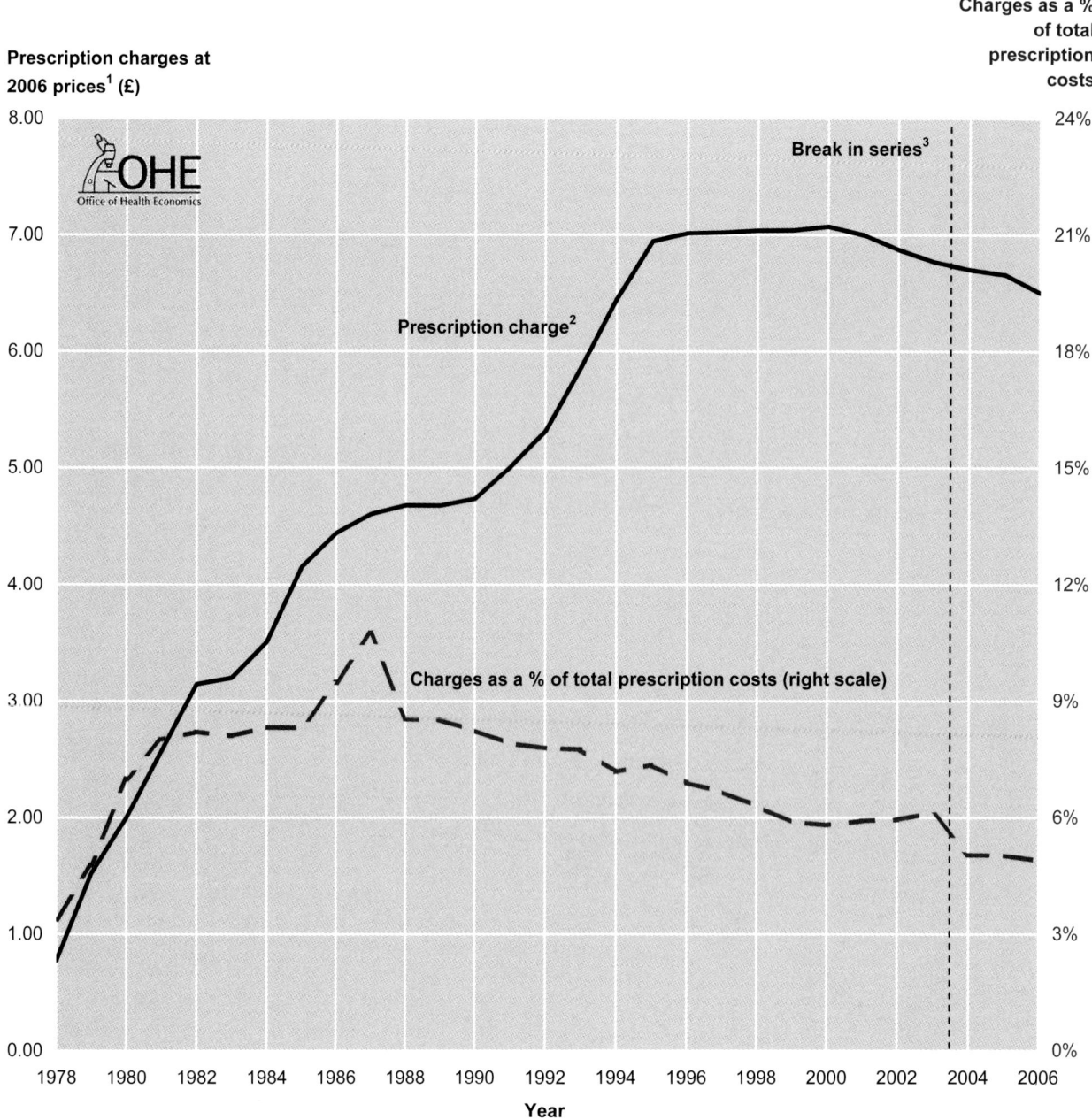

*Notes:*  1 As adjusted by the Gross Domestic Product (GDP) deflator at market prices.
2 The same prescription charge applied in all parts of the UK until March 2000.  Curve from then on is for England, Scotland and Northern Ireland. Charges in Wales were frozen at £6 in April 2000, reduced to £4 on 1st April 2005 and then made free from 1st April 2007.
3 Figures prior to 2004 are taken from the Annual Abstract of Statistics and relate to payments by patients for pharmaceutical services, this data was last published for 2003/2004. As such, comparable data are not available since 2003/04 and data shown for 2004 relate to prescription  charge revenue, including income received by pharmacists and dispensing doctors and income from the sale of pre-payment certificates.
Figures for charges as a % of total prescription costs relate to financial years ending the year shown on the x-axis and prescription charges are as at  1st April of the year shown.

*Sources:*  Prescription Pricing Authority, England.
Health of Wales Information Services.
Information Services Division of the NHS in Scotland.
Central Services Agency, Northern Ireland.
Health and Personal Social Services Statistics for England (DH).
Scottish Health Statistics (ISD).
Health Statistics Wales (NAW).
Annual Statistical Report (Northern Ireland CSA).
Annual Abstract of Statistics (ONS).
Economic Trends (ONS).

# FHS: General Pharmaceutical Services

Figure 4.17 **Revenue from prescription charges and as a percentage of General Pharmaceutical Services (GPS) cost, UK, 1951/52 - 2005/06**

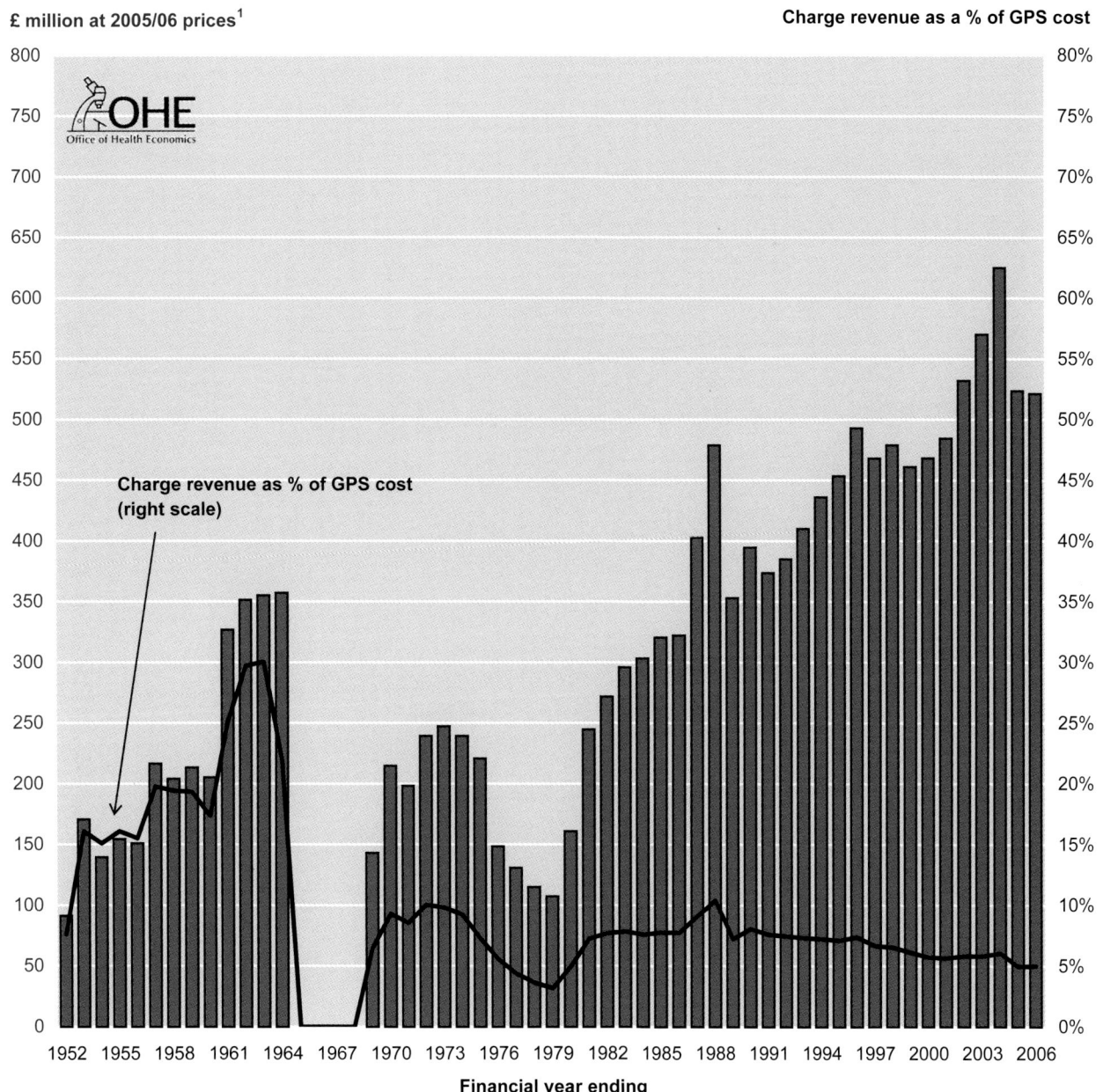

**£ million at 2005/06 prices**[1]

**Charge revenue as a % of GPS cost**

*Notes:* Charges were first introduced in 1952 and temporarily abolished between 1965 and 1968.

Same prescription charge applied in all parts of the UK until March 2000. Charges in Wales were frozen at £6 in April 2000, reduced to £4 on 1st April 2005 and then made free on 1st April 2007.

Figures prior to 2004/05 are taken from the Annual Abstract of Statistics and relate to payments by patients for pharmaceutical services, this data was last published for2003/2004. As such, comparable data is not available since 2003/04 and data shown relates to prescription charge revenue, including income received by pharmacists and dispensing doctors and income from the sale of pre-payment certificates.

1 As adjusted by the Gross Domestic Product (GDP) deflator at market prices.

Figure for 2004 is an OHE estimate.

*Sources:* Annual Abstract of Statistics (ONS).

The Government's Expenditure Plans (DH).

Health and Personal Social Services Statistics for England (DH).

Scottish Health Statistics (ISD).

Health Statistics Wales (NAW).

Annual Statistical Report (Northern Ireland CSA).

Figure 4.18  **Proportion of NHS prescriptions exempt from the prescription charge, England, 1984 - 2006**

**Number of prescriptions (million)**                                    **Per cent**

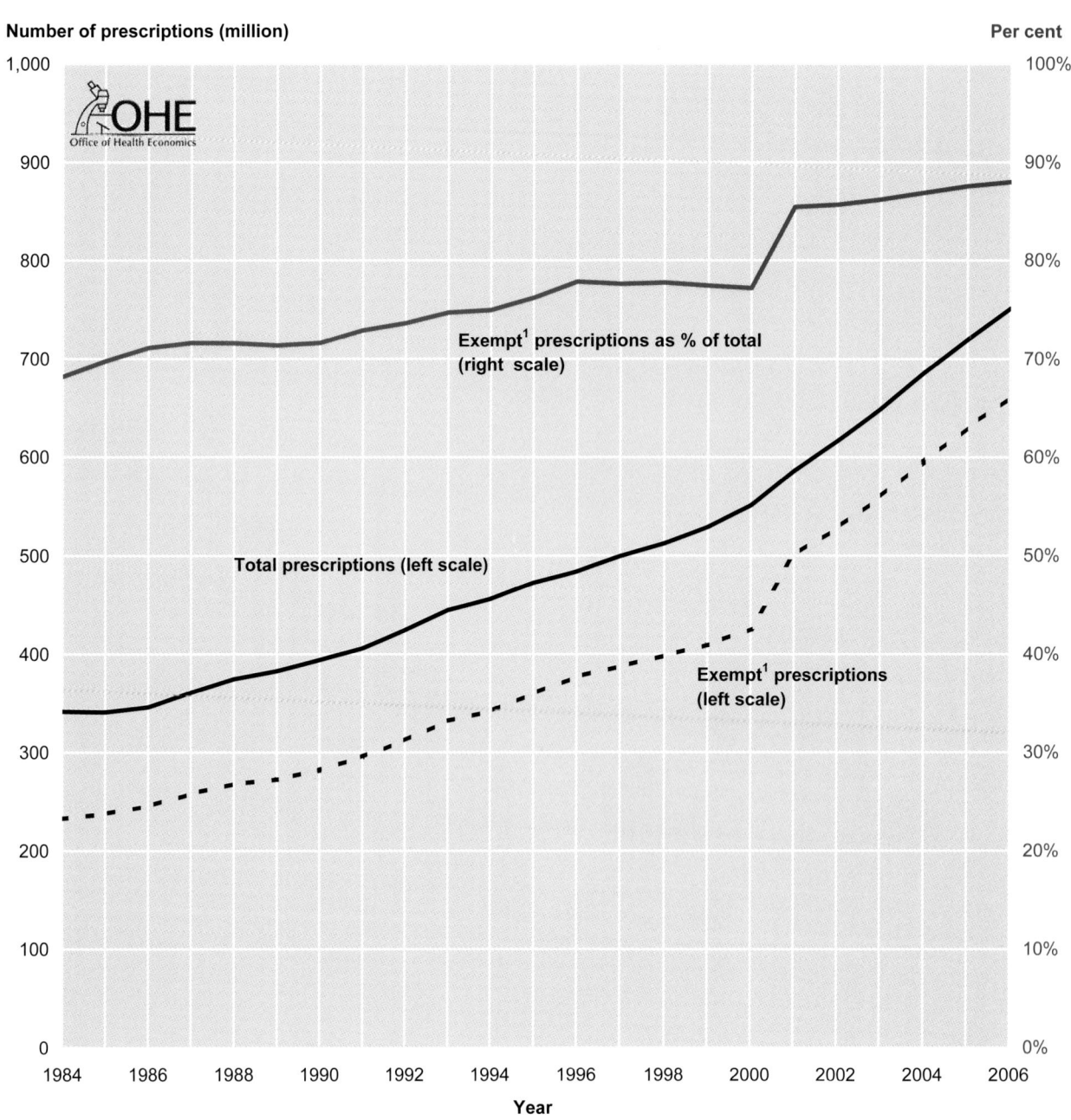

Exempt[1] prescriptions as % of total (right scale)

Total prescriptions (left scale)

Exempt[1] prescriptions (left scale)

**Year**

*Notes:*  Total prescriptions include those dispensed by chemists, dispensing doctors and for personal administration.  Exempt items also include prescribed contraceptives and personally administered items, which are free of charge.

Figures from 1991 onwards are based on the new PCA system and are based on items, they are not strictly comparable with previous years and may differ from those shown elsewhere in the Compendium.

Since 1991, figures relate to the total count of items written and dispensed, whereas earlier figures relate to the aggregate prescription fees. Prior to 2001 figures are based on a sample of 1 in 20 prescriptions dispensed by community pharmacists and appliance suppliers who are contracted to the NHS  only. From 2001 all  figures also include prescriptions dispensed by dispensing doctors and personally administered prescriptions which are free of charge.

From 1984 onwards figures for chargeable prescriptions include pre-payment certificates.

1 See Box 4.13 on page 224 for the categories of people exempt from prescription charges.

*Sources:*  Health and Personal Social Services Statistics for England (DH).

Prescriptions Dispensed in the Community Statistics: England  (DH).

Prescriptions Dispensed in the Community Statistics: England  (Information Centre (IC)).

# FHS: General Pharmaceutical Services

Table 4.27    Net ingredient cost (NIC) of NHS prescriptions ($R_x$s) dispensed[1], UK, 1949 - 2006

| Year | England £m | Wales £m | Scotland £m | Northern Ireland £m | United Kingdom £m | UK NIC Per capita £ | UK NIC Per $R_x$ £ |
|---|---|---|---|---|---|---|---|
| 1949 | 14[2] | - | - | - | 14[2] | 0.28 | 0.06 |
| 1950 | 18[2] | - | - | - | 18[2] | 0.35 | 0.07 |
| 1955 | 29[2] | - | - | - | 29[2] | 0.57 | 0.11 |
| 1960 | 52[2] | - | 5 | - | 57[3] | 1.09 | 0.23 |
| 1965 | 86[2] | - | 10 | - | 96[3] | 1.77 | 0.34 |
| 1966 | 99 | 8 | 11 | - | 118[3] | 2.15 | 0.39 |
| 1967 | 105 | 8 | 12 | - | 126[3] | 2.29 | 0.41 |
| 1968 | 111 | 9 | 12 | 7 | 139 | 2.51 | 0.45 |
| 1969 | 122 | 10 | 14 | 7 | 152 | 2.74 | 0.50 |
| 1970 | 134 | 10 | 15 | 8 | 166 | 2.99 | 0.54 |
| 1971 | 137 | 11 | 17 | 8 | 173 | 3.09 | 0.57 |
| 1972 | 155 | 12 | 19 | 9 | 196 | 3.49 | 0.62 |
| 1973 | 171 | 14 | 21 | 10 | 216 | 3.85 | 0.67 |
| 1974 | 205 | 16 | 25 | 12 | 258 | 4.59 | 0.77 |
| 1975 | 265 | 21 | 32 | 12 | 329 | 5.85 | 0.95 |
| 1976 | 343 | 27 | 42 | 15 | 427 | 7.59 | 1.18 |
| 1977 | 434 | 34 | 53 | 19 | 540 | 9.60 | 1.48 |
| 1978 | 518 | 39 | 63 | 22 | 642 | 11.43 | 1.70 |
| 1979 | 592 | 45 | 72 | 26 | 735 | 13.07 | 1.96 |
| 1980 | 716 | 54 | 86 | 31 | 888 | 15.76 | 2.37 |
| 1981 | 834 | 63 | 98 | 37 | 1,032 | 18.31 | 2.79 |
| 1982 | 977 | 72 | 112 | 43 | 1,204 | 21.39 | 3.14 |
| 1983 | 1,105 | 81 | 126 | 48 | 1,361 | 24.15 | 3.50 |
| 1984 | 1,181 | 87 | 136 | 52 | 1,456 | 25.79 | 3.68 |
| 1985 | 1,250 | 90 | 142 | 53 | 1,536 | 27.16 | 3.91 |
| 1986 | 1,366 | 99 | 154 | 57 | 1,676 | 29.57 | 4.22 |
| 1987 | 1,537 | 110 | 171 | 65 | 1,883 | 33.15 | 4.55 |
| 1988 | 1,737 | 125 | 193 | 73 | 2,129 | 37.41 | 4.98 |
| 1989 | 1,882 | 137 | 216 | 82 | 2,317 | 40.59 | 5.32 |
| 1990 | 2,079 | 151 | 240 | 92 | 2,563 | 44.78 | 5.74 |
| 1991 | 2,332 | 171 | 267 | 107 | 2,877 | 50.09 | 6.15 |
| 1992 | 2,637 | 193 | 304 | 123 | 3,257 | 56.56 | 6.67 |
| 1993 | 2,902 | 211 | 333 | 140 | 3,586 | 62.13 | 7.01 |
| 1994 | 3,340 | 241 | 375 | 158 | 4,114 | 71.11 | 7.34 |
| 1995 | 3,606 | 262 | 411 | 178 | 4,456 | 76.80 | 7.65 |
| 1996 | 3,921 | 283 | 447 | 195 | 4,847 | 83.33 | 8.10 |
| 1997 | 4,260 | 310 | 492 | 211 | 5,272 | 90.41 | 8.54 |
| 1998 | 4,594 | 333 | 528 | 223 | 5,678 | 97.10 | 8.94 |
| 1999 | 5,178 | 373 | 588 | 240 | 6,379 | 108.70 | 9.73 |
| 2000 | 5,454 | 399 | 639 | 250 | 6,741 | 114.48 | 9.89 |
| 2001 | 5,979 | 435 | 675 | 272 | 7,362 | 124.53 | 10.17 |
| 2002 | 6,701 | 489 | 746 | 299 | 8,235 | 138.81 | 10.80 |
| 2003 | 7,355 | 530 | 809 | 330 | 9,025 | 151.53 | 11.26 |
| 2004 | 7,908 | 566 | 850 | 365 | 9,690 | 161.91 | 11.46 |
| 2005 | 7,754 | 545 | 822 | 360 | 9,481 | 157.39 | 10.71 |
| 2006 | 8,037 | 564 | 869 | 374 | 9,844 | 162.48 | 10.62 |

*Notes:*    Net ingredient cost is the basic price of the ingredients before discount (which is calculated on the ingredient cost at a variable rate related to the total number of prescriptions dispensed by the contractors in each month).
1 Figures relate to prescriptions dispensed by community pharmacists and appliance suppliers who are contracted to the NHS and from 1994 include dispensing doctors.
2 Figures relate to England and Wales.
3 Figures relate to Great Britain.

*Sources:*    Prescription Pricing Authority, England.
Health of Wales Information Services.
Information Services Division of NHS in Scotland.
Central Services Agency, Northern Ireland.
Health and Personal Social Services Statistics for England (DH).
Scottish Health Statistics (ISD).
Health Statistics Wales (NAW).
Annual Statistical Report (Northern Ireland CSA).
Population Projections Database (GAD).

Table 4.28    **Average net ingredient cost per prescription dispensed and at constant prices [1] (1996=100) by country, UK, 1996 - 2006**

## Net ingredient cost per prescription dispensed

£ (cash)

| | Year | | | | | | | | | | |
|---|---|---|---|---|---|---|---|---|---|---|---|
| | **1996** | **1997** | **1998** | **1999** | **2000** | **2001** | **2002** | **2003** | **2004** | **2005** | **2006** |
| **United Kingdom** | 8.10 | 8.54 | 8.94 | 9.73 | 9.89 | 10.17 | 10.80 | 11.26 | 11.46 | 10.71 | 10.62 |
| **England** | 8.08 | 8.52 | 8.94 | 9.76 | 9.89 | 10.17 | 10.82 | 11.27 | 11.46 | 10.70 | 10.57 |
| **Wales** | 7.56 | 7.96 | 8.31 | 9.00 | 9.26 | 9.44 | 9.98 | 10.33 | 10.41 | 9.62 | 9.49 |
| **Scotland** | 8.20 | 8.71 | 9.02 | 9.75 | 10.08 | 10.31 | 10.85 | 11.33 | 11.45 | 10.76 | 11.04 |
| **Northern Ireland** | 9.24 | 9.64 | 9.93 | 10.33 | 10.56 | 11.10 | 11.76 | 12.51 | 13.37 | 12.87 | 12.81 |

## At constant prices [1] (1996=100)

| | Year | | | | | | | | | | |
|---|---|---|---|---|---|---|---|---|---|---|---|
| | **1996** | **1997** | **1998** | **1999** | **2000** | **2001** | **2002** | **2003** | **2004** | **2005** | **2006** |
| **United Kingdom** | 100 | 103 | 105 | 112 | 113 | 113 | 116 | 117 | 116 | 106 | 103 |
| **England** | 100 | 103 | 105 | 113 | 113 | 113 | 116 | 117 | 116 | 106 | 103 |
| **Wales** | 100 | 103 | 105 | 111 | 113 | 112 | 115 | 115 | 113 | 102 | 98 |
| **Scotland** | 100 | 103 | 105 | 111 | 114 | 113 | 115 | 116 | 114 | 105 | 106 |
| **Northern Ireland** | 100 | 102 | 102 | 105 | 106 | 108 | 111 | 114 | 119 | 112 | 109 |

*Notes:*     All figures relate to prescriptions dispensed by community pharmacists and appliance contractors who are contracted to the NHS in calendar years.
Net ingredient cost is the basic price of the ingredients before discount (which is calculated on the ingredient cost at a variable rate related to the total number of prescriptions dispensed by the contractors in each month).
1 As adjusted by the Gross Domestic Product (GDP) deflator at market prices.

*Sources:*     Prescription Pricing Authority, England.
Health of Wales Information Service.
Information Services Division of the NHS in Scotland.
Central Services Agency, Northern Ireland.
Economic Trends (ONS).

# FHS: General Pharmaceutical Services

Table 4.29   **Net ingredient cost (NIC) of prescriptions per capita and per household, UK, 1975 - 2006**

| Year | England | Wales | Scotland | Northern Ireland | UK | England | Wales | Scotland | Northern Ireland | UK |
|------|---------|-------|----------|------------------|-----|---------|-------|----------|------------------|-----|
| | | | | | **NIC per capita (£ cash)** | | | | | |
| | | | **(£ cash)** | | | | At constant prices[1] (Index 1975=100) | | | |
| 1975 | 6 | 8 | 6 | 8 | 6 | 100 | 100 | 100 | 100 | 100 |
| 1980 | 15 | 19 | 17 | 20 | 16 | 136 | 129 | 137 | 130 | 136 |
| 1985 | 27 | 32 | 28 | 34 | 27 | 172 | 157 | 166 | 158 | 171 |
| 1990 | 44 | 53 | 47 | 58 | 45 | 211 | 193 | 212 | 201 | 210 |
| 1991 | 49 | 60 | 53 | 67 | 50 | 223 | 206 | 224 | 220 | 223 |
| 1992 | 55 | 67 | 60 | 76 | 57 | 243 | 224 | 245 | 241 | 242 |
| 1993 | 60 | 73 | 65 | 86 | 62 | 259 | 238 | 261 | 265 | 259 |
| 1994 | 69 | 83 | 73 | 96 | 71 | 293 | 267 | 288 | 294 | 292 |
| 1995 | 75 | 91 | 81 | 108 | 77 | 307 | 282 | 308 | 320 | 307 |
| 1996 | 81 | 98 | 88 | 117 | 83 | 321 | 294 | 324 | 336 | 321 |
| 1997 | 88 | 107 | 97 | 126 | 90 | 339 | 313 | 348 | 352 | 340 |
| 1998 | 94 | 115 | 104 | 133 | 97 | 356 | 328 | 365 | 363 | 356 |
| 1999 | 106 | 129 | 116 | 143 | 109 | 393 | 361 | 400 | 383 | 392 |
| 2000 | 111 | 137 | 126 | 148 | 114 | 407 | 381 | 430 | 393 | 408 |
| 2001 | 121 | 150 | 133 | 161 | 125 | 432 | 404 | 443 | 415 | 432 |
| 2002 | 135 | 167 | 148 | 176 | 139 | 466 | 437 | 473 | 438 | 465 |
| 2003 | 148 | 181 | 160 | 194 | 152 | 494 | 457 | 497 | 468 | 492 |
| 2004 | 158 | 192 | 167 | 214 | 162 | 515 | 474 | 507 | 502 | 512 |
| 2005 | 154 | 185 | 161 | 209 | 157 | 490 | 445 | 478 | 480 | 487 |
| 2006 | 158 | 190 | 170 | 215 | 162 | 493 | 448 | 491 | 482 | 491 |
| | | | | | **NIC per household (£ cash)** | | | | | |
| | | | **(£ cash)** | | | | At constant prices[1] (Index 1975=100) | | | |
| 1975 | 16 | 22 | 18 | 25 | 17 | 100 | 100 | 100 | 100 | 100 |
| 1980 | 42 | 54 | 47 | 61 | 43 | 132 | 124 | 130 | 123 | 131 |
| 1985 | 70 | 85 | 73 | 102 | 72 | 159 | 144 | 148 | 150 | 157 |
| 1990 | 110 | 134 | 118 | 168 | 113 | 187 | 169 | 178 | 185 | 185 |
| 1991 | 122 | 150 | 131 | 194 | 126 | 197 | 180 | 187 | 203 | 195 |
| 1992 | 137 | 169 | 148 | 217 | 141 | 213 | 194 | 204 | 218 | 212 |
| 1993 | 150 | 183 | 160 | 244 | 155 | 227 | 205 | 215 | 239 | 225 |
| 1994 | 171 | 208 | 179 | 266 | 176 | 255 | 229 | 236 | 257 | 253 |
| 1995 | 184 | 225 | 195 | 299 | 190 | 267 | 241 | 251 | 281 | 265 |
| 1996 | 199 | 241 | 211 | 319 | 205 | 278 | 250 | 261 | 289 | 277 |
| 1997 | 215 | 263 | 230 | 365 | 222 | 294 | 265 | 278 | 323 | 292 |
| 1998 | 231 | 281 | 245 | 375 | 238 | 307 | 277 | 289 | 323 | 305 |
| 1999 | 258 | 314 | 272 | 394 | 266 | 338 | 304 | 315 | 334 | 335 |
| 2000 | 270 | 333 | 293 | 401 | 278 | 349 | 319 | 337 | 336 | 347 |
| 2001 | 291 | 360 | 308 | 434 | 300 | 367 | 335 | 344 | 353 | 364 |
| 2002 | 323 | 400 | 338 | 469 | 332 | 394 | 359 | 364 | 370 | 389 |
| 2003 | 352 | 429 | 363 | 512 | 361 | 415 | 373 | 380 | 391 | 410 |
| 2004 | 375 | 454 | 378 | 559 | 384 | 432 | 386 | 385 | 416 | 425 |
| 2005 | 364 | 433 | 362 | 544 | 372 | 410 | 359 | 361 | 396 | 403 |
| 2006 | 373 | 444 | 379 | 560 | 382 | 410 | 360 | 369 | 398 | 404 |

*Notes:*   NIC is the basic price of the ingredients before discount (which is calculated on the ingredient cost at a variable rate related to the number of prescriptions dispensed by contractors each month).

Figures relate to prescriptions dispensed by community pharmacists and appliance suppliers who are contracted to the NHS and from 1994 include dispensing doctors.

1 At constant prices, as adjusted by the Gross Domestic Product (GDP) deflator at market prices.

*Sources:*   Prescription Pricing Authorities in England, Wales, Scotland and Northern Ireland.
Health and Personal Social Services Statistics for England (DH).
Scottish Health Statistics (ISD).
Health Statistics Wales (NAW).
Annual Statistical Report (Northern Ireland CSA).
Economic Trends (ONS).
Population Projections Database (GAD).
Household Estimates and projections (DCLG).
Household projections (GROS).
Household data (NISRA).

Table 4.30    **Net ingredient cost[1] of prescriptions and cost per capita by age group, England, 1978 - 2006**

| Calendar year | Net ingredient cost (£ million cash): | | | Percentage breakdown: | |
|---|---|---|---|---|---|
| | Total | Under 16[4] | Elderly[3] | Under 16[4] | Elderly[3] |
| 1978 | 518 | 38 | 182 | 7 | 35 |
| 1980 | 716 | 52 | 276 | 7 | 39 |
| 1985 | 1,334 | 86 | 515 | 6 | 39 |
| 1986 | 1,459 | 90 | 568 | 6 | 39 |
| 1987 | 1,644 | 101 | 642 | 6 | 39 |
| 1988 | 1,865 | 121 | 734 | 6 | 39 |
| 1989 | 2,027 | 133 | 800 | 7 | 39 |
| 1990 | 2,243 | 145 | 884 | 6 | 39 |
| 1991 | 2,520 | 167 | 1,003 | 7 | 40 |
| 1992 | 2,859 | 192 | 1,124 | 7 | 39 |
| 1993 | 3,159 | 218 | 1,234 | 7 | 39 |
| 1994 | 3,405 | 238 | 1,326 | 7 | 39 |
| 1995 | 3,681 | 260 | 1,464 | 7 | 40 |
| 1996 | 4,007 | 266 | 1,724 | 7 | 43 |
| 1997 | 4,368 | 277 | 1,906 | 6 | 44 |
| 1998 | 4,702 | 282 | 2,060 | 6 | 44 |
| 1999 | 5,291 | 288 | 2,420 | 5 | 46 |
| 2000 | 5,585 | 284 | 2,621 | 5 | 47 |
| 2001[2] | 6,117 | 313 | 3,120 | 5 | 51 |
| 2002 | 6,847 | 325 | 3,561 | 5 | 52 |
| 2003 | 7,510 | 339 | 3,989 | 5 | 53 |
| 2004 | 8,080 | 354 | 4,334 | 4 | 54 |
| 2005 | 7,937 | 380 | 4,180 | 5 | 53 |
| 2006 | 8,197 | 413 | 4,402 | 5 | 54 |

**Net ingredient cost per capita**

| Calendar year | Net ingredient cost per person (£ cash): | | | Real[5] index (1978=100) | | |
|---|---|---|---|---|---|---|
| | Total | Under 16[4] | Elderly[3] | Total | Under 16[4] | Elderly[3] |
| 1978 | 11.20 | 3.70 | 22.50 | 100 | 100 | 100 |
| 1980 | 15.30 | 5.40 | 33.40 | 101 | 108 | 110 |
| 1985 | 26.50 | 10.30 | 60.10 | 127 | 150 | 144 |
| 1986 | 28.80 | 10.80 | 65.80 | 134 | 153 | 153 |
| 1987 | 32.40 | 12.20 | 73.70 | 144 | 164 | 163 |
| 1988 | 36.50 | 13.80 | 84.00 | 152 | 174 | 174 |
| 1989 | 39.40 | 14.80 | 91.10 | 152 | 173 | 175 |
| 1990 | 43.30 | 16.20 | 100.60 | 155 | 176 | 180 |
| 1991 | 48.40 | 15.90 | 113.10 | 165 | 164 | 191 |
| 1992 | 54.50 | 18.00 | 126.50 | 178 | 178 | 206 |
| 1993 | 59.80 | 20.10 | 138.70 | 191 | 194 | 220 |
| 1994 | 64.00 | 21.70 | 149.40 | 201 | 206 | 233 |
| 1995 | 76.07 | 26.04 | 164.87 | 233 | 241 | 251 |
| 1996 | 82.59 | 26.66 | 171.88 | 243 | 238 | 252 |
| 1997 | 89.75 | 27.71 | 189.56 | 258 | 241 | 271 |
| 1998 | 96.30 | 28.18 | 203.83 | 270 | 239 | 285 |
| 1999 | 107.91 | 28.76 | 238.37 | 298 | 240 | 327 |
| 2000 | 113.43 | 28.42 | 257.10 | 309 | 234 | 349 |
| 2001[2] | 123.69 | 31.55 | 304.98 | 328 | 253 | 403 |
| 2002 | 137.91 | 32.99 | 346.13 | 353 | 256 | 441 |
| 2003 | 150.64 | 34.56 | 384.05 | 374 | 260 | 475 |
| 2004 | 161.29 | 36.25 | 412.57 | 390 | 265 | 497 |
| 2005 | 157.37 | 39.07 | 392.52 | 372 | 280 | 462 |
| 2006 | 162.53 | 42.48 | 413.31 | 376 | 297 | 475 |

*Notes:*    These figures differ from those shown in Table 4.27 due to differences in definition.
1 Net ingredient cost is the basic price of the ingredients before discount (which is calculated on the ingredient cost at a variable rate related to the total number of prescriptions dispensed by the contractors in each month).
2 Prior to 2001 all figures are based on a sample of 1 in 20 prescriptions dispensed by community pharmacists and appliance contractors who are contracted to the NHS only.  From 2001 all figures also include prescriptions dispensed by dispensing doctors and personally administered prescriptions.
See footnotes to Table 4.25 for changes in the data.
3 Prior to 20th October 1995 "elderly people" includes men aged 65 years and over and women aged 60 and over.  After this date "elderly people" includes men and women aged 60 years and over.
4 Figures relate to children aged under 16 and others aged under 19 and still in full-time education.
5 As adjusted by the Gross Domestic Product (GDP) deflator at market prices.

*Sources:*    Prescriptions Dispensed in the Community Statistics: England (DH Statistical Bulletin).
Economic Trends: Annual Supplement (ONS).

# FHS: General Pharmaceutical Services

Figure 4.19  **Net ingredient cost[1] (NIC) per elderly person[2], England, 1978 - 2006**

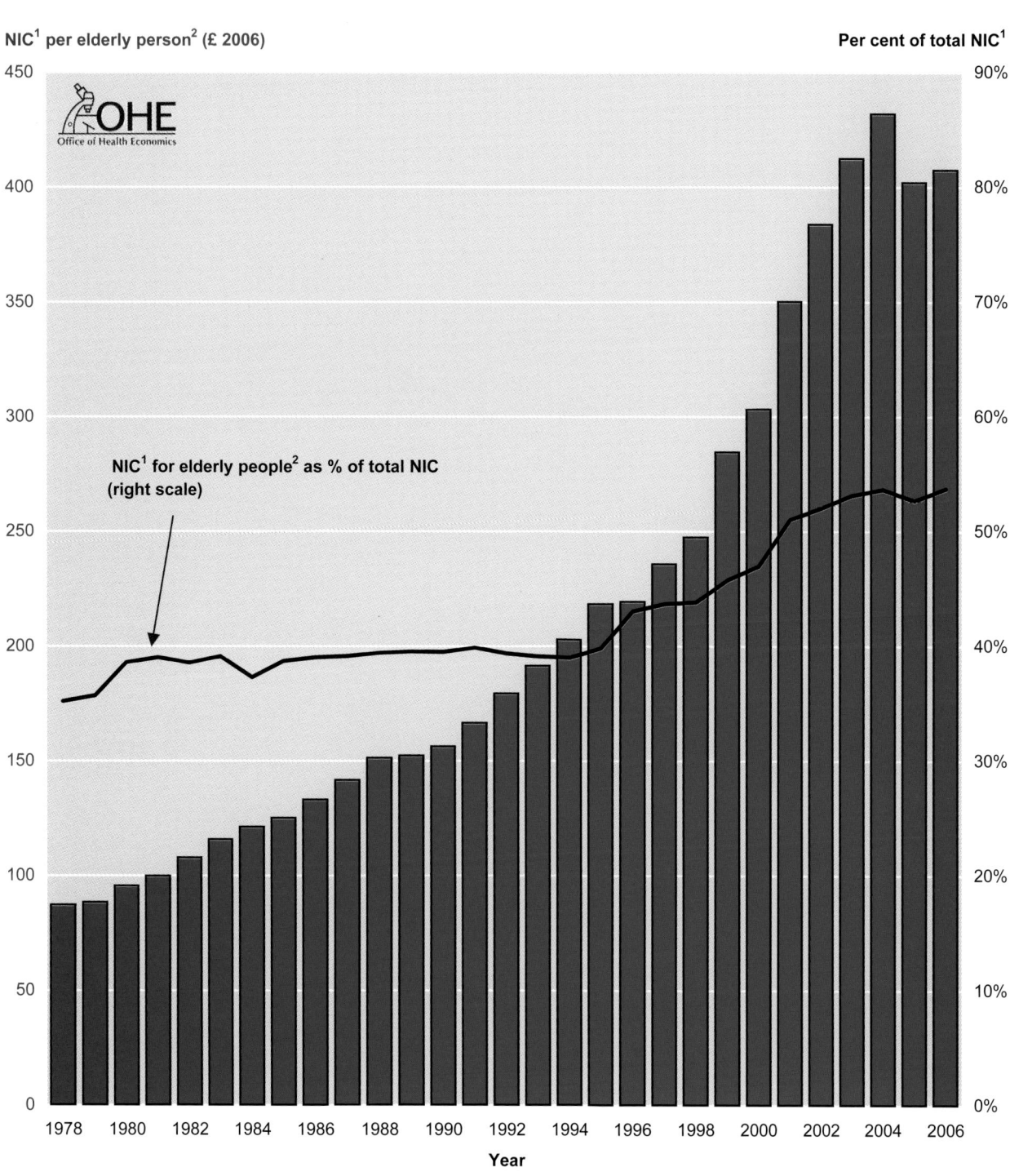

NIC[1] per elderly person[2] (£ 2006)

Per cent of total NIC[1]

NIC[1] for elderly people[2] as % of total NIC (right scale)

Year

*Notes:*   1 At 2006 prices, as adjusted by the Gross Domestic Product (GDP) deflator at market prices.
2 Until 1995 figures relate to men aged 65 years and over and women aged 60 years and over.  From 20 October 1995, includes men aged over 60 years.

*Sources:*   Prescriptions Dispensed in the Community Statistics: England (DH Statistical Bulletin).
Prescriptions Dispensed in the Community Statistics: England (Information Centre IC).
Economic Trends: Annual Supplement (ONS).

Figure 4.20 **Prescription items per capita dispensed by community pharmacists[1], by major therapeutic group, UK, 1996 - 2006**

**Number of prescription items per capita**

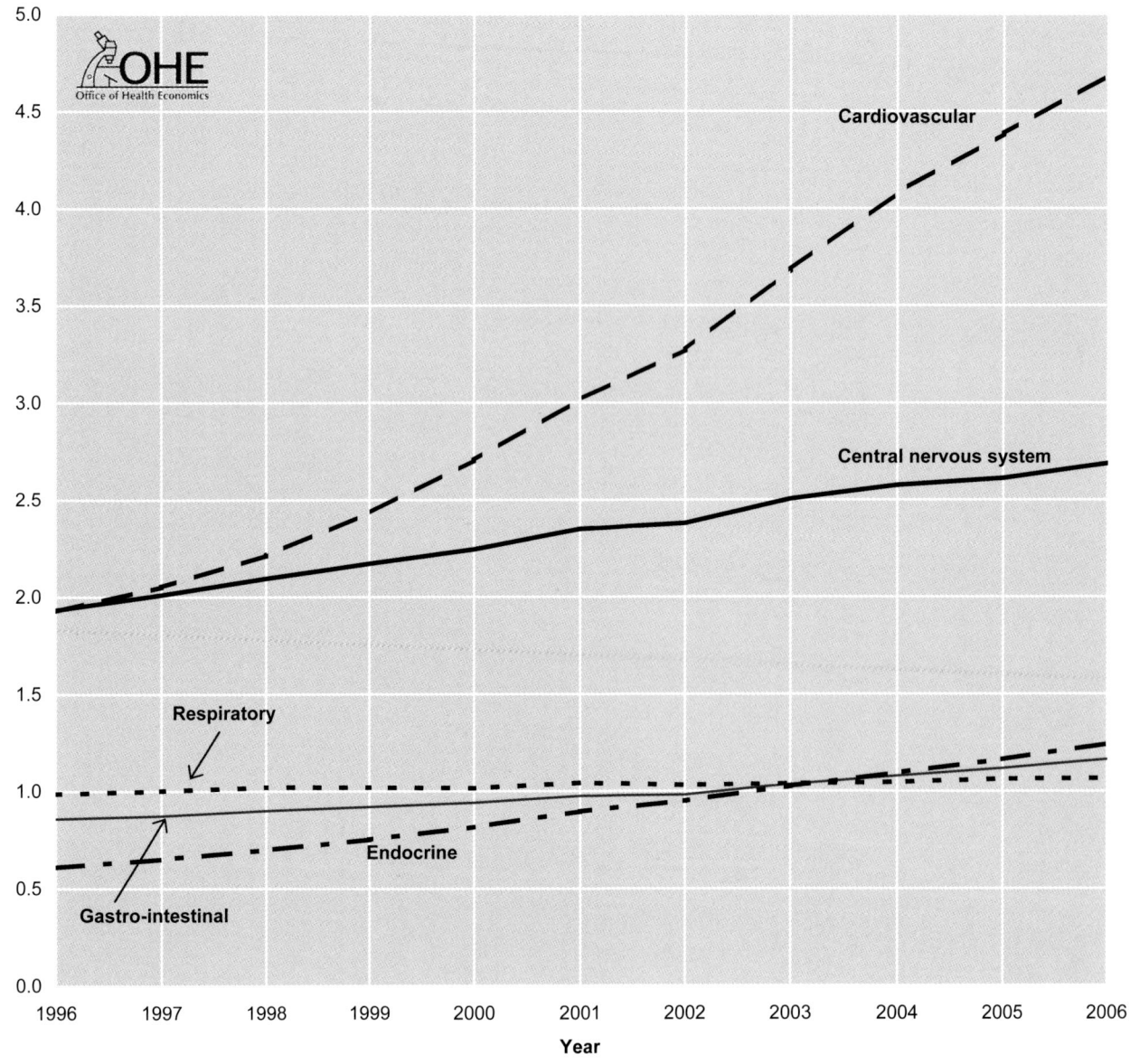

*Note:* 1 Figures relate to community pharmacists and appliance contractors who are contracted to the NHS.
*Sources:* Prescription Cost Analysis, England (DH).
Prescription Cost Analysis, Wales (HOWIS).
Prescription Cost Analysis, Scotland (ISD).
Prescription Cost Analysis, Northern Ireland (CSA).
Population Projections Database (GAD).

Figure 4.21  **Net ingredient cost (NIC) per capita, by major therapeutic group, UK, 1996 - 2006**

**NIC per capita (£ at 2006 prices[1])**

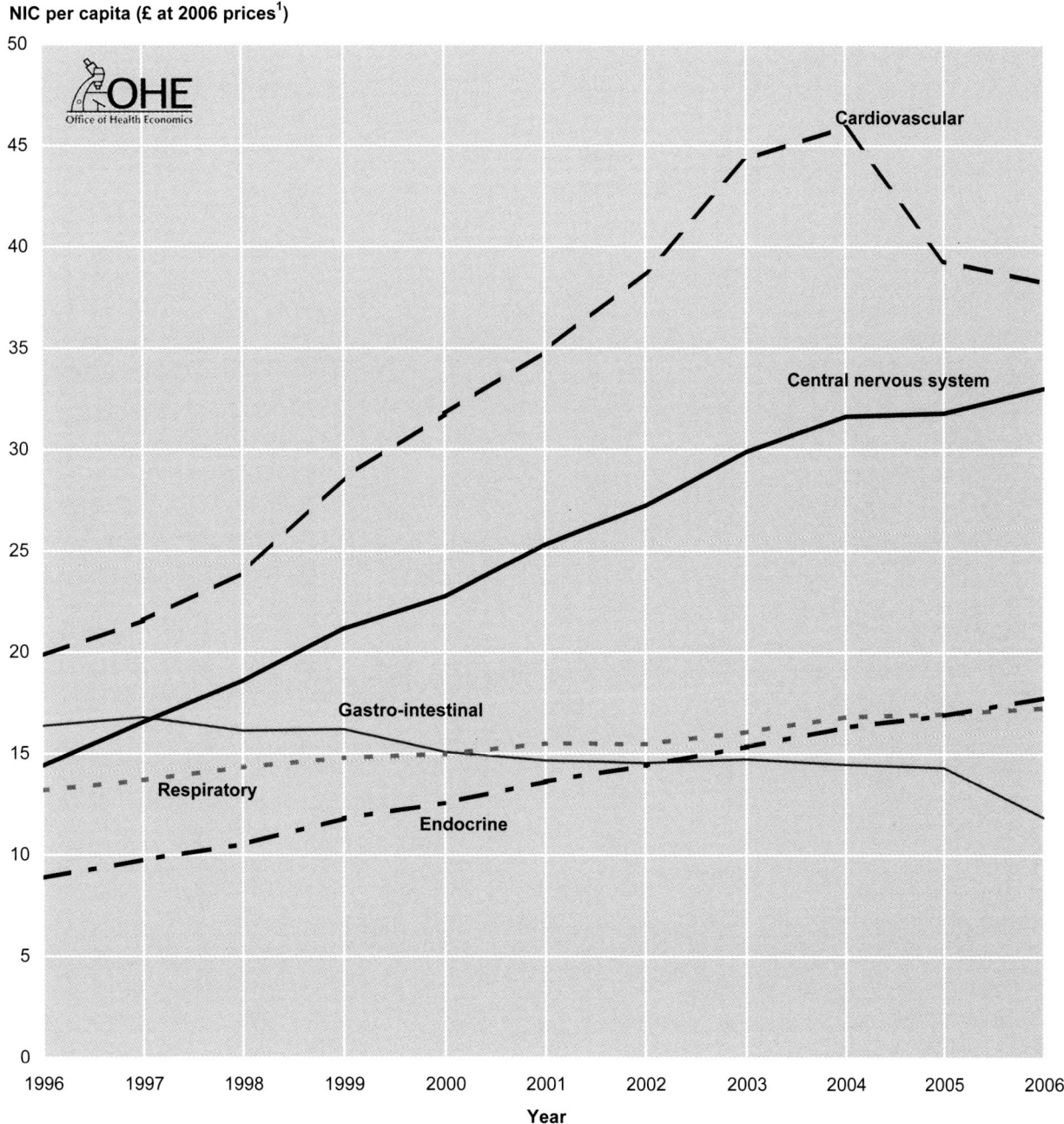

Note:       1 At 2006 prices as adjusted by the Gross Domestic Product (GDP) deflator at market prices.
Sources:   Prescription Cost Analysis, England (DH).
             Prescription Cost Analysis, Wales (HOWIS).
             Prescription Cost Analysis, Scotland (ISD).
             Prescription Cost Analysis, Northern Ireland (CSA).
             Population Projections Database (GAD).

Table 4.31  Number and net ingredient cost (NIC) of prescriptions by therapeutic group, UK, 1996 - 2006

| BNF | Therapeutic group | Prescription items (millions): | | | | | NIC of prescriptions (£m): | | | | |
|---|---|---|---|---|---|---|---|---|---|---|---|
| | | 1996 | 2001 | 2004 | 2005 | 2006 | 1996 | 2001 | 2004 | 2005 | 2006 |
| | Total | 596.7 | 721.9 | 840.9 | 881.1 | 918.6 | 4,955.7 | 7,532.6 | 9,947.1 | 9,809.1 | 10,111.0 |
| 1 | Gastro-intestinal system | 49.9 | 57.4 | 64.4 | 67.3 | 70.4 | 749.0 | 754.9 | 827.2 | 842.5 | 718.2 |
| 1.3 | Ulcer-healing drugs | 17.6 | 24.5 | 31.3 | 34.0 | 36.9 | 561.6 | 550.1 | 606.2 | 612.9 | 468.8 |
| 1.6 | Laxatives | 13.5 | 15.2 | 15.9 | 16.3 | 16.5 | 55.5 | 53.2 | 55.6 | 61.3 | 70.1 |
| 2 | Cardiovascular system | 112.1 | 177.4 | 243.3 | 264.0 | 283.5 | 910.4 | 1,797.2 | 2,624.3 | 2,311.3 | 2,314.5 |
| 2.2 | Diuretics | 28.4 | 36.9 | 44.4 | 45.5 | 45.5 | 63.4 | 75.8 | 78.7 | 89.9 | 105.9 |
| 2.4 | Beta-adrenoceptor blocking drugs | 17.7 | 25.0 | 32.1 | 33.3 | 33.3 | 97.8 | 103.3 | 123.6 | 119.0 | 127.2 |
| 2.5 | Anti-hypertensive therapy | 14.5 | 29.8 | 45.9 | 50.6 | 56.0 | 266.8 | 500.8 | 728.6 | 598.8 | 611.1 |
| 2.6 | Nitrates/calcium channel blockers | 27.6 | 33.3 | 37.7 | 39.4 | 41.9 | 342.1 | 454.5 | 506.6 | 458.7 | 393.4 |
| 2.12 | Lipid lowering drugs | 3.8 | 16.6 | 35.6 | 42.4 | 49.7 | 113.7 | 543.3 | 939.9 | 785.4 | 780.0 |
| 3 | Respiratory system | 57.3 | 61.3 | 62.6 | 64.0 | 64.5 | 602.9 | 798.0 | 961.8 | 998.0 | 1,045.9 |
| 3.1 | Bronchodilators | 28.4 | 30.7 | 30.6 | 30.7 | 30.8 | 231.4 | 297.2 | 317.4 | 326.0 | 333.6 |
| 3.2 | Corticosteroids (inhaled) | 13.2 | 15.1 | 16.5 | 17.2 | 17.7 | 298.8 | 384.0 | 509.7 | 538.6 | 581.3 |
| 4 | Central nervous system | 112.4 | 138.2 | 153.9 | 157.1 | 162.6 | 664.0 | 1,308.5 | 1,808.8 | 1,870.5 | 1,998.7 |
| 4.2 | Drugs used in psychoses & related dis. | 5.9 | 7.0 | 8.1 | 8.4 | 8.8 | 38.5 | 164.1 | 270.6 | 276.6 | 302.4 |
| 4.3 | Antidepressant drugs | 18.3 | 30.2 | 36.1 | 36.5 | 38.3 | 243.3 | 435.4 | 515.3 | 448.9 | 389.4 |
| 4.7 | Analgesics | 50.1 | 56.3 | 59.3 | 60.8 | 62.4 | 192.8 | 300.0 | 381.8 | 447.4 | 551.8 |
| 5 | Infections | 62.5 | 52.0 | 51.0 | 52.1 | 52.3 | 279.6 | 274.3 | 296.8 | 287.4 | 281.0 |
| 5.1 | Antibacterial drugs | 57.3 | 46.5 | 44.8 | 45.6 | 45.6 | 216.6 | 203.4 | 211.2 | 202.0 | 212.2 |
| 6 | Endocrine system | 35.5 | 52.7 | 65.3 | 70.0 | 75.2 | 406.9 | 701.5 | 933.2 | 994.1 | 1,075.7 |
| 6.1 | Drugs used in diabetes | 12.7 | 21.5 | 29.1 | 31.3 | 33.5 | 148.9 | 333.2 | 538.8 | 591.3 | 667.4 |
| 6.4 | Sex hormones | 8.3 | 9.1 | 6.6 | 6.2 | 6.1 | 157.3 | 199.8 | 139.8 | 116.0 | 112.4 |
| 7 | Obstetrics and gynaecology[1] | 14.7 | 17.2 | 19.5 | 20.2 | 21.0 | 94.4 | 197.0 | 283.7 | 304.9 | 309.5 |
| 7.3 | Contraceptives | 10.4 | 10.2 | 10.3 | 10.3 | 10.3 | 49.7 | 60.0 | 76.4 | 79.3 | 85.3 |
| 8 | Malignant disease[2] | 3.1 | 4.1 | 4.8 | 3.9 | 4.1 | 143.8 | 258.6 | 349.6 | 327.0 | 360.0 |
| 8.3 | Sex hormones and antagonists | 2.0 | 2.2 | 2.4 | 2.4 | 2.5 | 86.9 | 168.7 | 234.1 | 224.9 | 247.4 |
| 9 | Nutrition and blood | 16.3 | 19.9 | 26.1 | 28.6 | 31.8 | 150.0 | 260.8 | 354.5 | 389.4 | 443.6 |
| 9.4 | Oral nutrition | 3.2 | 4.2 | 5.0 | 5.3 | 8.8 | 94.2 | 154.2 | 198.7 | 214.3 | 240.8 |
| 10 | Musculo-skeletal and joint disease | 31.8 | 34.1 | 36.6 | 35.3 | 34.7 | 249.9 | 294.2 | 385.9 | 274.0 | 268.3 |
| 10.1 | Rheumatic diseases and gout | 24.8 | 27.6 | 30.1 | 28.8 | 28.0 | 206.4 | 249.7 | 336.8 | 232.9 | 226.8 |
| 11 | Eye preparations | 14.5 | 16.8 | 18.8 | 19.2 | 19.7 | 60.0 | 106.9 | 132.3 | 140.5 | 152.4 |
| 12 | Ear, nose and oropharynx | 11.4 | 11.8 | 11.6 | 11.8 | 12.0 | 54.2 | 63.4 | 72.2 | 70.5 | 76.2 |
| 13 | Skin | 43.1 | 43.0 | 43.3 | 43.4 | 43.0 | 215.4 | 234.6 | 262.4 | 263.8 | 278.0 |
| 13.4 | Topical corticosteroids | 15.4 | 15.4 | 15.0 | 14.9 | 14.9 | 49.0 | 55.9 | 59.8 | 59.9 | 70.9 |
| 14 | Immunological products | 11.6 | 13.8 | 14.7 | 17.3 | 14.6 | 100.7 | 126.5 | 144.4 | 166.6 | 147.1 |
| 14.4 | Vaccines and antisera | 11.4 | 13.8 | 14.7 | 17.1 | 14.6 | 97.1 | 123.0 | 141.0 | 162.1 | 143.4 |
| 15 | Anaesthesia | 0.9 | 0.9 | 0.9 | 1.0 | 1.0 | 2.2 | 3.4 | 4.5 | 4.9 | 5.4 |
| | Others including dressings and appliances | 19.6 | 21.4 | 23.8 | 25.3 | 27.1 | 292.1 | 390.1 | 507.3 | 561.0 | 620.6 |

Notes:  All figures are based on the British National Formulary (BNF).  Figures below the BNF heading relate to chapters and sub-sections of the BNF.
Figures relate to prescriptions dispensed by community pharmacists and appliances contractors who are contracted to the NHS, dispensing
doctors and personal administration.
1 Including urinary tract disorders.
2 Including immunosuppression.

Sources: Prescription Cost Analysis, England (DH).
Prescription Cost Analysis, Wales (HOWIS).
Prescription Cost Analysis, Scotland (ISD).
Prescription Cost Analysis, Northern Ireland (CSA).

Table 4.32 **Number and net ingredient cost (NIC) of prescriptions by therapeutic group, England, 1996 - 2006**

| BNF | Therapeutic group | Prescription items (millions): | | | | | NIC of prescriptions (£m): | | | | |
|---|---|---|---|---|---|---|---|---|---|---|---|
| | | 1996 | 2001 | 2004 | 2005 | 2006 | 1996 | 2001 | 2004 | 2005 | 2006 |
| | Total | 484.9 | 587.0 | 686.1 | 720.3 | 752.0 | 4,007.0 | 6,116.6 | 8,079.6 | 7,936.6 | 8,196.8 |
| 1 | **Gastro-intestinal system** | 39.5 | 45.4 | 51.1 | 53.6 | 56.3 | 578.9 | 584.3 | 647.7 | 656.1 | 562.2 |
| 1.3 | Ulcer-healing drugs | 13.4 | 19.0 | 24.5 | 26.9 | 29.6 | 427.0 | 418.9 | 469.4 | 470.8 | 352.9 |
| 1.6 | Laxatives | 11.1 | 12.5 | 13.1 | 13.4 | 13.6 | 45.5 | 42.8 | 45.1 | 50.2 | 57.6 |
| 2 | **Cardiovascular system** | 91.2 | 145.1 | 200.6 | 218.0 | 234.8 | 740.1 | 1,464.2 | 2,151.1 | 1,872.7 | 1,885.1 |
| 2.2 | Diuretics | 23.1 | 30.2 | 36.5 | 37.6 | 37.6 | 51.7 | 61.9 | 65.6 | 75.8 | 88.5 |
| 2.4 | Beta-adrenoceptor blocking drugs | 14.4 | 20.4 | 26.4 | 27.5 | 27.4 | 79.3 | 81.6 | 98.6 | 93.4 | 101.8 |
| 2.5 | Anti-hypertensive therapy | 12.1 | 25.0 | 38.6 | 42.9 | 47.7 | 224.0 | 420.6 | 610.0 | 484.0 | 501.5 |
| 2.6 | Nitrates/calcium channel blockers | 22.0 | 26.8 | 30.7 | 32.3 | 34.7 | 270.1 | 366.7 | 412.4 | 369.0 | 313.5 |
| 2.12 | Lipid lowering drugs | 3.1 | 13.5 | 29.4 | 35.6 | 42.1 | 92.9 | 438.8 | 769.2 | 625.0 | 622.3 |
| 3 | **Respiratory system** | 46.6 | 49.9 | 50.8 | 52.0 | 52.3 | 485.8 | 641.6 | 772.9 | 801.4 | 837.8 |
| 3.1 | Bronchodilators | 23.0 | 24.9 | 24.8 | 24.9 | 24.9 | 185.5 | 238.5 | 253.6 | 261.0 | 266.3 |
| 3.2 | Corticosteroids (inhaled) | 10.9 | 12.4 | 13.5 | 14.1 | 14.6 | 241.0 | 308.7 | 410.7 | 436.1 | 473.3 |
| 4 | **Central nervous system** | 89.3 | 109.1 | 121.9 | 124.6 | 129.1 | 527.6 | 1,034.8 | 1,431.6 | 1,473.8 | 1,580.6 |
| 4.2 | Drugs used in psychoses & related disorders | 4.8 | 5.7 | 6.6 | 6.9 | 7.2 | 31.0 | 132.8 | 219.2 | 223.6 | 244.9 |
| 4.3 | Antidepressant drugs | 15.0 | 24.3 | 29.0 | 29.4 | 31.0 | 191.2 | 341.7 | 400.7 | 338.5 | 291.5 |
| 4.7 | Analgesics | 39.3 | 44.0 | 46.6 | 47.9 | 49.4 | 152.2 | 234.4 | 298.7 | 355.2 | 449.1 |
| 5 | **Infections** | 50.9 | 42.4 | 41.5 | 42.5 | 42.6 | 225.5 | 222.1 | 240.2 | 231.5 | 226.2 |
| 5.1 | Antibacterial drugs | 46.6 | 37.9 | 36.5 | 37.2 | 37.2 | 174.4 | 162.8 | 170.9 | 162.0 | 171.0 |
| 6 | **Endocrine system** | 29.7 | 43.8 | 54.2 | 58.2 | 62.6 | 337.5 | 580.2 | 772.2 | 821.7 | 890.1 |
| 6.1 | Drugs used in diabetes | 10.7 | 18.1 | 24.5 | 26.5 | 28.4 | 123.7 | 278.6 | 450.6 | 495.3 | 562.5 |
| 6.4 | Sex hormones | 7.0 | 7.6 | 5.5 | 5.2 | 5.1 | 129.5 | 164.9 | 114.9 | 94.3 | 91.4 |
| 7 | **Obstetrics and gynaecology[1]** | 12.2 | 14.3 | 16.2 | 16.8 | 17.5 | 77.7 | 159.3 | 230.4 | 247.8 | 251.2 |
| 7.3 | Contraceptives | 8.7 | 8.6 | 8.7 | 8.7 | 8.7 | 41.6 | 50.0 | 63.8 | 66.3 | 71.7 |
| 8 | **Malignant disease[2]** | 2.6 | 3.4 | 4.0 | 3.2 | 3.3 | 118.1 | 213.6 | 292.1 | 272.8 | 300.5 |
| 8.3 | Sex hormones and antagonists | 1.6 | 1.9 | 2.0 | 2.0 | 2.1 | 71.1 | 140.0 | 196.0 | 186.7 | 206.2 |
| 9 | **Nutrition and blood** | 13.1 | 16.1 | 21.2 | 23.3 | 26.1 | 122.5 | 216.4 | 294.4 | 323.4 | 367.9 |
| 9.4 | Oral nutrition | 2.5 | 3.3 | 4.0 | 4.2 | 7.7 | 75.5 | 125.1 | 163.4 | 177.2 | 200.8 |
| 10 | **Musculo-skeletal and joint disease** | 25.9 | 27.7 | 29.6 | 28.6 | 28.2 | 200.8 | 232.4 | 305.0 | 216.0 | 214.1 |
| 10.1 | Rheumatic diseases and gout | 20.3 | 22.5 | 24.4 | 23.2 | 22.7 | 165.7 | 196.1 | 265.6 | 177.6 | 175.0 |
| 11 | **Eye preparations** | 12.1 | 14.1 | 15.8 | 16.1 | 16.5 | 50.3 | 91.0 | 113.0 | 120.2 | 130.2 |
| 12 | **Ear, nose and oropharynx** | 9.4 | 9.7 | 9.5 | 9.7 | 9.7 | 44.3 | 51.7 | 59.0 | 57.7 | 62.4 |
| 13 | **Skin** | 34.9 | 34.6 | 35.0 | 35.2 | 34.8 | 171.8 | 184.1 | 210.3 | 212.3 | 224.2 |
| 13.4 | Topical corticosteroids | 12.7 | 12.6 | 12.2 | 12.2 | 12.2 | 39.8 | 45.2 | 48.0 | 48.2 | 57.5 |
| 14 | **Immunological products** | 10.7 | 12.9 | 13.8 | 16.1 | 13.6 | 88.8 | 110.3 | 126.0 | 146.4 | 129.1 |
| 14.4 | Vaccines and antisera | 10.5 | 12.9 | 13.8 | 16.1 | 13.6 | 85.4 | 107.0 | 122.7 | 143.5 | 126.2 |
| 15 | **Anaesthesia** | 0.8 | 0.8 | 0.8 | 0.9 | 0.9 | 1.8 | 2.8 | 3.6 | 3.8 | 4.2 |
| | **Others including dressings and appliances** | 15.9 | 17.8 | 20.1 | 21.5 | 23.5 | 235.3 | 327.9 | 430.1 | 478.9 | 531.1 |

*Notes:* All figures are based on the British National Formulary (BNF). Figures below the BNF heading relate to chapters and sub-sections of the BNF.
Figures relate to prescriptions dispensed by community pharmacists and appliances contractors who are contracted to the NHS, dispensing doctors and personal administration.
1 Including urinary tract disorders.
2 Including immunosuppression.

*Source:* Prescription Cost Analysis, England (DH).

Table 4.33  Number and net ingredient cost (NIC) of prescriptions by therapeutic group, Wales, 1996 - 2006

| BNF | Therapeutic group | Prescription items (millions): | | | | | NIC of prescriptions (£m): | | | | |
|---|---|---|---|---|---|---|---|---|---|---|---|
| | | 1996 | 2001 | 2004 | 2005 | 2006 | 1996 | 2001 | 2004 | 2005 | 2006 |
| | Total | 37.0 | 46.0 | 54.0 | 56.6 | 58.9 | 288.4 | 443.8 | 577.0 | 560.0 | 574.0 |
| 1 | Gastro-intestinal system | 3.1 | 3.6 | 4.1 | 4.3 | 4.5 | 43.3 | 44.9 | 47.9 | 48.3 | 40.6 |
| 1.3 | Ulcer-healing drugs | 1.1 | 1.6 | 2.1 | 2.1 | 2.1 | 33.2 | 33.6 | 35.6 | 35.6 | 35.6 |
| 1.6 | Laxatives | 0.7 | 0.8 | 0.9 | 0.9 | 0.9 | 3.0 | 3.0 | 3.0 | 3.0 | 3.0 |
| 2 | Cardiovascular system | 7.7 | 11.9 | 16.7 | 18.1 | 19.3 | 55.2 | 104.2 | 152.2 | 130.1 | 130.5 |
| 2.2 | Diuretics | 1.9 | 2.4 | 3.0 | 3.0 | 3.0 | 4.1 | 4.4 | 4.5 | 4.5 | 4.5 |
| 2.4 | Beta-adrenoceptor blocking drugs | 1.1 | 1.5 | 2.0 | 2.0 | 2.0 | 5.6 | 5.8 | 7.0 | 7.0 | 7.0 |
| 2.5 | Anti-hypertensive therapy | 1.0 | 2.0 | 3.1 | 3.1 | 3.1 | 15.6 | 28.7 | 40.5 | 40.5 | 40.5 |
| 2.6 | Nitrates/calcium channel blockers | 1.9 | 2.3 | 2.6 | 2.6 | 2.6 | 23.6 | 26.9 | 29.5 | 29.5 | 29.5 |
| 2.12 | Lipid lowering drugs | 0.2 | 1.1 | 2.6 | 2.6 | 2.6 | 5.9 | 30.9 | 55.7 | 55.7 | 55.7 |
| 3 | Respiratory system | 3.5 | 3.8 | 4.0 | 4.1 | 4.1 | 37.5 | 52.2 | 62.7 | 64.8 | 67.4 |
| 3.1 | Bronchodilators | 1.8 | 2.0 | 2.0 | 2.0 | 2.0 | 15.1 | 19.6 | 20.9 | 20.9 | 20.9 |
| 3.2 | Corticosteroids (inhaled) | 0.8 | 0.9 | 1.1 | 1.1 | 1.1 | 18.3 | 26.0 | 34.1 | 34.1 | 34.1 |
| 4 | Central nervous system | 7.6 | 9.6 | 10.5 | 10.7 | 11.0 | 40.0 | 80.9 | 108.5 | 109.9 | 116.8 |
| 4.2 | Drugs used in psychoses & related disorders | 0.3 | 0.4 | 0.5 | 0.5 | 0.5 | 2.3 | 9.9 | 16.2 | 16.2 | 16.2 |
| 4.3 | Antidepressant drugs | 1.1 | 1.9 | 2.3 | 2.3 | 2.3 | 14.9 | 27.1 | 31.0 | 31.0 | 31.0 |
| 4.7 | Analgesics | 3.5 | 3.9 | 4.1 | 4.1 | 4.1 | 11.2 | 19.0 | 24.4 | 24.4 | 24.4 |
| 5 | Infections | 3.3 | 2.9 | 2.8 | 2.9 | 2.9 | 14.6 | 15.3 | 15.8 | 15.2 | 15.1 |
| 5.1 | Antibacterial drugs | 3.0 | 2.6 | 2.5 | 2.5 | 2.5 | 11.6 | 11.6 | 11.5 | 11.5 | 11.5 |
| 6 | Endocrine system | 2.1 | 3.2 | 4.1 | 4.5 | 4.8 | 21.5 | 37.9 | 51.8 | 54.9 | 58.9 |
| 6.1 | Drugs used in diabetes | 0.8 | 1.3 | 1.8 | 1.8 | 1.8 | 8.8 | 17.9 | 29.5 | 29.5 | 29.5 |
| 6.4 | Sex hormones | 0.4 | 0.5 | 0.4 | 0.4 | 0.4 | 8.0 | 10.5 | 7.4 | 7.4 | 7.4 |
| 7 | Obstetrics and gynaecology[1] | 0.7 | 0.9 | 1.1 | 1.1 | 1.2 | 4.8 | 10.6 | 15.4 | 16.5 | 16.5 |
| 7.3 | Contraceptives | 0.5 | 0.5 | 0.5 | 0.5 | 0.5 | 2.2 | 3.0 | 3.9 | 3.9 | 3.9 |
| 8 | Malignant disease[2] | 0.2 | 0.3 | 0.3 | 0.3 | 0.3 | 8.8 | 14.7 | 19.5 | 17.9 | 20.0 |
| 8.3 | Sex hormones and antagonists | 0.1 | 0.1 | 0.1 | 0.1 | 0.1 | 5.4 | 9.8 | 13.7 | 13.7 | 13.7 |
| 9 | Nutrition and blood | 1.0 | 1.3 | 1.7 | 1.9 | 2.1 | 8.5 | 15.1 | 21.1 | 23.0 | 25.8 |
| 9.4 | Oral nutrition | 0.2 | 0.2 | 0.3 | 0.3 | 0.3 | 5.4 | 8.9 | 10.6 | 10.6 | 10.6 |
| 10 | Musculo-skeletal and joint disease | 2.0 | 2.2 | 2.3 | 2.2 | 2.2 | 15.4 | 19.1 | 23.1 | 16.4 | 15.9 |
| 10.1 | Rheumatic diseases and gout | 1.5 | 1.8 | 1.9 | 1.9 | 1.9 | 12.7 | 16.3 | 20.2 | 20.2 | 20.2 |
| 11 | Eye preparations | 0.9 | 1.0 | 1.1 | 1.2 | 1.2 | 3.6 | 6.3 | 8.0 | 8.4 | 9.1 |
| 12 | Ear, nose and oropharynx | 0.6 | 0.7 | 0.7 | 0.7 | 0.7 | 2.7 | 3.6 | 4.2 | 4.1 | 4.6 |
| 13 | Skin | 2.4 | 2.5 | 2.4 | 2.3 | 2.3 | 11.5 | 13.0 | 14.4 | 14.2 | 14.6 |
| 13.4 | Topical corticosteroids | 0.7 | 0.8 | 0.8 | 0.8 | 0.8 | 2.4 | 3.1 | 3.2 | 3.2 | 3.2 |
| 14 | Immunological products | 0.6 | 0.7 | 0.7 | 0.9 | 0.7 | 4.6 | 5.5 | 6.2 | 7.8 | 6.8 |
| 14.4 | Vaccines and antisera | 0.6 | 0.7 | 0.7 | 0.7 | 0.7 | 4.5 | 5.5 | 6.1 | 6.1 | 6.1 |
| 15 | Anaesthesia | 0.0 | 0.1 | 0.1 | 0.1 | 0.1 | 0.1 | 0.2 | 0.4 | 0.5 | 0.7 |
| | Others including dressings and appliances | 1.2 | 1.3 | 1.4 | 1.5 | 1.6 | 16.4 | 20.2 | 25.9 | 28.0 | 30.8 |

Notes:  All figures are based on the British National Formulary (BNF). Figures below the BNF heading relate to chapters and sub-sections of the BNF. Figures relate to prescriptions dispensed by community pharmacists and appliances contractors who are contracted to the NHS, dispensing doctors and personal administration.
1 Including urinary tract disorders.
2 Including immunosuppression.

Source:  Prescription Cost Analysis, Wales (HOWIS).

Table 4.34    **Number and net ingredient cost (NIC) of prescriptions by therapeutic group, Scotland, 1996 - 2006**

| BNF | Therapeutic group | Prescription items (millions): | | | | | NIC of prescriptions (£m): | | | | |
|---|---|---|---|---|---|---|---|---|---|---|---|
| | | 1996 | 2001 | 2004 | 2005 | 2006 | 1996 | 2001 | 2004 | 2005 | 2006 |
| | Total | 53.7 | 64.5 | 73.4 | 76.2 | 78.8 | 464.4 | 704.4 | 925.2 | 951.6 | 967.0 |
| 1 | Gastro-intestinal system | 5.2 | 6.1 | 6.6 | 6.8 | 7.0 | 90.3 | 92.4 | 95.5 | 101.6 | 83.8 |
| 1.3 | Ulcer-healing drugs | 2.3 | 2.9 | 3.5 | 3.7 | 3.9 | 72.1 | 71.6 | 73.4 | 78.1 | 57.6 |
| 1.6 | Laxatives | 1.2 | 1.4 | 1.4 | 1.5 | 1.5 | 4.9 | 5.3 | 5.4 | 6.0 | 7.0 |
| 2 | Cardiovascular system | 10.3 | 15.7 | 20.0 | 21.4 | 22.6 | 83.3 | 169.6 | 230.5 | 223.0 | 213.3 |
| 2.2 | Diuretics | 2.7 | 3.3 | 3.8 | 3.9 | 3.9 | 5.5 | 7.2 | 6.5 | 7.5 | 10.0 |
| 2.4 | Beta-adrenoceptor blocking drugs | 1.7 | 2.4 | 2.9 | 3.0 | 3.0 | 8.7 | 9.9 | 11.2 | 11.8 | 12.2 |
| 2.5 | Anti-hypertensive therapy | 1.0 | 2.0 | 3.1 | 3.5 | 3.9 | 20.3 | 37.7 | 56.7 | 54.6 | 50.4 |
| 2.6 | Nitrates/calcium channel blockers | 2.8 | 3.2 | 3.4 | 3.5 | 3.6 | 35.5 | 46.3 | 48.5 | 45.1 | 37.0 |
| 2.12 | Lipid lowering drugs | 0.3 | 1.5 | 2.7 | 3.3 | 3.8 | 10.8 | 56.3 | 82.0 | 74.6 | 70.6 |
| 3 | Respiratory system | 4.9 | 5.4 | 5.6 | 5.7 | 5.8 | 54.7 | 76.1 | 92.4 | 96.9 | 103.0 |
| 3.1 | Bronchodilators | 2.6 | 2.8 | 2.8 | 2.8 | 2.8 | 21.5 | 28.6 | 32.4 | 33.5 | 35.2 |
| 3.2 | Corticosteroids (inhaled) | 1.1 | 1.4 | 1.4 | 1.5 | 1.5 | 27.0 | 36.2 | 47.0 | 49.9 | 53.7 |
| 4 | Central nervous system | 10.8 | 13.5 | 15.0 | 15.3 | 15.7 | 68.4 | 139.2 | 193.1 | 208.1 | 217.0 |
| 4.2 | Drugs used in psychoses & related disorders | 0.5 | 0.6 | 0.6 | 0.6 | 0.7 | 3.5 | 14.5 | 23.6 | 24.9 | 27.9 |
| 4.3 | Antidepressant drugs | 1.7 | 2.8 | 3.4 | 3.5 | 3.6 | 26.5 | 48.0 | 58.6 | 55.9 | 46.5 |
| 4.7 | Analgesics | 5.0 | 5.8 | 6.3 | 6.4 | 6.5 | 20.8 | 34.6 | 44.7 | 52.6 | 60.0 |
| 5 | Infections | 5.7 | 4.7 | 4.7 | 4.7 | 4.8 | 27.9 | 26.4 | 29.7 | 30.2 | 28.8 |
| 5.1 | Antibacterial drugs | 5.3 | 4.2 | 4.1 | 4.1 | 4.2 | 21.1 | 20.9 | 20.4 | 20.9 | 21.6 |
| 6 | Endocrine system | 3.0 | 4.3 | 5.2 | 5.5 | 5.9 | 36.9 | 63.5 | 80.2 | 86.5 | 91.7 |
| 6.1 | Drugs used in diabetes | 0.9 | 1.6 | 2.1 | 2.2 | 2.4 | 13.1 | 27.4 | 42.5 | 48.1 | 54.3 |
| 6.4 | Sex hormones | 0.7 | 0.7 | 0.6 | 0.5 | 0.5 | 15.1 | 19.0 | 13.2 | 10.8 | 10.2 |
| 7 | Obstetrics and gynaecology[1] | 1.3 | 1.5 | 1.6 | 1.7 | 1.8 | 8.9 | 20.7 | 28.3 | 30.5 | 31.2 |
| 7.3 | Contraceptives | 0.9 | 0.8 | 0.8 | 0.8 | 0.8 | 4.6 | 5.4 | 6.5 | 6.7 | 6.9 |
| 8 | Malignant disease[2] | 0.3 | 0.3 | 0.4 | 0.3 | 0.3 | 12.1 | 22.7 | 27.7 | 26.8 | 28.9 |
| 8.3 | Sex hormones and antagonists | 0.2 | 0.2 | 0.2 | 0.2 | 0.2 | 7.3 | 13.8 | 17.4 | 17.7 | 19.8 |
| 9 | Nutrition and blood | 1.4 | 1.7 | 2.2 | 2.4 | 2.6 | 12.3 | 20.3 | 25.8 | 29.4 | 34.1 |
| 9.4 | Oral nutrition | 0.3 | 0.4 | 0.5 | 0.5 | 0.5 | 8.5 | 13.4 | 14.6 | 16.1 | 17.3 |
| 10 | Musculo-skeletal and joint disease | 2.9 | 3.0 | 3.3 | 3.3 | 3.1 | 23.8 | 30.1 | 39.1 | 29.2 | 26.2 |
| 10.1 | Rheumatic diseases and gout | 2.3 | 2.5 | 2.8 | 2.8 | 2.5 | 20.1 | 26.5 | 34.6 | 24.8 | 21.8 |
| 11 | Eye preparations | 1.1 | 1.3 | 1.4 | 1.4 | 1.5 | 4.6 | 7.5 | 8.8 | 9.2 | 10.1 |
| 12 | Ear, nose and oropharynx | 1.0 | 1.0 | 1.1 | 1.1 | 1.1 | 5.4 | 6.3 | 6.9 | 6.7 | 7.1 |
| 13 | Skin | 3.9 | 4.1 | 4.1 | 4.1 | 4.1 | 21.2 | 25.9 | 26.4 | 26.4 | 27.8 |
| 13.4 | Topical corticosteroids | 1.5 | 1.5 | 1.5 | 1.5 | 1.5 | 5.1 | 5.9 | 6.5 | 6.6 | 8.0 |
| 14 | Immunological products | 0.3 | 0.2 | 0.2 | 0.2 | 0.2 | 5.9 | 7.7 | 10.2 | 9.7 | 9.4 |
| 14.4 | Vaccines and antisera | 0.3 | 0.2 | 0.2 | 0.2 | 0.2 | 5.9 | 7.7 | 10.2 | 9.7 | 9.4 |
| 15 | Anaesthesia | 0.0 | 0.0 | 0.0 | 0.0 | 0.0 | 0.2 | 0.3 | 0.4 | 0.4 | 0.4 |
| | Others including dressings and appliances | 1.6 | 1.7 | 1.8 | 1.8 | 1.4 | 28.5 | 33.3 | 38.4 | 40.4 | 43.8 |

*Notes:*    All figures are based on the British National Formulary (BNF).  Figures below the BNF heading relate to chapters and sub-sections of the BNF.
Figures relate to prescriptions dispensed by community pharmacists and appliances contractors who are contracted to the NHS, dispensing
doctors and personal administration.
1 Including urinary tract disorders.
2 Including immunosuppression.
0.0 non zero but <0.05.

*Source:*  Prescription Cost Analysis, Scotland (ISD).

Table 4.35   Number and net ingredient cost (NIC) of prescriptions by therapeutic group, Northern Ireland, 1996 - 2006

| BNF | Therapeutic group | Prescription items (millions): | | | | | NIC of prescriptions (£m): | | | | |
|---|---|---|---|---|---|---|---|---|---|---|---|
| | | 1996 | 2001 | 2004 | 2005 | 2006 | 1996 | 2001 | 2004 | 2005 | 2006 |
| | Total | 21.1 | 24.3 | 27.1 | 27.7 | 28.8 | 195.8 | 267.8 | 365.4 | 360.9 | 373.3 |
| 1 | Gastro-intestinal system | 2.1 | 2.3 | 2.5 | 2.6 | 2.6 | 36.5 | 33.3 | 36.1 | 36.5 | 31.6 |
| 1.3 | Ulcer-healing drugs | 0.8 | 1.0 | 1.2 | 1.3 | 1.4 | 29.3 | 25.9 | 27.8 | 28.4 | 22.7 |
| 1.6 | Laxatives | 0.5 | 0.5 | 0.5 | 0.5 | 0.5 | 2.1 | 2.1 | 2.1 | 2.1 | 2.5 |
| 2 | Cardiovascular system | 2.8 | 4.6 | 6.0 | 6.4 | 6.8 | 31.7 | 59.3 | 90.6 | 85.5 | 85.6 |
| 2.2 | Diuretics | 0.6 | 0.9 | 1.0 | 1.0 | 1.0 | 2.0 | 2.3 | 2.0 | 2.0 | 2.9 |
| 2.4 | Beta-adrenoceptor blocking drugs | 0.5 | 0.7 | 0.9 | 0.9 | 0.9 | 4.2 | 6.0 | 6.9 | 6.8 | 6.2 |
| 2.5 | Anti-hypertensive therapy | 0.3 | 0.7 | 1.0 | 1.1 | 1.2 | 6.9 | 13.7 | 21.4 | 19.6 | 18.7 |
| 2.6 | Nitrates/calcium channel blockers | 0.8 | 1.0 | 1.0 | 1.0 | 1.0 | 12.9 | 14.7 | 16.1 | 15.1 | 13.4 |
| 2.12 | Lipid lowering drugs | 0.1 | 0.5 | 0.9 | 1.0 | 1.2 | 4.2 | 17.3 | 32.9 | 30.0 | 31.4 |
| 3 | Respiratory system | 2.2 | 2.2 | 2.2 | 2.2 | 2.3 | 24.8 | 28.1 | 33.7 | 34.8 | 37.7 |
| 3.1 | Bronchodilators | 1.0 | 1.0 | 1.0 | 1.0 | 1.0 | 9.2 | 10.5 | 10.5 | 10.6 | 11.2 |
| 3.2 | Corticosteroids (inhaled) | 0.4 | 0.4 | 0.5 | 0.5 | 0.5 | 12.4 | 13.1 | 17.8 | 18.6 | 20.2 |
| 4 | Central nervous system | 4.7 | 6.0 | 6.4 | 6.5 | 6.7 | 28.0 | 53.5 | 75.6 | 78.7 | 84.3 |
| 4.2 | Drugs used in psychoses & related disorders | 0.3 | 0.3 | 0.3 | 0.4 | 0.4 | 1.7 | 6.8 | 11.6 | 11.9 | 13.3 |
| 4.3 | Antidepressant drugs | 0.6 | 1.1 | 1.3 | 1.4 | 1.4 | 10.7 | 18.7 | 25.0 | 23.4 | 20.4 |
| 4.7 | Analgesics | 2.3 | 2.5 | 2.4 | 2.5 | 2.5 | 8.6 | 12.0 | 14.0 | 15.2 | 18.4 |
| 5 | Infections | 2.5 | 2.0 | 1.9 | 2.0 | 2.0 | 11.6 | 10.6 | 11.2 | 10.5 | 11.0 |
| 5.1 | Antibacterial drugs | 2.3 | 1.9 | 1.7 | 1.7 | 1.8 | 9.5 | 8.2 | 8.4 | 7.7 | 8.2 |
| 6 | Endocrine system | 0.8 | 1.3 | 1.7 | 1.8 | 2.0 | 11.0 | 19.8 | 28.9 | 31.1 | 35.0 |
| 6.1 | Drugs used in diabetes | 0.2 | 0.5 | 0.8 | 0.8 | 0.9 | 3.2 | 9.3 | 16.2 | 18.4 | 21.1 |
| 6.4 | Sex hormones | 0.2 | 0.2 | 0.2 | 0.2 | 0.2 | 4.7 | 5.4 | 4.2 | 3.5 | 3.4 |
| 7 | Obstetrics and gynaecology[1] | 0.4 | 0.5 | 0.6 | 0.6 | 0.6 | 3.1 | 6.5 | 9.5 | 10.0 | 10.7 |
| 7.3 | Contraceptives | 0.3 | 0.3 | 0.3 | 0.3 | 0.3 | 1.3 | 1.6 | 2.3 | 2.4 | 2.7 |
| 8 | Malignant disease[2] | 0.1 | 0.1 | 0.1 | 0.1 | 0.1 | 4.9 | 7.6 | 10.3 | 9.5 | 10.5 |
| 8.3 | Sex hormones and antagonists | 0.0 | 0.0 | 0.1 | 0.1 | 0.1 | 3.1 | 5.1 | 7.0 | 6.8 | 7.7 |
| 9 | Nutrition and blood | 0.8 | 0.8 | 0.9 | 1.0 | 1.1 | 6.7 | 9.1 | 13.3 | 13.6 | 15.8 |
| 9.4 | Oral nutrition | 0.2 | 0.2 | 0.3 | 0.3 | 0.3 | 4.8 | 6.9 | 10.0 | 10.4 | 12.1 |
| 10 | Musculo-skeletal and joint disease | 1.0 | 1.1 | 1.3 | 1.2 | 1.2 | 9.9 | 12.6 | 18.7 | 12.4 | 12.1 |
| 10.1 | Rheumatic diseases and gout | 0.7 | 0.9 | 1.0 | 0.9 | 0.9 | 8.0 | 10.7 | 16.5 | 10.2 | 9.9 |
| 11 | Eye preparations | 0.4 | 0.4 | 0.4 | 0.5 | 0.5 | 1.5 | 2.1 | 2.6 | 2.7 | 3.0 |
| 12 | Ear, nose and oropharynx | 0.5 | 0.4 | 0.4 | 0.4 | 0.4 | 1.9 | 1.8 | 2.2 | 2.0 | 2.1 |
| 13 | Skin | 2.0 | 1.8 | 1.7 | 1.7 | 1.7 | 11.0 | 11.7 | 11.2 | 10.9 | 11.5 |
| 13.4 | Topical corticosteroids | 0.5 | 0.5 | 0.5 | 0.5 | 0.5 | 1.7 | 1.8 | 2.0 | 1.9 | 2.2 |
| 14 | Immunological products | 0.1 | 0.1 | 0.0 | 0.1 | 0.1 | 1.4 | 2.9 | 2.1 | 2.7 | 1.7 |
| 14.4 | Vaccines and antisera | 0.1 | 0.1 | 0.0 | 0.1 | 0.1 | 1.4 | 2.8 | 2.0 | 2.7 | 1.7 |
| 15 | Anaesthesia | 0.0 | 0.0 | 0.0 | 0.0 | 0.0 | 0.1 | 0.1 | 0.1 | 0.1 | 0.2 |
| | Others including dressings and appliances | 0.8 | 0.5 | 0.6 | 0.6 | 0.6 | 11.9 | 8.7 | 13.0 | 13.7 | 14.9 |

Notes:   All figures are based on the British National Formulary (BNF). Figures below the BNF heading relate to chapters and sub-sections of the BNF. Figures relate to prescriptions dispensed by community pharmacists and appliances contractors who are contracted to the NHS, dispensing doctors and personal administration.
1 Including urinary tract disorders.
2 Including immunosuppression.

Source:   Prescription Cost Analysis, Northern Ireland (CSA).

Table 4.36  **Percentage of total number and net ingredient cost (NIC) of prescriptions by therapeutic group, UK, 1996 - 2006**

| BNF | Therapeutic group | Prescription items (millions): | | | | | NIC of prescriptions (£m): | | | | |
|---|---|---|---|---|---|---|---|---|---|---|---|
| | | 1996 | 2001 | 2004 | 2005 | 2006 | 1996 | 2001 | 2004 | 2005 | 2006 |
| | Total | 597 | 722 | 841 | 881 | 919 | 4,956 | 7,533 | 9,947 | 9,809 | 10,111 |
| | | | | | | Percentage of annual total | | | | | |
| 1 | **Gastro-intestinal system** | 8.4 | 7.9 | 7.7 | 7.6 | 7.7 | 15.1 | 10.0 | 8.3 | 8.6 | 7.1 |
| 1.3 | Ulcer-healing drugs | 2.9 | 3.4 | 3.7 | 3.9 | 4.0 | 11.3 | 7.3 | 6.1 | 6.2 | 4.6 |
| 1.6 | Laxatives | 2.3 | 2.1 | 1.9 | 1.8 | 1.8 | 1.1 | 0.7 | 0.6 | 0.6 | 0.7 |
| 2 | **Cardiovascular system** | 18.8 | 24.6 | 28.9 | 30.0 | 30.9 | 18.4 | 23.9 | 26.4 | 23.6 | 22.9 |
| 2.2 | Diuretics | 4.8 | 5.1 | 5.3 | 5.2 | 4.9 | 1.3 | 1.0 | 0.8 | 0.9 | 1.0 |
| 2.4 | Beta-adrenoceptor blocking drugs | 3.0 | 3.5 | 3.8 | 3.8 | 3.6 | 2.0 | 1.4 | 1.2 | 1.2 | 1.3 |
| 2.5 | Anti-hypertensive therapy | 2.4 | 4.1 | 5.5 | 5.7 | 6.1 | 5.4 | 6.6 | 7.3 | 6.1 | 6.0 |
| 2.6 | Nitrates/calcium channel blockers | 4.6 | 4.6 | 4.5 | 4.5 | 4.6 | 6.9 | 6.0 | 5.1 | 4.7 | 3.9 |
| 2.12 | Lipid lowering drugs | 0.6 | 2.3 | 4.2 | 4.8 | 5.4 | 2.3 | 7.2 | 9.4 | 8.0 | 7.7 |
| 3 | **Respiratory system** | 9.6 | 8.5 | 7.4 | 7.3 | 7.0 | 12.2 | 10.6 | 9.7 | 10.2 | 10.3 |
| 3.1 | Bronchodilators | 4.8 | 4.3 | 3.6 | 3.5 | 3.3 | 4.7 | 3.9 | 3.2 | 3.3 | 3.3 |
| 3.2 | Corticosteroids (inhaled) | 2.2 | 2.1 | 2.0 | 2.0 | 1.9 | 6.0 | 5.1 | 5.1 | 5.5 | 5.7 |
| 4 | **Central nervous system** | 18.8 | 19.1 | 18.3 | 17.8 | 17.7 | 13.4 | 17.4 | 18.2 | 19.1 | 19.8 |
| 4.2 | Drugs used in psychoses & related disorders | 1.0 | 1.0 | 1.0 | 0.9 | 1.0 | 0.8 | 2.2 | 2.7 | 2.8 | 3.0 |
| 4.3 | Antidepressant drugs | 3.1 | 4.2 | 4.3 | 4.1 | 4.2 | 4.9 | 5.8 | 5.2 | 4.6 | 3.9 |
| 4.7 | Analgesics | 8.4 | 7.8 | 7.1 | 6.9 | 6.8 | 3.9 | 4.0 | 3.8 | 4.6 | 5.5 |
| 5 | **Infections** | 10.5 | 7.2 | 6.1 | 5.9 | 5.7 | 5.6 | 3.6 | 3.0 | 2.9 | 2.8 |
| 5.1 | Antibacterial drugs | 9.6 | 6.4 | 5.3 | 5.2 | 5.0 | 4.4 | 2.7 | 2.1 | 2.1 | 2.1 |
| 6 | **Endocrine system** | 6.0 | 7.3 | 7.8 | 7.9 | 8.2 | 8.2 | 9.3 | 9.4 | 10.1 | 10.6 |
| 6.1 | Drugs used in diabetes | 2.1 | 3.0 | 3.5 | 3.6 | 3.6 | 3.0 | 4.4 | 5.4 | 6.0 | 6.6 |
| 6.4 | Sex hormones | 1.4 | 1.3 | 0.8 | 0.7 | 0.7 | 3.2 | 2.7 | 1.4 | 1.2 | 1.1 |
| 7 | **Obstetrics and gynaecology[1]** | 2.5 | 2.4 | 2.3 | 2.3 | 2.3 | 1.9 | 2.6 | 2.9 | 3.1 | 3.1 |
| 7.3 | Contraceptives | 1.7 | 1.4 | 1.2 | 1.2 | 1.1 | 1.0 | 0.8 | 0.8 | 0.8 | 0.8 |
| 8 | **Malignant disease[2]** | 0.5 | 0.6 | 0.6 | 0.4 | 0.4 | 2.9 | 3.4 | 3.5 | 3.3 | 3.6 |
| 8.3 | Sex hormones and antagonists | 0.3 | 0.3 | 0.3 | 0.3 | 0.3 | 1.8 | 2.2 | 2.4 | 2.3 | 2.4 |
| 9 | **Nutrition and blood** | 2.7 | 2.8 | 3.1 | 3.2 | 3.5 | 3.0 | 3.5 | 3.6 | 4.0 | 4.4 |
| 9.4 | Oral nutrition | 0.5 | 0.6 | 0.6 | 0.6 | 1.0 | 1.9 | 2.0 | 2.0 | 2.2 | 2.4 |
| 10 | **Musculo-skeletal and joint disease** | 5.3 | 4.7 | 4.4 | 4.0 | 3.8 | 5.0 | 3.9 | 3.9 | 2.8 | 2.7 |
| 10.1 | Rheumatic diseases and gout | 4.2 | 3.8 | 3.6 | 3.3 | 3.1 | 4.2 | 3.3 | 3.4 | 2.4 | 2.2 |
| 11 | **Eye preparations** | 2.4 | 2.3 | 2.2 | 2.2 | 2.1 | 1.2 | 1.4 | 1.3 | 1.4 | 1.5 |
| 12 | **Ear, nose and oropharynx** | 1.9 | 1.6 | 1.4 | 1.3 | 1.3 | 1.1 | 0.8 | 0.7 | 0.7 | 0.8 |
| 13 | **Skin** | 7.2 | 6.0 | 5.1 | 4.9 | 4.7 | 4.3 | 3.1 | 2.6 | 2.7 | 2.7 |
| 13.4 | Topical corticosteroids | 2.6 | 2.1 | 1.8 | 1.7 | 1.6 | 1.0 | 0.7 | 0.6 | 0.6 | 0.7 |
| 14 | **Immunological products** | 2.0 | 1.9 | 1.8 | 2.0 | 1.6 | 2.0 | 1.7 | 1.5 | 1.7 | 1.5 |
| 14.4 | Vaccines and antisera | 1.9 | 1.9 | 1.7 | 1.9 | 1.6 | 2.0 | 1.6 | 1.4 | 1.7 | 1.4 |
| 15 | **Anaesthesia** | 0.1 | 0.1 | 0.1 | 0.1 | 0.1 | 0.0 | 0.0 | 0.0 | 0.0 | 0.1 |
| | **Others including dressings and appliances** | 3.3 | 3.0 | 2.8 | 2.9 | 3.0 | 5.9 | 5.2 | 5.1 | 5.7 | 6.1 |

*Notes:*  All figures are based on the British National Formulary (BNF).  Figures below the BNF heading relate to chapters and sub-sections of the BNF.
Figures relate to prescriptions dispensed by community pharmacists and appliances contractors who are contracted to the NHS, dispensing doctors and personal administration.
1 Including urinary tract disorders.
2 Including immunosuppression.
0.0 non zero but <0.05.

*Sources:*  Prescription Cost Analysis, England (DH).
Prescription Cost Analysis, Wales (HOWIS).
Prescription Cost Analysis, Scotland (ISD).
Prescription Cost Analysis, Northern Ireland (CSA).

Table 4.37 **Percentage of total number and net ingredient cost (NIC) of prescriptions by therapeutic group, England 1996 - 2006**

| BNF | Therapeutic group | Prescription items (millions): | | | | | NIC of prescriptions (£m): | | | | |
|---|---|---|---|---|---|---|---|---|---|---|---|
| | | 1996 | 2001 | 2004 | 2005 | 2006 | 1996 | 2001 | 2004 | 2005 | 2006 |
| | Total | 485 | 587 | 686 | 720 | 752 | 4,007 | 6,117 | 8,080 | 7,937 | 8,197 |
| | | Percentage of annual total | | | | | | | | | |
| 1 | **Gastro-intestinal system** | 8.1 | 7.7 | 7.5 | 7.4 | 7.5 | 14.4 | 9.6 | 8.0 | 8.3 | 6.9 |
| 1.3 | *Ulcer-healing drugs* | 2.8 | 3.2 | 3.6 | 3.7 | 3.9 | 10.7 | 6.8 | 5.8 | 5.9 | 4.3 |
| 1.6 | *Laxatives* | 2.3 | 2.1 | 1.9 | 1.9 | 1.8 | 1.1 | 0.7 | 0.6 | 0.6 | 0.7 |
| 2 | **Cardiovascular system** | 18.8 | 24.7 | 29.2 | 30.3 | 31.2 | 18.5 | 23.9 | 26.6 | 23.6 | 23.0 |
| 2.2 | *Diuretics* | 4.8 | 5.1 | 5.3 | 5.2 | 5.0 | 1.3 | 1.0 | 0.8 | 1.0 | 1.1 |
| 2.4 | *Beta-adrenoceptor blocking drugs* | 3.0 | 3.5 | 3.8 | 3.8 | 3.6 | 2.0 | 1.3 | 1.2 | 1.2 | 1.2 |
| 2.5 | *Anti-hypertensive therapy* | 2.5 | 4.3 | 5.6 | 6.0 | 6.3 | 5.6 | 6.9 | 7.6 | 6.1 | 6.1 |
| 2.6 | *Nitrates/calcium channel blockers* | 4.5 | 4.6 | 4.5 | 4.5 | 4.6 | 6.7 | 6.0 | 5.1 | 4.6 | 3.8 |
| 2.12 | *Lipid lowering drugs* | 0.6 | 2.3 | 4.3 | 4.9 | 5.6 | 2.3 | 7.2 | 9.5 | 7.9 | 7.6 |
| 3 | **Respiratory system** | 9.6 | 8.5 | 7.4 | 7.2 | 7.0 | 12.1 | 10.5 | 9.6 | 10.1 | 10.2 |
| 3.1 | *Bronchodilators* | 4.7 | 4.2 | 3.6 | 3.5 | 3.3 | 4.6 | 3.9 | 3.1 | 3.3 | 3.2 |
| 3.2 | *Corticosteroids (inhaled)* | 2.3 | 2.1 | 2.0 | 2.0 | 1.9 | 6.0 | 5.0 | 5.1 | 5.5 | 5.8 |
| 4 | **Central nervous system** | 18.4 | 18.6 | 17.8 | 17.3 | 17.2 | 13.2 | 16.9 | 17.7 | 18.6 | 19.3 |
| 4.2 | *Drugs used in psychoses & related disorders* | 1.0 | 1.0 | 1.0 | 1.0 | 1.0 | 0.8 | 2.2 | 2.7 | 2.8 | 3.0 |
| 4.3 | *Antidepressant drugs* | 3.1 | 4.1 | 4.2 | 4.1 | 4.1 | 4.8 | 5.6 | 5.0 | 4.3 | 3.6 |
| 4.7 | *Analgesics* | 8.1 | 7.5 | 6.8 | 6.6 | 6.6 | 3.8 | 3.8 | 3.7 | 4.5 | 5.5 |
| 5 | **Infections** | 10.5 | 7.2 | 6.1 | 5.9 | 5.7 | 5.6 | 3.6 | 3.0 | 2.9 | 2.8 |
| 5.1 | *Antibacterial drugs* | 9.6 | 6.5 | 5.3 | 5.2 | 4.9 | 4.4 | 2.7 | 2.1 | 2.0 | 2.1 |
| 6 | **Endocrine system** | 6.1 | 7.5 | 7.9 | 8.1 | 8.3 | 8.4 | 9.5 | 9.6 | 10.4 | 10.9 |
| 6.1 | *Drugs used in diabetes* | 2.2 | 3.1 | 3.6 | 3.7 | 3.8 | 3.1 | 4.6 | 5.6 | 6.2 | 6.9 |
| 6.4 | *Sex hormones* | 1.4 | 1.3 | 0.8 | 0.7 | 0.7 | 3.2 | 2.7 | 1.4 | 1.2 | 1.1 |
| 7 | **Obstetrics and gynaecology**[1] | 2.5 | 2.4 | 2.4 | 2.3 | 2.3 | 1.9 | 2.6 | 2.9 | 3.1 | 3.1 |
| 7.3 | *Contraceptives* | 1.8 | 1.5 | 1.3 | 1.2 | 1.2 | 1.0 | 0.8 | 0.8 | 0.8 | 0.9 |
| 8 | **Malignant disease**[2] | 0.5 | 0.6 | 0.6 | 0.4 | 0.4 | 2.9 | 3.5 | 3.6 | 3.4 | 3.7 |
| 8.3 | *Sex hormones and antagonists* | 0.3 | 0.3 | 0.3 | 0.3 | 0.3 | 1.8 | 2.3 | 2.4 | 2.4 | 2.5 |
| 9 | **Nutrition and blood** | 2.7 | 2.7 | 3.1 | 3.2 | 3.5 | 3.1 | 3.5 | 3.6 | 4.1 | 4.5 |
| 9.4 | *Oral nutrition* | 0.5 | 0.6 | 0.6 | 0.6 | 1.0 | 1.9 | 2.0 | 2.0 | 2.2 | 2.4 |
| 10 | **Musculo-skeletal and joint disease** | 5.3 | 4.7 | 4.3 | 4.0 | 3.8 | 5.0 | 3.8 | 3.8 | 2.7 | 2.6 |
| 10.1 | *Rheumatic diseases and gout* | 4.2 | 3.8 | 3.6 | 3.2 | 3.0 | 4.1 | 3.2 | 3.3 | 2.2 | 2.1 |
| 11 | **Eye preparations** | 2.5 | 2.4 | 2.3 | 2.2 | 2.2 | 1.3 | 1.5 | 1.4 | 1.5 | 1.6 |
| 12 | **Ear, nose and oropharynx** | 1.9 | 1.6 | 1.4 | 1.3 | 1.3 | 1.1 | 0.8 | 0.7 | 0.7 | 0.8 |
| 13 | **Skin** | 7.2 | 5.9 | 5.1 | 4.9 | 4.6 | 4.3 | 3.0 | 2.6 | 2.7 | 2.7 |
| 13.4 | *Topical corticosteroids* | 2.6 | 2.2 | 1.8 | 1.7 | 1.6 | 1.0 | 0.7 | 0.6 | 0.6 | 0.7 |
| 14 | **Immunological products** | 2.2 | 2.2 | 2.0 | 2.2 | 1.8 | 2.2 | 1.8 | 1.6 | 1.8 | 1.6 |
| 14.4 | *Vaccines and antisera* | 2.2 | 2.2 | 2.0 | 2.2 | 1.8 | 2.1 | 1.7 | 1.5 | 1.8 | 1.5 |
| 15 | **Anaesthesia** | 0.2 | 0.1 | 0.1 | 0.1 | 0.1 | 0.0 | 0.0 | 0.0 | 0.0 | 0.1 |
| | **Others including dressings and appliances** | 3.3 | 3.0 | 2.9 | 3.0 | 3.1 | 5.9 | 5.4 | 5.3 | 6.0 | 6.5 |

*Notes:* All figures are based on the British National Formulary (BNF). Figures below the BNF heading relate to chapters and sub-sections of the BNF. Figures relate to prescriptions dispensed by community pharmacists and appliances contractors who are contracted to the NHS, dispensing doctors and personal administration.
1 Including urinary tract disorders.
2 Including immunosuppression.
0.0 non zero but <0.05.

*Source:* Prescription Cost Analysis, England (DH).

Table 4.38 **Percentage of total number and net ingredient cost (NIC) of prescriptions by therapeutic group, Wales, 1996 - 2006**

| BNF | Therapeutic group | Prescription items (millions): | | | | | NIC of prescriptions (£m): | | | | |
|---|---|---|---|---|---|---|---|---|---|---|---|
| | | 1996 | 2001 | 2004 | 2005 | 2006 | 1996 | 2001 | 2004 | 2005 | 2006 |
| | Total | 37 | 46 | 54 | 57 | 59 | 288 | 444 | 577 | 560 | 574 |
| | | | | | | Percentage of annual total | | | | | |
| 1 | **Gastro-intestinal system** | **8.3** | **7.9** | **7.6** | **7.6** | **7.6** | **15.0** | **10.1** | **8.3** | **8.6** | **7.1** |
| 1.3 | Ulcer-healing drugs | 3.0 | 3.6 | 3.9 | 3.7 | 3.6 | 11.5 | 7.6 | 6.2 | 6.4 | 6.2 |
| 1.6 | Laxatives | 2.0 | 1.8 | 1.6 | 1.6 | 1.5 | 1.0 | 0.7 | 0.5 | 0.5 | 0.5 |
| 2 | **Cardiovascular system** | **20.9** | **25.9** | **30.9** | **31.9** | **32.8** | **19.2** | **23.5** | **26.4** | **23.2** | **22.7** |
| 2.2 | Diuretics | 5.3 | 5.3 | 5.5 | 5.3 | 5.1 | 1.4 | 1.0 | 0.8 | 0.8 | 0.8 |
| 2.4 | Beta-adrenoceptor blocking drugs | 3.0 | 3.3 | 3.7 | 3.5 | 3.4 | 1.9 | 1.3 | 1.2 | 1.2 | 1.2 |
| 2.5 | Anti-hypertensive therapy | 2.7 | 4.4 | 5.8 | 5.5 | 5.3 | 5.4 | 6.5 | 7.0 | 7.2 | 7.1 |
| 2.6 | Nitrates/calcium channel blockers | 5.2 | 5.0 | 4.8 | 4.6 | 4.4 | 8.2 | 6.1 | 5.1 | 5.3 | 5.1 |
| 2.12 | Lipid lowering drugs | 0.7 | 2.4 | 4.8 | 4.5 | 4.4 | 2.0 | 7.0 | 9.7 | 10.0 | 9.7 |
| 3 | **Respiratory system** | **9.5** | **8.4** | **7.3** | **7.2** | **6.9** | **13.0** | **11.8** | **10.9** | **11.6** | **11.8** |
| 3.1 | Bronchodilators | 4.9 | 4.3 | 3.7 | 3.5 | 3.4 | 5.2 | 4.4 | 3.6 | 3.7 | 3.6 |
| 3.2 | Corticosteroids (inhaled) | 2.1 | 2.1 | 2.0 | 1.9 | 1.8 | 6.3 | 5.9 | 5.9 | 6.1 | 5.9 |
| 4 | **Central nervous system** | **20.5** | **20.9** | **19.4** | **18.9** | **18.7** | **13.9** | **18.2** | **18.8** | **19.6** | **20.4** |
| 4.2 | Drugs used in psychoses & related disorders | 0.9 | 1.0 | 1.0 | 0.9 | 0.9 | 0.8 | 2.2 | 2.8 | 2.9 | 2.8 |
| 4.3 | Antidepressant drugs | 3.0 | 4.2 | 4.3 | 4.1 | 3.9 | 5.2 | 6.1 | 5.4 | 5.5 | 5.4 |
| 4.7 | Analgesics | 9.4 | 8.6 | 7.5 | 7.2 | 6.9 | 3.9 | 4.3 | 4.2 | 4.4 | 4.2 |
| 5 | **Infections** | **9.0** | **6.3** | **5.2** | **5.1** | **4.9** | **5.1** | **3.4** | **2.7** | **2.7** | **2.6** |
| 5.1 | Antibacterial drugs | 8.2 | 5.6 | 4.6 | 4.3 | 4.2 | 4.0 | 2.6 | 2.0 | 2.1 | 2.0 |
| 6 | **Endocrine system** | **5.8** | **7.0** | **7.7** | **7.9** | **8.2** | **7.5** | **8.5** | **9.0** | **9.8** | **10.3** |
| 6.1 | Drugs used in diabetes | 2.1 | 2.8 | 3.3 | 3.1 | 3.0 | 3.1 | 4.0 | 5.1 | 5.3 | 5.1 |
| 6.4 | Sex hormones | 1.1 | 1.0 | 0.7 | 0.6 | 0.6 | 2.8 | 2.4 | 1.3 | 1.3 | 1.3 |
| 7 | **Obstetrics and gynaecology**[1] | **2.0** | **2.0** | **2.0** | **2.0** | **2.0** | **1.7** | **2.4** | **2.7** | **2.9** | **2.9** |
| 7.3 | Contraceptives | 1.3 | 1.1 | 0.9 | 0.9 | 0.9 | 0.8 | 0.7 | 0.7 | 0.7 | 0.7 |
| 8 | **Malignant disease**[2] | **0.5** | **0.6** | **0.6** | **0.6** | **0.6** | **3.0** | **3.3** | **3.4** | **3.2** | **3.5** |
| 8.3 | Sex hormones and antagonists | 0.3 | 0.3 | 0.3 | 0.3 | 0.3 | 1.9 | 2.2 | 2.4 | 2.4 | 2.4 |
| 9 | **Nutrition and blood** | **2.8** | **2.8** | **3.2** | **3.3** | **3.5** | **2.9** | **3.4** | **3.7** | **4.1** | **4.5** |
| 9.4 | Oral nutrition | 0.5 | 0.5 | 0.5 | 0.5 | 0.5 | 1.9 | 2.0 | 1.8 | 1.9 | 1.8 |
| 10 | **Musculo-skeletal and joint disease** | **5.3** | **4.8** | **4.3** | **3.9** | **3.7** | **5.3** | **4.3** | **4.0** | **2.9** | **2.8** |
| 10.1 | Rheumatic diseases and gout | 4.1 | 3.8 | 3.6 | 3.4 | 3.3 | 4.4 | 3.7 | 3.5 | 3.6 | 3.5 |
| 11 | **Eye preparations** | **2.4** | **2.2** | **2.1** | **2.1** | **2.1** | **1.2** | **1.4** | **1.4** | **1.5** | **1.6** |
| 12 | **Ear, nose and oropharynx** | **1.6** | **1.5** | **1.2** | **1.2** | **1.2** | **0.9** | **0.8** | **0.7** | **0.7** | **0.8** |
| 13 | **Skin** | **6.4** | **5.3** | **4.4** | **4.1** | **3.9** | **4.0** | **2.9** | **2.5** | **2.5** | **2.5** |
| 13.4 | Topical corticosteroids | 2.0 | 1.8 | 1.4 | 1.4 | 1.3 | 0.8 | 0.7 | 0.6 | 0.6 | 0.6 |
| 14 | **Immunological products** | **1.5** | **1.5** | **1.3** | **1.6** | **1.3** | **1.6** | **1.2** | **1.1** | **1.4** | **1.2** |
| 14.4 | Vaccines and antisera | 1.5 | 1.5 | 1.3 | 1.3 | 1.2 | 1.6 | 1.2 | 1.1 | 1.1 | 1.1 |
| 15 | **Anaesthesia** | **0.1** | **0.1** | **0.1** | **0.1** | **0.1** | **0.0** | **0.0** | **0.1** | **0.1** | **0.1** |
| | **Others including dressings and appliances** | **3.4** | **2.9** | **2.6** | **2.6** | **2.7** | **5.7** | **4.6** | **4.5** | **5.0** | **5.4** |

Notes: All figures are based on the British National Formulary (BNF). Figures below the BNF heading relate to chapters and sub-sections of the BNF. Figures relate to prescriptions dispensed by community pharmacists and appliances contractors who are contracted to the NHS, dispensing doctors and personal administration.
1 Including urinary tract disorders.
2 Including immunosuppression.
0.0 non zero but <0.05.

Source: Prescription Cost Analysis, Wales (HOWIS).

Table 4.39  **Percentage of total number and net ingredient cost (NIC) of prescriptions by therapeutic group, Scotland, 1996 - 2006**

| BNF | Therapeutic group | Prescription items (millions): | | | | | NIC of prescriptions (£m): | | | | |
|---|---|---|---|---|---|---|---|---|---|---|---|
| | | 1996 | 2001 | 2004 | 2005 | 2006 | 1996 | 2001 | 2004 | 2005 | 2006 |
| | Total | 54 | 64 | 73 | 76 | 79 | 464 | 704 | 925 | 952 | 967 |
| | | Percentage of annual total | | | | | | | | | |
| 1 | Gastro-intestinal system | 9.7 | 9.4 | 9.0 | 9.0 | 8.9 | 19.4 | 13.1 | 10.3 | 10.7 | 8.7 |
| 1.3 | Ulcer-healing drugs | 4.2 | 4.5 | 4.7 | 4.8 | 4.9 | 15.5 | 10.2 | 7.9 | 8.2 | 6.0 |
| 1.6 | Laxatives | 2.2 | 2.1 | 2.0 | 1.9 | 1.9 | 1.1 | 0.8 | 0.6 | 0.6 | 0.7 |
| 2 | Cardiovascular system | 19.3 | 24.4 | 27.2 | 28.1 | 28.7 | 17.9 | 24.1 | 24.9 | 23.4 | 22.1 |
| 2.2 | Diuretics | 5.1 | 5.2 | 5.2 | 5.1 | 4.9 | 1.2 | 1.0 | 0.7 | 0.8 | 1.0 |
| 2.4 | Beta-adrenoceptor blocking drugs | 3.3 | 3.7 | 3.9 | 3.9 | 3.8 | 1.9 | 1.4 | 1.2 | 1.2 | 1.3 |
| 2.5 | Anti-hypertensive therapy | 1.8 | 3.2 | 4.3 | 4.6 | 4.9 | 4.4 | 5.4 | 6.1 | 5.7 | 5.2 |
| 2.6 | Nitrates/calcium channel blockers | 5.2 | 5.0 | 4.6 | 4.6 | 4.5 | 7.6 | 6.6 | 5.2 | 4.7 | 3.8 |
| 2.12 | Lipid lowering drugs | 0.5 | 2.3 | 3.6 | 4.3 | 4.8 | 2.3 | 8.0 | 8.9 | 7.8 | 7.3 |
| 3 | Respiratory system | 9.2 | 8.3 | 7.6 | 7.4 | 7.4 | 11.8 | 10.8 | 10.0 | 10.2 | 10.6 |
| 3.1 | Bronchodilators | 4.8 | 4.3 | 3.8 | 3.7 | 3.6 | 4.6 | 4.1 | 3.5 | 3.5 | 3.6 |
| 3.2 | Corticosteroids (inhaled) | 2.1 | 2.1 | 2.0 | 2.0 | 2.0 | 5.8 | 5.1 | 5.1 | 5.2 | 5.6 |
| 4 | Central nervous system | 20.2 | 20.9 | 20.4 | 20.1 | 19.9 | 14.7 | 19.8 | 20.9 | 21.9 | 22.4 |
| 4.2 | Drugs used in psychoses & related disorders | 0.9 | 0.9 | 0.9 | 0.8 | 0.8 | 0.7 | 2.1 | 2.6 | 2.6 | 2.9 |
| 4.3 | Antidepressant drugs | 3.1 | 4.4 | 4.7 | 4.6 | 4.5 | 5.7 | 6.8 | 6.3 | 5.9 | 4.8 |
| 4.7 | Analgesics | 9.4 | 9.1 | 8.5 | 8.4 | 8.2 | 4.5 | 4.9 | 4.8 | 5.5 | 6.2 |
| 5 | Infections | 10.7 | 7.2 | 6.4 | 6.2 | 6.1 | 6.0 | 3.7 | 3.2 | 3.2 | 3.0 |
| 5.1 | Antibacterial drugs | 9.8 | 6.5 | 5.6 | 5.4 | 5.3 | 4.5 | 3.0 | 2.2 | 2.2 | 2.2 |
| 6 | Endocrine system | 5.5 | 6.7 | 7.1 | 7.2 | 7.4 | 7.9 | 9.0 | 8.7 | 9.1 | 9.5 |
| 6.1 | Drugs used in diabetes | 1.8 | 2.4 | 2.8 | 2.9 | 3.1 | 2.8 | 3.9 | 4.6 | 5.1 | 5.6 |
| 6.4 | Sex hormones | 1.3 | 1.2 | 0.8 | 0.7 | 0.6 | 3.2 | 2.7 | 1.4 | 1.1 | 1.1 |
| 7 | Obstetrics and gynaecology[1] | 2.4 | 2.3 | 2.2 | 2.2 | 2.2 | 1.9 | 2.9 | 3.1 | 3.2 | 3.2 |
| 7.3 | Contraceptives | 1.6 | 1.3 | 1.1 | 1.1 | 1.0 | 1.0 | 0.8 | 0.7 | 0.7 | 0.7 |
| 8 | Malignant disease[2] | 0.5 | 0.5 | 0.5 | 0.4 | 0.4 | 2.6 | 3.2 | 3.0 | 2.8 | 3.0 |
| 8.3 | Sex hormones and antagonists | 0.3 | 0.3 | 0.2 | 0.2 | 0.2 | 1.6 | 2.0 | 1.9 | 1.9 | 2.0 |
| 9 | Nutrition and blood | 2.6 | 2.7 | 3.1 | 3.2 | 3.3 | 2.6 | 2.9 | 2.8 | 3.1 | 3.5 |
| 9.4 | Oral nutrition | 0.6 | 0.6 | 0.6 | 0.6 | 0.6 | 1.8 | 1.9 | 1.6 | 1.7 | 1.8 |
| 10 | Musculo-skeletal and joint disease | 5.3 | 4.7 | 4.5 | 4.3 | 3.9 | 5.1 | 4.3 | 4.2 | 3.1 | 2.7 |
| 10.1 | Rheumatic diseases and gout | 4.3 | 3.9 | 3.8 | 3.6 | 3.2 | 4.3 | 3.8 | 3.7 | 2.6 | 2.3 |
| 11 | Eye preparations | 2.1 | 2.0 | 1.9 | 1.9 | 1.9 | 1.0 | 1.1 | 0.9 | 1.0 | 1.0 |
| 12 | Ear, nose and oropharynx | 1.8 | 1.6 | 1.5 | 1.4 | 1.4 | 1.2 | 0.9 | 0.7 | 0.7 | 0.7 |
| 13 | Skin | 7.2 | 6.3 | 5.6 | 5.4 | 5.2 | 4.6 | 3.7 | 2.9 | 2.8 | 2.9 |
| 13.4 | Topical corticosteroids | 2.8 | 2.4 | 2.1 | 2.0 | 1.9 | 1.1 | 0.8 | 0.7 | 0.7 | 0.8 |
| 14 | Immunological products | 0.5 | 0.3 | 0.3 | 0.2 | 0.3 | 1.3 | 1.1 | 1.1 | 1.0 | 1.0 |
| 14.4 | Vaccines and antisera | 0.5 | 0.3 | 0.3 | 0.2 | 0.3 | 1.3 | 1.1 | 1.1 | 1.0 | 1.0 |
| 15 | Anaesthesia | 0.0 | 0.0 | 0.0 | 0.1 | 0.1 | 0.0 | 0.0 | 0.0 | 0.0 | 0.0 |
| | Others including dressings and appliances | 3.0 | 2.7 | 2.4 | 2.3 | 1.8 | 6.1 | 4.7 | 4.1 | 4.2 | 4.5 |

*Notes:*  All figures are based on the British National Formulary (BNF).  Figures below the BNF heading relate to chapters and sub-sections of the BNF.
Figures relate to prescriptions dispensed by community pharmacists and appliances contractors who are contracted to the NHS, dispensing doctors and personal administration.
1 Including urinary tract disorders.
2 Including immunosuppression.
0.0 non zero but <0.05.

*Source:*  Prescription Cost Analysis, Scotland (ISD).

Table 4.40   **Percentage of total number and net ingredient cost (NIC) of prescriptions by therapeutic group, Northern Ireland, 1996 - 2006**

| BNF | Therapeutic group | Prescription items (millions): | | | | | NIC of prescriptions (£m): | | | | |
|---|---|---|---|---|---|---|---|---|---|---|---|
| | | 1996 | 2001 | 2004 | 2005 | 2006 | 1996 | 2001 | 2004 | 2005 | 2006 |
| | Total | 21 | 24 | 27 | 28 | 29 | 196 | 268 | 365 | 361 | 373 |
| | | Percentage of annual total | | | | | | | | | |
| 1 | **Gastro-intestinal system** | 9.9 | 9.6 | 9.3 | 9.2 | 9.0 | 18.6 | 12.4 | 9.9 | 10.1 | 8.5 |
| 1.3 | Ulcer-healing drugs | 3.6 | 4.2 | 4.5 | 4.6 | 4.7 | 15.0 | 9.7 | 7.6 | 7.9 | 6.1 |
| 1.6 | Laxatives | 2.3 | 2.0 | 1.9 | 1.8 | 1.8 | 1.1 | 0.8 | 0.6 | 0.6 | 0.7 |
| 2 | **Cardiovascular system** | 13.5 | 19.1 | 22.1 | 22.9 | 23.5 | 16.2 | 22.1 | 24.8 | 23.7 | 22.9 |
| 2.2 | Diuretics | 3.0 | 3.6 | 3.7 | 3.6 | 3.5 | 1.0 | 0.9 | 0.6 | 0.6 | 0.8 |
| 2.4 | Beta-adrenoceptor blocking drugs | 2.2 | 2.9 | 3.2 | 3.2 | 3.2 | 2.1 | 2.2 | 1.9 | 1.9 | 1.7 |
| 2.5 | Anti-hypertensive therapy | 1.5 | 2.9 | 3.8 | 4.1 | 4.3 | 3.5 | 5.1 | 5.9 | 5.4 | 5.0 |
| 2.6 | Nitrates/calcium channel blockers | 4.0 | 3.9 | 3.6 | 3.6 | 3.6 | 6.6 | 5.5 | 4.4 | 4.2 | 3.6 |
| 2.12 | Lipid lowering drugs | 0.6 | 1.9 | 3.3 | 3.7 | 4.2 | 2.2 | 6.5 | 9.0 | 8.3 | 8.4 |
| 3 | **Respiratory system** | 10.5 | 9.0 | 8.1 | 8.0 | 8.0 | 12.7 | 10.5 | 9.2 | 9.7 | 10.1 |
| 3.1 | Bronchodilators | 4.8 | 4.2 | 3.7 | 3.6 | 3.5 | 4.7 | 3.9 | 2.9 | 2.9 | 3.0 |
| 3.2 | Corticosteroids (inhaled) | 1.9 | 1.8 | 1.8 | 1.8 | 1.9 | 6.4 | 4.9 | 4.9 | 5.1 | 5.4 |
| 4 | **Central nervous system** | 22.3 | 24.6 | 23.5 | 23.4 | 23.3 | 14.3 | 20.0 | 20.7 | 21.8 | 22.6 |
| 4.2 | Drugs used in psychoses & related disorders | 1.3 | 1.3 | 1.2 | 1.3 | 1.3 | 0.9 | 2.5 | 3.2 | 3.3 | 3.6 |
| 4.3 | Antidepressant drugs | 2.8 | 4.5 | 4.9 | 4.8 | 4.9 | 5.5 | 7.0 | 6.9 | 6.5 | 5.5 |
| 4.7 | Analgesics | 11.0 | 10.4 | 8.9 | 8.8 | 8.6 | 4.4 | 4.5 | 3.8 | 4.2 | 4.9 |
| 5 | **Infections** | 12.0 | 8.4 | 7.1 | 7.0 | 6.9 | 5.9 | 4.0 | 3.1 | 2.9 | 2.9 |
| 5.1 | Antibacterial drugs | 11.1 | 7.6 | 6.4 | 6.2 | 6.2 | 4.9 | 3.0 | 2.3 | 2.1 | 2.2 |
| 6 | **Endocrine system** | 3.8 | 5.5 | 6.3 | 6.5 | 6.8 | 5.6 | 7.4 | 7.9 | 8.6 | 9.4 |
| 6.1 | Drugs used in diabetes | 1.0 | 2.1 | 2.8 | 3.0 | 3.1 | 1.7 | 3.5 | 4.4 | 5.1 | 5.7 |
| 6.4 | Sex hormones | 1.0 | 1.0 | 0.7 | 0.6 | 0.6 | 2.4 | 2.0 | 1.2 | 1.0 | 0.9 |
| 7 | **Obstetrics and gynaecology[1]** | 2.1 | 2.2 | 2.2 | 2.2 | 2.2 | 1.6 | 2.4 | 2.6 | 2.8 | 2.9 |
| 7.3 | Contraceptives | 1.2 | 1.2 | 1.1 | 1.1 | 1.0 | 0.7 | 0.6 | 0.6 | 0.7 | 0.7 |
| 8 | **Malignant disease[2]** | 0.3 | 0.4 | 0.4 | 0.4 | 0.4 | 2.5 | 2.8 | 2.8 | 2.6 | 2.8 |
| 8.3 | Sex hormones and antagonists | 0.2 | 0.2 | 0.2 | 0.2 | 0.2 | 1.6 | 1.9 | 1.9 | 1.9 | 2.1 |
| 9 | **Nutrition and blood** | 3.6 | 3.4 | 3.4 | 3.4 | 3.6 | 3.4 | 3.4 | 3.6 | 3.8 | 4.2 |
| 9.4 | Oral nutrition | 0.8 | 0.9 | 1.0 | 1.0 | 1.2 | 2.5 | 2.6 | 2.7 | 2.9 | 3.3 |
| 10 | **Musculo-skeletal and joint disease** | 4.7 | 4.7 | 4.8 | 4.3 | 4.1 | 5.0 | 4.7 | 5.1 | 3.4 | 3.2 |
| 10.1 | Rheumatic diseases and gout | 3.4 | 3.6 | 3.8 | 3.3 | 3.0 | 4.1 | 4.0 | 4.5 | 2.8 | 2.6 |
| 11 | **Eye preparations** | 1.8 | 1.7 | 1.6 | 1.6 | 1.6 | 0.8 | 0.8 | 0.7 | 0.8 | 0.8 |
| 12 | **Ear, nose and oropharynx** | 2.2 | 1.7 | 1.6 | 1.5 | 1.5 | 1.0 | 0.7 | 0.6 | 0.6 | 0.6 |
| 13 | **Skin** | 9.3 | 7.6 | 6.3 | 6.2 | 6.0 | 5.6 | 4.4 | 3.1 | 3.0 | 3.1 |
| 13.4 | Topical corticosteroids | 2.3 | 2.0 | 1.7 | 1.7 | 1.6 | 0.9 | 0.7 | 0.5 | 0.5 | 0.6 |
| 14 | **Immunological products** | 0.3 | 0.3 | 0.2 | 0.2 | 0.2 | 0.7 | 1.1 | 0.6 | 0.8 | 0.5 |
| 14.4 | Vaccines and antisera | 0.3 | 0.3 | 0.2 | 0.2 | 0.2 | 0.7 | 1.1 | 0.5 | 0.8 | 0.5 |
| 15 | **Anaesthesia** | 0.0 | 0.0 | 0.0 | 0.0 | 0.0 | 0.0 | 0.0 | 0.0 | 0.0 | 0.0 |
| | **Others including dressings and appliances** | 3.8 | 2.0 | 2.0 | 2.0 | 2.0 | 6.1 | 3.3 | 3.6 | 3.8 | 4.0 |

Notes:   All figures are based on the British National Formulary (BNF).  Figures below the BNF heading relate to chapters and sub-sections of  the BNF.
Figures relate to prescriptions dispensed by community pharmacists and appliances contractors who are contracted to the NHS, dispensing doctors and personal administration.
1 Including urinary tract disorders.
2 Including immunosuppression.
0.0 non zero but <0.05.

Source:   Prescription Cost Analysis, Northern Ireland (CSA).

Table 4.41  **Net ingredient cost (NIC) per prescription item at 2006 prices[1] by therapeutic group, UK, 1996 - 2006**

| BNF | Therapeutic group | NIC per item (£ at 2006 prices) | | | | | At constant prices (Index 1996=100) | | | | |
|---|---|---|---|---|---|---|---|---|---|---|---|
| | | 1996 | 2001 | 2004 | 2005 | 2006 | 1996 | 2001 | 2004 | 2005 | 2006 |
| | Total | 10.59 | 11.97 | 12.38 | 11.40 | 11.01 | 100 | 113 | 117 | 108 | 104 |
| 1 | **Gastro-intestinal system** | 19.15 | 15.10 | 13.44 | 12.82 | 10.20 | 100 | 79 | 70 | 67 | 53 |
| 1.3 | Ulcer-healing drugs | 40.78 | 25.72 | 20.25 | 18.45 | 12.70 | 100 | 63 | 50 | 45 | 31 |
| 1.6 | Laxatives | 5.24 | 4.02 | 3.65 | 3.86 | 4.26 | 100 | 77 | 70 | 74 | 81 |
| 2 | **Cardiovascular system** | 10.36 | 11.62 | 11.29 | 8.96 | 8.16 | 100 | 112 | 109 | 87 | 79 |
| 2.2 | Diuretics | 2.85 | 2.36 | 1.86 | 2.02 | 2.33 | 100 | 83 | 65 | 71 | 82 |
| 2.4 | Beta-adrenoceptor blocking drugs | 7.05 | 4.74 | 4.03 | 3.66 | 3.82 | 100 | 67 | 57 | 52 | 54 |
| 2.5 | Anti-hypertensive therapy | 23.55 | 19.26 | 16.63 | 12.11 | 10.92 | 100 | 82 | 71 | 51 | 46 |
| 2.6 | Nitrates/calcium channel blockers | 15.83 | 15.67 | 14.06 | 11.92 | 9.39 | 100 | 99 | 89 | 75 | 59 |
| 2.12 | Lipid lowering drugs | 38.31 | 37.65 | 27.66 | 18.94 | 15.71 | 100 | 98 | 72 | 49 | 41 |
| 3 | **Respiratory system** | 13.42 | 14.93 | 16.09 | 15.97 | 16.22 | 100 | 111 | 120 | 119 | 121 |
| 3.1 | Bronchodilators | 10.40 | 11.11 | 10.86 | 10.87 | 10.85 | 100 | 107 | 104 | 105 | 104 |
| 3.2 | Corticosteroids (Inhaled) | 28.78 | 29.09 | 32.38 | 32.03 | 32.76 | 100 | 101 | 112 | 111 | 114 |
| 4 | **Central nervous system** | 7.54 | 10.87 | 12.31 | 12.19 | 12.30 | 100 | 144 | 163 | 162 | 163 |
| 4.2 | Drugs used in psychoses & related disorders | 8.26 | 26.79 | 34.93 | 33.84 | 34.40 | 100 | 325 | 423 | 410 | 417 |
| 4.3 | Antidepressant drugs | 16.95 | 16.54 | 14.96 | 12.58 | 10.16 | 100 | 98 | 88 | 74 | 60 |
| 4.7 | Analgesics | 4.91 | 6.11 | 6.74 | 7.54 | 8.84 | 100 | 124 | 137 | 154 | 180 |
| 5 | **Infections** | 5.71 | 6.06 | 6.10 | 5.65 | 5.37 | 100 | 106 | 107 | 99 | 94 |
| 5.1 | Antibacterial drugs | 4.82 | 5.01 | 4.94 | 4.54 | 4.65 | 100 | 104 | 102 | 94 | 96 |
| 6 | **Endocrine system** | 14.60 | 15.28 | 14.96 | 14.53 | 14.30 | 100 | 105 | 103 | 100 | 98 |
| 6.1 | Drugs used in diabetes | 15.00 | 17.78 | 19.38 | 19.32 | 19.91 | 100 | 119 | 129 | 129 | 133 |
| 6.4 | Sex hormones | 24.30 | 25.14 | 22.05 | 19.07 | 18.32 | 100 | 103 | 91 | 78 | 75 |
| 7 | **Obstetrics and gynaecology[2]** | 8.21 | 13.11 | 15.25 | 15.45 | 14.72 | 100 | 160 | 186 | 188 | 179 |
| 7.3 | Contraceptives | 6.12 | 6.74 | 7.75 | 7.87 | 8.26 | 100 | 110 | 127 | 129 | 135 |
| 8 | **Malignant disease[3]** | 59.25 | 72.09 | 76.97 | 84.87 | 87.24 | 100 | 122 | 130 | 143 | 147 |
| 8.3 | Sex hormones and antagonists | 55.81 | 86.70 | 103.63 | 95.07 | 98.37 | 100 | 155 | 186 | 170 | 176 |
| 9 | **Nutrition and blood** | 11.71 | 15.03 | 14.22 | 13.93 | 13.94 | 100 | 128 | 121 | 119 | 119 |
| 9.4 | Oral nutrition | 38.03 | 42.39 | 41.87 | 41.73 | 27.41 | 100 | 111 | 110 | 110 | 72 |
| 10.0 | **Musculo-skeletal and joint disease** | 10.03 | 9.90 | 11.03 | 7.95 | 7.74 | 100 | 99 | 110 | 79 | 77 |
| 10.1 | Rheumatic diseases and gout | 10.62 | 10.38 | 11.70 | 8.28 | 8.09 | 100 | 98 | 110 | 78 | 76 |
| 11 | **Eye preparations** | 5.29 | 7.31 | 7.36 | 7.49 | 7.75 | 100 | 138 | 139 | 142 | 146 |
| 12 | **Ear, nose and oropharynx** | 6.05 | 6.19 | 6.51 | 6.10 | 6.37 | 100 | 102 | 108 | 101 | 105 |
| 13 | **Skin** | 6.38 | 6.27 | 6.35 | 6.22 | 6.47 | 100 | 98 | 100 | 98 | 101 |
| 13.4 | Topical corticosteroids | 4.05 | 4.15 | 4.19 | 4.11 | 4.75 | 100 | 103 | 103 | 101 | 117 |
| 14 | **Immunological products** | 11.03 | 10.50 | 10.27 | 9.86 | 10.05 | 100 | 95 | 93 | 89 | 91 |
| 14.4 | Vaccines and antisera | 10.91 | 10.21 | 10.03 | 9.70 | 9.81 | 100 | 94 | 92 | 89 | 90 |
| 15 | **Anaesthesia** | 3.21 | 4.39 | 5.09 | 5.18 | 5.34 | 100 | 137 | 159 | 161 | 166 |
| | **Others including dressings and appliances** | 19.02 | 20.95 | 22.29 | 22.74 | 22.90 | 100 | 110 | 117 | 120 | 120 |

*Notes:*  All figures are based on the British National Formulary (BNF). Figures below the BNF heading relate to chapters and sub-sections of the BNF. Figures relate to prescriptions dispensed by community pharmacists and appliances contractors who are contracted to the NHS, dispensing doctors and personal administration.
1 At constant prices, as adjusted by the Gross Domestic Product (GDP) deflator at market prices.
2 Including urinary tract disorders.
3 Including immunosuppression.

*Sources:* Prescription Cost Analysis, England (DH).
Prescription Cost Analysis, Wales (HOWIS).
Prescription Cost Analysis, Scotland (ISD).
Prescription Cost Analysis, Northern Ireland (CSA).
Economic Trends (ONS).

# FHS: General Pharmaceutical Services

Table 4.42  Net ingredient cost (NIC) per prescription item at 2006 prices[1] by therapeutic group, England, 1996 - 2006

| BNF | Therapeutic group | NIC per item (£ at 2006 prices) | | | | | At constant prices (Index 1996=100) | | | | |
|---|---|---|---|---|---|---|---|---|---|---|---|
| | | 1996 | 2001 | 2004 | 2005 | 2006 | 1996 | 2001 | 2004 | 2005 | 2006 |
| | Total | 10.54 | 11.96 | 12.33 | 11.28 | 10.90 | 100 | 113 | 117 | 107 | 103 |
| 1 | Gastro-intestinal system | 18.68 | 14.77 | 13.26 | 12.53 | 9.99 | 100 | 79 | 71 | 67 | 53 |
| 1.3 | Ulcer-healing drugs | 40.63 | 25.37 | 20.03 | 17.88 | 11.93 | 100 | 62 | 49 | 44 | 29 |
| 1.6 | Laxatives | 5.22 | 3.94 | 3.60 | 3.84 | 4.24 | 100 | 75 | 69 | 73 | 81 |
| 2 | Cardiovascular system | 10.35 | 11.58 | 11.23 | 8.79 | 8.03 | 100 | 112 | 108 | 85 | 78 |
| 2.2 | Diuretics | 2.85 | 2.35 | 1.88 | 2.06 | 2.36 | 100 | 82 | 66 | 72 | 83 |
| 2.4 | Beta-adrenoceptor blocking drugs | 7.04 | 4.58 | 3.91 | 3.48 | 3.72 | 100 | 65 | 56 | 49 | 53 |
| 2.5 | Anti-hypertensive therapy | 23.56 | 19.27 | 16.55 | 11.56 | 10.50 | 100 | 82 | 70 | 49 | 45 |
| 2.6 | Nitrates/calcium channel blockers | 15.68 | 15.69 | 14.06 | 11.69 | 9.03 | 100 | 100 | 90 | 75 | 58 |
| 2.12 | Lipid lowering drugs | 37.75 | 37.24 | 27.35 | 17.99 | 14.78 | 100 | 99 | 72 | 48 | 39 |
| 3 | Respiratory system | 13.29 | 14.75 | 15.93 | 15.79 | 16.02 | 100 | 111 | 120 | 119 | 121 |
| 3.1 | Bronchodilators | 10.28 | 10.98 | 10.71 | 10.74 | 10.69 | 100 | 107 | 104 | 104 | 104 |
| 3.2 | Corticosteroids (Inhaled) | 28.15 | 28.54 | 31.89 | 31.58 | 32.43 | 100 | 101 | 113 | 112 | 115 |
| 4 | Central nervous system | 7.54 | 10.88 | 12.29 | 12.11 | 12.24 | 100 | 144 | 163 | 161 | 162 |
| 4.2 | Drugs used in psychoses & related disorder. | 8.21 | 26.87 | 34.72 | 33.38 | 33.84 | 100 | 327 | 423 | 407 | 412 |
| 4.3 | Antidepressant drugs | 16.31 | 16.10 | 14.47 | 11.79 | 9.39 | 100 | 99 | 89 | 72 | 58 |
| 4.7 | Analgesics | 4.94 | 6.11 | 6.71 | 7.60 | 9.09 | 100 | 124 | 136 | 154 | 184 |
| 5 | Infections | 5.65 | 6.01 | 6.06 | 5.58 | 5.31 | 100 | 106 | 107 | 99 | 94 |
| 5.1 | Antibacterial drugs | 4.77 | 4.93 | 4.91 | 4.45 | 4.60 | 100 | 103 | 103 | 93 | 96 |
| 6 | Endocrine system | 14.52 | 15.21 | 14.91 | 14.45 | 14.21 | 100 | 105 | 103 | 100 | 98 |
| 6.1 | Drugs used in diabetes | 14.70 | 17.64 | 19.26 | 19.14 | 19.78 | 100 | 120 | 131 | 130 | 135 |
| 6.4 | Sex hormones | 23.76 | 24.74 | 21.93 | 18.72 | 17.95 | 100 | 104 | 92 | 79 | 76 |
| 7 | Obstetrics and gynaecology[2] | 8.10 | 12.79 | 14.91 | 15.12 | 14.38 | 100 | 158 | 184 | 187 | 178 |
| 7.3 | Contraceptives | 6.08 | 6.67 | 7.68 | 7.82 | 8.25 | 100 | 110 | 126 | 129 | 136 |
| 8 | Malignant disease[3] | 58.62 | 71.18 | 76.61 | 87.17 | 89.70 | 100 | 121 | 131 | 149 | 153 |
| 8.3 | Sex hormones and antagonists | 55.23 | 85.95 | 103.28 | 93.64 | 96.99 | 100 | 156 | 187 | 170 | 176 |
| 9 | Nutrition and blood | 11.89 | 15.43 | 14.54 | 14.19 | 14.11 | 100 | 130 | 122 | 119 | 119 |
| 9.4 | Oral nutrition | 38.29 | 43.29 | 43.31 | 43.13 | 26.17 | 100 | 113 | 113 | 113 | 68 |
| 10.0 | Musculo-skeletal and joint disease | 9.87 | 9.61 | 10.77 | 7.74 | 7.59 | 100 | 97 | 109 | 78 | 77 |
| 10.1 | Rheumatic diseases and gout | 10.43 | 10.02 | 11.40 | 7.84 | 7.71 | 100 | 96 | 109 | 75 | 74 |
| 11 | Eye preparations | 5.31 | 7.43 | 7.48 | 7.63 | 7.89 | 100 | 140 | 141 | 144 | 148 |
| 12 | Ear, nose and oropharynx | 6.01 | 6.13 | 6.53 | 6.12 | 6.41 | 100 | 102 | 109 | 102 | 107 |
| 13 | Skin | 6.28 | 6.10 | 6.28 | 6.17 | 6.43 | 100 | 97 | 100 | 98 | 102 |
| 13.4 | Topical corticosteroids | 4.00 | 4.10 | 4.12 | 4.05 | 4.73 | 100 | 103 | 103 | 101 | 118 |
| 14 | Immunological products | 10.54 | 9.84 | 9.58 | 9.29 | 9.47 | 100 | 93 | 91 | 88 | 90 |
| 14.4 | Vaccines and antisera | 10.41 | 9.55 | 9.33 | 9.11 | 9.26 | 100 | 92 | 90 | 88 | 89 |
| 15 | Anaesthesia | 2.96 | 4.05 | 4.55 | 4.55 | 4.66 | 100 | 137 | 154 | 154 | 158 |
| | Others including dressings and appliances | 18.83 | 21.10 | 22.43 | 22.85 | 22.59 | 100 | 112 | 119 | 121 | 120 |

Notes:  All figures are based on the British National Formulary (BNF).  Figures below the BNF heading relate to chapters and sub-sections of the BNF.
Figures relate to prescriptions dispensed by community pharmacists and appliances contractors who are contracted to the NHS, dispensing doctors and personal administration.
1 At constant prices, as adjusted by the Gross Domestic Product (GDP) deflator at market prices.
2 Including urinary tract disorders.
3 Including immunosuppression.

Sources. Prescription Cost Analysis, England (DH).
Economic Trends (ONS).

Table 4.43  **Net ingredient cost (NIC) per prescription item at 2006 prices[1] by therapeutic group, Wales, 1996 - 2006**

| BNF | Therapeutic group | NIC per item (£ at 2006 prices) | | | | | At constant prices (Index 1996=100) | | | | |
|---|---|---|---|---|---|---|---|---|---|---|---|
| | | 1996 | 2001 | 2004 | 2005 | 2006 | 1996 | 2001 | 2004 | 2005 | 2006 |
| | Total | 9.95 | 11.06 | 11.19 | 10.12 | 9.74 | 100 | 111 | 112 | 102 | 98 |
| 1 | Gastro-intestinal system | 18.10 | 14.24 | 12.21 | 11.51 | 9.03 | 100 | 79 | 67 | 64 | 50 |
| 1.3 | Ulcer-healing drugs | 37.69 | 23.57 | 17.56 | 17.18 | 16.78 | 100 | 63 | 47 | 46 | 45 |
| 1.6 | Laxatives | 5.12 | 4.05 | 3.59 | 3.51 | 3.43 | 100 | 79 | 70 | 69 | 67 |
| 2 | Cardiovascular system | 9.12 | 10.02 | 9.56 | 7.37 | 6.76 | 100 | 110 | 105 | 81 | 74 |
| 2.2 | Diuretics | 2.68 | 2.10 | 1.59 | 1.55 | 1.52 | 100 | 78 | 59 | 58 | 57 |
| 2.4 | Beta-adrenoceptor blocking drugs | 6.45 | 4.42 | 3.67 | 3.59 | 3.50 | 100 | 69 | 57 | 56 | 54 |
| 2.5 | Anti-hypertensive therapy | 19.63 | 16.17 | 13.65 | 13.35 | 13.04 | 100 | 82 | 70 | 68 | 66 |
| 2.6 | Nitrates/calcium channel blockers | 15.61 | 13.49 | 11.85 | 11.59 | 11.32 | 100 | 86 | 76 | 74 | 73 |
| 2.12 | Lipid lowering drugs | 30.85 | 31.55 | 22.65 | 22.15 | 21.64 | 100 | 102 | 73 | 72 | 70 |
| 3 | Respiratory system | 13.65 | 15.57 | 16.56 | 16.27 | 16.50 | 100 | 114 | 121 | 119 | 121 |
| 3.1 | Bronchodilators | 10.66 | 11.22 | 10.89 | 10.65 | 10.40 | 100 | 105 | 102 | 100 | 98 |
| 3.2 | Corticosteroids (Inhaled) | 30.09 | 31.54 | 33.55 | 32.81 | 32.05 | 100 | 105 | 111 | 109 | 106 |
| 4 | Central nervous system | 6.73 | 9.64 | 10.82 | 10.53 | 10.63 | 100 | 143 | 161 | 157 | 158 |
| 4.2 | Drugs used in psychoses & related disorders | 8.61 | 25.81 | 31.94 | 31.24 | 30.51 | 100 | 300 | 371 | 363 | 355 |
| 4.3 | Antidepressant drugs | 17.26 | 16.19 | 14.07 | 13.76 | 13.44 | 100 | 94 | 82 | 80 | 78 |
| 4.7 | Analgesics | 4.11 | 5.53 | 6.28 | 6.14 | 6.00 | 100 | 134 | 153 | 149 | 146 |
| 5 | Infections | 5.59 | 6.05 | 5.86 | 5.35 | 5.18 | 100 | 108 | 105 | 96 | 93 |
| 5.1 | Antibacterial drugs | 4.87 | 5.12 | 4.88 | 4.77 | 4.66 | 100 | 105 | 100 | 98 | 96 |
| 6 | Endocrine system | 12.86 | 13.41 | 13.09 | 12.59 | 12.27 | 100 | 104 | 102 | 98 | 95 |
| 6.1 | Drugs used in diabetes | 14.67 | 15.89 | 17.41 | 17.03 | 16.63 | 100 | 108 | 119 | 116 | 113 |
| 6.4 | Sex hormones | 25.41 | 25.07 | 21.10 | 20.64 | 20.16 | 100 | 99 | 83 | 81 | 79 |
| 7 | Obstetrics and gynaecology[2] | 8.36 | 13.39 | 15.24 | 15.22 | 14.12 | 100 | 160 | 182 | 182 | 169 |
| 7.3 | Contraceptives | 5.85 | 6.78 | 7.92 | 7.75 | 7.57 | 100 | 116 | 135 | 132 | 129 |
| 8 | Malignant disease[3] | 55.68 | 63.96 | 67.69 | 58.76 | 60.93 | 100 | 115 | 122 | 106 | 109 |
| 8.3 | Sex hormones and antagonists | 55.15 | 78.65 | 96.31 | 94.20 | 92.01 | 100 | 143 | 175 | 171 | 167 |
| 9 | Nutrition and blood | 10.34 | 13.38 | 12.85 | 12.52 | 12.33 | 100 | 129 | 124 | 121 | 119 |
| 9.4 | Oral nutrition | 38.10 | 41.89 | 37.74 | 36.91 | 36.05 | 100 | 110 | 99 | 97 | 95 |
| 10.0 | Musculo-skeletal and joint disease | 10.07 | 10.03 | 10.32 | 7.63 | 7.35 | 100 | 100 | 103 | 76 | 73 |
| 10.1 | Rheumatic diseases and gout | 10.79 | 10.65 | 10.95 | 10.71 | 10.46 | 100 | 99 | 101 | 99 | 97 |
| 11 | Eye preparations | 5.26 | 7.12 | 7.32 | 7.29 | 7.42 | 100 | 135 | 139 | 139 | 141 |
| 12 | Ear, nose and oropharynx | 5.68 | 6.13 | 6.58 | 6.14 | 6.57 | 100 | 108 | 116 | 108 | 116 |
| 13 | Skin | 6.16 | 6.08 | 6.36 | 6.18 | 6.39 | 100 | 99 | 103 | 100 | 104 |
| 13.4 | Topical corticosteroids | 4.15 | 4.33 | 4.37 | 4.27 | 4.17 | 100 | 104 | 105 | 103 | 101 |
| 14 | Immunological products | 10.24 | 9.16 | 8.98 | 8.73 | 9.16 | 100 | 89 | 88 | 85 | 89 |
| 14.4 | Vaccines and antisera | 10.11 | 9.07 | 8.85 | 8.65 | 8.45 | 100 | 90 | 87 | 86 | 84 |
| 15 | Anaesthesia | 3.42 | 4.80 | 8.12 | 9.01 | 11.22 | 100 | 141 | 238 | 264 | 328 |
| | Others including dressings and appliances | 16.73 | 17.52 | 19.18 | 19.71 | 19.68 | 100 | 105 | 115 | 118 | 118 |

Notes:   All figures are based on the British National Formulary (BNF). Figures below the BNF heading relate to chapters and sub-sections of the BNF. Figures relate to prescriptions dispensed by community pharmacists and appliances contractors who are contracted to the NHS, dispensing doctors and personal administration.

1 At constant prices, as adjusted by the Gross Domestic Product (GDP) deflator at market prices.

2 Including urinary tract disorders.

3 Including immunosuppression.

Sources: Prescription Cost Analysis, Wales (HOWIS).
Economic Trends (ONS).

Table 4.44   **Net ingredient cost (NIC) per prescription item at 2006 prices [1] by therapeutic group, Scotland, 1996 - 2006**

| BNF | Therapeutic group | NIC per item (£ at 2006 prices) | | | | | At constant prices (Index 1996=100) | | | | |
|---|---|---|---|---|---|---|---|---|---|---|---|
| | | 1996 | 2001 | 2004 | 2005 | 2006 | 1996 | 2001 | 2004 | 2005 | 2006 |
| | **Total** | **11.03** | **12.53** | **13.19** | **12.79** | **12.28** | **100** | **114** | **120** | **116** | **111** |
| **1** | **Gastro-intestinal system** | **22.02** | **17.50** | **15.08** | **15.21** | **11.92** | **100** | **79** | **68** | **69** | **54** |
| 1.3 | Ulcer-healing drugs | 40.54 | 28.04 | 22.16 | 21.88 | 14.94 | 100 | 69 | 55 | 54 | 37 |
| 1.6 | Laxatives | 5.27 | 4.45 | 3.93 | 4.15 | 4.71 | 100 | 85 | 75 | 79 | 89 |
| **2** | **Cardiovascular system** | **10.28** | **12.38** | **12.08** | **10.65** | **9.43** | **100** | **121** | **118** | **104** | **92** |
| 2.2 | Diuretics | 2.59 | 2.48 | 1.78 | 1.97 | 2.56 | 100 | 95 | 69 | 76 | 99 |
| 2.4 | Beta-adrenoceptor blocking drugs | 6.34 | 4.77 | 4.07 | 4.07 | 4.07 | 100 | 75 | 64 | 64 | 64 |
| 2.5 | Anti-hypertensive therapy | 26.26 | 21.15 | 18.94 | 15.90 | 13.04 | 100 | 81 | 72 | 61 | 50 |
| 2.6 | Nitrates/calcium channel blockers | 16.08 | 16.40 | 14.89 | 13.31 | 10.39 | 100 | 102 | 93 | 83 | 65 |
| 2.12 | Lipid lowering drugs | 47.94 | 44.41 | 32.33 | 23.44 | 18.78 | 100 | 93 | 67 | 49 | 39 |
| **3** | **Respiratory system** | **14.16** | **16.29** | **17.27** | **17.49** | **17.73** | **100** | **115** | **122** | **123** | **125** |
| 3.1 | Bronchodilators | 10.76 | 11.87 | 12.10 | 12.24 | 12.49 | 100 | 110 | 112 | 114 | 116 |
| 3.2 | Corticosteroids (Inhaled) | 29.99 | 30.66 | 34.22 | 34.16 | 34.81 | 100 | 102 | 114 | 114 | 116 |
| **4** | **Central nervous system** | **8.06** | **11.87** | **13.46** | **13.91** | **13.84** | **100** | **147** | **167** | **173** | **172** |
| 4.2 | Drugs used in psychoses & related disorders | 8.66 | 27.52 | 39.22 | 40.69 | 42.93 | 100 | 318 | 453 | 470 | 496 |
| 4.3 | Antidepressant drugs | 20.43 | 19.34 | 17.93 | 16.39 | 13.06 | 100 | 95 | 88 | 80 | 64 |
| 4.7 | Analgesics | 5.29 | 6.78 | 7.49 | 8.44 | 9.28 | 100 | 128 | 142 | 160 | 176 |
| **5** | **Infections** | **6.21** | **6.48** | **6.64** | **6.56** | **5.97** | **100** | **104** | **107** | **106** | **96** |
| 5.1 | Antibacterial drugs | 5.11 | 5.73 | 5.21 | 5.20 | 5.15 | 100 | 112 | 102 | 102 | 101 |
| **6** | **Endocrine system** | **15.94** | **16.82** | **16.07** | **16.03** | **15.66** | **100** | **106** | **101** | **101** | **98** |
| 6.1 | Drugs used in diabetes | 17.66 | 20.06 | 21.46 | 21.95 | 22.51 | 100 | 114 | 122 | 124 | 127 |
| 6.4 | Sex hormones | 27.50 | 29.16 | 23.33 | 21.08 | 20.26 | 100 | 106 | 85 | 77 | 74 |
| **7** | **Obstetrics and gynaecology [2]** | **8.87** | **15.76** | **18.00** | **18.36** | **17.66** | **100** | **178** | **203** | **207** | **199** |
| 7.3 | Contraceptives | 6.60 | 7.49 | 8.16 | 8.30 | 8.47 | 100 | 113 | 124 | 126 | 128 |
| **8** | **Malignant disease [3]** | **59.32** | **80.80** | **82.24** | **87.84** | **89.67** | **100** | **136** | **139** | **148** | **151** |
| 8.3 | Sex hormones and antagonists | 53.19 | 92.65 | 103.49 | 102.54 | 108.49 | 100 | 174 | 195 | 193 | 204 |
| **9** | **Nutrition and blood** | **11.28** | **13.52** | **11.99** | **12.27** | **13.08** | **100** | **120** | **106** | **109** | **116** |
| 9.4 | Oral nutrition | 36.63 | 37.72 | 33.52 | 34.67 | 35.93 | 100 | 103 | 92 | 95 | 98 |
| **10.0** | **Musculo-skeletal and joint disease** | **10.58** | **11.40** | **12.33** | **9.06** | **8.49** | **100** | **108** | **116** | **86** | **80** |
| 10.1 | Rheumatic diseases and gout | 11.03 | 12.08 | 13.02 | 9.21 | 8.61 | 100 | 110 | 118 | 84 | 78 |
| **11** | **Eye preparations** | **5.09** | **6.58** | **6.54** | **6.58** | **6.87** | **100** | **129** | **128** | **129** | **135** |
| **12** | **Ear, nose and oropharynx** | **6.99** | **7.23** | **6.76** | **6.44** | **6.51** | **100** | **103** | **97** | **92** | **93** |
| **13** | **Skin** | **6.99** | **7.32** | **6.72** | **6.55** | **6.74** | **100** | **105** | **96** | **94** | **96** |
| 13.4 | Topical corticosteroids | 4.28 | 4.41 | 4.53 | 4.45 | 5.26 | 100 | 103 | 106 | 104 | 123 |
| **14** | **Immunological products** | **27.53** | **43.66** | **57.96** | **53.60** | **46.57** | **100** | **159** | **211** | **195** | **169** |
| 14.4 | Vaccines and antisera | 27.77 | 43.65 | 57.96 | 53.60 | 46.57 | 100 | 157 | 209 | 193 | 168 |
| **15** | **Anaesthesia** | **9.89** | **10.20** | **10.25** | **11.42** | **9.82** | **100** | **103** | **104** | **115** | **99** |
| | **Others including dressings and appliances** | **22.87** | **22.11** | **22.52** | **23.39** | **30.46** | **100** | **97** | **98** | **102** | **133** |

*Notes:*   All figures are based on the British National Formulary (BNF).  Figures below the BNF heading relate to chapters and sub-sections of the BNF.
Figures relate to prescriptions dispensed by community pharmacists and appliances contractors who are contracted to the NHS, dispensing doctors and personal administration.
1 At constant prices, as adjusted by the Gross Domestic Product (GDP) deflator at market prices.
2 Including urinary tract disorders.
3 Including immunosuppression.

*Sources:* Prescription Cost Analysis, Scotland (ISD).
Economic Trends (ONS).

# FHS: General Pharmaceutical Services

Table 4.45  Net ingredient cost (NIC) per prescription item at 2006 prices[1] by therapeutic group, Northern Ireland, 1996 - 2006

| BNF | Therapeutic group | NIC per item (£ at 2006 prices) | | | | | At constant prices (Index 1996=100) | | | | |
|---|---|---|---|---|---|---|---|---|---|---|---|
| | | 1996 | 2001 | 2004 | 2005 | 2006 | 1996 | 2001 | 2004 | 2005 | 2006 |
| | Total | 11.83 | 12.65 | 13.98 | 13.21 | 12.87 | 100 | 109 | 118 | 112 | 109 |
| 1 | Gastro-intestinal system | 22.29 | 16.43 | 14.85 | 14.60 | 12.09 | 100 | 73 | 67 | 65 | 54 |
| 1.3 | Ulcer-healing drugs | 48.82 | 29.17 | 23.75 | 22.76 | 16.75 | 100 | 58 | 49 | 47 | 34 |
| 1.6 | Laxatives | 5.71 | 4.82 | 4.24 | 4.27 | 4.81 | 100 | 81 | 74 | 75 | 84 |
| 2 | Cardiovascular system | 14.20 | 14.64 | 15.68 | 13.65 | 12.57 | 100 | 104 | 110 | 96 | 89 |
| 2.2 | Diuretics | 4.11 | 3.00 | 2.09 | 2.03 | 2.84 | 100 | 64 | 51 | 49 | 69 |
| 2.4 | Beta-adrenoceptor blocking drugs | 11.54 | 9.79 | 8.20 | 7.68 | 6.74 | 100 | 79 | 71 | 67 | 58 |
| 2.5 | Anti-hypertensive therapy | 27.29 | 22.53 | 21.47 | 17.55 | 15.01 | 100 | 81 | 79 | 64 | 55 |
| 2.6 | Nitrates/calcium channel blockers | 19.59 | 17.68 | 17.09 | 15.40 | 12.88 | 100 | 90 | 87 | 79 | 66 |
| 2.12 | Lipid lowering drugs | 45.22 | 43.50 | 38.64 | 29.38 | 25.62 | 100 | 103 | 85 | 65 | 57 |
| 3 | Respiratory system | 14.29 | 14.67 | 15.93 | 15.88 | 16.28 | 100 | 109 | 112 | 111 | 114 |
| 3.1 | Bronchodilators | 11.74 | 11.77 | 11.03 | 10.87 | 10.93 | 100 | 103 | 94 | 93 | 93 |
| 3.2 | Corticosteroids (Inhaled) | 40.45 | 34.56 | 37.78 | 36.80 | 37.07 | 100 | 86 | 93 | 91 | 92 |
| 4 | Central nervous system | 7.57 | 10.29 | 12.30 | 12.32 | 12.49 | 100 | 147 | 163 | 163 | 165 |
| 4.2 | Drugs used in psychoses & related disorders | 7.94 | 25.46 | 35.77 | 34.55 | 35.92 | 100 | 335 | 451 | 435 | 453 |
| 4.3 | Antidepressant drugs | 22.93 | 19.57 | 19.60 | 17.69 | 14.35 | 100 | 90 | 85 | 77 | 63 |
| 4.7 | Analgesics | 4.75 | 5.45 | 5.99 | 6.35 | 7.37 | 100 | 119 | 126 | 134 | 155 |
| 5 | Infections | 5.88 | 5.97 | 6.03 | 5.50 | 5.45 | 100 | 96 | 103 | 94 | 93 |
| 5.1 | Antibacterial drugs | 5.16 | 5.05 | 5.05 | 4.50 | 4.54 | 100 | 90 | 98 | 87 | 88 |
| 6 | Endocrine system | 17.30 | 17.11 | 17.69 | 17.46 | 17.81 | 100 | 105 | 102 | 101 | 103 |
| 6.1 | Drugs used in diabetes | 19.24 | 20.49 | 22.30 | 22.77 | 23.45 | 100 | 106 | 116 | 118 | 122 |
| 6.4 | Sex hormones | 29.49 | 25.73 | 23.37 | 20.07 | 19.38 | 100 | 94 | 79 | 68 | 66 |
| 7 | Obstetrics and gynaecology[2] | 9.01 | 13.76 | 16.76 | 16.80 | 16.77 | 100 | 138 | 186 | 186 | 186 |
| 7.3 | Contraceptives | 6.49 | 6.52 | 8.09 | 8.34 | 9.00 | 100 | 74 | 125 | 128 | 139 |
| 8 | Malignant disease[3] | 94.31 | 100.99 | 98.70 | 83.53 | 84.04 | 100 | 110 | 105 | 89 | 89 |
| 8.3 | Sex hormones and antagonists | 90.77 | 117.77 | 137.30 | 126.41 | 133.89 | 100 | 141 | 151 | 139 | 148 |
| 9 | Nutrition and blood | 11.30 | 12.86 | 14.81 | 14.48 | 15.04 | 100 | 116 | 131 | 128 | 133 |
| 9.4 | Oral nutrition | 36.58 | 37.75 | 39.36 | 37.68 | 36.19 | 100 | 102 | 108 | 103 | 99 |
| 10.0 | Musculo-skeletal and joint disease | 12.60 | 12.67 | 14.85 | 10.48 | 10.14 | 100 | 97 | 118 | 83 | 80 |
| 10.1 | Rheumatic diseases and gout | 14.18 | 14.09 | 16.71 | 11.43 | 11.17 | 100 | 96 | 118 | 81 | 79 |
| 11 | Eye preparations | 5.16 | 5.98 | 6.06 | 6.05 | 6.38 | 100 | 116 | 117 | 117 | 124 |
| 12 | Ear, nose and oropharynx | 5.27 | 5.13 | 5.38 | 4.84 | 4.84 | 100 | 100 | 102 | 92 | 92 |
| 13 | Skin | 7.15 | 7.31 | 6.79 | 6.49 | 6.63 | 100 | 103 | 95 | 91 | 93 |
| 13.4 | Topical corticosteroids | 4.42 | 4.36 | 4.39 | 4.13 | 4.69 | 100 | 96 | 99 | 94 | 106 |
| 14 | Immunological products | 31.36 | 50.91 | 44.34 | 46.12 | 28.03 | 100 | 161 | 141 | 147 | 89 |
| 14.4 | Vaccines and antisera | 30.72 | 50.06 | 44.02 | 45.99 | 28.03 | 100 | 161 | 143 | 150 | 91 |
| 15 | Anaesthesia | 7.44 | 11.52 | 12.71 | 11.26 | 11.44 | 100 | 167 | 171 | 151 | 154 |
| | Others including dressings and appliances | 18.74 | 20.69 | 24.41 | 24.65 | 25.19 | 100 | 108 | 130 | 132 | 134 |

Notes:  All figures are based on the British National Formulary (BNF). Figures below the BNF heading relate to chapters and sub-sections of the BNF. Figures relate to prescriptions dispensed by community pharmacists and appliances contractors who are contracted to the NHS, dispensing doctors and personal administration.
1 At constant prices, as adjusted by the Gross Domestic Product (GDP) deflator at market prices.
2 Including urinary tract disorders.
3 Including immunosuppression.

Sources: Prescription Cost Analysis, Northern Ireland (CSA).
Economic Trends (ONS).

# FHS: General Pharmaceutical Services

Figure 4.22 **Market share of branded and generic prescription items dispensed by community pharmacists[1], England, 1949 - 2006**

**Per cent of total items dispensed**

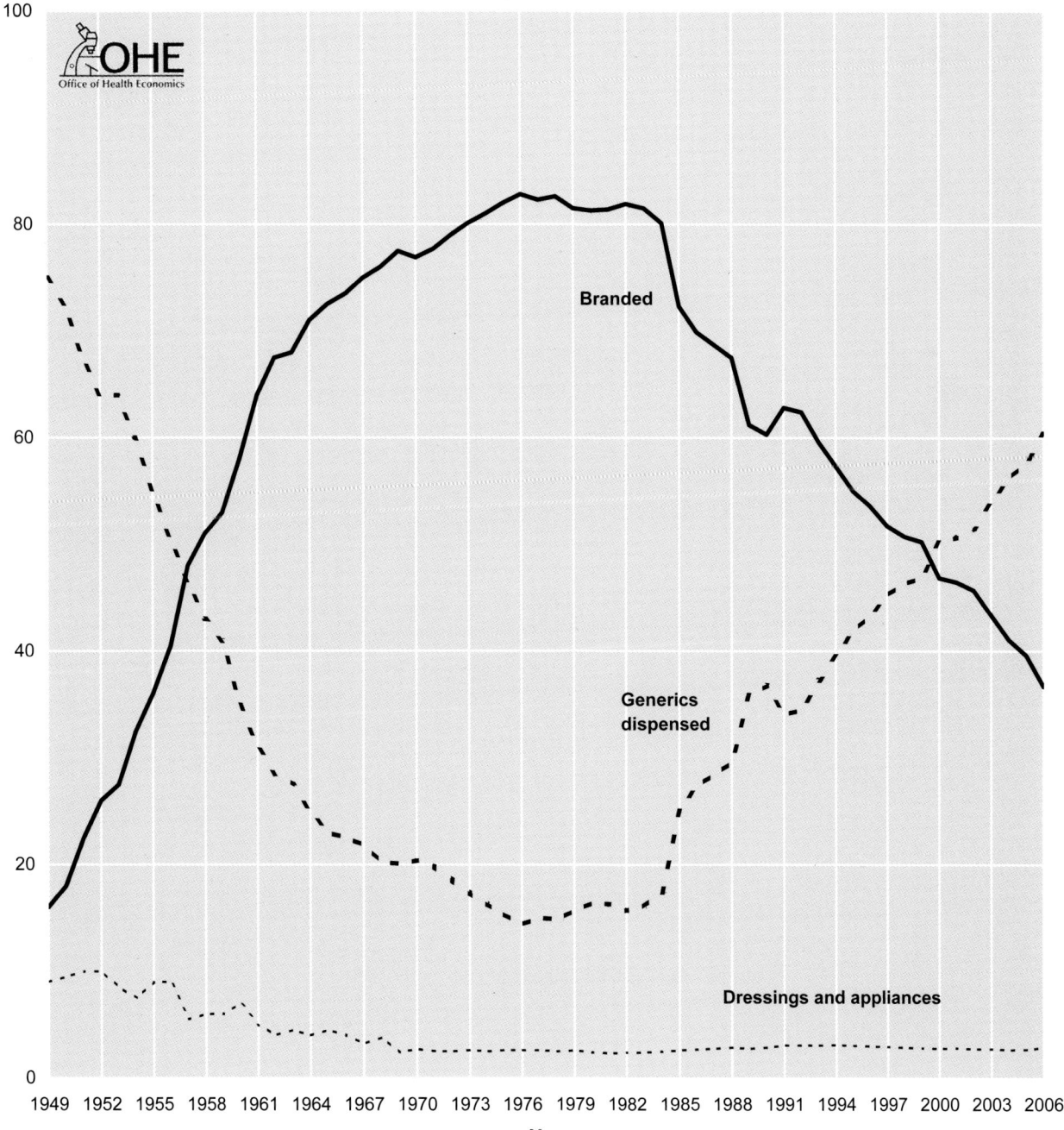

**Year**

*Notes:* 1 Figures relate to community pharmacists and appliance contractors contracted to the NHS.
   Data from 1994 have been revised, see DH Statistics Bulletin 2000/20.
*Sources:* Prescriptions Dispensed in the Community Statistics: England (DH Statistical Bulletin).
   Prescriptions Dispensed in the Community Statistics: England (Information Centre (IC)).

Figure 4.23  **Relationship between generic prescribing and generic dispensing, England, 2006**

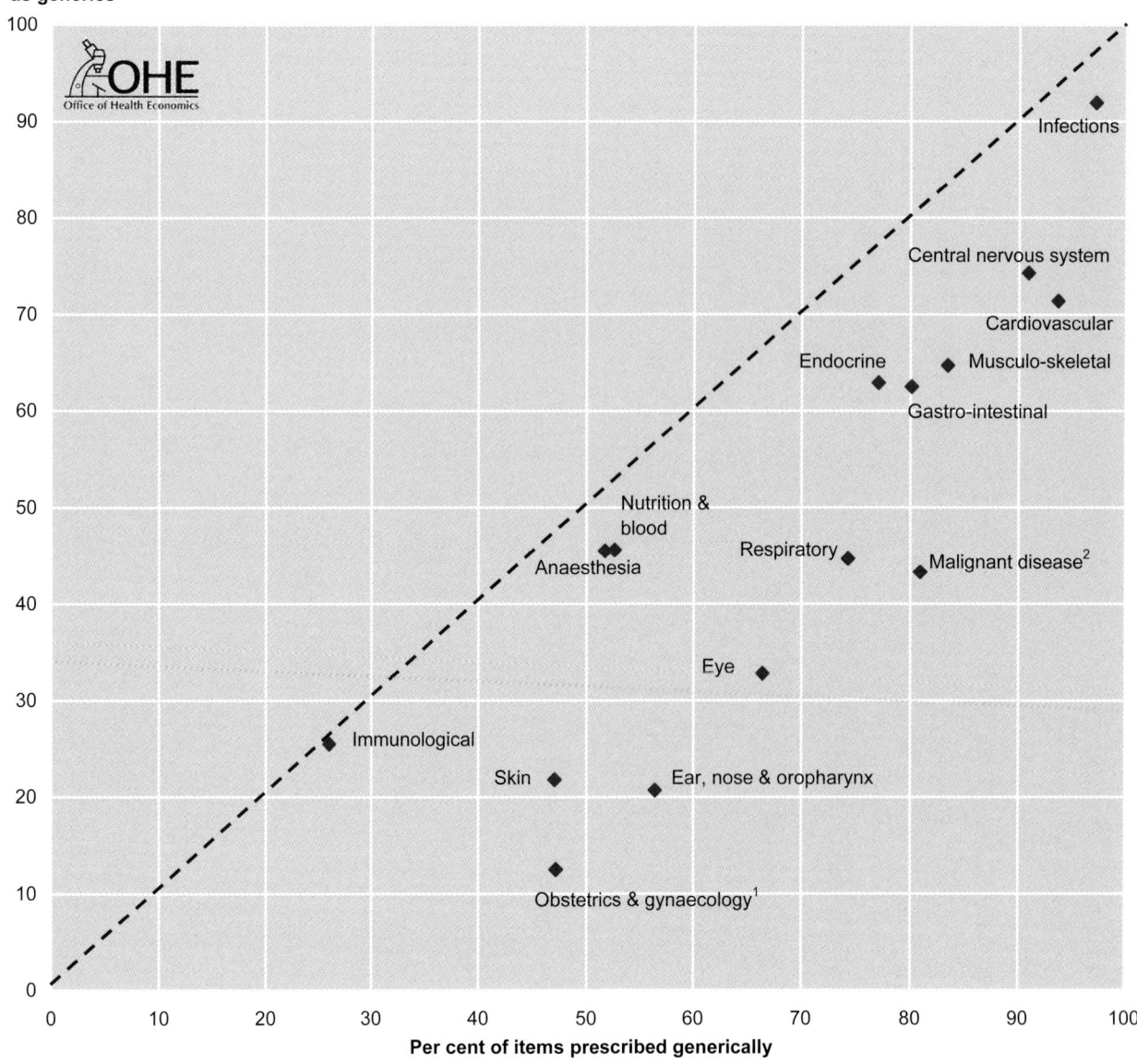

*Notes:*  The dashed line is a reference line showing equality between generic dispensing and prescribing.
1 Including urinary tract disorders.
2 Including immunosuppression.
Data points relate to British National Formulary chapters.
*Sources:* Prescriptions Dispensed in the Community Statistics: England (DH Statistical Bulletin).
Prescriptions Dispensed in the Community Statistics: England (Information Centre IC).

# FHS: General Pharmaceutical Services

Table 4.46  **Estimated total NHS expenditure on pharmaceuticals at manufacturers' prices[1], UK, 1969 - 2006**

£ million (cash)

| Year | Pharmaceutical services[1] | Dispensing doctors[1] | Hospital[1] | Total NHS medicines | NHS medicines cost: Per capita[2] £ (2006 prices) | NHS medicines cost: % total NHS cost | NHS medicines cost: % GDP |
|------|------|------|------|------|------|------|------|
| 1969 | 113 | 5 | 26 | 144 | 29.98 | 8.3 | 0.31 |
| 1970 | 124 | 6 | 29 | 159 | 30.39 | 8.0 | 0.31 |
| 1971 | 136 | 7 | 33 | 176 | 30.45 | 7.8 | 0.31 |
| 1972 | 142 | 7 | 37 | 185 | 29.52 | 7.1 | 0.29 |
| 1973 | 160 | 9 | 41 | 210 | 31.10 | 7.1 | 0.28 |
| 1974 | 176 | 10 | 50 | 236 | 30.05 | 6.2 | 0.28 |
| 1975 | 208 | 12 | 59 | 279 | 28.05 | 5.4 | 0.26 |
| 1976 | 266 | 14 | 73 | 353 | 30.94 | 5.8 | 0.28 |
| 1977 | 342 | 18 | 88 | 448 | 34.67 | 6.7 | 0.31 |
| 1978 | 439 | 24 | 121 | 584 | 40.16 | 7.7 | 0.35 |
| 1979 | 525 | 29 | 146 | 700 | 42.04 | 7.9 | 0.35 |
| 1980 | 613 | 35 | 178 | 826 | 41.88 | 7.3 | 0.36 |
| 1981 | 746 | 41 | 213 | 1,000 | 45.60 | 7.7 | 0.40 |
| 1982 | 872 | 49 | 247 | 1,168 | 50.19 | 8.3 | 0.42 |
| 1983 | 1,015 | 57 | 284 | 1,350 | 55.02 | 9.0 | 0.45 |
| 1984 | 1,141 | 66 | 317 | 1,524 | 59.22 | 9.5 | 0.47 |
| 1985 | 1,217 | 74 | 336 | 1,627 | 59.76 | 9.5 | 0.46 |
| 1986 | 1,269 | 80 | 357 | 1,706 | 60.76 | 9.2 | 0.45 |
| 1987 | 1,378 | 88 | 382 | 1,849 | 62.43 | 9.1 | 0.44 |
| 1988 | 1,554 | 99 | 420 | 2,074 | 65.55 | 8.8 | 0.44 |
| 1989 | 1,758 | 108 | 451 | 2,316 | 67.78 | 9.0 | 0.45 |
| 1990 | 1,918 | 121 | 495 | 2,533 | 68.68 | 8.9 | 0.45 |
| 1991 | 2,042 | 163 | 550 | 2,755 | 70.57 | 8.6 | 0.47 |
| 1992 | 2,309 | 192 | 688 | 3,189 | 78.47 | 9.0 | 0.52 |
| 1993 | 2,914 | 229 | 750 | 3,893 | 93.00 | 10.5 | 0.61 |
| 1994 | 3,141 | 259 | 827 | 4,227 | 99.19 | 10.6 | 0.62 |
| 1995 | 3,406 | 286 | 891 | 4,583 | 104.47 | 11.0 | 0.64 |
| 1996 | 3,749 | 241 | 890 | 4,880 | 107.01 | 11.2 | 0.64 |
| 1997 | 4,090 | 259 | 978 | 5,327 | 113.56 | 11.7 | 0.66 |
| 1998 | 4,409 | 291 | 1,107 | 5,807 | 120.52 | 12.1 | 0.67 |
| 1999 | 4,959 | 321 | 1,251 | 6,532 | 132.82 | 12.5 | 0.72 |
| 2000 | 5,244 | 336 | 1,390 | 6,969 | 139.53 | 12.2 | 0.73 |
| 2001 | 5,728 | 365 | 1,552 | 7,645 | 148.40 | 12.2 | 0.77 |
| 2002 | 6,409 | 407 | 1,764 | 8,580 | 160.31 | 12.3 | 0.82 |
| 2003 | 7,024 | 445 | 2,041 | 9,510 | 171.49 | 12.1 | 0.86 |
| 2004 | 7,540 | 480 | 2,340 | 10,360 | 181.21 | 12.0 | 0.88 |
| 2005 | 7,376 | 471 | 2,409 | 10,257 | 174.32 | 10.8 | 0.84 |
| 2006 | 7,657 | 491 | 2,575 | 10,723 | 176.98 | 10.5 | 0.83 |

*Notes:*  All figures exclude dressings and appliances.
GDP = Gross Domestic Product at market prices.
1 These figures have been obtained by deflating the net ingredient cost (before discount) of prescriptions dispensed during the year with a standard manufacturers' discount rate of 12.5 per cent (15 per cent prior to 1980). They are also known as 'NHS sales at manufacturer's prices'. These figures are representative of NHS expenditure on medicines, although the discount rate may differ slightly to that used by the NHS, which varies from year to year.
2 At 2006 prices, as adjusted by the GDP deflator at market prices.

*Sources:*  Prescription Pricing Authority Annual Reports.
Annual Abstract of Statistics (ONS).
Health and Personal Services Statistics for England (DH).
Health Statistics Wales (NAW).
Scottish Health Statistics (ISD).
Economic Trends (ONS).

Figure 4.24 **Estimated total NHS expenditure on medicines (at manufacturers' prices)** [1] **and per cent of gross NHS cost, UK, 1969 - 2006**

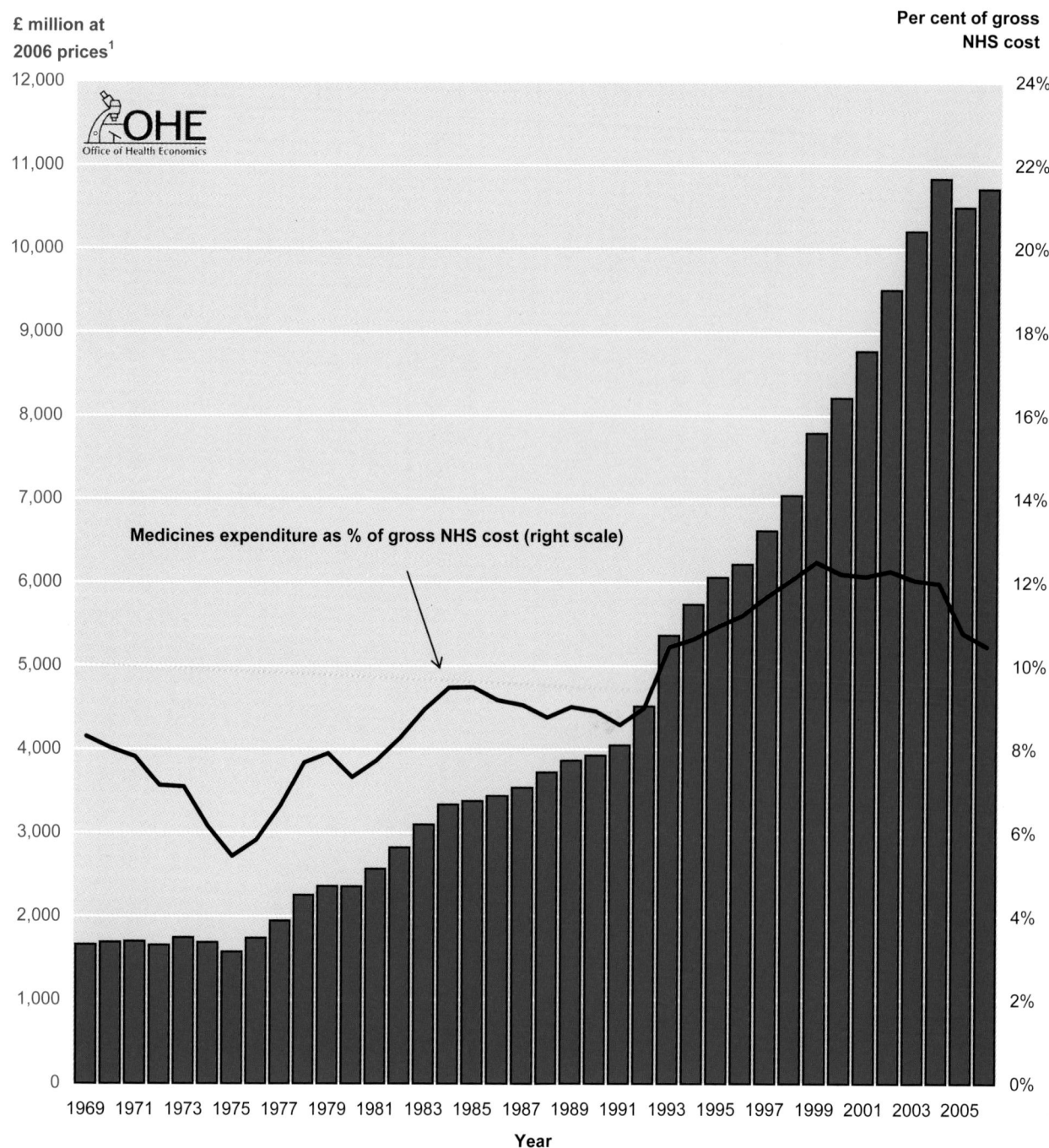

**£ million at 2006 prices** [1]

**Per cent of gross NHS cost**

Medicines expenditure as % of gross NHS cost (right scale)

**Year**

Notes:    All figures include medicines dispensed by chemists and dispensing doctors, and hospital purchases.
        1 As adjusted by the Gross Domestic Product (GDP) deflator at market prices.
Sources:  Prescription Pricing Authority Annual Reports.
        Annual Abstract of Statistics (ONS).
        Health and Personal Social Services Statistics for England (DH).
        Health Statistics Wales (NAW).
        Scottish Health Statistics (ISD).
        Economic Trends (ONS).

# FHS: General Dental Services

NHS dental care is mainly provided by general dental practitioners who contract with the NHS, although some treatment is carried out by salaried 'Personal Dental Services' (PDS) dentists, NHS community dental services and hospital dental departments. Community dental services are offered to pre-school and school age children, and to pregnant and nursing mothers attending community health clinics. Access to treatment at a dental hospital is usually by referral from a general dental practitioner, although patients may also present themselves at dental hospitals for emergency treatment. The activities of these two services are not included in this section of the Compendium.

Since the creation of the NHS in 1948, dentists working under contract to the NHS have been paid a fee for each item of treatment given. Under the dental contract, implemented on 1 October 1990, the remuneration of dentists by the NHS includes payment for preventive care as well as restorative treatments. A capitation fee was also paid covering most types of treatment for patients under the age of 18 registered with a NHS dentist. All NHS patients accepted by a dentist are now offered continuing care, emergency cover and guaranteed free replacement of dental treatments if they fail within a year. On 1$^{st}$ April 2006 a new dental contract came into effect in England and Wales, this introduced a different payment scheme for dentists' NHS work and places greater emphasis on preventative work. Dentists in Scotland and Northern Ireland are not subject to the new contract in England and Wales.

Although public funds continue to finance most GDS expenditure, part of funding across the UK comes from patient charges. In recent years the system of patient charges has undergone considerable change and is no longer consistent between the four countries. **Box 20** shows the new system of NHS dental charges introduced on 1$^{st}$ April 2006 in England and Wales.

Scotland introduced free dental examinations for all NHS registered patients on 1$^{st}$ April 2006, but those not exempt from NHS dental charges are still expected to pay 80% of the fees for other NHS dental treatments, up to a maximum of £384 for a single course of treatment (Health and Community care, Scottish Executive). In Northern Ireland the patient is also expected to pay 80% off the gross cost of treatments up to a maximum of £384 (Northern Ireland CSA). Exemptions exist in all four countries of the UK for those aged under 18, those aged 18 and in full time education, for patients who are pregnant or who have had a baby in the last 12 months, and for those on a low income (**Box 21**).

---

**Box 20 Dental charges in England & Wales[1]**

Those exempt from dental charges continue to receive treatment and care free of charge (see Box 21).

For those who pay for dental charges there are three standard charges in England and Wales, the amount charged will depend on the treatment needed.

Only one charge will be made for one treatment, even if more than one visit to the dentist is required to complete the course of treatment.

If more than one treatment is required at the same charge level within two months of seeing the dentist, the further treatment is free of charge.

| Levels of | treatment charges |
|---|---|
| £15.50[2] | • Examination, diagnosis and preventive care. If necessary, this includes X-rays, scale and polish, and planning for further treatment. |
| | • Urgent and out-of-hours care. |
| £42.40[2] | • This charge includes all treatment covered by the level one charge £15.50 PLUS additional treatment such as fillings, root canal treatment or extractions. |
| £189[2] | • This charge includes all treatments covered by the £15.50 and £42.40 charges PLUS more complex procedures such as crowns, dentures and bridges. |
| No charge | • Writing a prescription or removing stitches (usual charges apply for dispensing of prescription). |
| | • Repairs to dentures. |
| | • Referrals to sedation, orthodontic or home visit services (although a charge may be levied for treatment prior to referral and for the specialist service). |

**Referrals to another dentist**

Only one charge is made for one course of treatment even if this includes a referral to another dentist.

If a new course of treatment is required involving specialised services (sedation, orthodontics, and home visits) only one charge is paid to the dentist who provides the specialised service.

*Notes:* 1 NHS dental charges in England introduced on 1$^{st}$ April 2006.
2 In Wales, the three levels of charges are £12, £39 and £177.
*Sources:* NHS UK, Health of Wales information service, Scottish Executive Health.

---

In 2005/06 the gross cost of UK NHS General Dental Services (GDS) was £2,621 million, double in real terms the cost 30 years earlier (**Figure 4.25**). Growth in the current decade was similar to the decade before (**Box 22**). The average per capita outlay by the NHS on General Dental Services has risen over the past decade in the UK, standing at £43 in 2005/06. Per capita and per household expenditure are relatively similar across the four countries of the UK, but highest in Scotland of late (**Table 4.47**). Outlay by the NHS on General Dental Services is now less than there per cent of total NHS costs, compared to over 10% in 1949 (**Figure 4.25**).

Patient contributions (dental charges) amounted to about one quarter of the gross GDS cost in 2005/06 (**Figure 4.26**). After particularly large increases in the 1980s, the last decade has seen a slowdown in the rate of growth of patient contributions. **Figure 4.27** illustrates the increases in dental charges since they were introduced in 1951 and their impacts on the uptake of NHS General Dental Services. After the introduction of the new charging scheme as outlined above, charge income was not at the level expected, which resulted in a reduction in revenue in 2005 according to data published by the information centre, however, this was shown to increase again in 2006.[1]

Box 22 **Decadal percentage change in real[1] GDS expenditure, UK**

| | Real GDS expenditure | GDS per capita | Total NHS gross cost per capita |
|---|---|---|---|
| 1965 - 1975 | 38 | 33 | 62 |
| 1975 - 1985 | 23 | 22 | 22 |
| 1985 - 1995 | 28 | 25 | 51 |
| 1995 - 2005 | 28 | 23 | 69 |

*Note:* 1 As adjusted by GDP deflator at market prices.
*Sources:* Health and Personal Social Services Statistics for England (DH).
Health Statistics Wales (NAW).
Scottish Health Statistics (ISD).
Annual Statistical Report (Northern Ireland CSA).
Annual Abstract of Statistics (ONS).
Department of Health Departmental Report (DH).
NHS Board Operating Costs and Capital Expenditure (ISD Scotland).
Public Expenditure Statistical Analyses (HM Treasury).

There were 24,151 dentists (excluding assistants) working in the GDS in the UK in 2006, more than double the number in 1951. **Table 4.48** shows that growth in the numbers of NHS dentists stopped for a few years when a new dental contract was implemented in 1990. But an upward trend resumed in 1996. Amongst OECD countries, the UK has one of the lowest ratios of dentists to population (**Figure 4.28**).

Over the years, the general dental health of the population has improved markedly, with adults keeping more of their teeth longer and young adults having fewer fillings than their parents. Figures from the *General Household Survey* show a steady fall in the proportion of adults reporting no natural teeth, from 26% in 1983 to 10% in 2003 despite the ageing of the population (**Box 23**). Alternative information on dental health is available in the Adult Dental Health Survey, however, the most recent survey was conducted in 1998.

Box 23 **Percentage of adults with no natural teeth, Great Britain**

| | % without natural teeth | |
|---|---|---|
| Age group | 1983 | 2003 |
| All ages | 26 | 10 |
| 16 - 24 | 0 | 0 |
| 25 - 34 | 2 | 0 |
| 35 - 44 | 9 | 1 |
| 45 - 54 | 24 | 3 |
| 55 - 64 | 43 | 11 |
| 65 - 74 | 65 | 27 |
| over 75 | 82 | 47 |

*Notes:* There is no recent information available on the percentage having dental check ups.
From 1988 to 2004 the General Household Survey was on a financial year basis with interviews taking place from April to the following March.
*Source:* Living in Britain: Results from the General Household Survey (ONS).

References

1 Dental Statistics 1996-2006 Information centre for Health and Social Services (IC).

Table 4.47   **General Dental Services (GDS) gross expenditure per capita and per household, UK, 1975/76 - 2005/06**

| Year | England | Wales | Scotland | Northern Ireland | UK | England | Wales | Scotland | Northern Ireland | UK |
|---|---|---|---|---|---|---|---|---|---|---|
| | | | | | GDS expenditure per capita (£ cash) | | | | | |
| | | | (£ cash) | | | At constant prices[1] (Index 1975/76=100) | | | | |
| 1975/76 | 4 | 3 | 4 | 4 | 4 | 100 | 100 | 100 | 100 | 100 |
| 1980/81 | 9 | 8 | 8 | 8 | 9 | 114 | 135 | 101 | 101 | 114 |
| 1981/82 | 10 | 9 | 9 | 10 | 10 | 115 | 138 | 104 | 115 | 115 |
| 1982/83 | 12 | 10 | 10 | 10 | 11 | 129 | 144 | 108 | 108 | 118 |
| 1983/84 | 12 | 11 | 11 | 11 | 12 | 124 | 151 | 113 | 113 | 124 |
| 1984/85 | 14 | 12 | 12 | 12 | 14 | 137 | 156 | 117 | 117 | 137 |
| 1985/86 | 15 | 12 | 15 | 12 | 15 | 139 | 148 | 139 | 111 | 139 |
| 1986/87 | 16 | 14 | 17 | 14 | 16 | 144 | 168 | 153 | 126 | 144 |
| 1987/88 | 17 | 15 | 20 | 15 | 18 | 145 | 170 | 170 | 128 | 153 |
| 1988/89 | 20 | 18 | 19 | 17 | 20 | 159 | 191 | 151 | 135 | 159 |
| 1989/90 | 20 | 18 | 19 | 20 | 20 | 148 | 173 | 143 | 148 | 146 |
| 1990/91 | 22 | 20 | 20 | 22 | 22 | 150 | 183 | 135 | 151 | 148 |
| 1991/92 | 26 | 24 | 26 | 29 | 26 | 169 | 209 | 169 | 190 | 169 |
| 1992/93 | 27 | 26 | 26 | 29 | 27 | 171 | 215 | 165 | 184 | 170 |
| 1993/94 | 25 | 24 | 25 | 27 | 25 | 155 | 192 | 154 | 164 | 155 |
| 1994/95 | 27 | 24 | 25 | 29 | 26 | 160 | 196 | 152 | 172 | 159 |
| 1995/96 | 27 | 24 | 27 | 30 | 27 | 156 | 191 | 156 | 173 | 156 |
| 1996/97 | 27 | 25 | 27 | 31 | 27 | 154 | 192 | 153 | 175 | 154 |
| 1997/98 | 28 | 27 | 27 | 32 | 28 | 152 | 198 | 151 | 177 | 153 |
| 1998/99 | 30 | 29 | 31 | 34 | 30 | 158 | 206 | 164 | 182 | 159 |
| 1999/00 | 30 | 30 | 31 | 35 | 31 | 160 | 208 | 163 | 184 | 160 |
| 2000/01 | 32 | 31 | 32 | 37 | 32 | 166 | 217 | 164 | 189 | 166 |
| 2001/02 | 34 | 33 | 36 | 38 | 34 | 171 | 221 | 181 | 193 | 172 |
| 2002/03 | 35 | 34 | 39 | 39 | 36 | 173 | 223 | 189 | 191 | 174 |
| 2003/04 | 36 | 35 | 39 | 39 | 37 | 173 | 224 | 188 | 187 | 175 |
| 2004/05 | 39 | 36 | 43 | 39 | 39 | 180 | 221 | 198 | 182 | 181 |
| 2005/06 | 44 | 37 | 47 | 40 | 43 | 198 | 222 | 212 | 183 | 198 |
| | | | | | GDS expenditure per household (£ cash) | | | | | |
| | | | (£ cash) | | | At constant prices[1] (Index 1975/76=100) | | | | |
| 1975/76 | 11 | 9 | 12 | 12 | 11 | 100 | 100 | 100 | 100 | 100 |
| 1980/81 | 25 | 22 | 23 | 24 | 25 | 110 | 129 | 96 | 99 | 110 |
| 1981/82 | 27 | 25 | 25 | 32 | 27 | 110 | 131 | 97 | 118 | 110 |
| 1982/83 | 32 | 27 | 27 | 30 | 30 | 122 | 135 | 99 | 106 | 112 |
| 1983/84 | 32 | 30 | 30 | 33 | 32 | 116 | 141 | 103 | 111 | 116 |
| 1984/85 | 37 | 32 | 32 | 36 | 37 | 127 | 145 | 105 | 114 | 127 |
| 1985/86 | 39 | 32 | 39 | 36 | 39 | 129 | 136 | 123 | 108 | 128 |
| 1986/87 | 42 | 37 | 44 | 42 | 42 | 132 | 152 | 134 | 122 | 131 |
| 1987/88 | 44 | 39 | 51 | 45 | 47 | 131 | 153 | 147 | 123 | 139 |
| 1988/89 | 51 | 47 | 48 | 51 | 51 | 143 | 170 | 129 | 130 | 143 |
| 1989/90 | 50 | 45 | 48 | 59 | 50 | 132 | 153 | 121 | 140 | 130 |
| 1990/91 | 55 | 51 | 49 | 64 | 54 | 133 | 160 | 114 | 142 | 131 |
| 1991/92 | 65 | 61 | 65 | 85 | 65 | 149 | 182 | 142 | 178 | 148 |
| 1992/93 | 68 | 64 | 65 | 84 | 68 | 150 | 186 | 137 | 170 | 149 |
| 1993/94 | 63 | 59 | 62 | 76 | 63 | 136 | 166 | 127 | 150 | 135 |
| 1994/95 | 66 | 61 | 61 | 79 | 65 | 140 | 168 | 124 | 154 | 138 |
| 1995/96 | 66 | 61 | 64 | 82 | 66 | 136 | 163 | 127 | 154 | 135 |
| 1996/97 | 67 | 63 | 64 | 86 | 67 | 134 | 163 | 123 | 156 | 133 |
| 1997/98 | 68 | 66 | 65 | 92 | 68 | 132 | 168 | 120 | 164 | 131 |
| 1998/99 | 72 | 71 | 72 | 95 | 73 | 137 | 174 | 130 | 164 | 137 |
| 1999/00 | 74 | 72 | 73 | 96 | 75 | 138 | 175 | 129 | 163 | 137 |
| 2000/01 | 78 | 76 | 74 | 99 | 78 | 142 | 182 | 129 | 165 | 141 |
| 2001/02 | 81 | 79 | 82 | 102 | 82 | 145 | 183 | 141 | 167 | 145 |
| 2002/03 | 84 | 81 | 88 | 104 | 85 | 146 | 183 | 146 | 164 | 146 |
| 2003/04 | 87 | 84 | 89 | 103 | 87 | 146 | 184 | 143 | 159 | 146 |
| 2004/05 | 92 | 84 | 96 | 103 | 93 | 151 | 180 | 151 | 154 | 151 |
| 2005/06 | 103 | 86 | 105 | 105 | 103 | 166 | 179 | 160 | 154 | 163 |

*Notes:*   All figures include charges paid by patients.
1 As adjusted by the Gross Domestic Product (GDP) deflator at market prices.
*Sources:*   The Government's Expenditure Plans (DH).
Annual Abstract of Statistics (ONS).
Economic Trends (ONS).

Figure 4.25  **Gross cost[1] of General Dental Services (GDS) and per cent of gross NHS cost, UK, 1949/50 - 2005/06**

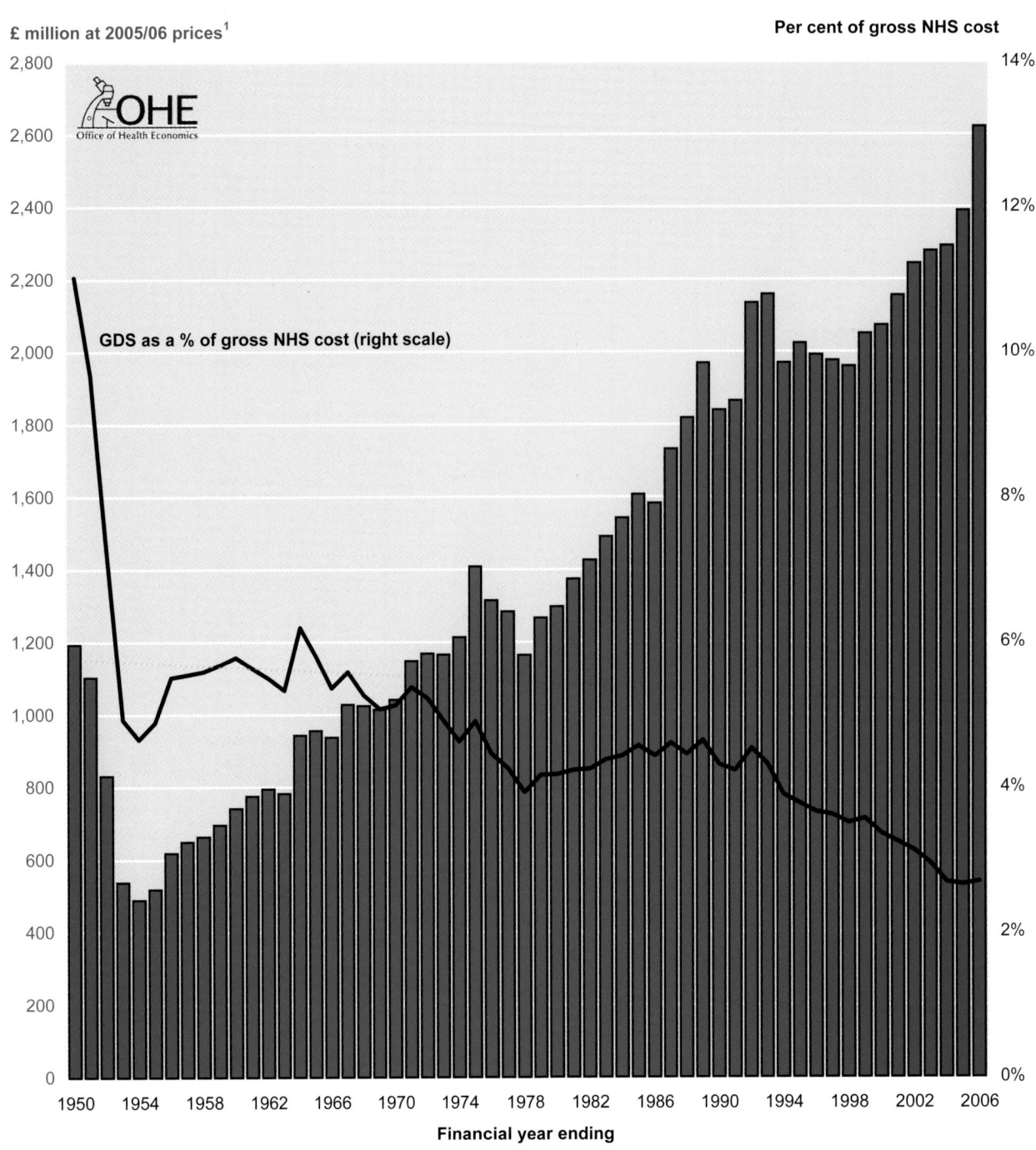

**£ million at 2005/06 prices[1]**

**Per cent of gross NHS cost**

GDS as a % of gross NHS cost (right scale)

**Financial year ending**

*Notes:*  Gross cost includes patient charges.
Figures are for financial year ending 31 March e.g 2000 = 1999/2000.
1 As adjusted by the Gross Domestic Product (GDP) deflator at market prices.

*Sources:*  Health and Personal Social Services Statistics for England (DH).
Health Statistics Wales (NAW).
Scottish Health Statistics (ISD).
Annual Statistical Report (Northern Ireland CSA).

Figure 4.26 **Patient dental charges and as a percentage of the gross cost of General Dental Services (GDS), UK, 1951/52 - 2005/06**

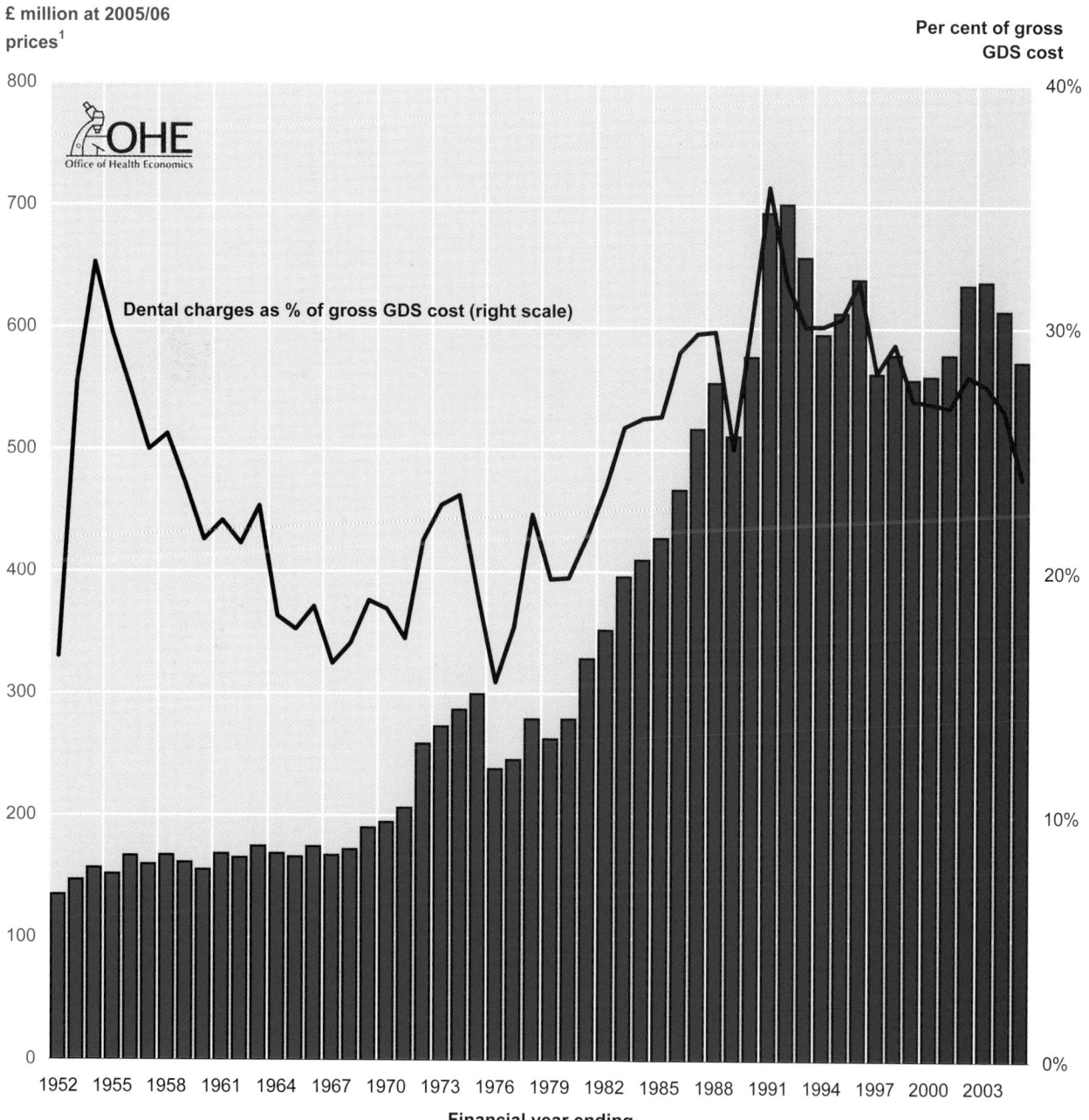

£ million at 2005/06 prices[1]

Per cent of gross GDS cost

Dental charges as % of gross GDS cost (right scale)

Financial year ending

*Notes:* Dental charges were first introduced in 1951. Data for 2001/02 onwards are OHE estimates based in part on available published data. Data for 2004/05 onwards are not strictly comparable with earlier data, as reliable data for PDS in England and Wales are not available before 2004/05 and therefore data prior to 2004/05 is based on GDS patient charges alone. In 2005/06 there was a shortfall in patient charge income, in part attributable to PDS pilots income being based on the old GDS system of patient charges in England and Wales. Figures are for financial years, ending the year shown on the x-axis.

1 At 2005/06 prices, as adjusted by the Gross Domestic Product (GDP) deflator at market prices.

*Sources:* Annual Abstract of Statistics (ONS).
Health and Personal Social Services Statistics for England (DH).
Health Statistics Wales (NAW).
Scottish Health Statistics (ISD).
Annual Statistical Report (Northern Ireland CSA).
Economic Trends (ONS).
Personal correspondance (DH).
HPSS Expenditure in Northern Ireland (DHSSPSNI).
Economic Data (HM Treasury).

# FHS: General Dental Services

Figure 4.27 **Courses[1] of dental treatment and per 1,000 people, UK, 1951 - 2004/05**

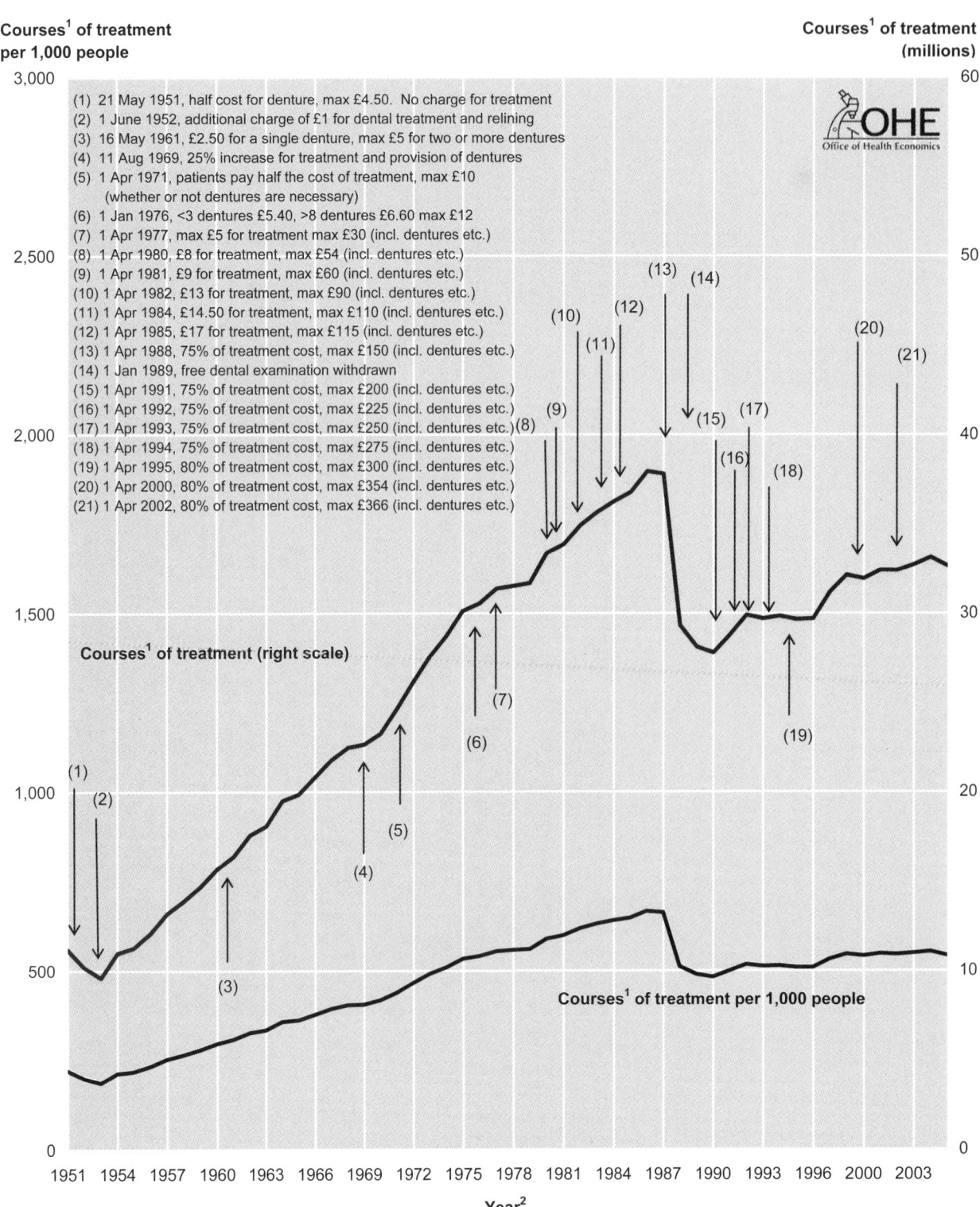

**Courses[1] of treatment
per 1,000 people**

**Courses[1] of treatment
(millions)**

(1) 21 May 1951, half cost for denture, max £4.50. No charge for treatment
(2) 1 June 1952, additional charge of £1 for dental treatment and relining
(3) 16 May 1961, £2.50 for a single denture, max £5 for two or more dentures
(4) 11 Aug 1969, 25% increase for treatment and provision of dentures
(5) 1 Apr 1971, patients pay half the cost of treatment, max £10
    (whether or not dentures are necessary)
(6) 1 Jan 1976, <3 dentures £5.40, >8 dentures £6.60 max £12
(7) 1 Apr 1977, max £5 for treatment max £30 (incl. dentures etc.)
(8) 1 Apr 1980, £8 for treatment, max £54 (incl. dentures etc.)
(9) 1 Apr 1981, £9 for treatment, max £60 (incl. dentures etc.)
(10) 1 Apr 1982, £13 for treatment, max £90 (incl. dentures etc.)
(11) 1 Apr 1984, £14.50 for treatment, max £110 (incl. dentures etc.)
(12) 1 Apr 1985, £17 for treatment, max £115 (incl. dentures etc.)
(13) 1 Apr 1988, 75% of treatment cost, max £150 (incl. dentures etc.)
(14) 1 Jan 1989, free dental examination withdrawn
(15) 1 Apr 1991, 75% of treatment cost, max £200 (incl. dentures etc.)
(16) 1 Apr 1992, 75% of treatment cost, max £225 (incl. dentures etc.)
(17) 1 Apr 1993, 75% of treatment cost, max £250 (incl. dentures etc.)
(18) 1 Apr 1994, 75% of treatment cost, max £275 (incl. dentures etc.)
(19) 1 Apr 1995, 80% of treatment cost, max £300 (incl. dentures etc.)
(20) 1 Apr 2000, 80% of treatment cost, max £354 (incl. dentures etc.)
(21) 1 Apr 2002, 80% of treatment cost, max £366 (incl. dentures etc.)

OHE
Office of Health Economics

Courses[1] of treatment (right scale)

Courses[1] of treatment per 1,000 people

**Year[2]**

*Notes:* Prior to 1988 figures relate to the number of treatments completed and emergency cases that were scheduled for payment. From 1988
onwards figures relate to the number of adult courses of treatments.
1 Including emergency cases.
2 Figures from 1998 onwards relate to financial years ending 31st March e.g. 2000 = 1999/2000.
Recent changes in dental charges can be found in the document section commencing on page 271.

*Sources:* Annual Abstract of Statistics (ONS).
Health and Personal Social Services Statistics for England (DH).
Health Statistics Wales (NAW).
Scottish Health Statistics (ISD).
Annual Statistical Report (Northern Ireland CSA).

Table 4.48  **Number of NHS dental practitioners[1], UK, 1951 - 2006**

30th September

| | Number of dental practitioners | | | | Per 100,000 population | | | |
|---|---|---|---|---|---|---|---|---|
| Year | England and Wales | Scotland | Northern Ireland[2] | United Kingdom | England and Wales | Scotland | Northern Ireland[2] | United Kingdom |
| 1951 | 9,694 | 1,254 | 331 | 11,279 | 22.1 | 24.6 | 24.1 | 22.4 |
| 1955 | 9,359 | 1,152 | 284 | 10,795 | 21.1 | 22.5 | 20.4 | 21.2 |
| 1960 | 9,853 | 1,064 | 296 | 11,213 | 21.5 | 20.5 | 20.8 | 21.4 |
| 1961 | 10,026 | 1,048 | 299 | 11,373 | 21.7 | 20.2 | 21.0 | 21.5 |
| 1962 | 10,540 | 1,046 | 304 | 11,890 | 22.6 | 20.1 | 21.2 | 22.3 |
| 1963 | 10,496 | 1,047 | 300 | 11,843 | 22.3 | 20.1 | 20.7 | 22.1 |
| 1964 | 10,414 | 1,065 | 309 | 11,788 | 22.0 | 20.4 | 21.2 | 21.8 |
| 1965 | 10,405 | 1,053 | 300 | 11,758 | 21.8 | 20.2 | 20.4 | 21.6 |
| 1966 | 10,416 | 1,134 | 317 | 11,867 | 21.7 | 21.8 | 21.5 | 21.7 |
| 1967 | 10,461 | 1,109 | 325 | 11,895 | 21.7 | 21.3 | 21.8 | 21.6 |
| 1968 | 10,593 | 1,102 | 334 | 12,029 | 22.0 | 21.2 | 22.2 | 21.9 |
| 1969 | 10,659 | 1,087 | 332 | 12,078 | 21.9 | 20.9 | 21.9 | 21.8 |
| 1970 | 10,843 | 1,091 | 329 | 12,263 | 22.2 | 20.9 | 21.5 | 22.0 |
| 1971 | 10,962 | 1,095 | 328 | 12,385 | 22.3 | 20.9 | 21.3 | 22.1 |
| 1972 | 11,209 | 1,120 | 322 | 12,651 | 22.7 | 21.4 | 20.9 | 22.6 |
| 1973 | 11,374 | 1,146 | 317 | 12,837 | 23.0 | 21.9 | 20.7 | 22.8 |
| 1974 | 11,528 | 1,176 | 320 | 13,024 | 23.3 | 22.4 | 21.0 | 23.2 |
| 1975 | 11,737 | 1,184 | 310 | 13,231 | 23.7 | 22.6 | 20.3 | 23.5 |
| 1976 | 12,054 | 1,194 | 309 | 13,557 | 24.4 | 22.8 | 20.3 | 24.1 |
| 1977 | 12,360 | 1,204 | 310 | 13,874 | 25.0 | 23.0 | 20.4 | 24.7 |
| 1978 | 12,517 | 1,223 | 309 | 14,049 | 25.3 | 23.5 | 20.3 | 25.0 |
| 1979 | 12,750 | 1,235 | 319 | 14,304 | 25.8 | 23.7 | 20.9 | 25.4 |
| 1980 | 13,039 | 1,280 | 336 | 14,655 | 26.3 | 24.6 | 21.9 | 26.0 |
| 1981 | 13,473 | 1,327 | 342 | 15,142 | 27.1 | 25.6 | 22.2 | 26.9 |
| 1982 | 13,936 | 1,387 | 363 | 15,686 | 28.1 | 26.8 | 23.6 | 27.9 |
| 1983 | 14,374 | 1,393 | 377 | 16,144 | 28.9 | 27.0 | 24.4 | 28.7 |
| 1984 | 14,780 | 1,434 | 394 | 16,608 | 29.7 | 27.9 | 25.3 | 29.4 |
| 1985 | 15,076 | 1,407 | 420 | 16,903 | 30.2 | 27.4 | 26.8 | 29.9 |
| 1986 | 15,256 | 1,488 | 428 | 17,172 | 30.5 | 29.1 | 27.2 | 30.3 |
| 1987 | 15,545 | 1,515 | 437 | 17,497 | 31.0 | 29.7 | 27.6 | 30.8 |
| 1988 | 15,868 | 1,523 | 460 | 17,851 | 31.6 | 30.0 | 29.0 | 31.4 |
| 1989 | 16,178 | 1,585 | 467 | 18,230 | 32.1 | 31.2 | 29.4 | 31.9 |
| 1990 | 15,901 | 1,645 | 519 | 18,065 | 31.4 | 32.4 | 32.5 | 31.6 |
| 1991 | 15,775 | 1,676 | 513 | 17,964 | 31.1 | 33.0 | 31.9 | 31.3 |
| 1992 | 15,698 | 1,702 | 523 | 17,923 | 30.9 | 33.5 | 32.2 | 31.1 |
| 1993 | 15,950 | 1,772 | 541 | 18,263 | 31.3 | 34.8 | 33.1 | 31.6 |
| 1994 | 15,885 | 1,763 | 569 | 18,217 | 31.1 | 34.6 | 34.6 | 31.5 |
| 1995 | 15,881 | 1,722 | 581 | 18,226 | 31.0 | 33.7 | 35.2 | 31.4 |
| 1996 | 16,114 | 1,721 | 596 | 18,431 | 31.3 | 33.8 | 35.9 | 31.7 |
| 1997 | 16,372 | 1,747 | 610 | 18,729 | 31.8 | 34.4 | 36.5 | 32.1 |
| 1998 | 16,699 | 1,789 | 633 | 19,121 | 32.3 | 35.2 | 37.7 | 32.7 |
| 1999 | 17,151 | 1,827 | 660 | 19,638 | 33.0 | 36.0 | 39.3 | 33.5 |
| 2000 | 17,500 | 1,823 | 674 | 19,997 | 33.6 | 36.0 | 40.0 | 34.0 |
| 2001 | 18,119 | 1,856 | 689 | 20,664 | 34.6 | 36.6 | 40.8 | 35.0 |
| 2002 | 18,283 | 1,881 | 689 | 20,853 | 34.8 | 37.2 | 40.6 | 35.2 |
| 2003 | 18,666 | 1,903 | 696 | 21,265 | 35.4 | 37.6 | 40.9 | 35.7 |
| 2004 | 19,398 | 1,919 | 720 | 22,037 | 36.6 | 37.8 | 42.1 | 36.8 |
| 2005 | 20,500 | 1,933 | 726 | 23,159 | 38.4 | 37.9 | 42.1 | 38.4 |
| 2006 | 21,366 | 2,025 | *760* | 24,151 | 39.8 | 39.6 | *43.6* | 39.9 |

*Notes:*   1 Figures exclude assistants.

2 Figures for Northern Ireland prior to 2005 relate to 31st December, for 2005 relate 1st April. 2006 figures are not yet available and relate to 31st October 2005.

The latest number for Northern Ireland shown in italics is for October 2006.

*Sources:*   Annual Abstract of Statistics (ONS).

Health and Personal Social Services Statistics for England (DH).

Health Statistics Wales (NAW).

Scottish Health Statistics (ISD).

Annual Statistical Report (Northern Ireland CSA).

Figure 4.28 **Number of practising dentists per 1,000 population in OECD countries, circa 2005**

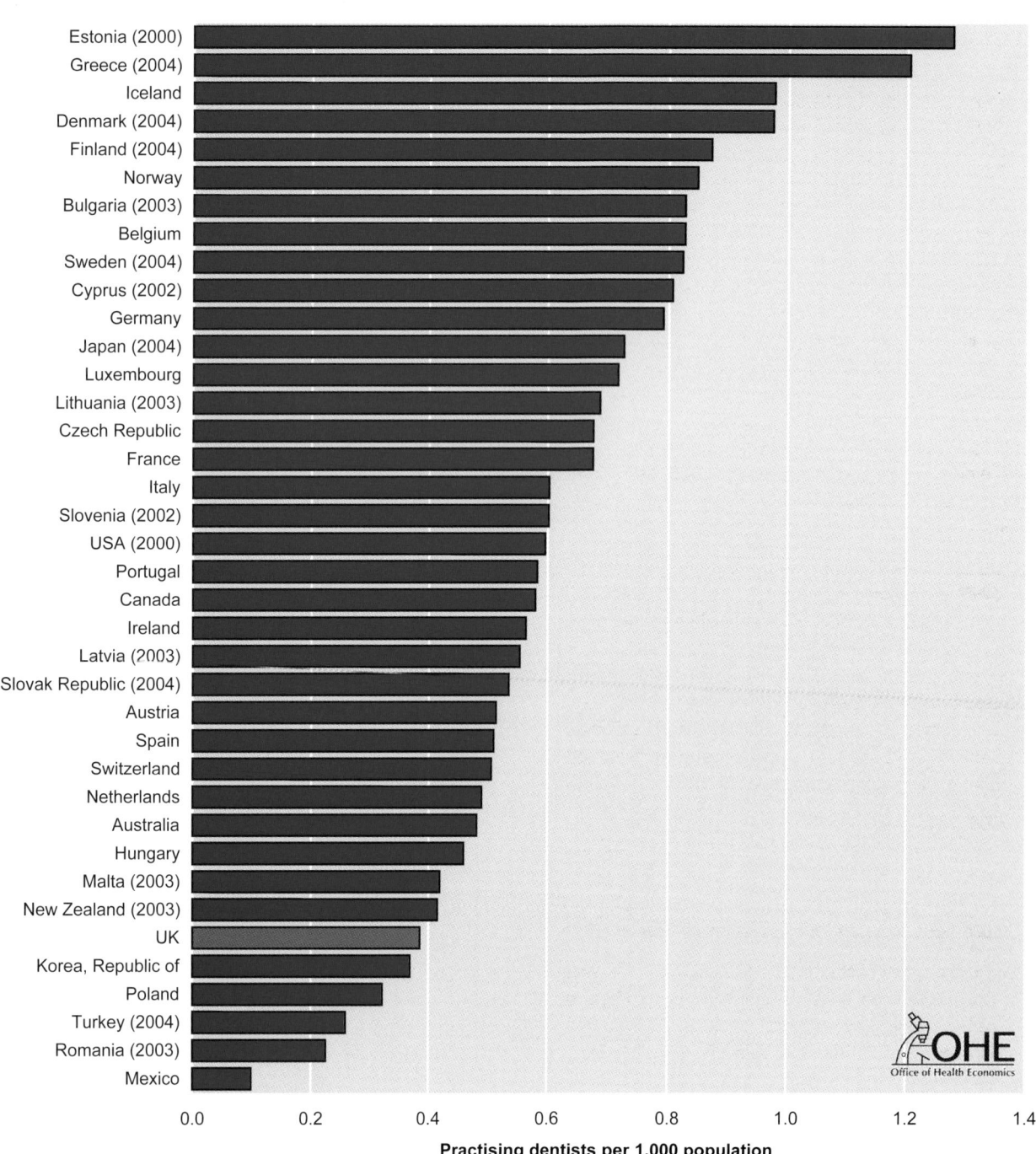

**Practising dentists per 1,000 population**

*Notes:*    Year is 2005 unless otherwise stated.
            UK number refers to dentists working for the NHS only.
*Sources:*  OECD Health Database.
            Annual Abstract of Statistics (ONS).
            Health and Personal Social Services Statistics for England (DH).
            Health Statistics Wales (NAW).
            Scottish Health Statistics (ISD).
            Annual Statistical Report (Northern Ireland CSA).
            Population Projections Database (GAD).

# FHS: General Ophthalmic Services

Until April 1989, the NHS General Ophthalmic Services (GOS) provided free sight tests to the whole population. Then access to these free services was restricted to children under 16 years, full-time students aged under 19 years, people who need complex lenses, diagnosed diabetics and glaucoma sufferers, those registered blind or partially-sighted, and people receiving income support or family credit. Free sight tests were reinstated from 1 April 1999 for those aged 60 or over throughout the UK, and reinstated in Scotland for all ages from 1<sup>st</sup> April 2006. Those not exempt are required to pay the full cost of sight tests and spectacles. In 2006/07 there were over 11 million sight tests paid for by the NHS in England and Wales, an increase of 50% over the previous decade, however this period encompasses the extension of eligibility to everyone aged 60 or older, see above (Ophthalmic Statistics, IC). Under the exemption scheme, a person requiring spectacles can exchange vouchers for a limited range of spectacles or contact lenses, or use them as partial payment for higher priced frames of their choice. The value of vouchers issued to exempt people varies from year to year and from one category of spectacle or lens to another.

There are two types of practitioners working under contract to the NHS ophthalmic services. These are ophthalmic medical practitioners (doctors who test sight and prescribe spectacles) and ophthalmic opticians who are not doctors but are qualified to test sight, prescribe and supply spectacles. In addition, there are dispensing opticians who dispense spectacles on NHS prescriptions, but their services are now provided on a private basis following the introduction of the voucher scheme in 1986

In 2005/06 there were 10,972 practising NHS ophthalmic opticians and practitioners in the UK, which represents an increase of 26% on the numbers in 1995/96. This is equivalent to an increase from 15.0 to 18.2 NHS opticians per 100,000 population over the same period (**Table 4.50**).

In 2005/06 the gross cost of the NHS GOS in the UK was £444 million, less than 0.5% of total NHS costs (**Figure 4.29**). **Table 4.49** shows that average per capita expenditure on GOS in the UK was £7.36 in 2005/06, being considerably lower in England than in the rest of the UK.

**Figure 4.30** illustrates the dramatic fall in the number of NHS funded sight tests following the abolition of free testing in 1989. With the re-introduction in April 1999 of free sight tests for people aged 60 and over, the number of tests picked up again somewhat.

# FHS: General Ophthalmic Services

Figure 4.29  **Gross cost[1] of General Ophthalmic Services (GOS) and per cent of gross NHS cost, UK, 1949/50 - 2005/06**

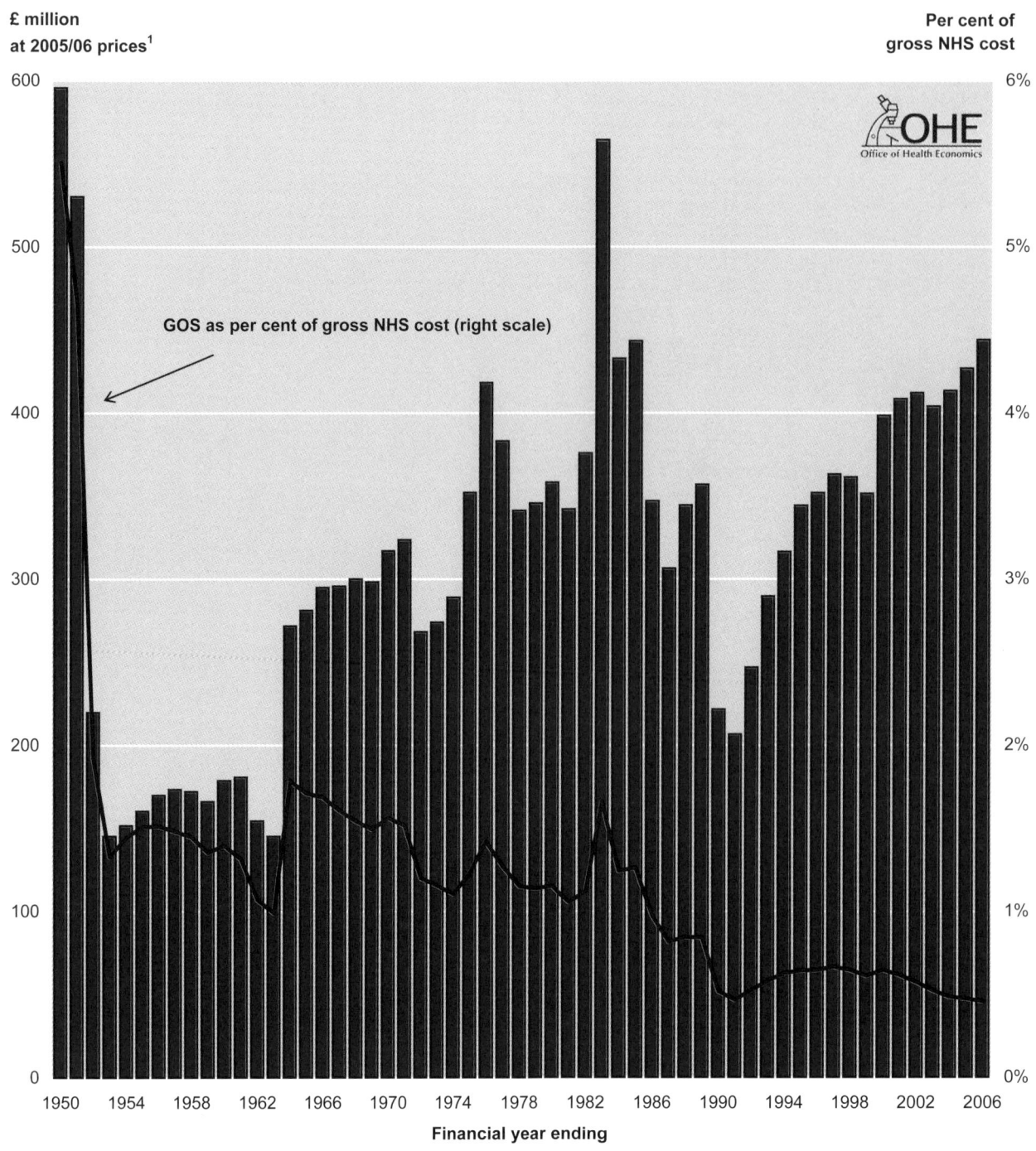

**£ million
at 2005/06 prices[1]**

**Per cent of
gross NHS cost**

GOS as per cent of gross NHS cost (right scale)

**Financial year ending**

*Notes:*  Figures include patient charges up to 1986 and, for 1983, contain an element of arrears payments.
Figures relate to financial year ending 31st March i.e. 2006=2005/06.
1 As adjusted using the Gross Domestic Product (GDP) deflator at market prices.
*Sources:*  Annual Abstract of Statistics (ONS).
Health and Personal Social Services Statistics for England (DH).
Health Statistics Wales (NAW).
Scottish Health Statistics (ISD).
Annual Statistical Report (Northern Ireland CSA).
Economic Trends (ONS).

Table 4.49  General Ophthalmic Services (GOS) expenditure per capita and per household, UK, 1975/76 - 2005/06

| Year | England | Wales | Scotland | Northern Ireland | UK | England | Wales | Scotland | Northern Ireland | UK |
|---|---|---|---|---|---|---|---|---|---|---|
| | | | | | GOS expenditure per capita (£ cash) | | | | | |
| | | | (£ cash) | | | At constant prices[1] (Index 1975/76=100) | | | | |
| 1975/76 | 1.00 | 1.00 | 1.00 | 1.00 | 1.00 | 100 | 100 | 100 | 100 | 100 |
| 1980/81 | 2.00 | 2.00 | 2.00 | 2.00 | 2.00 | 101 | 101 | 101 | 101 | 101 |
| 1983/84 | 3.00 | 4.00 | 3.00 | 3.00 | 3.00 | 124 | 165 | 124 | 124 | 124 |
| 1984/85 | 4.00 | 4.00 | 4.00 | 3.00 | 4.00 | 156 | 156 | 156 | 117 | 156 |
| 1985/86 | 3.00 | 3.00 | 3.00 | 2.00 | 3.00 | 111 | 111 | 111 | 74 | 111 |
| 1986/87 | 3.00 | 3.00 | 3.00 | 3.00 | 3.00 | 108 | 108 | 108 | 108 | 108 |
| 1987/88 | 3.00 | 3.00 | 3.00 | 3.00 | 3.00 | 102 | 102 | 102 | 102 | 102 |
| 1988/89 | 4.00 | 4.00 | 4.00 | 4.00 | 4.00 | 127 | 127 | 127 | 127 | 127 |
| 1989/90 | 2.27 | 3.01 | 2.85 | 2.88 | 2.38 | 67 | 89 | 85 | 85 | 70 |
| 1990/91 | 2.32 | 2.65 | 2.70 | 2.60 | 2.38 | 64 | 73 | 74 | 72 | 66 |
| 1991/92 | 2.94 | 3.48 | 3.23 | 3.48 | 3.01 | 76 | 90 | 84 | 90 | 78 |
| 1992/93 | 3.58 | 4.27 | 3.87 | 3.42 | 3.64 | 90 | 107 | 97 | 86 | 91 |
| 1993/94 | 3.99 | 4.68 | 4.36 | 4.50 | 4.07 | 98 | 115 | 107 | 110 | 100 |
| 1994/95 | 4.41 | 5.19 | 4.78 | 4.33 | 4.48 | 106 | 125 | 115 | 104 | 108 |
| 1995/96 | 4.61 | 5.54 | 5.06 | 5.19 | 4.71 | 108 | 130 | 118 | 121 | 110 |
| 1996/97 | 4.89 | 5.91 | 5.44 | 5.74 | 5.01 | 111 | 134 | 123 | 130 | 113 |
| 1997/98 | 4.96 | 6.19 | 5.73 | 6.05 | 5.12 | 109 | 136 | 126 | 133 | 113 |
| 1998/99 | 4.90 | 6.18 | 5.87 | 6.24 | 5.09 | 105 | 133 | 126 | 134 | 109 |
| 1999/00 | 5.72 | 6.92 | 6.31 | 6.76 | 5.86 | 120 | 145 | 133 | 142 | 123 |
| 2000/01 | 5.92 | 7.24 | 6.54 | 7.11 | 6.08 | 123 | 150 | 136 | 147 | 126 |
| 2001/02 | 6.10 | 7.50 | 6.66 | 7.39 | 6.25 | 124 | 152 | 135 | 150 | 127 |
| 2002/03 | 6 12 | 7.41 | 6.91 | 7.93 | 6.30 | 120 | 145 | 136 | 156 | 124 |
| 2003/04 | 6.45 | 7.50 | 7.10 | 8.20 | 6.61 | 123 | 143 | 135 | 156 | 126 |
| 2004/05 | 6.77 | 7.79 | 7.94 | 8.43 | 6.97 | 126 | 145 | 147 | 156 | 129 |
| 2005/06 | 7.10 | 8.01 | 8.97 | 8.96 | 7.36 | 129 | 146 | 163 | 163 | 134 |
| | | | | | GOS expenditure per household (£ cash) | | | | | |
| | | | (£ cash) | | | At constant prices[1] (Index 1975/76=100) | | | | |
| 1975/76 | 2.83 | 2.90 | 2.97 | 3.10 | 2.85 | 100 | 100 | 100 | 100 | 100 |
| 1980/81 | 5.46 | 5.57 | 5.63 | 6.10 | 5.50 | 97 | 97 | 96 | 99 | 97 |
| 1983/84 | 7.97 | 10.83 | 8.07 | 9.10 | 8.01 | 116 | 154 | 112 | 121 | 116 |
| 1984/85 | 10.55 | 10.73 | 10.63 | 9.05 | 10.60 | 146 | 145 | 140 | 114 | 145 |
| 1985/86 | 7.85 | 7.97 | 7.88 | 6.01 | 7.89 | 103 | 102 | 99 | 72 | 103 |
| 1986/87 | 7.79 | 7.90 | 7.79 | 8.99 | 7.83 | 99 | 98 | 94 | 104 | 99 |
| 1987/88 | 7.72 | 7.83 | 7.71 | 8.96 | 7.76 | 93 | 92 | 88 | 98 | 92 |
| 1988/89 | 10.20 | 10.33 | 10.16 | 11.89 | 10.24 | 114 | 113 | 109 | 122 | 114 |
| 1989/90 | 5.73 | 7.71 | 7.18 | 8.46 | 6.03 | 60 | 79 | 72 | 81 | 63 |
| 1990/91 | 5.84 | 6.74 | 6.73 | 7.57 | 6.00 | 57 | 64 | 62 | 67 | 58 |
| 1991/92 | 7.35 | 8.78 | 8.01 | 10.08 | 7.54 | 67 | 79 | 70 | 84 | 69 |
| 1992/93 | 8.91 | 10.72 | 9.55 | 9.76 | 9.08 | 79 | 93 | 81 | 79 | 80 |
| 1993/94 | 9.89 | 11.69 | 10.67 | 12.71 | 10.12 | 85 | 99 | 88 | 100 | 87 |
| 1994/95 | 10.90 | 12.91 | 11.63 | 11.98 | 11.10 | 93 | 107 | 95 | 93 | 94 |
| 1995/96 | 11.35 | 13.70 | 12.20 | 14.34 | 11.62 | 94 | 111 | 96 | 108 | 95 |
| 1996/97 | 12.01 | 14.57 | 13.01 | 15.86 | 12.33 | 96 | 114 | 99 | 116 | 98 |
| 1997/98 | 12.17 | 15.19 | 13.58 | 17.39 | 12.57 | 94 | 115 | 101 | 123 | 97 |
| 1998/99 | 12.01 | 15.13 | 13.82 | 17.46 | 12.46 | 91 | 112 | 100 | 121 | 94 |
| 1999/00 | 13.98 | 16.86 | 14.76 | 18.53 | 14.31 | 104 | 122 | 105 | 126 | 105 |
| 2000/01 | 14.39 | 17.55 | 15.17 | 19.18 | 14.74 | 105 | 126 | 106 | 128 | 107 |
| 2001/02 | 14.68 | 18.01 | 15.32 | 19.81 | 15.03 | 105 | 126 | 105 | 130 | 107 |
| 2002/03 | 14.64 | 17.65 | 15.78 | 21.08 | 15.06 | 101 | 120 | 104 | 134 | 104 |
| 2003/04 | 15.37 | 17.76 | 16.09 | 21.61 | 15.72 | 104 | 117 | 104 | 133 | 105 |
| 2004/05 | 16.10 | 18.38 | 17.90 | 22.05 | 16.53 | 106 | 118 | 112 | 132 | 108 |
| 2005/06 | 16.82 | 18.75 | 20.10 | 23.38 | 17.38 | 108 | 118 | 123 | 137 | 111 |

Notes:  Figures prior to 1986 include patient charges.
1 At constant prices, as adjusted by the Gross domestic Product (GDP) deflator at market prices.

Sources:  Annual Abstract of Statistics (ONS).
Health and Personal Social Services Statistics for England (DH).
Health Statistics Wales (NAW).
Scottish Health Statistics (ISD).
Annual Statistical Report (Northern Ireland CSA).
Economic Data (HM Treasury).

Figure 4.30  **Numbers of NHS sight tests and pairs of glasses[1] supplied per 1,000 population, UK, 1965 - 2006/07**

**Per 1,000 population**

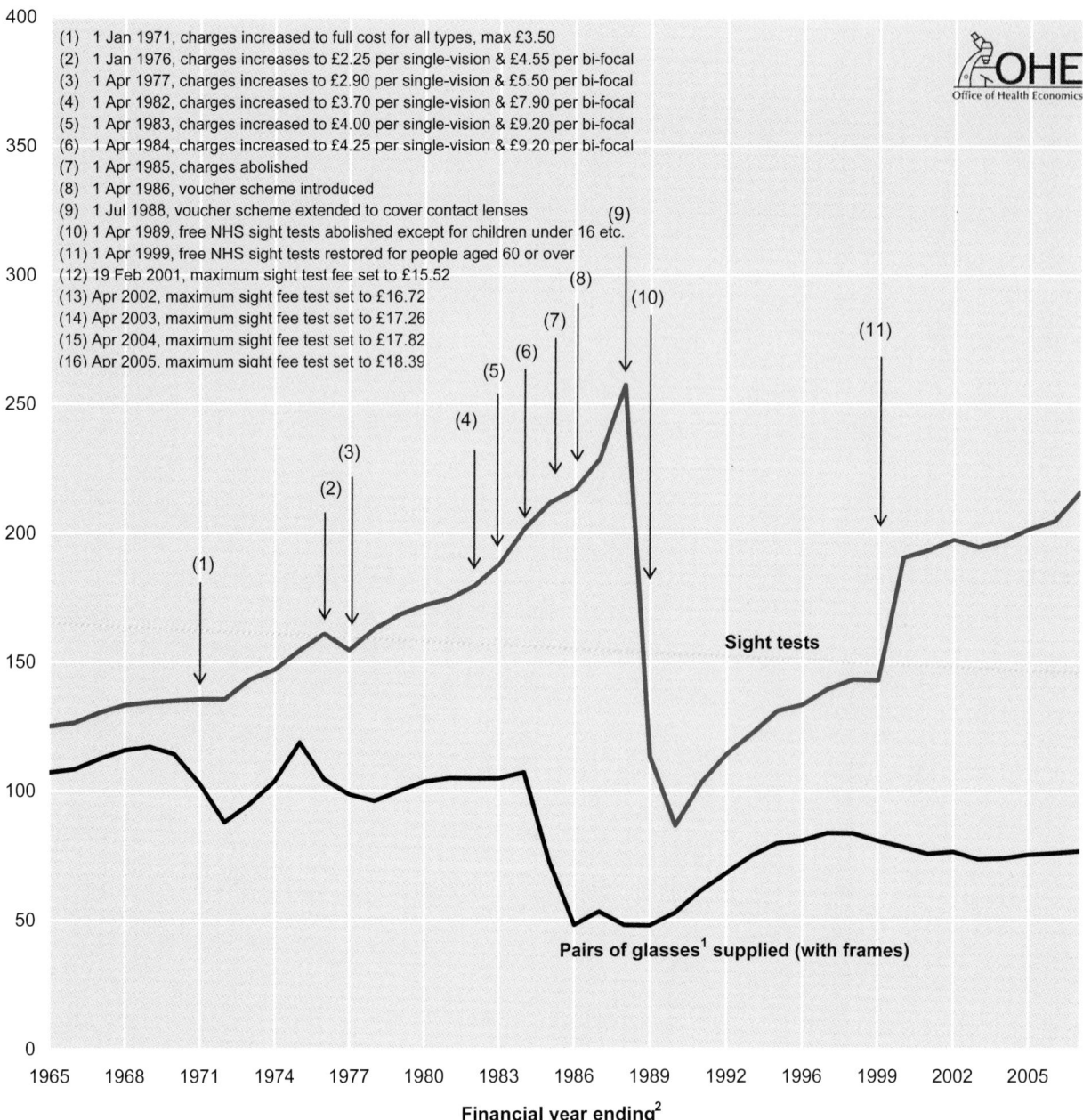

(1)  1 Jan 1971, charges increased to full cost for all types, max £3.50
(2)  1 Jan 1976, charges increases to £2.25 per single-vision & £4.55 per bi-focal
(3)  1 Apr 1977, charges increases to £2.90 per single-vision & £5.50 per bi-focal
(4)  1 Apr 1982, charges increased to £3.70 per single-vision & £7.90 per bi-focal
(5)  1 Apr 1983, charges increased to £4.00 per single-vision & £9.20 per bi-focal
(6)  1 Apr 1984, charges increased to £4.25 per single-vision & £9.20 per bi-focal
(7)  1 Apr 1985, charges abolished
(8)  1 Apr 1986, voucher scheme introduced
(9)  1 Jul 1988, voucher scheme extended to cover contact lenses
(10) 1 Apr 1989, free NHS sight tests abolished except for children under 16 etc.
(11) 1 Apr 1999, free NHS sight tests restored for people aged 60 or over
(12) 19 Feb 2001, maximum sight test fee set to £15.52
(13) Apr 2002, maximum sight fee test set to £16.72
(14) Apr 2003, maximum sight fee test set to £17.26
(15) Apr 2004, maximum sight fee test set to £17.82
(16) Apr 2005, maximum sight fee test set to £18.39

**Sight tests**

**Pairs of glasses[1] supplied (with frames)**

**Financial year ending[2]**

Notes:    1 From April 1989, figures relate to numbers of vouchers paid for.
          2 From 1993/94 onwards figures relate to financial year, ending 31st March of year shown on the x-axis (e.g. 2000 = 1999/2000).
          See text for changes in patient charges since 2005.
Sources:  Annual Abstract of Statistics (ONS).
          Health and Personal Social Services Statistics for England (DH).
          Health Statistics Wales (NAW).
          Scottish Health Statistics (ISD).
          Annual Statistical Report (Northern Ireland CSA).

Table 4.50 **Number of opticians and per 100,000 population, UK, 1949 - 2005/06**

31 March

| Year | Number of: | | | | Per 100,000 population | | | |
|---|---|---|---|---|---|---|---|---|
| | Ophthalmic practitioners[3] | Ophthalmic opticians[4] | Dispensing opticians[5] | Total | Ophthalmic practitioners[3] | Ophthalmic opticians[4] | Dispensing opticians[5] | Total |
| 1949[1] | 996 | 5,739 | 599 | 7,334 | 2.3 | 13.2 | 1.4 | 16.9 |
| 1950[1] | 983 | 6,179 | 639 | 7,801 | 2.3 | 14.2 | 1.5 | 17.9 |
| 1955[2] | 984 | 7,231 | 799 | 9,014 | 2.0 | 14.6 | 1.6 | 18.2 |
| 1960[2] | 976 | 7,150 | 1,032 | 9,158 | 1.9 | 14.0 | 2.0 | 18.0 |
| 1965[2] | 887 | 6,197 | 1,120 | 8,204 | 1.7 | 11.7 | 2.1 | 15.5 |
| 1966[2] | 953 | 5,846 | 1,098 | 7,897 | 1.8 | 11.0 | 2.1 | 14.9 |
| 1967[2] | 939 | 5,814 | 1,142 | 7,895 | 1.8 | 10.9 | 2.1 | 14.8 |
| 1968[2] | 931 | 5,679 | 1,118 | 7,728 | 1.7 | 10.6 | 2.1 | 14.5 |
| 1969 | 963 | 5,684 | 1,185 | 7,832 | 1.7 | 10.2 | 2.1 | 14.1 |
| 1970 | 986 | 5,594 | 1,274 | 7,854 | 1.8 | 10.1 | 2.3 | 14.1 |
| 1971 | 1,001 | 5,504 | 1,320 | 7,825 | 1.8 | 9.8 | 2.4 | 14.0 |
| 1972 | 1,000 | 5,397 | 1,367 | 7,764 | 1.8 | 9.6 | 2.4 | 13.8 |
| 1973 | 992 | 5,335 | 1,401 | 7,728 | 1.8 | 9.5 | 2.5 | 13.7 |
| 1974 | 992 | 5,256 | 1,386 | 7,634 | 1.8 | 9.3 | 2.5 | 13.6 |
| 1975 | 967 | 5,300 | 1,518 | 7,785 | 1.7 | 9.4 | 2.7 | 13.8 |
| 1976 | 959 | 5,332 | 1,610 | 7,901 | 1.7 | 9.5 | 2.9 | 14.1 |
| 1977 | 958 | 5,346 | 1,732 | 8,036 | 1.7 | 9.5 | 3.1 | 14.3 |
| 1978 | 933 | 5,391 | 1,886 | 8,210 | 1.7 | 9.6 | 3.4 | 14.6 |
| 1979 | 940 | 5,538 | 2,057 | 8,535 | 1.7 | 9.8 | 3.7 | 15.2 |
| 1980 | 965 | 5,679 | 2,232 | 8,876 | 1.7 | 10.1 | 4.0 | 15.8 |
| 1981 | 972 | 5,689 | 2,372 | 9,033 | 1.7 | 10.1 | 4.2 | 16.0 |
| 1982 | 978 | 5,772 | 2,501 | 9,251 | 1.7 | 10.3 | 4.4 | 16.4 |
| 1983 | 972 | 5,880 | 2,599 | 9,451 | 1.7 | 10.4 | 4.6 | 16.8 |
| 1984 | 988 | 6,024 | 2,766 | 9,778 | 1.7 | 10.7 | 4.9 | 17.3 |
| 1985 | 1,010 | 6,217 | 2,859 | 10,086 | 1.8 | 11.0 | 5.0 | 17.8 |
| 1986 | 1,048 | 6,318 | 2,979 | 10,345 | 1.8 | 11.1 | 5.2 | 18.2 |
| 1987/88 | 1,028 | 6,464 | - | 7,492 | 1.8 | 11.4 | - | 13.2 |
| 1988/89 | 1,003 | 6,691 | - | 7,694 | 1.8 | 11.7 | - | 13.5 |
| 1989/90 | 954 | 6,841 | - | 7,795 | 1.7 | 12.0 | - | 13.6 |
| 1990/91 | 944 | 6,990 | - | 7,934 | 1.6 | 12.1 | - | 13.8 |
| 1991/92 | 920 | 7,234 | - | 8,154 | 1.6 | 12.5 | - | 14.2 |
| 1992/93 | 897 | 7,416 | - | 8,313 | 1.5 | 12.8 | - | 14.4 |
| 1993/94 | 860 | 7,482 | - | 8,342 | 1.5 | 12.9 | - | 14.4 |
| 1994/95 | 802 | 7,578 | - | 8,380 | 1.4 | 13.1 | - | 14.5 |
| 1995/96 | 807 | 7,884 | - | 8,691 | 1.4 | 13.6 | - | 15.0 |
| 1996/97 | 832 | 8,094 | - | 8,926 | 1.4 | 13.9 | - | 15.3 |
| 1997/98 | 852 | 8,362 | - | 9,214 | 1.5 | 14.3 | - | 15.8 |
| 1998/99 | 879 | 8,711 | - | 9,589 | 1.5 | 14.9 | - | 16.4 |
| 1999/00 | 842 | 8,979 | - | 9,820 | 1.4 | 15.3 | - | 16.7 |
| 2000/01 | 797 | 8,950 | - | 9,746 | 1.4 | 15.2 | - | 16.5 |
| 2001/02 | 787 | 9,308 | - | 10,095 | 1.3 | 15.7 | - | 17.1 |
| 2002/03 | 720 | 9,467 | - | 10,187 | 1.2 | 15.9 | - | 17.2 |
| 2003/04 | 673 | 9,825 | - | 10,498 | 1.1 | 16.5 | - | 17.6 |
| 2004/05 | 639 | 10,112 | - | 10,751 | 1.1 | 16.9 | - | 17.9 |
| 2005/06 | 520 | 10,452 | - | 10,972 | 0.9 | 17.3 | - | 18.2 |

*Notes:* Prior to 1987/88 figures relate to various points of the year.
From 1987/88 figures for England, Wales and Scotland relate to 31 March and for Northern Ireland to 1 July.
From 1995 figures relate to 31st December for England, Wales and Scotland and to October for Northern Ireland.
1 Figures relate to England and Wales only.
2 Figures relate to Great Britain only.
3 An ophthalmic medical practitioner is a medically qualified optician who is entitled to test sight and prescribe (but not dispense) glasses.
4 An ophthalmic optician is entitled to test sight and dispense glasses.
5 A dispensing optician is entitled only to dispense glasses. As a result of the introduction of voucher scheme on 1 July 1986,
which led to the cessation of dispensing opticians' contracts, figures are no longer available from 1987 onwards.

*Sources:* Health and Personal Social Services Statistics for England (DH).
Health Statistics Wales (NAW).
Scottish Health Statistics (ISD).
Annual Statistical Report (Northern Ireland CSA).
Annual Abstract of Statistics (ONS).

**ABPI**  Association of the British Pharmaceutical Industry.

**Acute ill health**  A term used in the Compendium to describe a restriction of normal activities, as a result of illness or injury, for a period of at least two weeks.

**Acute services**  Surgical and non-surgical interventions provided in hospitals.

**AGR**  Average annual growth rate expressed in percentage terms.

**ASR**  Age standardised rate (See Section 1).

**Average**  defined as the arithmetic mean.

**BMI**  Body mass index.  A measure that takes weight divided by height in metres squared.

**BNF**  British National Formulary.  A classification of medicines according to their action on the human body. The BNF is joint publication of the British Medical Association and the Royal Pharmaceutical Society of Great Britain. It is revised twice a year.

**Cash limit**  Limit on the amount of money the Government plans to spend on certain services in a financial year as a means of control over cash spending in the year ahead. Cash limits were first introduced in 1976.

**CNS**  Central nervous system.

**Chronic ill health**  A term used in the Compendium to describe longstanding illness, disability or infirmity.

**Consultant**  A specialist hospital medical practitioner.

**Crude death rate**  The total number of deaths in a given time period divided by the population at the midpoint of the time period. Crude death rates are often expressed as "deaths per 100,000 population".

**CSA**  Northern Ireland Central Services Agency.

**Day case**  Day case patients are those admitted electively to a hospital ward for investigation or treatment and who do not occupy a bed overnight.

**DCLG**  Department for Communities and Local Government.

**Decadal**  Relating to a period of ten years. Decadal change is the change in a quantity over a period of ten years.

**Dependency ratio**  The ratio of the non-working age population to the working age population. Non-working age in the UK is taken as below 16 and above 65 years.

**Discharges and deaths**  Patients who have received hospital inpatient treatment and are subsequently discharged or have died in hospital.

**Dispensing doctor**  A general medical practitioner (GP) licensed to dispense medicines. Dispensing doctors are usually found in rural areas, where pharmacies are few.

**DH**  Department of Health for England.

**DHSSPS**  Northern Ireland Department of Health, Social Services and Public Safety.

**Drug Tariff**  A monthly publication of the DoH and the Welsh Office, giving price and other information for prescription medicines.

**DSS**  Department of Social Security.

**Elderly**  The Compendium of Health Statistics uses this term to describe people over the age of 64 years (i.e. 65 years and over).

**EU**  European Union. Comprised 15 members in 2003: Austria, Belgium, Denmark, Finland, France, Germany, Greece, Ireland, Italy, Luxembourg, The Netherlands, Portugal, Spain, Sweden and the UK. On 1 May 2004, under the EU extension programme, ten new members joined: Cyprus (Greek part), the Czech Republic, Estonia, Hungary, Latvia, Lithuania, Malta, Poland, Slovakia and Slovenia. 1 January 2007 enlarged to include Bulgaria and Romania.

**EU-15**  The group of 15 countries which formed the EU before 1 May 2004.

**EU-27**  The group of 27 countries which have formed the EU since 1 January 2007.

**Exempt prescriptions**  Prescriptions that do not attract an NHS prescription charge. Roughly half of the UK population receive free NHS prescription medicines.  See Box 13 of Section 4 for further details and a list of exemption categories.

**FCE**  Finished consultant episode. Measure of hospital inpatient activity, used in England since 1987/88. The period of time that one hospital inpatient spends under the care and responsibility of one consultant within one care provider. If a patient is transferred from the care of one consultant to another, even within the same hospital or ward, it constitutes a new FCE. The birth of a (live) infant in hospital also constitutes a FCE.

**FHS** Family Health Services include the General Medical (GMS), General Pharmaceutical (GPS), General Dental (GDS) and General Ophthalmic (GOS) services.

# Glossary

**Financial year**  The UK government's financial year ends on 31 March. For example, the financial year 2000/01 begins on 1 April 2000 and ends on 31 March 2001. Definitions of financial year vary from country to country.

**FTE**  Full-time equivalent. A measure of the work of part-time staff. For example, one part-timer working three days per week is equivalent to 0.6 (i.e. 3/5) FTE.

**GAD**  Government Actuary's Department.

**Generic**  An off-patent medicine. Until the patent expires, only the company that discovered a new medicine or their licensees may produce it. After patent expiry any company may produce the same generic compound.

**GB**  Great Britain. Comprises England, Scotland and Wales.

**GDP**  Gross Domestic Product. The value of all goods and services produced by UK residents, usually measured on an annual basis.

**GDP deflator**  An index showing the average growth of the prices of all items included in GDP. The GDP deflator is derived by dividing GDP in current prices by GDP in constant prices, and expressing it in index form. For example, the series may be scaled by taking the 1990 value to be 100.

**GHS**  General Household Survey. An annual survey carried out by the ONS, providing data on health, population characteristics, education and economic activity.

**GP**  General medical practitioner.

**GROS**  General Register Office of Scotland

**HCHS**  Hospital and Community Health Services.

**HES**  Hospital Episode Statistics

**HOWIS**  Health of Wales Information Services.

**HRG**  Healthcare Resource Group. A system for grouping treatment episodes which are similar in resource use and clinical response.

**HSE**  Health and Safety Executive.

**IC**  The NHS in England Information Centre for Health and Social Care.

**ICD**  International Classification of Diseases. An internationally defined system for classifying diseases and related health problems. The ICD undergoes periodic revision and is managed by the World Health Organisation. The latest edition is the 10$^{th}$ Revision (ICD10) published in 1992.

**ISD**  The NHS in Scotland Information and Statistics Division.

**Index number**  A statistical measure designed to show changes in a quantity with respect to time, location, or some other characteristic.

**Infant mortality rate**  The death rate amongst children under the age of one year, expressed per 1,000 live births.

**Inpatient**  A person occupying a hospital bed for at least one night.

**Life expectancy**  The average further number of years that a person at a specified age may expect to live.

**List size**  The number of people registered with a GP.

**MBD**  Marketing and Business Development.

**Median**  A measure of the central value of a set of observations. The median is the value in a set of ranked numbers that divides the data into two equal parts. For example, for the set of numbers 1, 2, 2, 5, 6, 10, 13, the median is 5. For an even number of observations, the median is defined as the mean of the two central observations.

**Mean**  A measure of the central value of a set of observations. The arithmetic mean of a set of n observations $x_1, x_2, x_3, ...., x_n$, is defined as the sum of all the $x_i$ divided by the number of observations, n. The geometric mean (not used in the Compendium) is defined as the n$^{th}$ root of the product of the $x_i$.

**Medical practitioner**  GP contracted to the NHS to provide the full range of general medical services.

**Morbidity**  Relating to illness or disease.

**Mortality**  Relating to death.

**NHS**  National Health Service of the UK.

**NIC**  Net Ingredient Cost refers to the cost of the drug before discounts and does not include any dispensing costs or fees. (See Section 4).

**NISRA**  Northern Ireland Statistics and Research Agency

**OECD**  Organisation for Economic Co-operation and Development. (See Section 1).

**OHE**  Office of Health Economics.

**ONS**  Office for National Statistics.

**Ordinary admission**  An admission where the patient is expected to remain in hospital for at least one night.

**OTC** Over the counter. A medicine available without a prescription.

**Outpatient** A patient attending a hospital for consultation without staying there overnight.

**PACT** Prescribing Analysis and Cost System. Prescribing doctors receive regular PACT reports from the PPA giving details of their recent prescribing, comparing them with local and national averages.

**Patient charges** This term is used in the Compendium to describe payments made by patients for various aspects of NHS treatment. Such charges include the prescription charge, payments made for amenity beds in NHS hospital wards, and charges for some types of dental treatment.

**PCT** Primary Care Trust. PCTs in England are statutory bodies which replaced the Health Authorities in April 2002 taking over the responsibility of identifying the health needs of their community, developing primary and community services, commissioning secondary services as well as providing directly a range of community health services.

**Per capita** Per person.

**PMI** Private medical insurance.

**PPA** Prescription Pricing Authority.

**PPRS** Pharmaceutical Price Regulation Scheme. The PPRS is a non-statutory agreement between the UK government and the research-based pharmaceutical industry operating in the UK, represented by the ABPI. It limits the rate of profit earned by pharmaceutical manufacturers from sales of branded medicines to the NHS.

**Prescription charge** A charge made to patients for NHS prescription medicines.

**Real** (terms, growth, etc.) A monetary amount adjusted to remove the effect of inflation. The Compendium usually uses the GDP deflator to make this adjustment, but other methods are possible. For example, the *all items Retail Price Index* may be appropriate in some circumstances.

**Sampling error** A numerical measure of the uncertainty associated with a quantity estimated from a sample of data. Sampling error decreases with increasing sample size.

**Throughput** A measure of hospital activity. The number of patients treated in a given time per bed.

**UK** United Kingdom. The UK comprises England, Scotland, Wales and Northern Ireland.

**USA** United States of America.

**Very elderly** The Compendium uses this term to describe people aged 75 years and over.

**WHO** World Health Organisation. An agency of the United Nations with responsibility for international health matters. It promotes the development of health services and the prevention and control of diseases.

# References

This section contains details of all source documents used in compiling the Compendium. Where appropriate, frequency of publication and other information is shown in italics. Government publications are generally available from The Stationery Office (formerly Her Majesty's Stationery Office).

Most publications of the Department of Health in England are available from:

DH Publications Orderline
PO Box 777
London
SE1 6XH

Tel 0870 155 54 55

Fax 0162 372 45 24

Email dh@prolog.uk.com

Department of Communities and Local Government. *Household estimates and projections.* London.

Department of Health. *Bed Availability and Occupancy: England. (Annual).*

Department of Health. *Community pharmacies in England and Wales.* Statistical Bulletin *(Annual).*

Department of Health. *Elective Admissions and Patients Waiting: England.* Statistical Bulletin. *(Quarterly).*

Department of Health. *General Medical Services Statistics: England and Wales. (Annual).*

Department of Health. *General Pharmaceutical Services in England and Wales.* Statistical Bulletin. *(Annual).*

Department of Health. *The Government's Expenditure Plans: Departmental Report.* London: The Stationery Office. *(Annual).*

Department of Health. *Health and Personal Social Services Statistics for England.* London: The Stationery Office. *(Annual).*

Department of Health. *Hospital Episode Statistics.* London. *(Annual).*

Department of Health. *NHS Hospital, Public Health Medicine and Community Health Service Medical and Dental Workforce Census England. (Annual).*

Department of Health. *NHS Hospital Activity Statistics: England.* Statistical Bulletin. *(Annual).*

Department of Health. *NHS Hospital and Community Health Services Non-medical Staff in England.* Statistical Bulletin. *(Annual).*

Department of Health. *Payment by Results: England.* London. *(2003).*

Department of Health. *Prescription Cost Analysis: England.* London. *(Annual).*

Department of Health. *Programme Budgeting.* Leeds. *(Annual).*

Department of Health. *Reference Costs.* Leeds. *(Annual).*

Department of Health. *Statistics for General Medical Practitioners in England.* Statistical Bulletin. *(Annual).*

Department of Health. *Statistics of Prescriptions Dispensed in the Community: England.* Statistical Bulletin. *(Annual).*

Department of Health and Association of the British Pharmaceutical Industry. *Pharmaceutical Price Regulation Scheme: 2005 (November 2004).*

Department of Health and the Office of Population Censuses and Surveys. *Hospital Inpatient Enquiry: Inpatient and Day Case Trends. (Series MB4).* London: The Stationery Office. *(This publication has been superseded by Hospital Episode Statistics from 1988).*

General Register Office of Scotland. *Household estimates and projections.* Edinburgh. *(Annual).*

General Register Office of Scotland. *Vital Events Reference Tables.* Edinburgh. *(Annual).*

Government Actuary's Department. *Life Tables. (Annual).*

Government Actuary's Department. *Population Projections. (Annual).*

Health and Safety Executive. *Labour Force Survey.* Caerphilly.

Health of Wales Information Services. *Prescription Cost Analysis: Wales.* Cardiff: The National Assembly for Wales. *(Annual).*

HM Treasury. *2004 Spending Review – Public Spending Plans 2005-2008*: London: The Stationery Office.

HM Treasury. *Economic Data.* London.

HM Treasury. *Public Expenditure: Statistical Analyses.* London: The Stationery Office. *(Annual).*

HM Treasury. *Supply Estimates: Main Estimates.* London: The Stationery Office. *(Annual).*

House of Commons Health Committee. *Public Expenditure on Health and Personal Social Services*. London: The Stationery Office. *(Annual)*.

House of Commons. *NHS (England) Summarised Accounts*. London: The Stationery Office. *(Annual)*.

House of Commons. *NHS (England and Wales) Summarised Accounts*. London: The Stationery Office. *(Annual)*.

House of Commons. *NHS (Scotland) Summarised Accounts*. London: The Stationery Office. *(Annual)*.

House of Commons. *NHS (Wales) Summarised Accounts*. London: The Stationery Office. *(Annual)*.

Information and Statistics Division. *Cancer Statistics* Edinburgh: The NHS in Scotland. *(Annual)*.

Information and Statistics Division. *Community Pharmacies*. Edinburgh: The NHS in Scotland. *(Annual)*.

Information and Statistics Division. *Daycase and Inpatient Activity*. Edinburgh: The NHS in Scotland.

Information and Statistics Division. *Dental Statistics*. Edinburgh: The NHS in Scotland.

Information and Statistics Division. *Workforce Statistics*. Edinburgh: The NHS in Scotland.

Information and Statistics Division. *NHS Board Operating Costs and Capital Expenditure*. Edinburgh: The NHS in Scotland. *(Annual)*.

Information and Statistics Division. *Prescription Cost Analysis: Scotland*. Edinburgh: The NHS in Scotland. *(Annual)*.

Information and Statistics Division. *Scottish Health Service Costs*. Edinburgh: The NHS in Scotland. *(Annual)*.

Information and Statistics Division. *Scottish Health Statistics*. Edinburgh: The NHS in Scotland. *(Annual)*.

Laing and Buisson. *Laing's Healthcare Market Review*. London: Laing and Buisson Publications Ltd. *(Annual)*.

Information Centre, *Demographic Trends*. Wellington: New Zealand's Official Statistics Agency.

Marketing and Business Development *UK dentistry market research report*.

National Assembly for Wales *Welsh Health Circular: Programme Budgeting results*. Cardiff.

National Assembly for Wales. *Health Statistics Wales*. Cardiff. *(Annual)*.

National Assembly for Wales *StatsWales*.

NHS England Health and Social Care Information Centre *NHS HCHS non-medical staff in England*

NHS England Health and Social Care Information Centre *Hospital Episode Statistics*

NHS England Health and Social Care Information Centre *General and Personal Medical Service, Detailed results*

NHS England Health and Social Care Information Centre *NHS Staff*

NHS England Health and Social Care Information Centre *NHS HCHS medical and dental staff in England*.

NHS England Health and Social Care Information Centre *General and Personal Medical Services in England*. (Annual)

NHS England Health and Social Care Information Centre *General Pharmaceutical Services Annual Bulletin (Annual)*

NHS England Health and Social Care Information Centre *General Ophthalmic Services: Activity statistics for England and Wales (Annual)*.

NHS England Health and Social Care Information Centre *General Ophthalmic Services: Workforce statistics for England and Wales (Annual)*.

NHS England Health and Social Care Information Centre *NHS staff (Annual)*.

NHS England Health and Social Care Information Centre *Prescriptions Dispensed in the Community: England*.

Northern Ireland Cancer Registry *Cancer Statistics*.

Northern Ireland Department of Health, Social Services and Public Safety. *Annual Statistical Report*. Belfast: Central Services Agency.

Northern Ireland Department of Health, Social Services and Public Safety. *Community Statistics*. Belfast: Central Services Agency. *(Annual)*

Northern Ireland Department of Health, Social Services and Public Safety. *Hospital Statistics*. Belfast: Central Services Agency. *(Annual)*.

Northern Ireland Department of Health, Social Services and Public Safety. *Main Estimates*. Belfast: Central Services Agency. *(Annual)*.

# References

Northern Ireland Department of Health, Social Services and Public Safety. *Prescription Cost Analysis: Northern Ireland*. Belfast: Central Services Agency. *(Annual)*.

Northern Ireland Statistics and Research Agency. *Demographic Statistics*. Belfast.

Office for National Statistics. *Adult Dental Health Survey, 1998*. London: The stationery Office. (2000).

Office for National Statistics. *Annual Abstract of Statistics*. London: The Stationery Office. *(Annual)*.

Office for National Statistics. *Cancer Registration Statistics*. London: The Stationery Office. *(Annual)*.

Office for National Statistics. *Consumer Trends*. London: The Stationery Office. *(Annual)*.

Office for National Statistics. *Economic Trends (Annual Supplement)*. London: The Stationery Office. *(Annual)*.

Office for National Statistics. *Economic and Labour Market Review*. London: The Stationery Office. *(Monthly)*.

Office for National Statistics. *General Household Survey. (Living in Britain: Results from the General Household Survey)*. London: The Stationery Office. *(Annual)*.

Office for National Statistics. *Key Population and Vital Statistics*. London: The Stationery Office. *(Annual)*.

Office for National Statistics. *Mid-year Population Estimates*. Population and Health Monitors: PP1. London: The Stationery Office. *(Annual)*.

Office for National Statistics. *Mortality Statistics (England & Wales): Cause. (Series DH2)*. London: The Stationery Office. *(Annual)*.

Office for National Statistics. *Mortality Statistics (England & Wales): Childhood, Infant and Perinatal. (Series DH3)*. London: The Stationery Office. *(Annual)*.

Office for National Statistics. *Population Estimates and Projections*. The Stationery Office.

Office for National Statistics. *Population Projections. Population and Health Monitors: PP2*. London: The Stationery Office. *(Annual)*.

Office for National Statistics. *Population Trends*. London: The Stationery Office. *(Quarterly)*.

Office for National Statistics. *Regional Trends*. London: The Stationery Office. *(Quarterly)*.

Office for National Statistics. *UK Economic Accounts*. London: The Stationery Office. *(Quarterly)*.

Office for National Statistics. *United Kingdom National Accounts (The Blue Book)*. London: The Stationery Office. *(Annual)*.

OPCS and Department of Health. *Morbidity Statistics from General Practice. Royal College of General Practitioners*. London: The Stationery Office. *(This is a national study carried out every ten years. The most recent relates to 1991/92)*.

Organisation for Economic Co-operation and Development and Centre de Recherche, d'Etude et de Documentation en Economique de la Santé. *OECD Health Database*. Paris: OECD. *(Annual)*.

Prescription Pricing Authority. *PPA Annual Report*. Newcastle upon Tyne. *(Annual)*.

Royal College of General Practitioners. *RCGP Profile of UK practices*.

Royal Pharmaceutical Society of Great Britain. *Annual Workforce census*.

The United Nations. *World Population Prospects*. New York. *(Annual)*.

Welsh Cancer Intelligence and Surveillance Unit *Cancer Statistics*.

World Bank. *World Development Indicators*. *(Annual)*.

World Health Organisation. *Global InfoBase*. Geneva.

World Health Organisation (1992). *International Classification of Diseases, 10th Revision*. Geneva.

World Health Organisation. *Mortality Database*. Geneva. *(Annual)*.

World Health Organisation. *National Health Accounts Series*. Geneva.

World Health Organisation. *World Health Report: Core Health Indicators*. Geneva. *(Annual)*.

World Health Organisation. *World Health Statistics Annual*. Geneva. *(Annual)*.

acute illness. *See* illness, limiting longstanding

administrative and clerical staff, hospital, 146, 147

alcohol consumption

    *England, 71*

    *EU countries, 72*

    *Great Britain, 6, 70*

    *Northern Ireland, 71*

    *OECD countries, 72*

    *Scotland, 71*

    *UK, 72*

    *Wales, 71*

bed occupancy. *See* hospital bed occupancy

beds in NHS hospitals. *See* hospital available beds

birth rates, 33, 36

branded prescriptions, 267

branded prescriptions, cost, 226

breast cancer

    *England and Wales, 47, 54, 58*

    *EU countries, 54, 58*

    *Northern Ireland, 47, 54, 58*

    *OECD countries, 54, 58*

    *Scotland, 47, 54, 58*

cancer incidence, site, 59, 60

cerebrovascular disease

    *England and Wales, 47, 54, 56*

    *EU countries, 54, 56*

    *Northern Ireland, 47, 54, 56*

    *OECD countries, 54, 56*

    *Scotland, 47, 54, 56*

chemists. *See* pharmacies and appliance contractors

chemists' income. *See* pharmacies' income

childhood mortality

    *EU countries, 42, 43*

    *OECD countries, 42, 43*

    *UK, 33, 36*

chronic illness. *See* illness, longstanding

cigarette smoking. *See* smoking

community health services expenditure, 118, 119

consultants, hospital, 156

    *England, 157*

    *Great Britain, 157*

    *Scotland, 157*

    *Wales, 157*

consumer spending, 130, 131

coronary heart disease

    *England and Wales, 4, 47, 54, 55*

    *EU countries, 54, 55*

    *Northern Ireland, 47, 54, 55*

    *OECD countries, 54, 55*

    *Scotland, 47, 54, 55*

days off work, cause. *See* work related illness

dental charges, 271, 272, 275

dental health, 272

dental practitioners

    *England and Wales, 277*

    *Northern Ireland, 277*

    *OECD countries, 278*

    *Scotland, 277*

    *UK, 277*

dental treatment, numbers, 276

dependency ratio

    *EU countries, 21*

    *OECD countries, 21*

    *UK, 1, 12*

discharges/deaths, hospital

    *Northern Ireland, 149, 152, 163*

    *OECD countries, 165*

    *Scotland, 149, 152, 163*

    *Wales, 163*

dispensing doctors, 202

    *England, 221*

    *Northern Ireland, 221*

    *Scotland, 221*

    *UK, 221*

    *Wales, 221*

domestic ancillary staff, hospital, 146, 147

drinking. *See* alcohol consumption

drugs bill at manufacturers' price, 269, 270

Family Health Services (FHS) expenditure

    *England, 191, 199*

    *Northern Ireland, 191, 199*

    *OECD countries, 196*

    *Scotland, 191, 199*

    *UK, 99, 135, 140, 143, 191, 192, 193, 194, 195, 197, 198*

*Wales, 191, 199*

**fertility rate, UK, 36**

**finished consultant episode (FCE), 137**

*England, 163*

*England and Wales, 149, 152*

*UK, 149, 151, 152, 163*

**finished consultant episode (FCE), cause, 168**

*England, 169, 173*

*UK, 169*

**finished consultant episode, specialty, 164**

**GDP deflator, 80**

**General Dental Services (GDS) expenditure**

*England, 273*

*Northern Ireland, 273*

*Scotland, 273*

*UK, 118, 119, 192, 193, 195, 198, 271, 272, 273, 274, 275*

*Wales, 273*

**General Medical Practitioner.** *See* **GP and medical practitioners**

**General Medical Services (GMS) expenditure**

*England, 203*

*Northern Ireland, 203*

*Scotland, 203*

*UK, 118, 119, 192, 193, 195, 198, 200, 204*

*Wales, 203*

**General Ophthalmic Services**

*UK, 279*

**General Ophthalmic Services (GOS) expenditure**

*England, 281*

*Northern Ireland, 281*

*Scotland, 281*

*UK, 118, 119, 192, 193, 195, 198, 280, 281*

*Wales, 281*

**General Pharmaceutical Services (GPS) expenditure**

*England, 227, 228*

*Northern Ireland, 227, 228*

*Scotland, 227, 228*

*UK, 118, 119, 192, 193, 195, 198, 224, 227, 228, 243*

*Wales, 227, 228*

**generic prescriptions, 268**

*cost, 226*

*market share, 267*

**GP consultation**

*cost, 201*

**GP consultations**

*GB, 64*

*place, 202*

*UK by age and sex, 219, 220*

**GP practice size**

*England and Wales, 216, 218*

*Northern Ireland, 217*

*Scotland, 217*

*UK, 216*

**GP practice staff, 200, 201**

**GP registrars**

*England, 209*

*Northern Ireland, 209*

*Scotland, 209*

*UK, 209*

*Wales, 209*

**GP, age and sex, 215**

**GP, list size**

*England, 211, 212*

*Northern Ireland, 211, 212*

*Scotland, 211, 212*

*UK, 211, 212*

*Wales, 211, 212*

**GP, numbers**

*OECD countries, 206*

*UK, 200*

**Gross Domestic Product (GDP)**

*EU countries, 88, 89, 94, 98, 110*

*OECD countries, 88, 89, 94, 98, 110*

*UK, 76, 79, 98, 100, 101, 103, 104*

**health care expenditure, private**

*EU countries, 91, 92, 93, 132, 133, 134*

*OECD countries, 91, 92, 93, 132, 133, 134*

*UK, 77, 82, 127, 128, 130, 131*

**health care expenditure, public**

*EU countries, 90, 92, 93, 105, 106, 107, 108, 109, 110*

*OECD countries, 90, 92, 93, 105, 106, 107, 108, 109, 110*

**health care expenditure, total**

*EU countries, 83, 84, 85, 86, 87, 94, 95, 96, 97*

OECD countries, 83, 84, 85, 86, 87, 94, 95, 96, 97

UK, 76, 77, 78, 79

**hospital acute beds**

Great Britain, 159

OECD countries, 158, 162, 165

**Hospital and Community Health Services (HCHS) expenditure**

age group, 111, 112

per capita, 99

**hospital available beds**

England, 160, 161, 163

England and Wales, 149, 152, 158

Northern Ireland, 149, 152, 158

Scotland, 149, 152, 158, 163

UK, 136, 137, 149, 151, 152, 158

Wales, 163

wards, 160

**hospital bed days, cause, 172, 174**

**hospital bed occupancy**

England, 160, 161

Northern Ireland, 161

Scotland, 161

UK, 161

Wales, 161

wards, 160

**hospital day case, specialty, 182**

**hospital expenditure**

England, 141

Northern Ireland, 141

OECD countries, 144

Scotland, 141

UK, 118, 119, 135, 140, 141, 142, 143, 145, 197

Wales, 141

**hospital inpatient waiting time, 178, 179**

HRG, 180

**hospital length of stay**

cause, 171, 174

England, 167

England and Wales, 166

Northern Ireland, 166

Scotland, 166

UK, 138, 166

**hospital managers, NHS, 135**

**hospital medicines cost, 269**

**hospital operations, 175, 176, 177**

**hospital ordinary admissions, cause, 170**

**hospital outpatient attendances, new**

England and Wales, 189

Northern Ireland, 189

Scotland, 189

UK, 139, 189

**hospital outpatient attendances, total**

England and Wales, 188

Northern Ireland, 188

Scotland, 188

UK, 139, 188, 190

**hospital outpatient waiting time, 181**

**hospital workforce, NHS, 146, 147**

**illness, limiting longstanding**

prevalence, 61

socioeconomic groups, 63

**illness, limiting longstanding**

condition, 65

**illness, longstanding**

condition, 65

England, 6

Great Britain, 6, 61, 62

Scotland, 6

socioeconomic groups, 63

Wales, 6

**illness, longstanding**

England, 5

Great Britain, 5

Scotland, 5

Wales, 5

**infant mortality**

EU countries, 38, 39, 40, 41

OECD countries, 38, 39, 40, 41, 95, 96, 97

UK, 33, 36

**infant mortality, rates**

England and Wales, 95, 96, 97

EU countries, 95, 96, 97

Northern Ireland, 95, 96, 97

Scotland, 95, 96, 97

**inpatient cost. See hospital inpatient cost**

**inpatient waiting time.** *See* **hospital inpatient waiting time**

**life expectancy**

England, 2, 27

England and Wales, 28, 29

EU countries, 30, 31, 32, 95, 96

Northern Ireland, 2, 27

OECD countries, 30, 31, 32, 95, 96

Scotland, 2, 27

UK, 2, 27

Wales, 2, 27

**live births**

UK, 36

**lung cancer**

England and Wales, 47, 54, 57

EU countries, 54, 57

Northern Ireland, 47, 54, 57

OECD countries, 54, 57

Scotland, 47, 54, 57

**managers, hospital.** *See* **hospital managers, NHS**

**median age**

EU countries, 26

OECD countries, 26

UK, 2, 12

UK countries, 26

**medical and dental staff, hospital**

England, 155

Scotland, 155

Wales, 155

**medical and dental staff, hospital**

England and Wales, 148

grade, 153

Northern Ireland, 148

Scotland, 148

specialty, 154

UK, 136, 146, 147, 148, 151

**medical and dental staff, hospital**

Great Britain, 155

**medical practitioners**

England, 213, 214

England and Wales, 207, 208, 210

Northern Ireland, 207, 208, 210, 213, 214

Scotland, 207, 208, 210, 213, 214

UK, 207, 208, 210, 213, 214

Wales, 213, 214

**medical product expenditure, private, 131**

UK, 77, 82

**medical staff**

community, 205

hospital, 205

**medical staff**

NHS, 205

**medicines bill.** *See* **drugs bill**

**mortality rates**

EU countries, 37

OECD countries, 37

UK, 2, 3, 33, 46

**mortality rates, age specific**

UK, 44, 45

**mortality trend, female**

England and Wales, 35

Northern Ireland, 35

Scotland, 35

**mortality trend, males**

England and Wales, 34

Northern Ireland, 34

Scotland, 34

**mortality, cause**

England, 47

EU countries, 49, 50, 51, 52

Northern Ireland, 47

OECD countries, 4, 49, 50, 51, 52

Scotland, 47

UK, 4, 46, 47, 53

Wales, 47

**NHS expenditure**

England, 117, 125

Northern Ireland, 117

Scotland, 117

UK, 77, 81, 98, 99, 100, 101, 102, 103, 104, 117, 135

Wales, 117, 126

**NHS expenditure plans**

England, 124

**NHS inflation.** *See* **NHS pay and prices index**

**NHS pay and prices index, 80, 81**

**NHS revenue expenditure, 113, 114**

**NHS sources of finance, 120**

**nursing and midwifery staff, hospital**

*England and Wales, 150*

*Northern Ireland, 150*

*Scotland, 150*

*UK, 136, 146, 147, 150, 151*

**obesity**

*England, 74*

*EU countries, 75*

*Great Britain, 7, 73*

*Northern Ireland, 74*

*OECD countries, 75*

*Scotland, 74*

*Wales, 74*

**Ophthalmic Services.** *See* **General Ophthalmic Services**

**opticians, number, 283**

**outpatient attendances.** *See* **hospital outpatient attendances**

**outpatient waiting time.** *See* **hospital outpatient waiting time**

**overweight.** *See* **obesity**

**patient charges, 100, 121**

**pharmaceutical expenditure**

*OECD countries, 229, 230*

**pharmacies and appliance contractors, number**

*Northern Ireland, 231, 233*

*Scotland, 231, 233*

*UK, 231, 233*

*Wales, 231, 233*

**pharmacies and appliance contractors, number**

*England, 231*

**pharmacies and appliance contractors, number**

*England, 233*

**pharmacies' income, 224**

**pharmacists, number practising**

*OECD countries, 232*

**population**

*England, 15, 19*

*England and Wales, 13*

*EU countries, 20*

*Great Britain, 13*

*Northern Ireland, 13, 18, 19*

*OECD countries, 20*

*Scotland, 13, 17, 19*

*UK, 1, 8, 9, 11, 13, 14, 19*

*Wales, 16, 19*

**population projections**

*England and Wales, 13*

*EU countries, 20*

*Great Britain, 13*

*Northern Ireland, 13*

*OECD countries, 20*

*Scotland, 13*

*UK, 8, 9, 11, 13*

**population projections, elderly**

*EU countries, 22, 23, 24, 25*

*OECD countries, 22, 23, 24, 25*

*UK, 10*

**population, elderly**

*England, 19*

*EU countries, 22, 23, 24, 25*

*Northern Ireland, 19*

*OECD countries, 22, 23, 24, 25*

*Scotland, 19*

*UK, 10, 12, 19*

*Wales, 19*

**population, working age, 1**

**prescription charges, 223, 241, 242, 243, 244**

**prescription charges exemption, 223, 224, 244**

**prescription items, dispensing doctors**

*England, 221*

*Northern Ireland, 221*

*Scotland, 221*

*UK, 221*

*Wales, 221*

**prescription, by therapeutic group**

*UK, 250*

**prescription, chargeable, 237**

**prescription, cost, 240**

*England, 239*

*Northern Ireland, 239*

*Scotland, 239*

*UK, 239*

*Wales, 239*

**prescription, Net Ingredient Cost (NIC)**

*England, 245, 246, 247*

# Index

*Northern Ireland, 245, 246, 247*

*older people, 248, 249*

*Scotland, 245, 246, 247*

*UK, 225, 245, 246, 247*

*under 16, 248*

*Wales, 245, 246, 247*

**prescription, Net Ingredient Cost (NIC) by therapeutic group**

*England, 253, 258, 263*

*Northern Ireland, 256, 261, 266*

*Scotland, 255, 260, 265*

*UK, 251, 252, 257, 262*

*Wales, 254, 259, 264*

**prescription, number**

*England, 233, 234, 235, 236*

*Northern Ireland, 233, 234, 235, 236*

*Scotland, 233, 234, 235, 236*

*UK, 222, 233, 234, 235, 236*

*Wales, 233, 234, 235, 236*

**prescription, number by therapeutic group**

*England, 253, 258*

*Northern Ireland, 256, 261*

*Scotland, 255, 260*

*UK, 252, 257*

*Wales, 254, 259*

**prescription, older people, 237, 238**

**prescription, under 16, 237**

**primary care.** *See* **Family Health Services**

**Private health care expenditure, 92, 93, 131, 134**

**private medical insurance, 127, 128, 129**

**private medical products expenditure**

*UK, 130*

**professional and technical staff, hospital, 146, 147**

**Programme Budget, NHS Expenditure**

*England, 125*

*Wales, 126*

**public employees, 115, 116**

**public expenditure, 122, 123**

**Public health care expenditure, 92, 93**

**Reference Cost, day case**

*NHS provider, 185*

*non-NHS provider, 187*

**Reference Cost, elective**

*NHS provider, 183*

*non-NHS provider, 186*

**Reference Cost, non-elective**

*NHS provider, 184*

**sight tests, NHS, 282**

**smoking**

*England, 68*

*EU countries, 69*

*Great Britain, 6, 67*

*Northern Ireland, 68*

*OECD countries, 69*

*Scotland, 68*

*UK, 69*

*Wales, 68*

**spectacles, NHS, 282**

**staff, hospital medical and dental.** *See* **medical and dental staff, hospital**

**Total health care expenditure, 77, 78, 83, 84, 86, 92, 93**

**UK population**

*UK, 1, 2, 10, 11, 12*

**weight.** *See* **obesity**

**work related illness**

*days off work, 66*

**workforce, hospital.** *See* **hospital workforce, NHS**

**working age population, UK, 2**

**years of life lost**

*England and Wales, 48*

# Online Compendium of Health Statistics

# 19th Edition 2008

## Order From

The Compendium of Health Statistics is available on-line, providing all the information contained in the hard back and more.

This on-line access provides a powerful text search facility, and enables tables, charts and graphs to be downloaded directly into Microsoft excel, and also allows charts and graphs to be downloaded directly into Microsoft PowerPoint presentations. Additional intermediate years are provided for several series of data.

With the online Compendium:

- instantly access information anytime, anywhere

- analyse, search and download charts, tables and graphs into reports or presentations.

For current special offers and further information contact ohecompendium@ohe.org

To purchase your copy of the online Compendium please complete and return the order form below or contact Radcliffe direct on Tel: +44 (0)1235 528 820 Fax: + 44 (0)1235 528 830
E-mail: orders@radcliffemed.com

| Qty | ISBN | Title | Cost | |
|---|---|---|---|---|
| ..... | 9781846192821 | Online single* user Compendium of Health Statistics, 19e Public Sector licence | £199.00 Plus VAT £ 34.82 Total £233.82 | ........ |
| ..... | 7981846182814 | Online single* user Compendium of Health Statistics, 19e Private Sector licence | £799.00 Plus VAT £139.82 Total £938.82 | ........ |
| | | Postage and Packaging: - UK 10% or order value (up to a max of £6.00) - Worldwide 20% of order value | | ........ ........ |
| | | | **Total £** | ........ |

**\* Site licences for multiple users of the Online Compendium are available. Please contact Radcliffe Publishing for further details.**

Name: ..................................................... Job Title: ...........................................................

Delivery Address: ...................................................................................................................

..................................................................... Postcode: .............................

Country: ..................E-Mail: ........................................................ Tel: .............................

Please charge my Visa/MasterCard/Switch - Card Number: ..............................................................

Expiry Date: ......................... CVV2 No............ Switch Issue No: ........... with the sum of £...................

Signature: ................................................................. Date: .....................................

Radcliffe Publishing Ltd, 18 Marcham Road, Abingdon, Oxon OX14 1AA, United Kingdom
Tel: +44 (0)1235 528 820 Fax: + 44 (0)1235 528 830
E-mail: orders@radcliffemed.com Web: www.radcliffe-oxford.com

**MEDICAL LIBRARY**

**DUNCAN MacMILLAN HOUSE**